Portable RN

The **All-in-One** Nursing Reference

FIFTH EDITION

T0200220

Clinical Editor
Denise Linton, DNS, APRN, FNP-BC

Associate Professor
Dudley Joseph Plaisance, Sr. BORSF Professorship
in Nursing
University of Louisiana at Lafayette
College of Nursing and Allied Health Professions
Lafayette, Louisiana

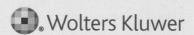. Wolters Kluwer

Philadelphia · Baltimore · New York · London
Buenos Aires · Hong Kong · Sydney · Tokyo

Acquisitions Editor: Nicole Dernoski
Editorial Coordinator: Ashley Pfeiffer
Marketing Manager: Linda Wetmore
Senior Production Project Manager: Alicia Jackson
Design Coordinator: Holly McLaughlin
Manufacturing Coordinator: Kathy Brown
Prepress Vendor: Absolute Service, Inc.

5th edition

9 8 7 6 5 4 3 2 1

Printed in China

Library of Congress Cataloging-in-Publication Data
ISBN: 978-1-975120-77-1
Library of Congress Control Number: 2019910439

Contents

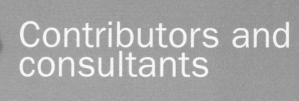

Contributors and consultants

Phyllis Adams, EdD, FNA-C, FAANP, FNAP
Associate Professor, Clinical
College of Nursing
University of Texas Arlington
Arlington, TX

Andrea Barnes Grant, PhD, ARNP-BC
Adjunct Professor
Department of Nursing
City University of New York-BMCC
New York, NY
Nurse Practitioner
Patient Care Services/Primary Care
Outpatient Clinic
VA New York Harbor Healthcare
System Brooklyn Campus
Brooklyn, NY

Paula Gray, DNP, CRNP, NP-C
Director of Family Program (Individual
Across the Lifespan)
Associate Professor of Nursing
School of Nursing
Widener University
Chester, PA

Marjorie Marie Grinam, BSN, MSN, CAPA
Senior Registered Nurse
Ambulatory Surgery Unit
Grady Health System
Atlanta, GA

Theresa Gunter Lawson, PhD, APRN, FNP-BC, CNE
Associate Professor
School of Nursing
Anderson University
Anderson, SC

Ashley H. Lee MSN, RN, CNE
Assistant Professor
Department of Nursing
Lander University
Greenwood, SC

Arlene McEachron, BSN, RN, CNOR
RN-CN1
Department of Nursing-Operating
Rooms
NewYork-Presbyterian Hospital
New York, NY

Sheryl Mitchell, DNP, APRN, FNP-BC, ACNP-BC
Director of Family Nurse Practitioner
Program
Clinical Assistant Professor
College of Nursing
University of South Carolina
Columbia, SC

Leslie MacTaggart Myers, DNP, APRN, ANP-BC, CNE
Senior Clinical Director
College of Nursing and Public Health
South University-Online
Savannah, GA

Ebony Watson, MSN, RN
Assistant Professor
Department of Nursing
University of Louisiana at Monroe
Monroe, LA

Reviewers

Ivolyn D. Grey, MSN, ANP-BC
Adult Nurse Practitioner Clinical
Advisor
UnitedHealthcare
Brooklyn, NY

Emily Hildreth, BSN, RN, SCRN
Clinical Nurse II
Neurosciences Intensive Care Unit
Duke University Hospital
Durham, NC

**John W. Howell II, AGACNP-BC,
MSN, BSN**
Neurology Hospitalist
Duke Raleigh Neurology Department
Duke Raleigh Hospital
Raleigh, NC

Sharonda Johnson, MSN, RN
Instructor
Department of Nursing
University of Louisiana at Lafayette
Lafayette, LA

**Timothy Nguyen, PharmD, BCPS,
FASCP**
Associate Professor of Pharmacy
Department of Pharmacy Practice
Arnold & Marie Schwartz College of
Pharmacy and Health Sciences
Long Island University
Brooklyn, NY

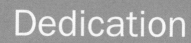

Dedication

This work is dedicated to my mother, the late Mrs. Monica Linton, who lovingly taught me the importance of an education, persistence, and hard work.

Preface

Portable RN: The All-in-One Nursing Reference, fifth edition, is a reference hand-book. The information is designed to assist you with caring for a variety of patients in different practice settings. As technology is evolving at a rapid rate, so are standards of care, management guidelines, and information about diseases and their treatment. Therefore, some web sites have been included so that you can access them and remain current on changes in areas such as screening guidelines.

Some changes that were made in this edition include:

- revised information about interviewing patients, physical examination, alerts, and the incorporation of *Diagnostic and Statistical Manual of Mental Disorders*, fifth edition, information
- updated reference ranges and age groups for some common laboratory tests
- substantial revision of common disorders
- revised therapeutic measures for pressure ulcers and preventing pressure ulcers sections
- updated list of Centers for Disease Control and Prevention nationally notifiable infectious diseases
- revised parenteral drug administration section
- extensive revision of aspects of recognizing and responding to drug hazards
- new information in end-of-life care.

1 Assessment

Reviewing the techniques

Reviewing assessment techniques

Performing a 10-minute assessment

You will not always want or need to assess a patient in 10 minutes. However, rapid assessment is crucial when you must intervene quickly—such as when a hospitalized patient has a change in his or her physical, mental, or emotional status.

You may also perform a rapid assessment to confirm a diagnostic finding. For example, if arterial blood gas analysis indicates a low oxygen content, you will quickly assess the patient for other signs of oxygen deprivation, such as increased respiratory rate and cyanosis.

General guidelines

Assess the patient quickly and systematically. To save time, cover some of the assessment components simultaneously. For example, make your general observations while checking the patient's vital signs or asking history questions.

Be flexible. You will not necessarily use the same sequence each time. Let the patient's chief complaint and your initial observations guide your assessment. You may be unable to obtain a quick history and instead will need to rely on your observations and the information on the patient's chart.

Keep the patient calm and cooperative. If you do not know the patient, first introduce yourself by name and title. Remain calm and reassure that you can help. If your demeanor can reduce the patient's anxiety, he or she will be more likely to give you accurate information.

Avoid drawing quick conclusions. In particular, do not assume that the patient's current symptom is related to the admitting diagnosis.

When every minute counts, follow these steps.

Assess airway, breathing, and circulation

As your first priority, this assessment may consist of just a momentary observation. However, when a patient appears to be unconscious or has difficulty breathing, you will assess more thoroughly to detect the problem and allow immediate intervention.

Make general observations

Note the patient's mental status, general appearance, and level of consciousness (LOC) for clues about the nature and severity of the condition.

Assess vital signs

Take the patient's body temperature, pulse, respiratory rate, and blood pressure. These provide a quick overview of physiologic condition as well as valuable information about the heart, lungs, and blood vessels. The seriousness of the chief complaint and your general observations of the patient's condition will determine how extensively you measure vital signs. Chief complaint is further discussed in chapter 2.

Conduct the health history

Use direct questions to explore the patient's perception of the chief complaint. Find out what is bothering him or her the most. Ask the patient to quantify the problem. For instance, does he or she feel worse today compared to yesterday? Such questions will help you to focus your assessment. If you are in a hurry or if the patient cannot respond, obtain information from other sources, such as family members, admission forms, the medical history, and the patient's chart.

Perform the physical examination

Begin by concentrating on areas related to the patient's chief complaint—the abdomen, for example, if the patient complains of abdominal pain. Compare the results with baseline data, if available.

You may have to perform a complete head-to-toe or body systems assessment—for instance, if a patient is unresponsive (yet has no breathing or circulatory problems) or is confused and, thus, unreliable. However, in most cases, the patient's chief complaint, your general observations, and your findings about the patient's vital signs will guide your assessment.

Guidelines for an effective interview

When you have time for a full assessment, begin by interviewing the patient. Developing an effective interviewing technique will help you to collect pertinent health history information efficiently. Use these guidelines to enhance your interviewing skills.

Be prepared

- Before the interview, review all available information. Read the current clinical records and, if applicable, previous records. This will focus the interview, prevent the patient from tiring, and save you time.

AGE ALERT

A patient's age, activity level, physical condition, and emotional state may affect vital signs. Compare with the patient's baseline, if available.

- Review with the patient what you have learned to ensure that the information is correct. Keep in mind that the patient's current complaint may be unrelated to the history.

Create a pleasant interviewing atmosphere

- Select a quiet, well-lit, and relaxing setting. Keep in mind that extraneous noise and activity can interfere with concentration, as can excessive or insufficient light. A relaxing atmosphere eases the patient's anxiety, promotes comfort, and conveys your willingness to listen.
- Ensure privacy. Some patients will not share personal information if they suspect that others can overhear. You may, however, let friends or family members remain if the patient requests it or if their help is needed.
- Make sure that the patient feels as comfortable as possible. If the patient is physically or emotionally distressed, provide care and reschedule the history taking if appropriate.
- Take your time. If you appear rushed, you may distract the patient. Give your undivided attention. If you have little time, focus on specific areas of interest and return later instead of hurrying through the entire interview.

Establish a good rapport

- Sit and chat with the patient for a few minutes before the interview. Standing may suggest that you are in a hurry, leading the patient to rush and omit important information.
- Explain the purpose of the interview. Emphasize how the patient benefits when the health care team has the information needed to diagnose and care for a health need.

- Show your concern for the patient's story. Maintain eye contact and occasionally repeat what the patient tells you. If you seem preoccupied or uninterested, he or she may choose not to confide in you.
- Encourage the patient to help you develop a realistic plan of care that will serve his or her perceived needs.

Set the tone and focus

- Encourage the patient to talk about the chief complaint. This helps you to focus on the most troublesome signs and symptoms and provides an opportunity to assess the patient's emotional state and level of understanding.
- Keep the interview informal but professional. Allow the patient time to answer questions fully and to add self-perceptions.
- Speak clearly and simply. Avoid using medical terms.

AGE ALERT

Make sure the patient hears and understands you, especially if he or she is elderly. If you think the patient misunderstands, ask him or her to restate what you have discussed.

ALERT

If there is a language barrier, identify a trained medical interpreter. Avoid using family members due to privacy concerns and the potential for misinterpretation.

- Pay close attention to the patient's words and actions, interpreting not only what is said but also what is not said.

Choose your words carefully

- Ask open-ended questions to encourage the patient to provide complete and pertinent information. Avoid yes-or-no questions.
- Listen carefully to the patient's answers. Use the patient's words in your subsequent questions to encourage elaboration on signs, symptoms, and other problems.

Take notes

- To decrease anxiety for the patient, explain the purpose of taking notes during the interview.
- Avoid documenting everything during the interview but make sure to jot down important information, such as dates, times, and key words or phrases. Use these to help you recall the complete history for the medical record.
- Face the patient directly, sitting at eye level during the interview. If using an electronic medical record, you may adjust your device so you can face the patient.
- Continue to make eye contact, even while documenting notes. This maintains rapport and allows you to observe nonverbal communication. If the patient discloses sensitive or traumatic information, cease your note taking to provide appropriate focus. If you are tape-recording the interview, obtain written consent from the patient.

Assessing overall health

For a quick look at the patient's overall health, ask these questions:

- Has your weight changed? Do your clothes, rings, and shoes fit?
- Do you have nonspecific signs and symptoms, such as weakness, fatigue, night sweats, or fever?
- Can you keep up with your normal daily activities?
- Have you had any unusual symptoms or problems recently?
- How many colds or other minor illnesses have you had in the last year?
- What prescription and over-the-counter medications, drugs, and supplements do you take?

Assessing activities of daily living

For a comprehensive look at the patient's health and health history, ask these questions:

Diet and elimination

- How would you describe your appetite?
- What do you normally eat in a 24-hour period?
- What foods do you like and dislike? Is your diet restricted at all?
- How much fluid do you drink during an average day?
- Are you allergic to any food?
- Do you prepare your meals, or does someone prepare them for you?
- Do you go to the grocery store, or does someone else shop for you?
- Do you snack and, if so, on what?
- Do you eat a variety of foods?
- Do you have enough money to purchase the groceries you need?
- Do you have any problems urinating?
- When do you usually have a bowel movement? Has this pattern changed recently?
- Do you take any foods, fluids, or drugs to maintain your normal bowel and urinary patterns?

(Text continues on page 10.)

Performing palpation techniques

Palpation uses pressure to assess structure size, placement, pulsation, and tenderness. Ballottement, a variation, involves bouncing tissues against the hand to assess rebound of floating structures. Ballottement can be used to assess a mass in a patient with ascites.

Light palpation

To perform light palpation, press gently on the skin, indenting it ½″ to ¾″ (1 to 2 cm). Use the lightest touch possible; too much pressure blunts your sensitivity. Close your eyes to concentrate on feeling.

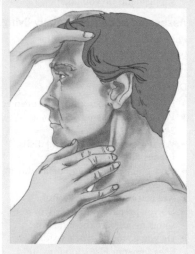

Deep palpation

To perform deep palpation, indent the skin about 1½″ (4 cm). Place your other hand on top of the palpating hand to control and guide your movements. To perform a variation of deep palpation that allows you to pinpoint an inflamed area, push down slowly and deeply and then lift your hand away quickly. If the patient complains of increased pain as you release the pressure, you have identified rebound tenderness.

Use both hands (bimanual palpation) to trap a deep, hard-to-palpate organ (such as the kidney or spleen) or to fix or stabilize an organ (such as the uterus) while palpating with the other hand.

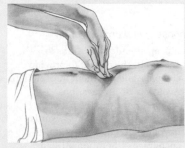

Light ballottement

To perform light ballottement, apply light, rapid pressure from quadrant to quadrant of the patient's abdomen. Keep your hand on the surface of the skin to detect tissue rebound.

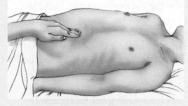

Deep ballottement

To perform deep ballottement, apply abrupt, deep pressure and then release, but maintain contact.

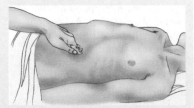

Performing percussion techniques

Percussion has two basic purposes: to produce percussion sounds and to elicit tenderness. It involves three types: indirect, direct, and blunt percussion.

Indirect percussion

The most commonly used method, indirect percussion, produces clear, crisp sounds when performed correctly. To perform indirect percussion, use the second finger of your nondominant hand as the pleximeter (the mediating device used to receive the taps) and the middle finger of your dominant hand as the plexor (the device used to tap the pleximeter). Place the pleximeter finger firmly against a body surface, such as the upper back or abdomen. With your wrist flexed loosely, use the tip of your plexor finger to deliver a crisp blow just beneath the distal joint of the pleximeter. Make sure you hold the plexor perpendicular to the pleximeter. Tap lightly and quickly, removing the plexor as soon as you have delivered each blow.

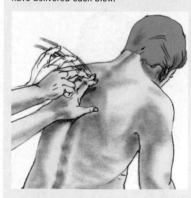

Direct percussion

To perform direct percussion, tap your hand or fingertip directly against the body surface as shown at the top of the next column. This method helps assess an adult's sinuses for tenderness.

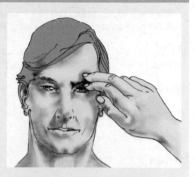

Blunt percussion

To perform blunt percussion, strike the ulnar surface of your fist against the body surface. Alternatively, you may use both hands by placing the palm of one hand over the area to be percussed and then making a fist with the other hand and using it to strike the back of the first hand. Both techniques aim to elicit tenderness—not to create a sound—over organs such as the kidneys. (Another blunt percussion method, used in the neurologic examination, involves tapping a rubber-tipped reflex hammer against a tendon to create a reflexive muscle contraction.)

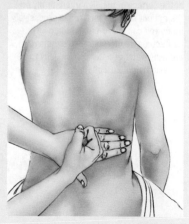

Identifying percussion sounds

Percussion produces sounds that vary according to the tissue being percussed. This chart includes common percussion sounds along with their characteristics and typical locations.

Sound	Intensity	Pitch	Duration
Resonance	Moderate to loud	Low	Moderate to long
Tympany	Loud	High	Moderate
Dullness	Soft to moderate	High	Long
Hyperresonance	Very loud	Very low	Long
Flatness	Soft	High	Short

Performing auscultation

Auscultation of body sounds—particularly those produced by the heart, lungs, blood vessels, stomach, and intestines—detects both high-pitched and low-pitched sounds. Although you can perform auscultation directly over a body area using only your ears, you will typically perform it indirectly, using a stethoscope.

Assessing high-pitched sounds

To assess high-pitched sounds, such as breath sounds and first and second heart sounds, use the diaphragm of the stethoscope. Make sure you place the entire surface of the diaphragm firmly on the patient's skin. If the area is excessively hairy, you can improve diaphragm contact and reduce extraneous noise by applying water or water-soluble jelly to the skin before auscultating.

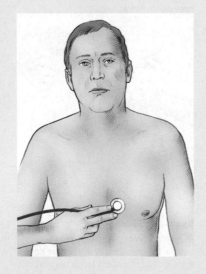

Quality	Source
Hollow	Normal lung
Drumlike	Gastric air bubble or intestinal air
Thudlike	Liver, full bladder, pregnant uterus, or spleen
Booming	Hyperinflated lung (as in emphysema)
Flat	Muscle, bone, or tumor

Assessing low-pitched sounds
To assess low-pitched sounds, such as heart murmurs and third and fourth heart sounds, lightly place the bell of the stethoscope on the appropriate area. Do not exert pressure. If you do, the patient's chest will act as a diaphragm and you will miss low-pitched sounds. If the patient is extremely thin or emaciated, use a stethoscope with a pediatric chest piece.

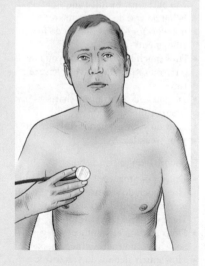

Exercise and sleep

- Do you do regular exercise? What types of exercise do you do? How often do you exercise? How do you feel after exercising?
- Do you fall asleep easily?
- How many hours do you sleep each day? When? Do you feel rested after sleeping?
- Do you take any medication/supplements or do anything to help you fall asleep?
- What do you do when you cannot sleep?
- Do you wake up during the night?
- Do you feel sleepy during the day? When?
- Do you routinely take naps?
- Do you have any recurrent, disturbing dreams?
- Have you ever been diagnosed with a sleep disorder, such as narcolepsy or sleep apnea?

Recreation and employment

- What type of paid work do you do? Do you work outside the home? Are you part-time or full-time?
- What do you do when you are not working? What do you do for enjoyment?
- How much leisure time do you have? Are you satisfied with your leisure time?
- Do you and your family share leisure time?
- How do your weekends differ from your weekdays?

Tobacco, alcohol, and drugs

- Do you use tobacco? If so, what kind? How much do you use each day? Each week? When did you start using it? Have you ever tried to stop?
- Do you drink alcoholic beverages? If so, what kind (beer, wine, whiskey)?
- How much alcohol do you drink each day? Each week? What time of day do you usually drink?
- Do you usually drink alone or with others?

- Do you drink more when you are under stress?
- Has drinking ever hampered your job performance or personal relationships?
- Do you or does anyone in your family worry about your drinking?
- Do you feel dependent on alcohol?
- Do you feel dependent on coffee, tea, or soft drinks? How much of these beverages do you drink in an average day?
- Do you use drugs that are not prescribed to you by a healthcare provider (marijuana, cocaine, heroin, methamphetamine, steroids, pain pills, sleeping pills, anxiety pills, etc.)?

Assessing the family

When assessing how and to what extent the patient's family fulfills its functions, remember to assess both the family into which the patient was born (family of origin) and, if different, the patient's current family.

Because the following questions target a nuclear family—that is, mother, father, and children—you may need to modify them somewhat for other types of families, such as single-parent families, families that include grandparents, patients who live alone, same-sex couples, or unrelated individuals who live as a family. Remember, you are assessing the *patient's perception* of family function. Do not make assumptions about the patient's identity or family structure.

Affective function

To assess how family members regard each other, ask these questions:
- How do the members of your family treat each other?
- How do they feel about each other?
- How do they regard each other's needs and wants?
- How are feelings expressed in your family?
- Can family members safely express both positive and negative feelings?

- What happens when family members disagree?
- How do family members deal with conflict?
- Do you feel safe in your environment?

Socialization and social placement

To assess the flexibility of family responsibilities, which aids discharge planning, ask these questions:

- How satisfied are you and your partner with your roles as a couple?
- How did you decide to have (or not have) children?
- Do you and your partner agree about how to bring up the children? If not, how do you work out differences?
- Do you and your partner agree on household responsibilities?
- Who is responsible for taking care of the children? Is this arrangement mutually satisfactory?
- How well do you feel your children are growing up?
- Are family roles negotiable within the limits of age and ability?
- Do you share cultural values and beliefs with your children?

Health care function

To identify the family caregiver and thus facilitate discharge planning, ask these questions:

- Who takes care of family members when they are sick? Who makes healthcare provider appointments?
- Are your children learning about personal hygiene, healthy eating, exercising, and the importance of adequate sleep and rest?
- How does your family adjust when a member is ill and unable to fulfill expected roles?

Family and social structure

To assess the value the patient places on family and other social structures, ask these questions:

- How important is your family to you?
- Do you have any friends whom you consider family?

- Does anyone other than your immediate family (for example, grandparents) live with you?
- Are you involved in community affairs? Do you enjoy the activities?

Economic function

To explore money issues and their relation to power roles within the family, ask these questions:

- Does your family income meet the family's basic needs?
- Who makes decisions about family money allocation?
- If you take prescription medications, do you have enough money to pay for them?

Assessing the cardiovascular system

Initial questions

- Ask the patient about cardiac problems, such as heart attack, palpitations, tachycardia or other irregular rhythms, chest pain, dyspnea on exertion, paroxysmal nocturnal dyspnea, and cough.
- Explore vascular problems. Does the patient experience pain, cyanosis, edema, ascites, intermittent claudication, cold extremities, or phlebitis? Has he or she ever had a stroke or symptoms of a stroke?
- Ask about postural hypotension, hypertension, rheumatic fever, varicose veins, and peripheral vascular diseases.
- Ask when, if ever, the patient had an electrocardiogram.

Inspecting the precordium

- First, place the patient in a supine position, with his or her head flat or elevated for respiratory comfort. If you are examining an obese patient or one with large breasts, have the patient sit upright. This position will

(*Text continues on page 16.*)

Positioning the patient for cardiac auscultation

During auscultation, you will typically stand to the right of the patient, who is in a supine position. The patient may lie flat or at a comfortable elevation.

If the heart sounds seem faint or undetectable, try repositioning the patient. Alternate positioning may enhance the sounds or make them seem louder by bringing the heart closer to the surface of the chest. Common alternate positions include the seated, forward-leaning position and the left-lateral decubitus position.

Forward-leaning position

The forward-leaning position is best for hearing high-pitched sounds related to semilunar valve problems, such as aortic and pulmonic valve murmurs. Aortic regurgitation is sometimes heard only in the forward-leaning position. To auscultate these sounds, help the patient into the forward-leaning position and place the diaphragm of the stethoscope over the aortic and pulmonic areas in the right and left second intercostal spaces.

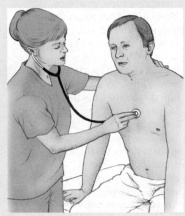

Auscultating heart sounds

Using a stethoscope with 10″ to 12″ (25- to 30-cm) tubing, follow these steps to auscultate heart sounds:

• Locate the four different auscultation sites, as illustrated at right.

In the aortic area, blood moves from the left ventricle during systole, crossing the aortic valve and flowing through the aortic arch. In the pulmonic area, blood ejected from the right ventricle during systole crosses the pulmonic valve and flows through the main pulmonary artery. In the tricuspid area, sounds reflect the movement of blood from the right atrium across the tricuspid valve, filling the right ventricle during diastole. In the mitral, or apical, area, sounds represent blood flow across the mitral valve and left ventricular filling during diastole.

• Begin auscultation in the aortic area, placing the stethoscope in the second intercostal space along the right sternal border.

• Then move to the pulmonic area, located in the second intercostal space at the left sternal border.

• Next, assess the tricuspid area, which lies in the fifth intercostal space along the left sternal border.

• Finally, listen in the mitral area, located in the fifth intercostal space near the midclavicular line.

Note: If the patient's heart is enlarged, the mitral area may be closer to the anterior axillary line.

Left-lateral decubitus position

The left-lateral decubitus position is best for hearing low-pitched sounds related to atrioventricular valve problems, such as mitral valve murmurs and extra heart sounds. A mitral stenosis murmur is sometimes heard only in the left-lateral position. A pericardial rub can be heard in this position and is an abnormal finding. To auscultate these sounds, help the patient into the left-lateral decubitus position and place the bell of the stethoscope over the apical area. If these positions do not enhance the heart sounds, try auscultating with the patient standing or squatting.

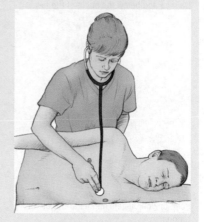

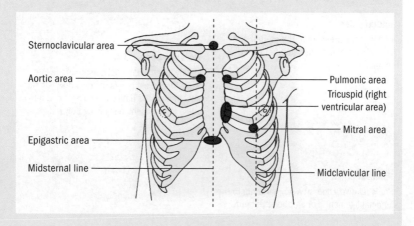

Palpating arterial pulses

To palpate the arterial pulses, you will apply pressure with your index and middle fingers positioned as shown here.

Carotid pulse

Lightly place your fingers just medial to the trachea and below the angle of the jaw.

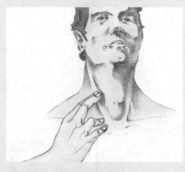

Brachial pulse

Position your fingers medial to the biceps tendon.

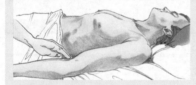

Radial pulse

Apply gentle pressure to the medial and ventral side of the wrist, just below the thumb.

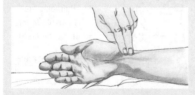

Femoral pulse

Press relatively hard at a point inferior to the inguinal ligament. For an obese patient, palpate in the crease of the groin, halfway between the pubic bone and the hip bone.

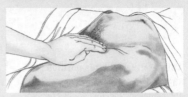

Popliteal pulse

Press firmly against the popliteal fossa at the back of the knee.

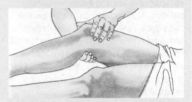

Posterior tibial pulse

Curve your fingers around the medial malleolus and feel the pulse in the groove between the Achilles tendon and the malleolus.

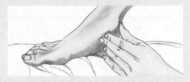

Dorsalis pedis pulse

Lightly touch the medial dorsum of the foot while the patient points the toes down. In this site, the pulse is difficult to palpate and may seem to be absent in some healthy patients.

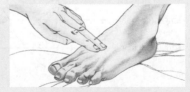

Evaluating edema

To assess pitting edema, press firmly for 5 to 10 seconds over a bony surface, such as the tibia, fibula, sacrum, or sternum. Then remove your finger and note how long the depression remains. Document your observation on a scale of +1 (barely detectable depression) to +4 (persistent pit as deep as 1″ [2.5 cm]).

In severe edema, tissue swells so much that fluid cannot be displaced, making pitting impossible. The surface feels rock-hard, and subcutaneous tissue becomes fibrotic. Brawny edema may develop eventually.

+1 pitting edema

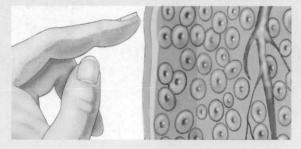

+4 pitting edema

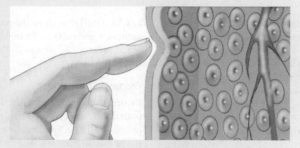

Brawny edema

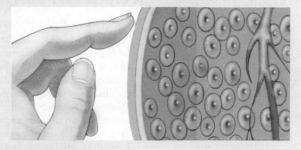

Palpating the thorax

Palpation of the anterior and posterior thorax can detect structural and skin abnormalities, areas of pain, and chest asymmetry. To perform this technique, use the fingertips and palmar surfaces of one or both hands to palpate systematically and in a circular motion. Alternate palpation from one side of the thorax to the other.

Anterior thorax

Begin palpation in the supraclavicular area (#1 in the diagram at right). Then palpate the anterior thorax in the following sequence: infraclavicular, sternal, xiphoid, rib, and axillary areas.

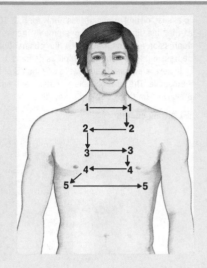

bring the heart closer to the anterior chest wall and make pulsations more visible. If time allows, you can use tangential lighting to cast shadows across the chest. This makes it easier to see abnormalities.

- Standing to the patient's right (unless you are left-handed), remove the clothing covering the chest wall. Quickly identify the following anatomic sites, named for their underlying structures: sternoclavicular, pulmonary, aortic, right ventricular, epigastric, and left ventricular areas.
- Make a visual sweep of the chest wall, watching for movement, pulsations, and exaggerated lifts or heaves (strong outward thrusts seen at the sternal border or apex during systole).

Measuring blood pressure

When you assess the patient's blood pressure, you are measuring the fluctuating force that blood exerts against arterial walls as the heart contracts and relaxes. To measure blood pressure accurately, follow these steps.

Preparing the patient

Before beginning, make sure that the patient is relaxed and warm and has not had caffeine, smoked, or exercised in the last 30 minutes. The patient can sit, stand, or lie down during standard blood pressure measurement.

Applying the cuff and stethoscope

- To obtain a reading in an arm (the most common measurement site), first choose an appropriately sized cuff. (The cuff should cover two-thirds of the upper arm length.) Then wrap the sphygmomanometer cuff snugly around the upper arm, above the antecubital area. Center the cuff bladder over the brachial artery.

Posterior thorax

Begin palpation in the supraclavicular area. Then move to the area between the scapulae (interscapular), then the area below the scapulae (infrascapular), and finally down to the lateral walls of the thorax.

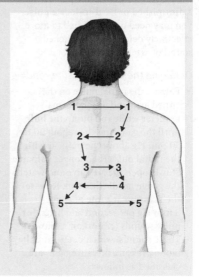

 AGE ALERT

Children should begin routine annual screening for blood pressure at age 3. When measuring blood pressure in an infant or child, an appropriate-sized cuff should cover two-thirds of the upper arm length. Because blood pressure may be inaudible in children younger than age 2, consider using an electronic stethoscope or Doppler to obtain a more accurate measurement.

placing it on a table or a chair arm or by supporting it with your hand. Rest a recumbent patient's arm at his or her side. Do not use the patient's muscle strength to hold up the arm; tension from muscle contraction can elevate systolic pressure and distort the findings.

- Palpate the brachial pulse, just below and slightly medial to the antecubital area. Place the earpieces of the stethoscope in your ears and position the stethoscope head over the brachial artery, just distal to the cuff or slightly beneath it.

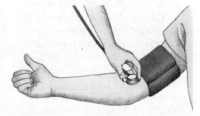

- Most cuffs have arrows that should be placed over the brachial artery.
- Place the sphygmomanometer level with the patient's arm. Keep the patient's arm level with the heart by

Generally, you will use the easy-to-handle, flat diaphragm to auscultate the pulse. However, if the patient has a diminished or hard-to-locate pulse, you may need to use the bell to more effectively detect the low-pitched sound of arterial blood flow.

Obtaining the blood pressure reading

- Palpate the radial pulse on the cuffed arm and watch the manometer while you pump the bulb until the gauge reaches about 20 to 30 mm Hg above the point at which the radial pulse is no longer palpable. Slowly open the air valve and watch the gauge needle descend. Release the pressure at a rate of about 3 mm Hg per second and listen for pulse sounds (Korotkoff's sounds). These sounds, which determine the blood pressure measurement, are classified as follows:

Phase I
A clear, faint tapping starts and increases in intensity to a thud or a louder tap.

Phase II
The tapping changes to a soft swishing sound.

Phase III
A clear, crisp tapping sound returns.

Phase IV (first diastolic sound)
The sound becomes muffled and takes on a blowing quality.

Phase V
The sound disappears.

- As soon as you hear blood begin to pulse through the brachial artery, note the reading on the aneroid dial. This sound reflects phase I (the first Korotkoff's sound) and coincides with the patient's systolic pressure. Continue to deflate the cuff, noting the point at which pulsations diminish or become muffled—phase IV (the fourth Korotkoff's sound), and

the point at which they disappear—phase V (the fifth Korotkoff's sound), which coincides with the patient's diastolic pressure. The American Heart Association and multiple other professional organizations recommend documenting phases I and V using the nearest even number. To avoid confusion and to make your measurements useful, follow this format for recording blood pressure: systolic/diastolic (for example, 120/76).

Assessing the respiratory system

Initial questions

- Inquire about dyspnea or shortness of breath. Are there breathing problems after physical exertion? Ask about pain, wheezing, paroxysmal nocturnal dyspnea, and orthopnea (for example, number of pillows used to sleep).
- Ask if the patient has cough, sputum production, hemoptysis, or night sweats.
- Ask if the patient has emphysema, pleurisy, bronchitis, tuberculosis, pneumonia, asthma, or frequent respiratory tract infections.

Inspecting the chest

Position the patient to allow access to the posterior and anterior chest. If his or her condition permits, have the patient sit on the edge of a bed, examination table, or chair, leaning forward with arms folded across the chest. If this is not possible, place the patient in semi-Fowler's position for the anterior chest examination. Then ask him or her to lean forward slightly and use the side rails or mattress for support while you quickly examine the posterior chest. If the patient cannot lean forward, place him or her in a lateral position or ask another staff member to help him or her to sit up.

Systematically compare one side of the chest with the other.

- First, inspect the patient's chest for obvious problems, such as draining, open wounds, bruises, abrasions, scars, and cuts. Also look for less obvious problems, such as rib deformities, fractures, lesions, or masses.
- Examine the shape of the patient's chest wall. Observe the anteroposterior and transverse diameters.
- Note the patient's respiratory pattern, watching for characteristics such as pursed-lip breathing.
- Observe the movement of the chest during respirations. The chest should move upward and outward symmetrically on inspiration. Factors that may affect movement include pain, poor positioning, and abdominal distention. Watch for paradoxical movement (possibly resulting from fractured ribs or flail chest) and asymmetrical expansion (atelectasis or underlying pulmonary disease).
- Check for use of the accessory muscles and retraction of the intercostal spaces during inspiration (possibly indicating respiratory distress). You may notice sudden, violent intercostal retraction (airway obstruction or tension pneumothorax); retraction of the abdominal muscles during expiration (chronic obstructive pulmonary disease and other obstructive disorders); inspiratory intercostal bulging (cardiac enlargement or aneurysm); or localized expiratory bulging (rib fracture or flail chest).

Palpating for tactile fremitus

Because sound travels more easily through solid structures than through air, assessing for tactile fremitus—which involves palpating for voice

vibrations—provides valuable information about the contents of the lungs. Follow this procedure:

- Place your open palm flat against the patient's chest without touching the chest with your fingers.

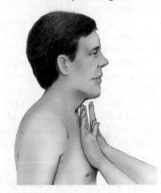

- Ask the patient to repeat a resonant phrase, such as "ninety-nine" or "blue moon," as you systematically move your hands over the chest from the central airways to the lung periphery and back. Always proceed systematically from the top of the suprascapular area to the interscapular, infrascapular, and hypochondriac areas (found at the levels of the 5th and 10th intercostal spaces to the right and left of the midline).
- Repeat this procedure on the posterior thorax. You should feel vibrations of equal intensity on either side of the chest. Fremitus normally occurs in the upper chest, close to the bronchi, and feels strongest at the second intercostal space on either side of the sternum. Little or no fremitus should occur in the lower chest. The intensity of the vibrations varies according to the thickness and structure of the patient's chest wall as well as the intensity and voice pitch.

Percussing the thorax

Percussion of the thorax helps to determine the boundaries of the lungs and the amount of gas, liquid, or solid in the lungs. Percussion can effectively assess structures as deep as 1¾" to 3" (4 to 8 cm).

To percuss a patient's thorax, always use indirect percussion, which involves striking one finger with another. Proceed systematically, percussing the anterior, lateral, and posterior chest over the intercostal spaces.

Avoid percussing over bones, such as the manubrium, sternum, xiphoid, clavicles, ribs, vertebrae, or scapulae. Because of their denseness, bones produce a dull sound on percussion and, therefore, yield no useful information.

Always follow the same sequence when performing percussion, comparing variations in sound from one side to the other. This helps to ensure consistency and prevents you from overlooking important findings.

Anterior thorax

Place your hands over the lung apices in the supraclavicular area. Then proceed downward, moving from side to side at intervals of 1½" to 2" (4 to 5 cm), as shown below. Anterior chest percussion should produce resonance from below the clavicle to the fifth intercostal space on the right (where dullness occurs close to the liver) and to the third intercostal space on the left (where dullness occurs near the heart).

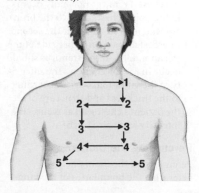

Posterior thorax

Progress in a zigzag fashion from the suprascapular to the interscapular to the infrascapular areas, avoiding the vertebral column and the scapulae, as shown below. Posterior percussion should sound resonant to the level of T10.

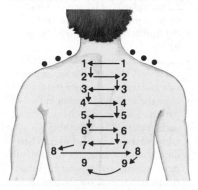

Lateral thorax

Starting at the axilla, move down the side of the rib cage, percussing between the ribs, as shown below. Percussion of the lateral chest should produce resonance to the sixth or eighth intercostal space.

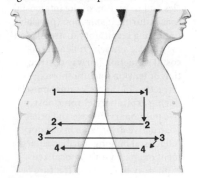

Auscultating breath sounds

Auscultating breath sounds is an important step in physical assessment. It helps you to detect abnormal accumulation of fluid or mucus and obstructed air passages.

To detect breath sounds, auscultate the anterior, lateral, and posterior thorax, following the same sequence that you used for percussion of the thorax. Begin at the upper lobes and move from side to side and down, comparing findings.

AGE ALERT

If the patient is a child, begin just below the right clavicle, moving to the midsternum, left clavicle, left nipple, and right nipple. Assess one full breath (inspiration and expiration) at each point.

Auscultate the lungs to detect normal, abnormal, and absent breath sounds. Classify breath sounds by their location, intensity, pitch, and duration during the inspiratory and expiratory phases.

Assessing the neurologic system

Initial questions

- Ask the patient to state his or her full name and the date, time, and place where he or she is now.
- Investigate the character of any headaches (frequency, intensity, location, and duration).
- Determine whether your patient has vertigo or syncope.
- Ask if there is a history of seizures or use of anticonvulsants.
- Explore cognitive disturbances, including recent or remote memory loss, hallucinations, disorientation, speech and language dysfunction, or inability to concentrate.
- Ask if the patient has a history of sensory disturbances, including tingling, numbness, and sensory loss.

- Explore motor problems, including problems with gait, balance, coordination, tremor, spasm, or paralysis.
- Ask if cognitive, sensory, or motor symptoms have interfered with activities of daily living.

Assessing neurologic vital signs

A supplement to routine measurement of temperature, pulse, and respirations, neurologic vital signs are used to evaluate the patient's LOC, pupillary activity, and level of orientation to time, place, person, and situation.

LOC reflects brain stem function and usually provides the first sign of central nervous system deterioration. Changes in pupillary activity may signal increased intracranial pressure (ICP). Level of orientation evaluates higher cerebral functions. Evaluating muscle strength and tone, reflexes, and posture may also help to identify nervous system damage. Finally, evaluating the respiratory rate and pattern can help to locate brain lesions and determine their size.

Equipment

Penlight • thermometer • stethoscope • sphygmomanometer • pupil size chart

Implementation

- Explain the procedure to the patient, even if he or she is unresponsive.
- Assess the patient's LOC.
- Ask the patient to state his or her full name. If he or she responds appropriately, assess orientation to time, place, and person. Assess the quality of the replies.
- Assess the patient's ability to understand and follow one-step commands that require a motor response. For example, opening and closing the eyes. Note whether he or she can maintain the LOC.
- If the patient does not respond to commands, squeeze the nail beds

on the fingers and toes with moderate pressure and note the response. Alternately, rub the upper portion of the sternum between the second and third intercostal spaces with your knuckles. Check the motor responses bilaterally to rule out monoplegia and hemiplegia.

Examine pupils and eye movement

- Ask the patient to open his or her eyes. If unresponsive, gently lift the upper eyelids. Inspect the pupils for size and shape and compare them for equality. To evaluate them more precisely, use a chart showing the various pupil sizes.
- Test the patient's direct light response. First, darken the room. Hold each eyelid open in turn, keeping the other eye covered. Swing the penlight from the patient's ear toward the midline of the face. Shine the light directly into the eye. Normally, the pupil constricts immediately when exposed to light and then dilates immediately when the light is removed. Wait 20 seconds before testing the other pupil to allow it to recover from reflex stimulation.
- Test consensual light response. Hold both eyelids open but shine the light into one eye only. Watch for constriction in the other pupil, which indicates proper nerve function.
- Brighten the room and ask the conscious patient to open his or her eyes. Observe the eyelids for ptosis or drooping. Then check the extraocular movements. Hold up one finger and ask the patient to follow it with his or her eyes as you move your finger up, down, laterally, and obliquely. See if the patient's eyes track together to follow your finger (conjugate gaze). Watch for involuntary jerking or oscillating

movements (nystagmus). A few beats of nystagmus in extreme lateral gaze are considered normal.

- Check accommodation. Hold up one finger midline to the patient's face and several feet away. Ask the patient to focus on your finger as you move it toward the nose. The eyes should converge, and the pupils should constrict equally.
- Test the corneal reflex with a wisp of cotton. Have the patient look straight ahead. Bring the cotton wisp in from the side to lightly touch the cornea. Observe the patient for bilateral blinking. Tearing will occur in the eye that is touched.
- If the patient is unconscious, test the oculocephalic (doll's eye) reflex. Hold the patient's eyelids open. Quickly but gently turn the patient's head to one side and then to the other. If the patient's eyes move in the opposite direction from the side to which you turn the head, the reflex is intact.

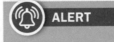

ALERT

Never test this reflex if you know or suspect that the patient has a cervical spine injury.

Evaluate motor function

- If the patient is conscious, test grip strength in both hands at the same time. Extend your hands, ask the patient to squeeze your fingers as hard as he or she can, and compare the strength of each hand. Grip strength is usually slightly stronger in the dominant hand.
- Test arm strength by having the patient close his or her eyes and hold arms straight out in front, with the

palms up. See if either arm drifts downward or pronates, which indicates weakness.

- Test leg strength by having the patient raise the legs, one at a time, against gentle downward pressure from your hand.
- If the patient is unconscious, exert pressure on each fingernail bed. If the patient withdraws, compare the strength of each limb.

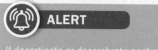

ALERT

If decorticate or decerebrate posturing develops in response to painful stimuli, notify the healthcare provider immediately. (See Comparing decerebrate and decorticate postures.)

- Flex and extend the extremities on both sides to evaluate muscle tone.
- Test the plantar reflex in all patients. Stroke the lateral aspect of the sole of the patient's foot with your thumbnail. Normally, this elicits flexion of all toes. Watch for a positive Babinski's sign—dorsiflexion of the great toe with fanning of the other toes—which indicates an upper motor neuron lesion.
- Test for Brudzinski's and Kernig's signs in patients suspected of having meningitis.

Complete the neurologic examination

- Take the patient's temperature, pulse rate, respiration rate, and blood pressure. Especially check pulse pressure—the difference between systolic and diastolic pressure—because widening pulse pressure can indicate increasing ICP.

Comparing decerebrate and decorticate postures

Decerebrate posture results from damage to the upper brain stem. In this posture, the arms are adducted and extended, with the wrists pronated and the fingers flexed. The teeth are clenched. The legs are stiffly extended, with plantar flexion of the feet.

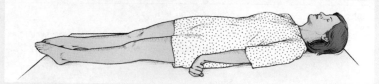

Decorticate posture results from damage to one or both corticospinal tracts. In this posture, the arms are adducted and flexed, with the wrists and fingers flexed on the chest. The legs are stiffly extended and rotated internally, with plantar flexion of the feet.

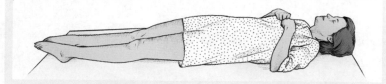

Special considerations

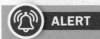

ALERT

If a patient's status was previously stable and there is a sudden change in neurologic or routine vital signs, assess his or her condition further and notify the healthcare provider immediately.

Assessing cerebellar function

To evaluate cerebellar function, you will test the patient's balance, whole-body coordination, and extremity coordination.

Heel-to-toe walking

To assess balance, ask the patient to walk heel to toe. Although he or she may be slightly unsteady, the patient should be able to walk and maintain balance.

Romberg's test

To perform this test, ask the patient to stand with feet together, eyes open, and arms at his or her side. Hold your outstretched arms on either side of the patient so you can provide support if he or she sways to one side or the other. Observe the patient's balance and then ask him or her to close his or her eyes. Note whether there is loss of balance or swaying. If the patient falls to one side, Romberg's test result is abnormal. Patients with cerebellar dysfunction have difficulty maintaining their balance with eyes closed because they cannot use the visual cues that orient them to the upright position.

Point-to-point movements

To evaluate the patient's extremity coordination, test finger-to-nose movements. Have the patient sit about 2′ (0.6 m) away from you. Hold your

Comparing delirium, dementia, and depression

This table highlights the distinguishing characteristics of delirium, dementia, and depression.

Clinical feature	Delirium
Onset	Acute, sudden
Course	Short, with diurnal fluctuations in symptoms; symptoms worse at night, in darkness, and on awakening
Progression	Abrupt
Duration	Hours to less than 1 month; seldom longer
Awareness	Reduced
Alertness	Fluctuates; lethargic or hypervigilant
Attention	Decreased

index finger up and have the patient touch the tip of his or her index finger to the tip of yours and then to touch his or her nose. Next, move your finger and ask the patient to repeat the maneuver. Gradually, increase the speed as you repeat the test. Then test the other side. Expect the patient to be more accurate with the dominant hand. A patient with cerebellar dysfunction will overshoot the target, and movements will be jerky.

To evaluate the lower extremities, test the heel-to-shin movements. Have the patient place his or her heel on the opposite knee and slide it down the shin. This should be repeated on the other side. Note the accuracy and smoothness of the movements.

Rapid alternating movements

To further evaluate the patient's extremity coordination, test rapid alternating movements. Ask the patient to touch the thumb of the right hand to the right index finger and then to each of the remaining fingers. Then instruct the patient to increase the speed. Observe movements for smoothness and accuracy. Repeat the test on the left hand.

To test the lower extremities, the patient should tap the ball of each foot on the floor as quickly as possible.

Assessing reflexes

Assessment of the deep tendon and superficial reflexes provides information about the intactness of the sensory receptor organ. It also evaluates how well the afferent nerve relays the sensory message to the spinal cord, the spinal cord or brain stem segment mediates the reflex, the lower motor neurons transmit messages to the muscles, and the muscles respond to motor messages.

Dementia	Depression
Gradual	Sudden or brief
Lifelong; symptoms progressive and irreversible	Diurnal effects, with symptoms typically worse in the morning; situational fluctuations but less than with acute confusion
Slow but uneven	Variable, rapid, or slow but even
Months to years	At least 2 weeks but can be several months to years *(Note: Diagnostic and Statistical Manual of Mental Disorders* [5th ed.] specifies duration of at least 2 weeks for diagnosis.)
Clear	Clear
Generally normal	Normal
Generally normal	May decrease temporarily

(continued)

Comparing delirium, dementia, and depression (continued)

Clinical feature	Delirium
Orientation	Generally impaired but reversible
Memory	Recent and immediate memory impaired
Thinking	Disorganized, distorted, and fragmented; incoherent speech, either slow or accelerated
Perception	Distorted, with illusions, delusions, and hallucinations; difficulty distinguishing between reality and misperceptions
Speech	Incoherent
Psychomotor behavior	Variable; hypokinetic, hyperkinetic, and mixed
Sleep and wake cycle	Altered
Affect	Variable affective anxiety, restlessness, and irritability; reversible
Findings on mental status testing	Distracted from task; numerous errors

To evaluate the patient's reflexes, test deep tendon and superficial reflexes and observe the patient for primitive reflexes.

Deep tendon reflexes

Before you test a deep tendon reflex, make sure that the limb is relaxed and the joint is in midposition; for instance, the knee or elbow should be flexed at a 45-degree angle. Then distract the patient by asking him or her to focus on an object across the room. If he or she focuses on the performance, the cerebral cortex may dampen his or her response. You can also distract the patient by using Jendrassik's maneuver to enhance the biceps response. Simply instruct the patient to clench his or her teeth or to squeeze his or her thigh. To enhance the patellar reflex, have the patient lock his or her fingers together and pull. Document which technique you used to distract the patient.

Always move from head to toe in testing deep tendon reflexes and compare contralateral reflexes. To elicit

Dementia	Depression
May be impaired as disease progresses	May be disoriented
Recent and remote memory impaired	Selective or patchy impairment
Difficulty with abstraction; impoverished thoughts and impaired judgment; words difficult to find	Intact, with themes of hopelessness, helplessness, or self-deprecation
Misperceptions usually absent	Intact, without delusions or hallucinations, except in severe cases
Dysphasia as disease progresses; aphasia	Normal, slow, or rapid
Normal; may have apraxia	Variable, with psychomotor retardation or agitation
Fragmented	Insomnia or somnolence
Superficial, inappropriate, and labile; attempts to conceal deficits in intellect; may show personality changes, aphasia, and agnosia; lacks insight	Depressed, dysphoric mood, with exaggerated and detailed symptoms; preoccupied with personal thoughts; insight present; verbal elaboration
Failings highlighted by family; struggles with test, with frequent "near-miss" answers; exerts great effort to find an appropriate reply; commonly requests feedback on performance	Failings highlighted by patient; commonly responds "do not know"; exerts little effort; commonly gives up; appears indifferent toward examination and does not care or attempt to find answer

the reflex, tap the tendon lightly but firmly with the reflex hammer. Then grade the briskness of the response: 0 (no response), 1+ (diminished), 2+ (normal), 3+ (brisker than average), 4+ (hyperactive).

Biceps reflex
Position the patient's arm so that the elbow is flexed at a 45-degree angle and the arm is relaxed. Place your thumb or index finger over the biceps tendon and your remaining fingers loosely over the triceps muscle. Strike your thumb or

index finger with the pointed tip of the reflex hammer and watch and feel for contraction of the biceps muscle and flexion of the forearm.

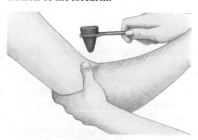

Triceps reflex

Have the patient abduct the arm and place the forearm across the chest. Strike the triceps tendon about 2″ (5 cm) above the olecranon process on the extensor surface of the upper arm. Watch for contraction of the triceps muscle and extension of the forearm.

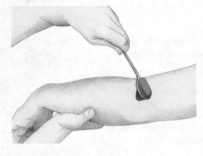

Brachioradialis reflex

Instruct the patient to rest the ulnar surface of the hand on the knee and to partially flex the elbow. With the tip of the hammer, strike the radius about 2″ (5 cm) proximal to the radial styloid. Watch for supination of the hand and flexion of the forearm at the elbow.

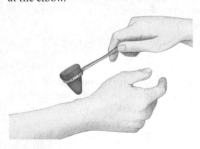

Patellar reflex

Have the patient sit on the side of the bed with legs dangling freely. If the patient cannot sit up, flex the knee at a 45-degree angle and place your non-dominant hand behind it for support. Strike the patellar tendon just below the patella and look for contraction of

the quadriceps muscle in the anterior thigh and for extension of the leg.

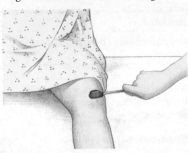

Achilles reflex

Slightly flex the foot and support the plantar surface. Using the pointed end of the reflex hammer, strike the Achilles tendon. Watch for plantar flexion of the foot and ankle.

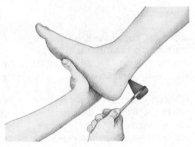

Superficial reflexes

Superficial reflexes include the abdominal, cremasteric, and plantar reflexes. To elicit these reflexes, stimulate the skin or mucous membranes. To document your findings, use a plus sign (+) to indicate that a reflex is present and a minus sign (−) to indicate that it is absent.

Abdominal reflex

Place the patient in the supine position, with arms at the sides and knees slightly flexed. Using the tip of the reflex hammer, a key, or an applicator stick, briskly stroke both sides of the abdomen above and below the umbilicus, moving from the periphery toward the midline. After each stroke, watch for contraction of the abdominal muscles and movement of the umbilicus toward the stimulus. If you are evaluating an obese patient, retract the umbilicus to the side opposite the stimulus and note whether it pulls toward the stimulus. Aging and disease of the upper and lower motor neurons can cause an absent abdominal reflex.

the great toe. You may also see a more pronounced response in which the other toes extend and abduct. In some cases, you may even see dorsiflexion of the ankle, knee, and hip.

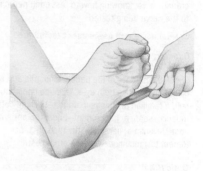

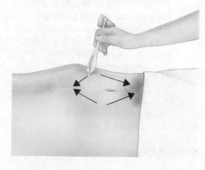

Cremasteric reflex

With a male patient, use an applicator stick to lightly stimulate the inner thigh. Watch for contraction of the cremaster muscle in the scrotum and prompt elevation of the testicle on the side of the stimulus. This reflex may be absent in patients with upper or lower motor neuron disease.

Plantar reflex

Using an applicator stick or a tongue depressor, slowly stroke the lateral side of the patient's sole, from the heel to the great toe and across the ball of the foot, forming an upside-down "J." The normal response is plantar flexion of the toes. In an elderly patient, this normal response may be diminished because of arthritic deformities of the toe or foot.

In patients with disorders of the pyramidal tract (such as stroke), Babinski's reflex, an abnormal response, is elicited. The patient responds to the stimulus with dorsiflexion of

Primitive reflexes

Although normal in infants, primitive reflexes are pathologic in adults.

Snout reflex

Tap lightly on the patient's upper lip. Lip pursing indicates frontal lobe damage. Cerebral degenerative disease may be the cause.

Sucking reflex

If the patient begins sucking while you are feeding him or her or suctioning his or her mouth, you have elicited a reflex that indicates cortical damage characteristic of advanced dementia.

Grasp reflex

Apply gentle pressure to the patient's palm with your fingers. If he or she grasps your fingers between the thumb and index finger, he or she may have cortical (premotor cortex) damage. This is the last of the reflexes to appear.

Glabellar reflex

Repeatedly tap the bridge of the patient's nose. A persistent blinking response indicates diffuse cortical dysfunction.

(Text continues on page 33.)

Assessing the cranial nerves

Assessment of the cranial nerves provides valuable information about the condition of the central nervous system, particularly the brain stem. Because a disorder can affect any cranial nerve, knowing how to test each nerve is important. The techniques vary according to the nerve being tested.

Cranial nerve and assessment technique	Normal findings
Olfactory (CN I)	
Check the patency of the patient's nostrils and ask him or her to close both eyes. Occlude one nostril and hold a familiar, pungent substance—such as coffee, tobacco, soap, or peppermint—under the patient's nose. Ask him or her to identify the substance. Repeat this technique with the other nostril.	The patient should be able to detect the smell and identify it correctly. If the patient detects the smell but cannot identify it, offer a choice, such as, "Do you smell lemon, coffee, or peppermint?"
Optic (CN II)	
Assess visual acuity with a Snellen's chart, visual fields by confrontation, and the retinal structures.	Visual acuity, visual fields, and optic structures intact
Oculomotor (CN III), trochlear (CN IV), and abducens (CN VI)	
Assess pupil size, pupil shape, and pupillary response to light and accommodation. Test the coordinated function of these three nerves by evaluating the patient's extraocular eye movement through cardinal fields of gaze.	The pupils should be equal, round, and reactive to light and accommodation. When assessing pupil size, look for trends. For example, watch for a gradual increase in the size of one pupil or the appearance of unequal pupils in a patient whose pupils previously were equal. The eyes should move smoothly and in a coordinated manner through all six directions of eye movement. Observe each eye for rapid oscillation (nystagmus), movement not in unison with that of the other eye, or inability to move in certain directions (ophthalmoplegia). Also note any double vision (diplopia).

Assessing the cranial nerves (continued)

Cranial nerve and assessment technique	Normal findings

Trigeminal (CN V)

To assess the sensory portion of the trigeminal nerve, gently touch the right and then the left side of the patient's forehead with a cotton ball while his or her eyes are closed. Instruct the patient to indicate when the cotton touches the area. Compare the patient's response on both sides. Repeat the technique bilaterally on the cheeks and jaw. Next, repeat the entire procedure using a sharp object. The cap of a disposable ballpoint pen can be used to test light touch (dull end) and sharp stimuli (sharp end). (If you detect an abnormality, also test for temperature sensation by touching the patient's skin with test tubes filled with hot and cold water and asking him or her to differentiate between them.)

A patient with a normal trigeminal nerve should report feeling both light touch and sharp stimuli in all three areas (forehead, cheek, and jaw) on both sides of the face.

To assess the motor portion of the trigeminal nerve, ask the patient to clench the jaws. Palpate the temporal and masseter muscles bilaterally, checking for symmetry. Try to open the patient's clenched jaws. Next, watch for symmetry as the patient opens and closes the mouth.

The jaws should clench symmetrically and remain closed against resistance.

Assess the corneal reflex by having the patient look up and away. Gently touch the cornea with a fine wisp of cotton.

The lids of both eyes should close when one cornea is touched.

(continued)

Assessing the cranial nerves *(continued)*

Cranial nerve and assessment technique	Normal findings
Facial (CN VII)	
To test the motor portion of the facial nerve, ask the patient to wrinkle the forehead, raise and lower the eyebrows, smile to show the teeth, and puff out the cheeks. With the patient's eyes closed tightly, attempt to open the eyelids. With each of these movements, observe closely for symmetry.	Normal facial movements and strength are symmetrical.
The sensory portion of the facial nerve supplies taste sensation to the anterior two-thirds of the tongue. Prepare four marked, closed containers containing (1) salt, (2) sugar, (3) vinegar (or lemon), and (4) quinine (or bitters). With the patient's eyes closed, place salt on the anterior two-thirds of the tongue using a cotton-tipped applicator or dropper. Ask him or her to identify the taste as sweet, salty, sour, or bitter. Rinse the patient's mouth with water. Repeat this procedure, alternating flavors and sides of the tongue until all four flavors have been tested on both sides. The glossopharyngeal nerve (CN IX) supplies taste sensations to the posterior one-third of the tongue; these are usually tested at the same time.	Normal taste sensations are symmetrical.
Acoustic (CN VIII)	
Test the patient's hearing acuity with the whispered voice test.	The patient should be able to hear a whispered voice in each ear.
The vestibular aspect of CN VIII is generally not tested unless there is a specific neurologic finding. For example, Romberg's test or extraocular movement testing may be used in these cases.	The patient should display normal eye movement and balance, with no dizziness or vertigo.
Glossopharyngeal (CN IX) and vagus (CN X)	
These nerves are assessed together due to their overlapping functions. Listen to the patient's voice for indications of a hoarse or nasal quality. Observe the patient's soft palate when he or she says "ah." Test the gag reflex after preparing the patient. To evoke this reflex, touch the posterior wall of the pharynx with a cotton-tipped applicator or tongue depressor.	The patient's voice should sound strong and clear. The soft palate and uvula should rise symmetrically when he or she says "ah," and the uvula should remain midline. The gag reflex should be intact. If results are abnormal, evaluate each side of the posterior wall of the pharynx to confirm the integrity of both cranial nerves.

Assessing the cranial nerves *(continued)*

Cranial nerve and assessment technique	Normal findings
Spinal accessory (CN XI)	
Apply downward pressure on the patient's shoulders as he or she attempts to shrug in resistance. Note shoulder strength and symmetry while inspecting and palpating the trapezius muscle. Place your hand on the side of the patient's face and ask the patient to turn his or her head against resistance. Note neck strength while inspecting and palpating the sternocleidomastoid muscle. Repeat for the opposite side.	Normally, both shoulders should overcome resistance with equal strength. The neck should overcome resistance in both directions.
Hypoglossal (CN XII)	
Observe the patient's protruded tongue for deviation from midline, atrophy, or fasciculations (very fine muscle movements indicative of lower motor neuron disease). Ask the patient to move the tongue rapidly from side to side with the mouth open and then curl the tongue up toward the nose and then down toward the chin. Use a tongue depressor to apply resistance to the protruded tongue and ask the patient to try to push it to one side. Repeat on the other side and note tongue strength. Listen to the patient's speech for the sounds D, L, N, and T. If general speech is not adequate for assessment, ask the patient to repeat a phrase or series of words containing these sounds.	Normally, the tongue should be midline and the patient should be able to move it equally right, left, up, and down. The pressure that the tongue exerts on the tongue depressor should be equal on both sides. Speech should be clear.

From Bickley, L. S., Szilagyi, P. G., & Hoffman, R. M. (2017). *Bates' guide to physical examination and history taking* (12th ed.). Philadelphia, PA: Wolters Kluwer.

Using the Glasgow Coma Scale

The Glasgow Coma Scale provides an objective way to evaluate a patient's LOC and to detect changes from the baseline. To use this scale, evaluate and score your patient's best eye opening response, verbal response, and motor response. A total score of 15 indicates that the patient is alert; oriented to time, place, and person; and can follow simple commands. A comatose patient will score 7 points or less. A score of 3 indicates a deep coma and a poor prognosis.

Eye opening response

- Open spontaneously (score: 4)
- Open to verbal command (score: 3)
- Open to pain (score: 2)
- No response (score: 1)

Verbal response

- Oriented and converses (score: 5)
- Disoriented and converses (score: 4)
- Uses inappropriate words (score: 3)
- Makes incomprehensible sounds (score: 2)
- No response (score: 1)

Assessing the pupils

Pupillary changes can signal different conditions. Use these illustrations and lists of causes to help you detect problems.

Bilaterally equal and reactive

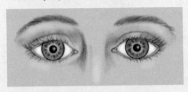

- Normal

Unilateral, dilated (4 mm), fixed, and nonreactive

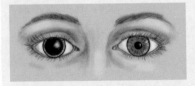

- Uncal herniation with oculomotor nerve damage
- Brain stem compression by an expanding lesion or an aneurysm
- Increased intracranial pressure
- Tentorial herniation
- Head trauma with subsequent subdural or epidural hematoma
- Normal in some people

Bilateral, dilated (4 mm), fixed, and nonreactive

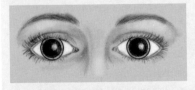

- Severe midbrain damage
- Cardiopulmonary arrest (hypoxia)
- Anticholinergic poisoning
- Deep anesthesia
- Dilating drops

Bilateral, midsized (2 mm), fixed, and nonreactive

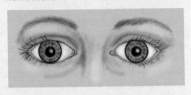

- Midbrain involvement caused by edema, hemorrhage, infarction, laceration, or contusion

Unilateral, small (1.5 mm), and nonreactive

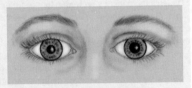

- Disruption of the sympathetic nerve supply to the head caused by a spinal cord lesion above T1

Bilateral, pinpoint (less than 1 mm), and usually nonreactive

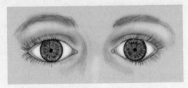

- Lesion of the pons, usually after hemorrhage, leading to blocked sympathetic impulses
- Opiates such as morphine (Pupils may be reactive.)
- Iritis
- Pilocarpine drugs

Motor response

- Obeys verbal command (score: 6)
- Localizes painful stimulus (score: 5)
- Flexion, withdrawal (score: 4)
- Flexion, abnormal—decorticate rigidity (score: 3)
- Extension—decerebrate rigidity (score: 2)
- No response (score: 1)

Assessing the GI system

Initial questions

- Explore signs and symptoms, such as appetite and weight changes, dysphagia, nausea, vomiting, heartburn, stomach or abdominal pain, frequent belching or flatulence, hematemesis, and jaundice. Has the patient had ulcers?
- Determine whether the patient frequently uses laxatives. Ask about hemorrhoids, rectal bleeding, character of stools (color, odor, and consistency), and changes in bowel habits. Is there a history of diarrhea, constipation, irritable bowel syndrome, Crohn's disease, colitis, diverticulitis, or cancer?
- Ask if he or she has had hernias, gallbladder disease, or liver disease such as hepatitis or cirrhosis.
- Ask if he or she has had abdominal swelling or ascites.
- If the patient is older than age 50, ask about the date and results of the last Hemoccult test and screening colonoscopy.

Inspecting the abdomen

Place the patient in the supine position, with arms at the sides and head on a pillow to help relax the abdominal muscles.

Mentally divide the abdomen into quadrants or regions. Systematically inspect all areas, if time and the patient's condition permit, concluding with the symptomatic area.

Examine the patient's entire abdomen, observing the overall contour, color, and skin integrity. Look for rashes, scars, or incisions from past surgeries. Observe the umbilicus for protrusions or discoloration.

Note visible abdominal asymmetry, masses, pulsations, or peristalsis. You can detect masses—especially hepatic and splenic masses—more easily by inspecting the areas while the patient takes a deep breath and holds it. This forces the diaphragm downward, increasing intra-abdominal pressure and reducing the size of the abdominal cavity.

Finally, examine the rectal area for redness, irritation, or hemorrhoids.

 ALERT

If the patient is pregnant, vary the position used for assessment depending on the stage of pregnancy. For example, if the patient is in the final weeks, avoid the supine position because it may impair respiratory excursion and blood flow. To enhance comfort, have the patient lie on her side or assume semi-Fowler's position. Also, during the assessment, remember the normal variations associated with pregnancy: increased pigmentation of the abdominal midline, purplish striae, and upward displacement of the abdominal organs and umbilicus.

Auscultating bowel sounds

Auscultate the abdomen to detect sounds that provide information about bowel motility and the condition of the abdominal vessels and organs. It is important to auscultate the abdomen prior to palpation or percussion to avoid distorting the bowel sounds.

To auscultate bowel sounds, which result from the movement of air and fluid through the bowel, press the diaphragm of the stethoscope against the abdomen and listen carefully. Auscultate the four quadrants systematically.

The movement of air and fluid through the bowel by peristalsis normally creates soft, bubbling sounds with no regular pattern, commonly with soft clicks and gurgles interspersed. Loud, rapid, high-pitched, gurgling bowel sounds are hyperactive and may occur normally in a hungry patient. Sounds occurring at a rate of one every minute or longer are hypoactive and normally occur after bowel surgery or after the colon has filled with feces.

When describing bowel sounds, be specific—for example, indicate whether they are hypoactive, normoactive, hyperactive, or borborygmi (audible stomach growling).

In a routine complete assessment, auscultate for a full 5 minutes before determining that bowel sounds are absent. However, if you are pressed for time, perform a rapid assessment. If you cannot hear bowel sounds within 2 minutes, suspect a serious problem. Even if subsequent palpation stimulates peristalsis, report a long silence in that quadrant.

Before you report absent bowel sounds, however, make sure that the patient's bladder is empty. A full bladder may obscure the sounds. Gently pressing on the abdominal surface may initiate peristalsis and audible bowel sounds, as will having the patient eat or drink.

Next, lightly apply the bell of the stethoscope to each quadrant to auscultate for vascular sounds, such as bruits and venous hums, and for friction rubs. Normally, you should not hear vascular sounds.

Percussing the abdomen

Abdominal percussion helps to determine the size and location of abdominal organs and helps you identify areas of tenderness, gaseous distention, ascites, or solid masses.

To perform this technique, percuss in all four quadrants, moving clockwise to the percussion sites in each quadrant, as shown below. Keep appropriate organ locations in mind as you progress. However, if the patient has pain in a particular quadrant, adjust the percussion sequence to percuss that quadrant last. When tapping, move your right finger away quickly to avoid inhibiting vibrations.

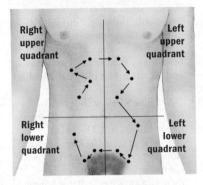

When assessing a tender abdomen, have the patient cough and then lightly percuss the area where the cough produced the pain, helping to localize the involved area. As you percuss, note areas of dullness, tympany, and flatness as well as patient complaints of tenderness.

Percussion sounds vary depending on the density of underlying structures; usually, you will detect dull notes over solids and tympanic notes over air. The predominant abdominal percussion sound is tympany, which is created by percussion over an air-filled stomach or intestine. Dull sounds normally occur over the liver and spleen, a lower intestine filled with feces, and a bladder filled with urine. Distinguishing abdominal percussion notes may be difficult in obese patients.

ALERT

Abdominal percussion or palpation is contraindicated in patients with abdominal organ transplants or suspected leaking abdominal aortic aneurysm. It should be performed cautiously in patients with suspected appendicitis.

Palpating the abdomen

Abdominal palpation provides useful clues about the character of the abdominal wall; the size, condition, and consistency of the abdominal organs; the presence and nature of abdominal masses; and the presence, degree, and location of abdominal pain. For a rapid assessment, palpate primarily to detect areas of pain and tenderness, guarding, rebound tenderness, and costovertebral angle tenderness.

AGE ALERT

An abdominal mass in a child may be a nephroblastoma. Do not palpate it to avoid spreading tumor cells.

Light palpation

Use light palpation to detect tenderness, areas of muscle spasm or rigidity, and superficial masses. To palpate for superficial masses in the abdominal wall, have the patient raise the head and shoulders to tighten the abdominal muscles. Tension obscures a deep mass, but a wall mass remains palpable. Palpate using the finger pads or palmar surface of three to four fingers. Depress ½″ to 1″ (1 to 2.5 cm) using circular motions.

This technique may also help you to determine whether pain originates from the abdominal muscles or from deeper structures.

If you detect tenderness, check for involuntary guarding or abdominal rigidity. As the patient exhales, palpate the abdominal rectus muscles. Normally, they soften and relax on exhalation; note abnormal muscle tension or inflexibility. Involuntary guarding points to peritoneal irritation. In generalized peritonitis, rigidity is severe and diffuse, commonly described as a "boardlike" abdomen.

A tense or ticklish patient may exhibit voluntary guarding. Help the patient relax with deep breathing with inhalation through the nose and exhalation through the mouth.

If a patient has abdominal pain, check for rebound tenderness. Because this maneuver can be painful, perform it near the end of the abdominal assessment. Press your fingertips into the site where the patient reports pain or tenderness. As you quickly release the pressure, the abdominal tissue will rebound. If the patient reports pain as the tissue springs back, you have elicited rebound tenderness.

Deep palpation

If time permits, perform deep abdominal palpation to detect deep tenderness or masses and evaluate organ size. Press 1″ to 3″ (2.5 to 8 cm), assessing for tenderness and masses. If you feel a mass, note its size, shape, consistency, and location. If the patient has pain or tenderness, note if the location is generalized or localized. Note guarding that the patient exhibits during deep palpation. You may feel tensing of a small or large area of abdominal musculature directly below your fingers.

Eliciting abdominal pain

Rebound tenderness and the iliopsoas and obturator signs can indicate conditions consistent with an acute abdomen requiring urgent attention. These include appendicitis, cholecystitis, pancreatitis, diverticulitis, pelvic inflammatory disease, ruptured cyst, ruptured ectopic pregnancy, and peritoneal injury.

Rebound tenderness

Place the patient in the supine position with the knees flexed to relax the abdominal muscles. Place your hands gently on the right lower quadrant at McBurney's point, located about midway between the umbilicus and the anterior superior iliac spine. Slowly and deeply dip your fingers into the area.

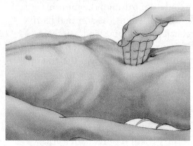

Now release the pressure quickly in a smooth motion. Pain on release—rebound tenderness—is a positive sign of an acute abdomen. The pain may radiate to the umbilicus. *Caution:* Do not repeat this maneuver to minimize the risk of rupturing an inflamed appendix.

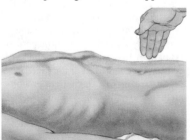

Iliopsoas sign

Place the patient in the supine position with the legs straight. Instruct the patient to raise the right leg upward as you exert slight downward pressure with your hand.

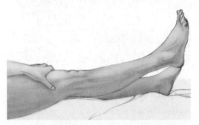

Repeat the maneuver with the left leg. Increased abdominal pain with testing on either leg is a positive result, indicating irritation of the psoas muscle.

Obturator sign

Place the patient in the supine position with the right leg flexed 90 degrees at the hip and knee. Hold the patient's leg just above the knee and at the ankle and then rotate the leg laterally and medially. Increased pain is a positive sign, indicating irritation of the obturator muscle.

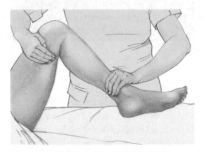

Percussing, palpating, and hooking the liver

You can estimate the size and position of the liver through percussion and palpation (or, in some cases, hooking).

The following illustrations show the correct hand positions for these three techniques.

Liver percussion

Begin by percussing the abdomen along the right midclavicular line, starting below the level of the umbilicus. Move upward until the percussion notes change from tympany to dullness, usually at or slightly below the costal margin. Mark the point of change with a felt-tip pen.

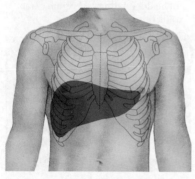

Percuss along the right midclavicular line, starting above the nipple. Move downward until the percussion notes change from normal lung resonance to dullness, usually at the fifth to seventh intercostal space. Again, mark the point of change with a felt-tip pen. Estimate the size of the liver by measuring the distance between the two marks.

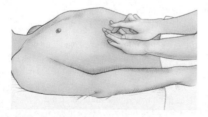

Liver palpation

Place one hand on the patient's back at the approximate height of the liver.

Place your other hand below your mark of liver fullness on the right lateral abdomen. Point your fingers toward the right costal margin and press gently in and up as the patient inhales deeply. As the diaphragm lowers, this maneuver may bring the liver edge down to a palpable position.

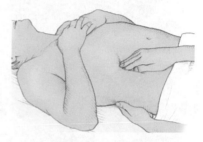

Liver hooking

If liver palpation is unsuccessful, try hooking the liver. Stand on the patient's right side, below the area of liver dullness, as shown below. As the patient inhales deeply, press your fingers inward and upward, attempting to feel the liver with the fingertips of both hands.

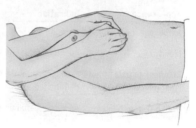

Palpating for indirect inguinal hernia

To check for an indirect inguinal hernia, examine the patient while he stands. Then examine him in a supine position. Place your gloved index finger on the neck of his scrotum and gently push upward into the inguinal canal, as shown in the next page.

If you meet resistance or if the patient complains of pain, stop the examination. When you have inserted your finger as far as possible, ask him to bear down and cough. A hernia will feel like a mass of tissue that withdraws when met by the finger.

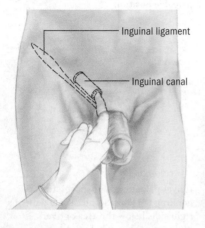

Inguinal ligament

Inguinal canal

Assessing the urinary system

Initial questions

- Ask about urine color, oliguria, and nocturia. (See *Evaluating urine color*.) Does your patient experience incontinence, dysuria, frequency, urgency, or difficulty with the urinary stream (such as reduced flow or dribbling)?
- Ask about pyuria, urine retention, and passage of calculi.
- Ask the patient if there is a history of bladder, kidney, or urinary tract infections.

AGE ALERT

If your patient is a child, ask the parents if they have had problems with his or her toilet training or bed-wetting.

Evaluating urine color

For important clues about your patient's health, ask about changes in urine color. Such changes can result from fluid intake, medications, dietary factors, and various disorders.

Appearance	Indication
Amber or straw color	Normal
Cloudy	Infection, inflammation, glomerulonephritis, vegetarian diet
Colorless or pale straw color (dilute urine)	Excess fluid intake, chronic renal disease, diabetes insipidus, diuretic therapy
Dark brown or black	Acute glomerulonephritis, drugs (such as nitrofurantoin, metronidazole, and antimalarials)
Dark yellow or amber (concentrated urine)	Low fluid intake, dehydration, acute febrile disease, vomiting or diarrhea causing fluid loss, food (such as carrots)
Green-brown	Bile duct obstruction
Orange	Urobilinuria, drugs (such as phenazopyridine and rifampin), obstructive jaundice (tea-colored urine)
Red	Hemorrhage (hematuria), injury to urinary tract, cancer, kidney stones, drugs (such as phenazopyridine and doxorubicin), food (such as beets)

Inspecting the urethral meatus

Put on gloves before examining the urethral meatus.

To inspect a male patient's urethral meatus, have him lie in the supine position and drape him, exposing only his penis. Then compress the tip of the glans to open the urethral meatus, which should be located in the center of the glans. Check for swelling, discharge, signs of urethral infection, and ulcerations, which can signal a sexually transmitted disease (STD).

To inspect a female patient's urethral meatus, help her into the dorsal lithotomy position and drape her, exposing only the area to be assessed. Spread the labia and look for the urethral meatus. It should be a pink, irregular, slitlike opening located at the midline, just above the vagina. Check for swelling, discharge, signs of urethral infection, cystocele, and ulcerations, which may signal an STD.

Percussing the urinary organs

Percuss the kidneys to elicit pain or tenderness and percuss the bladder to elicit percussion sounds. Before you start, tell the patient what you are going to do. Otherwise, the patient may be startled and you could mistake the reaction for a feeling of acute tenderness.

Kidney percussion

With the patient sitting upright, percuss each costovertebral angle (the angle over each kidney whose borders are formed by the lateral and downward curve of the lowest rib and the spinal column). To perform direct percussion, place your left palm over the costovertebral angle and gently strike it with your right fist, as shown in the next column. Use just enough force to cause a painless but perceptible thud. To perform indirect percussion, gently strike your fist over each costovertebral angle. Make sure to percuss both sides of the body to assess both kidneys. A patient normally feels a thudding sensation or pressure during percussion. Pain or tenderness suggests a kidney infection.

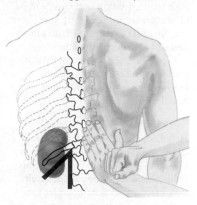

Bladder percussion

Before you percuss the bladder, have the patient urinate. Then ask the patient to lie in the supine position. Next, directly percuss the area over the bladder, beginning 2″ (5 cm) above the symphysis pubis, as shown below. To detect differences in sound, percuss toward the base of the bladder. Percussion normally produces a tympanic sound. A dull sound is produced over a urine-filled bladder.

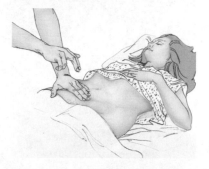

Palpating the urinary organs

Bimanual palpation of the kidneys and bladder may detect tenderness, lumps, and masses. In the normal adult, the kidneys usually cannot be palpated because of their location deep within the abdomen. However, they may be palpable in a thin patient or in a patient with reduced abdominal muscle mass. (The right kidney is slightly lower, so it may be easier to palpate.) Both kidneys descend with deep inhalation.

If palpable, the bladder normally feels firm and relatively smooth. However, an adult's bladder may not be palpable.

Kidney palpation

Help the patient into the supine position and expose the abdomen from the xiphoid process to the symphysis pubis. Standing at the patient's right side, place your left hand under the back, midway between the lower costal margin and the iliac crest, as shown below.

Next, place your right hand on the patient's abdomen, directly above your left hand. Angle your right hand slightly toward the costal margin. To palpate the right lower edge of the right kidney, press your right fingertips about 1½" (4 cm) above the right iliac crest at the midinguinal line; press your left fingertips upward into the right costovertebral angle, as shown below.

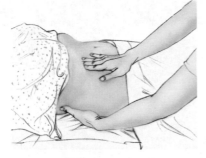

Instruct the patient to inhale deeply so that the lower portion of the right kidney can move down between your hands. If it does, note the shape and size of the kidney. Normally, it feels smooth, solid, and firm, yet elastic. Ask the patient if palpation causes tenderness.

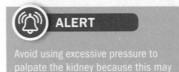

Avoid using excessive pressure to palpate the kidney because this may cause intense pain.

To assess the left kidney, move to the patient's left side and position your hands as described earlier, but with this change: Place your right hand 2" (5 cm) above the left iliac crest. Then apply pressure with both hands as the patient inhales. If the left kidney can be palpated, compare it with the right kidney; it should be the same size.

Bladder palpation

Before you palpate the bladder, make sure that the patient has voided. Then locate the edge of the bladder by pressing deeply in the midline about 1" to 2" (2.5 to 5 cm) above the symphysis pubis, as shown below.

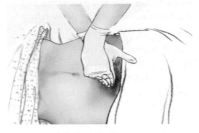

As you palpate the bladder, note its size and location and check for lumps, masses, and tenderness. The bladder normally feels firm and relatively smooth. (Keep in mind that an adult's bladder may not be palpable.) During deep palpation, the patient may report the urge to urinate—a normal response.

Assessing the male reproductive system

Initial questions

- Ask the patient about penile discharge or lesions and testicular pain or lumps.
- Ask if the patient performs testicular self-examinations. Has he had a vasectomy?
- Ask about the patient's sexual history, including sexual orientation, type of activity, frequency, number of partners, safe sex practices, and condom use.
- Ask about STDs and other infections. Assess the patient's knowledge of how to prevent STDs, including AIDS.
- Find out if the patient has a history of prostate problems.
- Ask if he is satisfied with his sexual function. Does he have any concerns about erectile dysfunction or sterility? Also inquire about his contraceptive practices.

Inspecting and palpating the male genitalia

It is recommended to have a chaperone during examination of the genitalia. First, ask the patient to disrobe from the waist down and to cover himself with a drape. Then put on gloves and examine his penis, scrotum, testicles, inguinal and femoral areas, and prostate gland (if applicable).

Penis

Observe the penis. Its size will depend on the patient's age and overall development. The penile skin should be slightly wrinkled and pink to light brown in a white patient and light brown to dark brown in a dark-skinned patient. Check the penile shaft and glans for lesions, nodules, inflammation, and swelling. Also check the glans for smegma, a cheesy secretion.

Gently compress the glans and inspect the urethral meatus for discharge, inflammation, and lesions, specifically genital warts. If you note a discharge, obtain a culture specimen for sexually transmitted infections, such as gonorrhea and chlamydia.

Using your thumb and forefinger, palpate the entire penile shaft. It should be somewhat firm, and the skin should be smooth and movable. Note swelling, nodules, or indurations.

Scrotum and testicles

Have the patient hold his penis away from his scrotum so that you can observe the general size and appearance of the scrotum. The skin will be darker than the rest of the body. Spread the surface of the scrotum and examine the skin for swelling, nodules, redness, ulceration, and distended veins. You will probably see some sebaceous cysts—firm, white-to-yellow, nontender cutaneous lesions. Also check for pitting edema, a sign of cardiovascular disease. Spread the pubic hair and check the skin for lesions and parasites.

Gently palpate both testicles between your thumb and first two fingers. Assess their size, shape, and response to pressure (typically, deep visceral pain). The testicles should be equal in size. They should feel firm, smooth, and rubbery, and they should move freely in the scrotal sac. If you note hard, irregular areas or lumps, transilluminate the testicle by darkening the room and pressing the head of a flashlight against the scrotum, behind the lump. The testicle will appear as an opaque shadow, as will lumps, masses, warts, or blood-filled areas. Transilluminate the other testicle to compare your findings.

Next, palpate the epididymis, which is normally located in the posterolateral area of the testicle. It should be smooth, discrete, nontender, and free from swelling or induration.

Finally, palpate each spermatic cord, located above each testicle. Begin palpating at the base of the epididymis and continue to the inguinal canal. The vas deferens is a smooth, movable cord inside the spermatic cord. If you feel swelling, irregularity, or nodules, transilluminate the problem area, as described earlier. If serous fluid is present, you will see a red glow; if tissue and blood are present, you will not see this glow.

Prostate gland

Usually, a physician performs prostate palpation as part of a rectal examination. However, if the patient has not scheduled a separate rectal examination, you may palpate the prostate during the reproductive system assessment. Because palpation of the prostate usually is uncomfortable and may embarrass the patient, begin by explaining the procedure and reassuring the patient that the procedure should not be painful.

Have the patient urinate to empty the bladder and reduce discomfort during the examination. Then ask him to stand at the end of the examination table, with his elbows flexed and his upper body resting on the table. If he cannot assume this position because he is unable to stand, have him lie on his left side with his right knee and hip flexed or with both knees drawn up toward his chest.

Inspect the skin of the perineal, anal, and posterior scrotal surfaces. The skin should appear smooth and unbroken, with no protruding masses.

Apply water-soluble lubricant to your gloved index finger. Then introduce the finger, pad down, into the patient's rectum. Instruct the patient to relax to ease passage of the finger through the anal sphincter.

Using the pad of your index finger, gently palpate the prostate on the anterior rectal wall, located just past the anorectal ring. The prostate should feel smooth and rubbery. Normal size varies but usually is about that of a walnut. The prostate should not protrude into the rectum lumen. Identify the two lateral lobes and the median sulcus.

Assessing the female reproductive system

Initial questions

- Ask your patient about her age at menarche and the character of her menses (frequency, regularity, and duration). What was the date of her last period? Does she have a history of menorrhagia, metrorrhagia, dysmenorrhea, or amenorrhea? If she is postmenopausal, determine the date of menopause.
- Assess for obstetric and gynecologic surgical history.
- Ask if she has irregular or painful vaginal bleeding, dyspareunia, or frequent vaginal infections.
- Ask about her type of sexual practices, frequency, number of partners, safe sex practices, and condom use.
- Ask about her obstetric history, including the total number of pregnancies (gravida), number of births after 20 weeks (para), number of premature births, number of abortions or miscarriages, and number of living children. Has she had any problems with fertility?
- Has she experienced sexual assault or abuse?
- Assess the current birth control method.
- Determine the dates of her last gynecologic examination and Papanicolaou (Pap) test.

- Ask about STDs and other infections. Assess her knowledge of how to prevent STDs, including HIV.
- Ask the patient about her satisfaction with her sexual function.

Palpating the breasts and axillae

Have the patient put on a gown. Assess the patient's breast history, including tumors, cancer, cysts, trauma, surgery, galactorrhea, and implants. Ask about mammograms. Ask about lumps, pain, breast changes, and discharge.

It is advised to have a chaperone present during examination of the breasts. Begin the breast examination with the patient sitting with her arms at her sides. Inspect the breasts with the patient's arms over her head and then when she is leaning forward with her hands pressed into her hips. Visually note any abnormalities such as skin dimpling or retractions. Palpate each breast using the pads of your fingers. Use a specific pattern, such as spiraling outward, a circular motion, or moving vertically across the breast. Include the tail of Spence and axilla. Then examine the breast with the patient supine. Place a pillow under the side you are examining and have the patient raise her arm above her head and place her hand behind her head. Proceed to palpate each breast as described earlier.

Note the consistency of the breast tissue. Check for nodules or unusual tenderness. Nodularity may increase before menstruation, and tenderness may result from premenstrual fullness, cysts, or cancer. Any lump or mass that feels different from the rest of the breast may represent a pathologic change.

Palpate the areola and nipple and gently compress the nipple between your thumb and index finger to detect discharge. If you see discharge, note the color, consistency, and quantity.

With the patient seated, palpate the axillae. Palpate the right axilla with the middle three fingers of one hand while supporting the patient's arm with your other hand. You may palpate one or more soft, small, nontender central nodes. If the nodes feel large, hard, or tender, or if the patient has a suspicious-looking lesion, palpate the other groups of lymph nodes.

Inspecting the female genitalia

Before you begin the examination, ask the patient to urinate. Next, help her into the dorsal lithotomy position and drape her. It is advised to have a chaperone present during any genital examination regardless of gender. After putting on gloves, examine the patient's external and internal genitalia, as appropriate.

Inspecting the external genitalia

Observe the skin and hair distribution of the mons pubis. Spread the hair with your fingers to check for lesions and parasites.

Next, inspect the skin of the labia majora, spreading the hair to examine for lesions, parasites, and genital warts. The skin should be slightly darker than the rest of the body, and the labia majora should be round and full. Examine the labia minora, which should be dark pink and moist. In nulliparous women, the labia majora and minora are close together; in women who have experienced vaginal deliveries, they may gape open.

Closely observe each vulvar structure for syphilitic chancres, ulcerations, and cancerous lesions. Examine the area of Bartholin's and Skene's glands and ducts for swelling, erythema, enlargement, or discharge. Next, inspect the urethral opening. It should be slitlike and the same color as the mucous membranes. Look for erythema, polyps, and discharge.

Inspecting the internal genitalia

First, select a speculum that is appropriate for the patient. In most cases, you will use a Graves' speculum. However, if the patient is a virgin or nulliparous or has a contracted introitus as a result of menopause, you should use a Pedersen's speculum.

Hold the blades of the speculum under warm running water. This warms the blades and helps to lubricate them, making insertion easier and more comfortable for the patient. Do not use commercial lubricants—they are bacteriostatic and will distort cells on Pap tests. Sit or stand at the foot of the examination table. Tell the patient that she will feel your touch on her skin and some pressure when you insert the speculum.

Separate the labia with the fingers and gently pull down on the posterior aspect to open the introitus. With the speculum closed, insert the blades so that the width is almost vertical. Gently push downward and rotate the blade width to horizontal. Follow the canal to the cervix. Open the blades and position them with the cervix in view.

While inserting and withdrawing the speculum, note the color, texture, and mucosal integrity of the vagina and vaginal secretions. A thin, white, odorless discharge is normal.

With the speculum in place, examine the cervix for color, position, size, shape, mucosal integrity, and discharge. The cervix should be smooth, round, rosy pink, and free from ulcerations and nodules. The cervical opening, or so, may appear differently based on pregnancy history. It may be small and round or slitlike. The cervix can have benign lesions such as nabothian cysts or visible columnar epithelium. A clear, watery discharge is normal during ovulation; a slightly bloody discharge is normal just before menstruation. Obtain a culture specimen of any other discharge. After you inspect the cervix, obtain a specimen for a Pap test.

When you have completed your examination, unlock the speculum blades and close them slowly while you begin to withdraw the instrument. Close the blades completely before they reach the introitus and withdraw the speculum from the vagina.

Palpating the uterus

To palpate the uterus bimanually, insert the index and middle fingers of one gloved hand into the patient's vagina and place your other hand on the abdomen between the umbilicus and symphysis pubis. Press the abdomen in and down while you elevate the cervix and uterus with your two fingers, as shown on the next page. Try to grasp the uterus between your hands. Note cervical motion tenderness—this can indicate pelvic infection. Next, place your abdominal hand in the left lower quadrant and elevate the left ovary with your gloved fingers. Repeat the technique on the right side. Each ovary should be small and almond-shaped. Document any tenderness or mass.

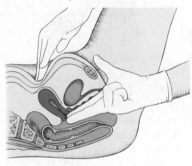

Slide your fingers farther into the anterior fornix and palpate the body of the uterus between your hands. Note its size, shape, surface characteristics, consistency, and mobility. Note tenderness of the uterine body and fundus. Also note fundal position.

Assessing the musculoskeletal system

Initial questions

- Ask if the patient has muscle pain, joint pain, swelling, tenderness, or difficulty with balance or gait. Is there any joint stiffness? If so, find out when it occurs and how long it lasts.
- Ask whether the patient has noticed noise with joint movement.
- Is there a history of arthritis or gout?
- Ask about a history of fractures, injuries, back problems, surgeries, or deformities. Ask about weakness and paralysis.

- Explore limitations on walking, running, or participation in sports. Do muscle or joint problems interfere with activities of daily living?

AGE ALERT

If the patient is an infant or a toddler, ask the parents if the patient has achieved developmental milestones—such as sitting up, crawling, and walking.

Assessing range of motion

Assess the patient's posture, gait, and stance. Assessment of joint range of motion (ROM) tests joint function. To assess joint ROM, ask the patient to move specific joints through the normal ROM. If the patient cannot do so, move the joints through passive ROM.

The following figures show each joint and illustrate the tests for ROM, including the expected degree of motion for each joint.

Shoulders

To assess forward flexion and backward extension, have the patient bring the straightened arm forward and up and then behind him or her.

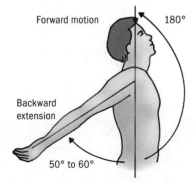

Forward motion   180°

Backward
extension

50° to 60°

Assess abduction and adduction by asking the patient to bring the straightened arm to the side and up and then in front of him or her.

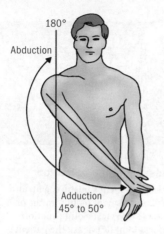

180°

Abduction

Adduction
45° to 50°

To assess external and internal rotation, have the patient abduct the arm with the elbow bent. Then ask the patient to place his or her hand first behind the head and then behind the small of his or her back.

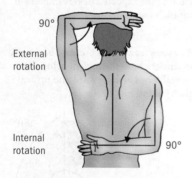

90°

External
rotation

Internal
rotation

90°

Elbows

Assess flexion by having the patient bend his or her arm and attempt to touch his or her shoulder. Assess extension by having him or her straighten the arm.

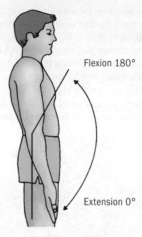

Flexion 180°

Extension 0°

To assess pronation and supination, hold the patient's elbow in a flexed position and ask him or her to rotate the arm until the palm faces the floor. Then rotate the hand back until the palm faces upward.

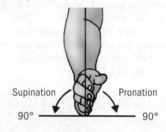

Supination   Pronation

90° —————————— 90°

Wrists

To assess flexion, ask the patient to bend the wrist downward; assess extension by having him or her straighten the wrist. To assess hyperextension, ask him or her to bend the wrist upward.

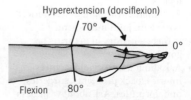

Hyperextension (dorsiflexion)

70°

0°

Flexion   80°

Assess radial and ulnar deviation by asking the patient to move his or her hand first toward the radial side and then toward the ulnar side.

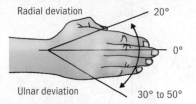

Radial deviation 20°

0°

Ulnar deviation 30° to 50°

Fingers

To assess abduction and adduction, have the patient first spread the fingers and then bring them together. In abduction, there should be 20 degrees between the fingers; in adduction, the fingers should touch.

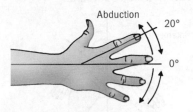

Abduction 20°

0°

To assess extension and flexion, ask the patient first to straighten the fingers and then to make a fist with the thumb remaining straight.

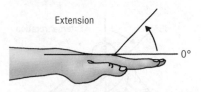

Extension

0°

Flexion

0°

90°

Thumbs

Assess extension by having the patient straighten the thumb. To assess flexion, have him or her bend the thumb at the top joint and then at the bottom.

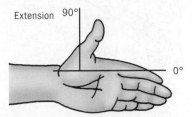

Extension 90°

0°

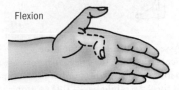

Flexion

Assess adduction by having the patient extend the hand, bringing the thumb first to the index finger and then to the little finger.

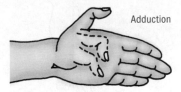

Adduction

Hips

Assess flexion by asking the patient to bend the knee to the chest while keeping the back straight. If the patient has undergone total hip replacement, do not perform this movement without the surgeon's permission; motion can dislocate the prosthesis.

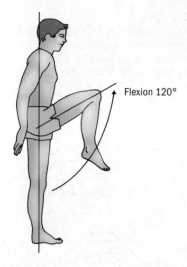

Flexion 120°

Assess extension by having the patient straighten the knee. To assess hyperextension, ask him or her to extend the leg straight back. This motion can be performed with the patient in the prone or standing position.

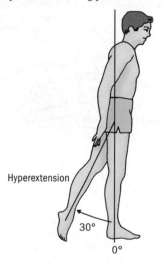

Hyperextension

30°

0°

To assess abduction, have the patient move the straightened leg away from the midline.

To assess adduction, instruct the patient to move the straightened leg from the midline toward the opposite leg.

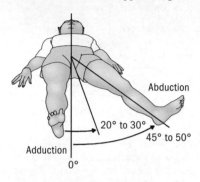

Abduction

20° to 30°

45° to 50°

Adduction

0°

To assess internal and external rotation, ask the patient to bend the knee and turn the leg inward. Then have him or her turn the leg outward.

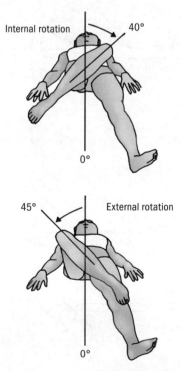

Internal rotation

40°

0°

45°

External rotation

0°

Knees

Ask the patient to straighten his or her leg at the knee to show extension; ask him or her to bend the knee and bring the foot up to touch his or her buttock to demonstrate flexion.

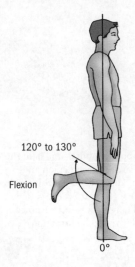

120° to 130°

Flexion

0°

Toes

Assess extension and flexion by asking the patient to straighten and then curl the toes. Then check hyperextension by asking him or her to straighten the toes and point them upward.

Hyperextension (dorsiflexion)

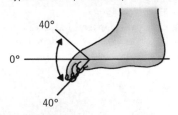

40°

0°

40°

Ankles and feet

Have the patient show plantar flexion by bending the foot downward. Ask the patient to show hyperextension by bending the foot upward.

Hyperextension (dorsiflexion)

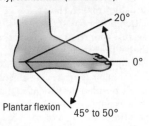

20°

0°

Plantar flexion 45° to 50°

To assess eversion and inversion, ask the patient to point the toes. Have him or her turn the foot inward and then outward.

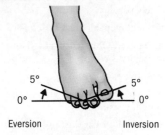

5°   5°
0°   0°

Eversion   Inversion

To assess forefoot adduction and abduction, stabilize the patient's heel while he or she turns the foot first inward and then outward.

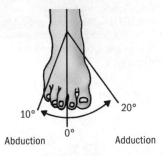

10°   20°
0°

Abduction   Adduction

Testing muscle strength

Assess motor function by testing the patient's strength in the affected limb. Before you begin the muscle strength tests, find out whether the patient is right- or left-handed. The dominant arm is usually stronger. Have the patient attempt normal ROM movements against your resistance. Note the strength that the patient exerts. If the muscle group is weak, lessen your resistance to permit an accurate assessment. If necessary, position the patient so that the limb does not have to resist gravity and repeat the test.

To minimize subjective interpretations of the test findings, rate muscle strength on a scale of 0 to 5, as follows:

0 = No visible or palpable contraction felt; paralysis

1 = Slight palpable contraction felt

2 = Passive ROM maneuvers when gravity is removed

3 = Active ROM against gravity

4 = Active ROM against gravity and light resistance

5 = Active ROM against full resistance; normal strength

Deltoid

With your patient's arm fully extended, place one hand over the deltoid muscle and the other hand on the wrist. Have him or her abduct the arm to a horizontal position against your resistance; palpate for deltoid contraction.

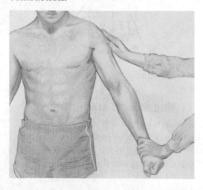

Biceps

With your hand on the patient's fist, have him or her flex the forearm against your resistance; observe for biceps contraction.

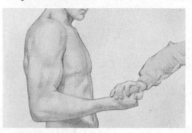

Triceps

Have the patient abduct and hold the arm midway between flexion and extension. Hold and support his or her arm at the wrist and ask the patient to extend it against your resistance. Observe for triceps contraction.

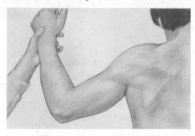

Dorsal interosseous

Have the patient extend and spread the fingers and resist your attempt to squeeze them together.

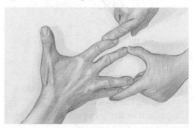

Forearm and hand (grip)

Have the patient grasp your middle and index fingers and squeeze them as hard as he or she can.

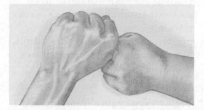

Psoas

Support the patient's leg and have him or her raise the knee and flex the hip against your resistance (as shown below). Observe for psoas contraction.

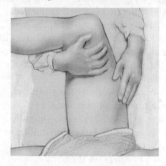

Quadriceps

Have the patient bend the knee slightly while you support the lower leg. Then ask him or her to extend his or her knee against your resistance; as he or she is doing so, palpate for quadriceps contraction.

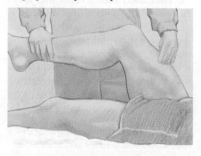

Gastrocnemius

With the patient in the prone position, support the foot and ask him or her to plantar flex the ankle against your resistance. Palpate for gastrocnemius contraction.

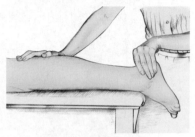

Anterior tibialis

With the patient sitting on the side of the examination table with legs dangling, place your hand on the foot and ask him or her to dorsiflex the ankle against your resistance.

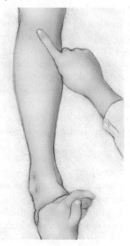

Extensor hallucis longus

With your fingers on the patient's great toe, have him or her dorsiflex the toe against your resistance. Palpate for extensor hallucis contraction.

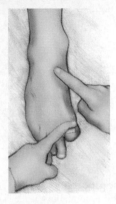

Assessing the skin

Initial questions

- Determine if your patient has any known skin disease, such as psoriasis, acne, eczema, or hives.
- Ask the patient to describe any changes in skin pigmentation, temperature, moisture, or hair distribution.
- Examine the skin for itching, rashes, or scaling. Is the skin excessively dry or oily?
- How does the skin react to hot or cold weather?
- Ask the patient about skin care, sun exposure, use of sun protection factor (SPF) products and SPF number used, and use of protective clothing.
- Ask if your patient has noticed easy bruising or bleeding, changes in warts or moles, or lumps. Ask about the presence and location of scars, sores, and ulcers.

Inspecting and palpating the skin

Before you begin your examination, make sure that the lighting is adequate for inspection. Put on a pair of gloves. To examine the patient's skin, you will use both inspection and palpation—sometimes simultaneously. During your examination, focus on such skin tissue characteristics as color, texture, turgor, moisture, and temperature. Evaluate skin lesions, edema, hair distribution, and fingernails and toenails.

Color

Begin by systematically inspecting the overall appearance of the skin. Remember, skin color reflects the patient's nutritional, hematologic, cardiovascular, and pulmonary status.

Observe the patient's general coloring and pigmentation, keeping in mind racial differences as well as normal variations from one part of the body to another. Examine all exposed areas of the skin, including the face, ears, back of the neck, axillae, and backs of the hands and arms.

Note the location of any bruising, discoloration, or erythema. Look for pallor, a dusky appearance, jaundice, and cyanosis. Ask the patient if he or she has noticed any changes in skin color anywhere on the body.

Texture

Inspect and palpate the texture of the skin, noting thickness and mobility. Does the skin feel rough, smooth, thick, fragile, or thin? Changes can indicate local irritation or trauma, or they may be a result of problems in other body systems. For example, rough, dry skin is common in hypothyroidism; soft, moist skin is common in hyperthyroidism. To determine if the skin over a joint is supple or taut, have the patient bend the joint as you palpate.

Turgor

Assessing the turgor, or elasticity, of the patient's skin helps you to evaluate hydration. To assess turgor, gently squeeze the skin on the forearm. If it quickly returns to its original shape, the patient has normal turgor. If it resumes its original shape slowly or maintains a tented shape, the skin has poor turgor.

AGE ALERT

Decreased turgor occurs with dehydration as well as with aging. Increased turgor is associated with progressive systemic sclerosis.

To accurately assess skin turgor in an elderly patient, try squeezing the skin of the sternum or forehead instead of the forearm. In an elderly patient, the skin of the forearm tends to be paper-thin, dry, and wrinkled, so it does not accurately represent the patient's hydration status.

Moisture

Observe the skin for excessive dryness or moisture. If the patient's skin is too dry, you may see reddened or flaking areas. Elderly patients commonly have dry, itchy skin. Moisture that appears shiny may result from oiliness.

If the patient is overhydrated, the skin may be edematous and spongy. Localized edema can occur in response to trauma or skin abnormalities such as ulcers. When you palpate local edema, document associated discoloration or lesions.

Temperature

To assess skin temperature, touch the surface with the back of your hand. Inflamed skin will feel warm because of increased blood flow. Cool skin results from vasoconstriction. With hypovolemic shock, for instance, the skin feels cool and clammy.

Make sure to distinguish between generalized and localized warmth or coolness. Generalized warmth, or hyperthermia, is associated with fever stemming from a systemic infection or viral illness. Localized warmth occurs with a burn or localized infection. Generalized coolness occurs with hypothermia; localized coolness, with arteriosclerosis.

Skin lesions

During your inspection, you may note vascular changes in the form of red, pigmented lesions. Among the most common lesions are hemangiomas, telangiectases, petechiae, purpura, and ecchymoses. These lesions may indicate medical conditions. For instance, you can see telangiectases in pregnant patients and in those with hepatic cirrhosis.

Assessing dark skin

Be prepared for certain color variations when assessing dark-skinned patients. For example, some dark-skinned patients have a pigmented line, called Futcher's line, extending diagonally and symmetrically from the shoulder to the elbow on the lateral edge of the bicep muscle. This line is normal. Deeply pigmented ridges in the palms are also a normal variation.

To detect color variations in dark-skinned patients, examine the sclerae, conjunctivae, buccal mucosa, tongue, lips, nail beds, palms, and soles. A yellow-brown or ash-gray color in dark-skinned patients indicates pallor, which results from a lack of the underlying pink and red tones normally present in dark skin.

Among dark-skinned patients, yellowish pigmentation is not necessarily an indication of jaundice. To detect jaundice in these patients, examine the hard palate and the sclerae.

Look for petechiae by examining areas with lighter pigmentation, such as the abdomen, gluteal areas, and the palmar aspect of the forearm. To distinguish petechiae and ecchymoses from erythema in dark-skinned patients, apply pressure to the area. Erythematous areas will blanch, but petechiae or ecchymoses will not. Erythema is commonly associated with increased skin warmth.

When you assess edema in dark-skinned patients, remember that the affected area may have decreased color because fluid expands the distance between the pigmented layers and the external epithelium. When you palpate the affected area, it may feel tight.

Cyanosis can be difficult to identify due to skin tones. Because certain factors, such as cold, affect the lips and nail beds, make sure to assess the conjunctivae, palms, soles, buccal mucosa, and tongue as well.

To detect rashes in dark-skinned patients, palpate the area to identify changes in skin texture.

Evaluating skin color variations

Color	Distribution	Possible Cause
Absent	Small, circumscribed areas	Vitiligo
	Generalized	Albinism
Blue	Around lips (circumoral pallor) or generalized	Cyanosis (*Note:* In dark-skinned patients, bluish gingivae are normal.)
Deep red	Generalized	Polycythemia vera (increased red blood cell count)
Pink	Local or generalized	Erythema (superficial capillary dilation and congestion)
Tan to brown	Facial patches	Chloasma of pregnancy or butterfly rash of lupus erythematosus
Tan to brown-bronze	Generalized (not related to sun exposure)	Addison's disease
Yellow	Sclera or generalized	Jaundice from liver dysfunction (*Note:* In dark-skinned patients, yellow-brown pigmentation of the sclera is normal.)
Yellow-orange	Palms, soles, and face; not sclera	Carotenemia (carotene in the blood)
Multiple colors	Asymmetrical irregular lesions	Melanoma

Assessing the eyes, ears, nose, and throat

Initial questions

Eyes

- Ask the patient about vision problems, such as myopia, hyperopia, blurred vision, or double vision. Does the patient use corrective lenses?
- Determine the date of the last eye examination.
- Are there any visual disturbances, such as rainbows around lights, blind spots, flashing lights, or loss of vision?
- Is there any excessive tearing, dry eyes, itching, burning, pain, inflammation, swelling, color blindness, or photophobia?
- Elicit any history of eye infections, eye trauma, glaucoma, cataracts, detached retina, or other eye disorders.
- If he or she is older than age 50 or has a family history of glaucoma, ask about the date and results of his or her last test for glaucoma.

Ears

- Find out if the patient has hearing problems, such as deafness, poor hearing, tinnitus, or vertigo. Is he or she abnormally sensitive to noise? Has there been a recent change in hearing?
- Ask about ear discharge, pain, or tenderness behind the ears.
- Ask about frequent or recent ear infections or ear surgery.
- Ask the date and result of the last hearing test.
- Does the patient use a hearing aid?
- Determine ear-care habits, including the use of cotton-tipped applicators to remove ear wax.
- Ask about exposure to loud noise, including the use of protective earplugs or headphones.

Nose

- Ask about nasal problems, including allergies, sinusitis, discharge, colds, rhinitis, trauma, and frequent sneezing.
- Determine whether your patient has an obstruction, breathing problems, or an inability to smell. Have there been any nosebleeds? Has he or she had a change in appetite or the sense of smell? Has the patient used nasal sprays?
- Ask about surgery on the nose or sinuses. If so, ask when, why, and what type.

Mouth and throat

- Investigate whether your patient has sores in the mouth or on the tongue. Is there a history of oral herpes infection?
- Ask if he or she has toothaches, bleeding gums, loss of taste, voice changes, dry mouth, or frequent sore throats.
- If the patient has frequent sore throats, ask when they occur. Are they associated with fever or difficulty swallowing? How have the sore throats been treated medically?
- Ask if the patient has ever had a problem swallowing. If so, does he or she have trouble swallowing solids or liquids? Is the problem constant or intermittent? What precipitates the difficulty? What makes it go away?
- Determine whether there are dental caries or tooth loss. Does the patient wear dentures or bridges?
- Ask about the date and result of the last dental examination.
- Ask about his or her dental hygiene practices, including the use of fluoride toothpaste, waterpik, and/or floss.

Inspecting the conjunctivae

Inferior palpebral conjunctiva

While wearing gloves, gently evert the patient's lower eyelid with the thumb and index finger, as shown below. Ask the patient to look up, down, to the left, and to the right as you examine the palpebral conjunctiva. It should be clear and shiny.

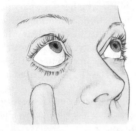

Superior palpebral conjunctiva

Check the superior palpebral conjunctiva only if you suspect a foreign body or if the patient has eyelid pain. To perform this examination, ask the patient to look down while you gently pull the medial eyelashes forward and upward with your thumb and index finger.

While holding the eyelashes, press on the tarsal border with a cotton-tipped applicator to evert the eyelid, as shown below. Hold the lashes against the brow and examine the conjunctiva, which should be pink, with no swelling.

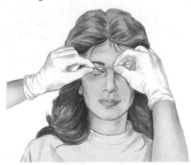

To return the eyelid to its normal position, release the eyelashes and ask the patient to look upward. If this does not invert the eyelid, grasp the eyelashes and gently pull them forward.

Testing the pupillary response and cardinal positions of gaze

The pupillary response to light should be tested before the cardinal positions of gaze. Shine a bright light in the eye and bring the light in from the side. Watch the response of the pupil to light in that eye and also in the opposite eye. Repeat the test on the other eye. Test for near accommodation by having the patient focus on an object in the distance and then shift focus to an object close to the face. Normal pupils will constrict with vision shift from distant to near object.

The cardinal positions of gaze test evaluate the oculomotor, trigeminal, and abducens nerves as well as the extraocular muscles. To perform the test, sit directly in front of the patient and ask him or her to remain still. Hold a small object, such as a pencil, directly in front of the nose at a distance of about 18″ (46 cm). Ask the patient to follow the object with only the eyes without moving the head.

Next, move the object to each of the six cardinal positions, returning it to the midpoint after each movement. The patient's eyes should remain parallel as they move. Document abnormal findings, such as nystagmus or the failure of one eye to follow the object. *Note*: When the eyes are in extreme lateral positions, a few unsustained beats of nystagmus are normal.

Test each of the six cardinal positions of gaze: left superior, left lateral, left inferior, right inferior, right lateral, and right superior. The following illustrations show testing of the three left positions.

Left superior

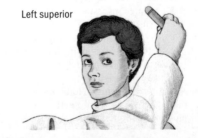

Left lateral

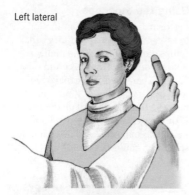

Left inferior

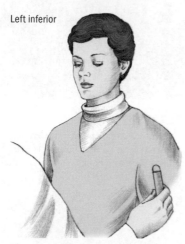

Performing an ophthalmoscopic examination

To use an ophthalmoscope to identify abnormalities of the inner eye, follow these steps.

- Place the patient in a darkened room.
- Sit or stand in front of the patient with your head about 18″ (46 cm) in front of and about 15 degrees to the right of the patient's line of vision in the right eye. Hold the ophthalmoscope in your right hand with the viewing aperture as close to your right eye as possible. Place your left thumb on the patient's

right eyebrow to keep from hitting him or her with the ophthalmoscope as you move in close. Keep your right index finger on the lens selector to adjust the lens as necessary, as shown below. To examine the left eye, perform these steps on the patient's left side. Use your left eye to examine the left eye.

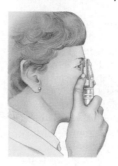

- Instruct the patient to look straight ahead at a fixed point on the wall. Next, approaching from an oblique angle about 15″ (38 cm) out and with the diopter set at 0, focus a small circle of light on the pupil, as shown below.

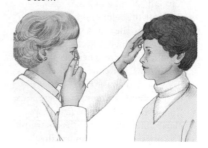

Look for the orange-red glow of the red reflex, which should be sharp and distinct through the pupil. The red reflex indicates that the lens is free from structural abnormalities and clouding.

- Move closer to the patient, changing the lens selector with your forefinger to keep the retinal structures in focus, as shown in the next page.

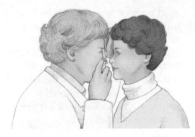

- View the vitreous humor, observing for opacity.
- Look for a retinal blood vessel and follow that vessel toward the patient's nose, rotating the lens selector to keep the vessel in focus. Carefully examine all of the retinal structures, including the retinal vessels, optic disk, retinal background, macula, and fovea centralis retinae.
- Examine the vessels for color, size ratio of arterioles to veins, arteriole light reflex, and arteriovenous (AV) crossing. The crossing points should be smooth, without nicks or narrowing. The vessels should be free from exudate, bleeding, and narrowing. Retinal vessels normally have an AV ratio of 2:3 or 4:5.
- Evaluate the color of the retinal structures. The retina should be light yellow to orange, and the background should be free from hemorrhages, aneurysms, and exudates. The optic disk, located on the nasal side of the retina, should be orange-red with distinct margins. Note the size, shape, clarity, and color of the disk margins. The physiologic cup is normally yellow-white and readily visible.
- Examine the macula last, and as briefly as possible, because it is very light sensitive. The macula, which is darker than the rest of the retinal background, is free from vessels and located temporally to the optic disk. The fovea centralis retina is a slight depression in the center of the macula.

Using the otoscope

Perform an otoscopic examination to assess the external auditory canal, tympanic membrane, and malleus. Before you insert the speculum into the patient's ear, check the canal opening for foreign particles or discharge. Palpate the tragus and pull up the auricle. If this area is tender, the patient may have external otitis, and inserting the speculum could be painful.

AGE ALERT

A pneumatic otoscope may be used in pediatric patients to assess mobility of the tympanic membrane in otitis media with effusion.

If the ear canal is clear, straighten the canal by grasping the auricle and pulling it up and back, as shown below. Then insert the speculum.

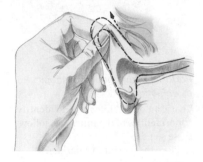

AGE ALERT

For an infant or a toddler, to straighten the canal, grasp the auricle and pull it down and back.

Hold the otoscope as shown below, with your hands parallel to the patient's head and the handle of the otoscope facing up. This position ensures that gentle pressure is exerted. Avoid hitting the ear canal with the speculum. *Note:* Some providers prefer holding the otoscope with handle facing down in young pediatric patients to accommodate the position of the canal.

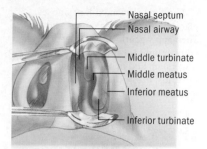

Nasal septum
Nasal airway
Middle turbinate
Middle meatus
Inferior meatus
Inferior turbinate

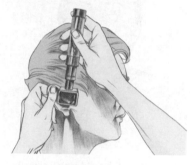

Inspecting the nostrils

To perform direct inspection of the nostrils, you will need a nasal speculum and a small flashlight or penlight.

Have the patient sit in front of you and tilt the head back. Insert the tip of the closed speculum into one of the nostrils until you reach the point where the blade widens. Slowly open the speculum as wide as you can without causing discomfort. Shine the flashlight into the nostril to illuminate the area. The illustration below shows proper placement of the nasal speculum. The inset shows the structures that should be visible during examination of the left nostril.

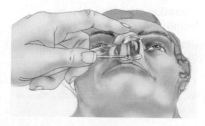

Note the color and patency of the nostril and the presence of exudate. The mucosa should be moist, pink to red, and free from lesions and polyps. Normally, you would not see drainage, edema, or inflammation of the nasal mucosa, although some tissue enlargement is normal in a pregnant patient.

You should see the choana (posterior air passage), cilia, and the middle and inferior turbinates. Below each turbinate is a groove, or meatus, where the paranasal sinuses drain.

When you have completed your inspection of one nostril, close the speculum and remove it. Then inspect the other nostril.

Inspecting and palpating the frontal and maxillary sinuses

During an inspection, you will be able to examine the frontal and maxillary sinuses but not the ethmoidal and sphenoidal sinuses. However, if the frontal and maxillary sinuses are infected, you can assume that the ethmoidal and sphenoidal are infected as well.

Begin by checking for swelling around the eyes, especially over the sinus area. Then palpate the frontal and maxillary sinuses for tenderness and warmth.

To palpate the frontal sinuses, place your thumb above the patient's eyes, just under the bony ridges of the upper orbits, and press up. Place your fingertips on the forehead and apply gentle pressure.

To palpate the maxillary sinuses, place your thumbs as shown below. Then apply gentle pressure by pressing your thumbs (or index and middle fingers) up and in on each side of the nose, just below the zygomatic bone (cheekbone).

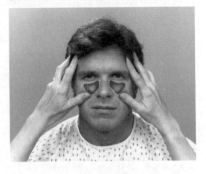

Inspecting and palpating the thyroid gland

To locate the thyroid gland, observe the lower third of the patient's anterior neck. With the patient's neck extended slightly, look for masses or asymmetry in the gland. Ask the patient to sip water, with the neck still slightly extended. Watch the thyroid rise and fall with the trachea. You should see slight, symmetrical movement. A fixed thyroid lobe may indicate a mass.

Palpate the thyroid gland while standing in front of the patient. Locate the cricoid cartilage first and then move one hand to each side to palpate the thyroid lobes. The lobes can be difficult to feel because of their location and the presence of overlying tissues.

Another way to test the thyroid is to stand behind the patient and place the fingers of both hands on the neck, just below the cricoid cartilage. Have the patient swallow and feel the rise of the thyroid isthmus. Move your fingers down and to the sides to feel the lateral lobes.

To evaluate the size and texture of the thyroid gland, ask the patient to tilt the head to the right. Gently displace the thyroid toward the right. Have the patient swallow as you palpate the lateral lobes of the thyroid, as shown below. Displace the thyroid toward the left to examine the left side.

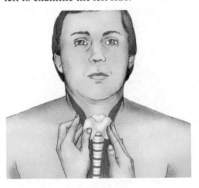

An enlarged thyroid may feel well-defined and finely lobulated. Thyroid nodules feel like a knot, protuberance, or swelling. A firm, fixed nodule may be a tumor. Do not confuse thick neck muscles with an enlarged thyroid or goiter.

Inspecting the mouth and throat

To perform direct inspection of the mouth and throat, you will need a flashlight or penlight and a tongue depressor. Assess the lips, tongue, teeth, gums, oral mucosa, tonsils, and throat. Many nurses combine the oral assessment with the cranial nerve assessments for glossopharyngeal, vagus, and hypoglossal nerves.

Palpating the cervical lymph nodes

Use the pads of your fingertips in a circular motion to perform light palpation. Palpate each cervical lymph node area bilaterally and simultaneously for comparison. Document any masses or tenderness.

Selected references

American Psychiatric Association. (2013). *Diagnostic and statistical manual of mental disorders* (5th ed.). Arlington, VA: Author.

Bickley, L. S., Szilagyi, P. G., & Hoffman, R. M. (2017). *Bates' guide to physical examination and history taking* (12th ed.). Philadelphia, PA: Wolters Kluwer.

Flynn, J. T., Kaelber, D. C., Baker-Smith, C. M., Blowey, D., Carroll, A. E., Daniels, S. R., . . . Urbina, E. M. (2017). Clinical practice guideline for screening and management of high blood pressure in children and adolescents. *Pediatrics, 140*(3), e20171904.

Whelton, P., Carey, R., Aronow, W., Casey, D., Jr., Collins, K., Himmelfrab, C., . . . Wright, J., Jr. (2018). 2017 ACC/AHA/AAPA/ABC/ACPM/AGS/APhA/ASH/ASPC/NMA/PCNA guideline for the prevention, detection, evaluation, and management of high blood pressure in adults: A report of the American College of Cardiology/American Heart Association Task Force on Clinical Practice Guidelines. *Hypertension, 71*(6), e13–e115.

2

Assessment Findings

Distinguishing health from disease

Normal findings

To distinguish between health and disease, you must be able to recognize normal assessment findings in each part of the body. When you perform a physical examination, use this head-to-toe roster of normal findings as a reference. It is designed to help you quickly zero in on physical abnormalities and evaluate your patient's overall condition.

Head and neck

Inspection

Head

- A symmetrical, lesion-free skull
- Symmetrical facial structures with normal variations in skin texture and pigmentation
- An ability to shrug the shoulders, a sign of an adequately functioning cranial nerve XI (accessory nerve)

Neck

- Unrestricted range of motion in the neck
- No bulging of the thyroid
- Symmetrical lymph nodes with no swelling
- Flat jugular veins

Palpation

Head

- No lumps or tenderness on the head
- Symmetrical strength in the facial muscles, a sign of adequately functioning cranial nerves V and VII (trigeminal and facial nerves)
- Symmetrical sensation when you stroke a wisp of cotton on each cheek

Neck

- Mobile, soft lymph nodes less than ½″ (1 cm) with no tenderness
- Symmetrical pulses in the carotid arteries
- A palpable, symmetrical, lesion-free thyroid with no tenderness
- Midline location of the trachea and absence of tracheal tenderness
- No crepitus, tenderness, or lesions in the cervical spine
- Symmetrical muscle strength in the neck

Auscultation

Head

- Auscultate the temporal artery.

Neck

- Auscultate for carotid bruits.
- Auscultate for thyroid bruits.

Eyes

Inspection

- No edema, scaling, or lesions on eyelids
- Eyelids completely covering corneas when closed
- Eyelid color the same as surrounding skin color
- Palpebral fissures of equal height
- Margin of the upper lid falling between the superior pupil margin and the superior limbus
- Symmetrical, lesion-free upper eyelids that do not sag or droop when the patient opens his or her eyes
- Evenly distributed eyelashes that curve outward
- Globe of the eye neither protruding from nor sunken into the orbit

- Eyebrows with equal size, color, and distribution
- Absence of nystagmus
- Clear conjunctiva with visible small blood vessels and no signs of drainage
- White sclera visible through the conjunctiva
- A transparent anterior chamber that contains no visible material when you shine a penlight into the side of the eye
- Transparent, smooth, and bright cornea with no visible irregularities or lesions
- Closing of the lids of both eyes when you stroke each cornea with a wisp of cotton, a test of cranial nerve V (trigeminal nerve)
- Round, equal-sized pupils that react to light and accommodation
- Constriction of both pupils when you shine a light on one
- Lacrimal structures free from exudate, swelling, and excessive tearing
- Proper eye alignment
- Parallel eye movement in each of the six cardinal fields of gaze

Palpation
- No eyelid swelling or tenderness
- Globes that feel equally firm but not overly hard or spongy
- Lacrimal sacs that do not regurgitate fluid

Ears

Inspection
- Bilaterally symmetrical, proportionately sized auricles with a vertical measurement of 1½″ to 4″ (4 to 10 cm)
- Tip of ear crossing eye–occiput line (an imaginary line extending from the lateral aspect of the eye to the occipital protuberance)
- Long axis of the ear perpendicular to (or no more than 10 degrees from perpendicular to) the eye–occiput line

- Color match between the ears and facial skin
- No signs of inflammation, lesions, or nodules
- No cracking, thickening, scaling, or lesions behind the ear when you bend the auricle forward
- No visible discharge from the auditory canal
- A patent external meatus
- Skin color on the mastoid process that matches the skin color of the surrounding area
- No redness or swelling
- Normal drum landmarks and a bright reflex, with no canal inflammation or drainage, seen on otoscopic examination

Palpation
- No masses or tenderness on the auricle
- No tenderness on the auricle or tragus during manipulation
- Either small, nonpalpable lymph nodes on the auricle or discrete, mobile lymph nodes with no signs of tenderness
- Well-defined, bony edges on the mastoid process with no signs of tenderness

Nose and mouth

Inspection

Nose
- Symmetrical, lesion-free nose with no deviation of the septum or discharge
- Little or no nasal flaring
- Nonedematous frontal and maxillary sinuses
- Ability to identify familiar odors
- Pink-red nasal mucosa with no visible lesions and no purulent drainage
- No evidence of foreign bodies or dried blood in the nose

Mouth
- Pink lips with no dryness, cracking, lesions, or cyanosis
- Symmetrical facial structures

- Ability to purse the lips and puff out the cheeks, a sign of an adequately functioning cranial nerve VII (facial nerve)
- Ability to open and close the mouth easily
- Light pink, moist oral mucosa with no ulcers or lesions
- Visible salivary ducts with no inflammation
- White, hard palate
- Pink, soft palate
- Pink gums with no tartar, inflammation, hemorrhage, or leukoplakia
- All teeth intact, with no signs of occlusion, caries, or breakage
- Pink tongue that protrudes symmetrically and has no swelling, coating, ulcers, or lesions
- Ability to move the tongue easily and without tremor, a sign of a properly functioning cranial nerve XII (hypoglossal nerve)
- No swelling or inflammation on the anterior and posterior arches
- No lesions or inflammation on the posterior pharynx
- Lesion-free tonsils that are the appropriate size for the patient's age
- An uvula that moves upward when the patient says "ah" and a gag reflex that occurs when a tongue blade touches the posterior pharynx. These are signs of properly functioning cranial nerves IX and X (glossopharyngeal and vagus nerve) .

Palpation

Nose

- No structural deviation, tenderness, or swelling on the external nose
- No tenderness or edema on the frontal and maxillary sinuses

Mouth

- Lips free from pain and induration
- No tenderness on the posterior and lateral surfaces of the tongue
- No tenderness or nodules on the floor of the mouth

Lungs
Inspection

- Symmetrical side-to-side configuration of the chest
- Anteroposterior diameter less than the transverse diameter, with a 1:2 ratio in an adult
- Normal chest shape, with no deformities, such as a barrel chest, kyphosis, retraction, sternal protrusion, or depressed sternum
- Costal angle less than 90 degrees, with the ribs joining the spine at a 45-degree angle
- Quiet, unlabored respirations with no use of accessory neck, shoulder, or abdominal muscles. You should also see no intercostal, substernal, or supraclavicular retractions.
- Symmetrically expanding chest wall during respirations
- Normal adult respiratory rate of 12 to 20 breaths/minute, with some variation depending on the patient's age
- Regular respiratory rhythm, with expiration taking about twice as long as inspiration. Men and children breathe diaphragmatically, whereas women breathe thoracically.
- Skin color that matches the rest of the body's complexion

Palpation

- Warm, dry skin
- No tender spots or bulges in the chest
- No asymmetrical expansion, fremitus, or subcutaneous crepitation

Percussion

- Resonant percussion sounds over the lungs

Auscultation

- Loud, high-pitched bronchial breath sounds over the trachea
- Intense, medium-pitched bronchovesicular breath sounds over the mainstem bronchi, between the scapulae, and below the clavicles

- Soft, breezy, low-pitched vesicular breath sounds over most of the peripheral lung fields

Heart

Inspection

- No visible pulsations, except at the point of maximum impulse (PMI)
- No lifts (heaves) or retractions in the four valve areas of the chest wall

Palpation

- No detectable vibrations or thrills
- No lifts (heaves)
- No pulsations, except at the PMI and epigastric area. At the PMI, a localized (less than ½″ [1 cm] in diameter) tapping pulse may be felt at the start of systole. In the epigastric area, pulsation from the abdominal aorta may be palpable.

Auscultation

- A first heart sound (S_1)—the *lub* sound heard best with the diaphragm of the stethoscope over the mitral area when the patient is in a left lateral position. It sounds longer, lower, and louder there than second heart sounds (S_2). S_1 splitting may be audible in the tricuspid area.
- An S_2 sound—the *dub* sound heard best with the diaphragm of the stethoscope in the aortic area while the patient sits and leans forward. It sounds shorter, sharper, higher, and louder there than S_1 sounds. Normal S_2 splitting may be audible in the pulmonic area on inspiration.
- A third heart sound (S_3). This sound is normal in children and slender, young adults with no cardiovascular disease. It usually disappears when adults reach ages 25 to 35. However, in an older adult, it may signify ventricular failure. S_3 may be heard best with the bell of the stethoscope over the mitral area with the patient in a supine position and exhaling. It sounds short, dull, soft, and low.

- A murmur, which may be functional in children and young adults but is abnormal in older adults. Innocent murmurs are soft and short, and they vary with respirations and patient's position. They occur in early systole and are heard best in the pulmonic or mitral area with the patient in a supine position.

Abdomen

Inspection

- Skin free from vascular lesions, jaundice, surgical scars, and rashes
- Faint venous patterns (except in thin patients)
- Flat, round, or scaphoid abdominal contour
- Symmetrical abdomen
- Umbilicus positioned midway between the xiphoid process and the symphysis pubis, with a flat or concave hemisphere
- No variations in skin color
- No apparent bulges
- Abdominal movement apparent with respirations
- Pink or silver-white striae from pregnancy or weight loss

Auscultation

- High-pitched, gurgling bowel sounds, heard every 5 to 15 seconds through the diaphragm of the stethoscope in all four quadrants of the abdomen
- Vascular sounds heard through the bell of the stethoscope
- Venous hum over the inferior vena cava
- No bruits, murmurs, friction rubs, or other venous hums

Percussion

- Tympany predominantly over hollow organs, including the stomach, intestines, bladder, abdominal aorta, and gallbladder
- Dullness over solid masses, including the liver, spleen, pancreas, kidneys, uterus, and a full bladder

Palpation

- No tenderness or masses
- Abdominal musculature free from tenderness and rigidity
- No guarding, rebound tenderness, distention, or ascites
- Unpalpable liver except in children (If palpable, the liver edge is regular, sharp, and nontender and is felt no more than ¾″ [2 cm] below the right costal margin.)
- Unpalpable spleen
- Unpalpable kidneys except in thin patients or those with a flaccid abdominal wall (The right kidney is felt more commonly than the left.)

Arms and legs

Inspection

- No gross deformities
- Symmetrical body parts
- Good body alignment
- No involuntary movements
- Smooth gait
- Full range of motion in all muscles and joints
- No pain with full range of motion
- No visible swelling or inflammation of joints or muscles
- Equal bilateral limb length and symmetrical muscle mass

Palpation

- Normal shape with no swelling or tenderness
- Equal bilateral muscle tone, texture, and strength
- No involuntary contractions or twitching
- Equally strong bilateral pulses

Exploring the most common chief complaints

A patient's chief complaint is the starting point for almost every initial assessment. You may be the patient's first contact, so you must recognize the condition and determine the need for medical or nursing intervention. To thoroughly evaluate the patient's chief complaint, you must ask the right questions about the patient's health history, conduct a physical examination based on the history data you collect, and analyze possible causes of the problem.

The following list examines the most common chief complaints encountered in nursing practice. For each one, you will find a concise description, detailed questions to ask during the history, areas to focus on during the physical examination, and common causes to consider.

Anxiety

A subjective reaction to a real or imagined threat, anxiety is a nonspecific feeling of uneasiness or dread. It may be mild to moderate or severe. Mild to moderate anxiety may cause slight physical or psychological discomfort. Severe anxiety may be incapacitating or even life-threatening.

Anxiety is a normal response to actual danger, prompting the body (through stimulation of the sympathetic nervous system) to purposeful action. It is also a normal response to physical and emotional stress, which virtually any illness can produce. Anxiety may also be precipitated or exacerbated by many nonpathologic factors, including lack of sleep, poor diet, and excessive intake of caffeine or other stimulants. However, excessive, unwarranted anxiety may indicate an underlying psychological problem.

Health history

- What are you anxious about? When did the anxiety first occur? What were the circumstances? What do you think caused it?
- Is the anxiety constant or sporadic? Do you notice any precipitating factors?
- How intense is the anxiety on a scale of 0 to 10, with 10 being the worst? What decreases it?
- Do you smoke? Do you use caffeine? Alcohol? Drugs? What medications do you take?

Physical examination

Perform a complete physical examination, focusing on complaints that the anxiety may trigger or aggravate.

Causes

Asthma

In allergic asthma attacks, acute anxiety occurs with dyspnea, wheezing, productive cough, accessory muscle use, hyperresonant lung fields, diminished breath sounds, coarse crackles, cyanosis, tachycardia, and diaphoresis.

Conversion disorder

Chronic anxiety is characteristic of conversion disorder, along with one or two somatic complaints that have no physiologic basis. Common complaints are dizziness, chest pain, palpitations, a lump in the throat, and choking.

Hyperthyroidism

Acute anxiety may be an early sign of hyperthyroidism. Classic signs include heat intolerance, weight loss despite increased appetite, nervousness, tremor, palpitations, sweating, an enlarged thyroid, and diarrhea. Exophthalmos may occur as well.

Hyperventilation syndrome

Hyperventilation syndrome produces acute anxiety, pallor, circumoral and peripheral paresthesia, and, occasionally, carpopedal spasms.

Mitral valve prolapse

Panic may occur in patients with mitral valve prolapse, which is referred to as the click-murmur syndrome. The disorder may also cause paroxysmal palpitations accompanied by sharp, stabbing, or aching precordial pain. Its hallmark is a midsystolic click followed by an apical systolic murmur.

Mood disorder

In the depressive form of mood disorder, chronic anxiety occurs with varying severity. The hallmark is depression on awakening that abates during the day. Associated findings include dysphoria; anger; insomnia or hypersomnia; decreased libido, interest, energy, and concentration; appetite disturbance; multiple somatic complaints; and suicidal thoughts.

Obsessive-compulsive disorder

Chronic anxiety occurs in obsessive-compulsive disorder, along with recurrent, unshakable thoughts or impulses to perform ritualistic acts. The patient recognizes these acts as irrational but cannot control them. Anxiety builds if he or she cannot perform these acts and diminishes after he or she does.

Phobias

In phobias, chronic anxiety occurs along with persistent fear of an object, activity, or situation that results in a compelling desire to avoid it. The patient recognizes the fear as irrational but cannot suppress it.

Postconcussion syndrome

Postconcussion syndrome may produce chronic anxiety or periodic attacks of acute anxiety. Associated symptoms include irritability, insomnia, dizziness, and mild headache. The anxiety is usually most pronounced in situations that demand attention, judgment, or comprehension.

Posttraumatic stress disorder

Posttraumatic stress disorder produces chronic anxiety of varying severity and is accompanied by intrusive, vivid memories and thoughts of the traumatic event. The patient also relives the event in dreams and nightmares. Insomnia, depression, and feelings of numbness and detachment are common.

Somatoform disorder

Most common in adolescents and young adults, somatoform disorder is characterized by chronic anxiety and various somatic complaints that have no physiologic basis. Anxiety and depression may be prominent or hidden by dramatic, flamboyant, or seductive behavior.

Other causes
Angina pectoris, chronic obstructive pulmonary disease, heart failure, hypochondriacal neurosis, hypoglycemia, myocardial infarction (MI), pheochromocytoma, pneumothorax, and pulmonary embolism can cause anxiety. Certain drugs cause anxiety, especially sympathomimetics and central nervous system stimulants. Also, many antidepressants can cause paradoxical anxiety.

Cough (nonproductive)

A nonproductive cough is a noisy, forceful expulsion of air from the lungs that does not yield sputum or blood. One of the most common signs of a respiratory disorder, a nonproductive cough can be infective and cause damage, such as airway collapse, rupture of the alveoli, or blebs.

A nonproductive cough that later becomes productive is a classic sign of a progressive respiratory disease. An acute nonproductive cough has a sudden onset and may be self-limiting. A nonproductive cough that persists beyond 1 month is considered chronic; this type of cough commonly results from cigarette smoking.

Health history
- When did the cough begin? Does a certain body position or a specific activity relieve or exacerbate it? Does it get better or worse at certain times of the day? How does the cough sound? Does it occur often? Is it paroxysmal?
- Does pain accompany the cough?
- Have you noticed any recent changes in your appetite, energy level, exercise tolerance, or weight? Have you had surgery recently? Do you have any allergies? Do you smoke? Have you been exposed recently to fumes or chemicals?
- What medications are you taking?

Physical examination
Note whether the patient appears agitated, anxious, confused, diaphoretic, flushed, lethargic, nervous, pale, or restless. Is his or her skin cold or warm, clammy or dry?

Observe the rate and depth of his or her respirations, noting abnormal patterns. Then examine his or her chest configuration and chest wall motion.

Check the patient's nose and mouth for congestion, drainage, inflammation, and signs of infection. Then inspect his or her neck for jugular vein distention and tracheal deviation.

As you palpate the patient's neck, note enlarged lymph nodes or masses. Next, percuss his or her chest while listening for dullness, flatness, and tympany. Finally, auscultate his or her lungs for crackles, decreased or absent breath sounds, pleural friction rubs, rhonchi, and wheezes.

Causes
Asthma
Typically, an asthma attack occurs at night, starting with a nonproductive cough and mild wheezing. Then it progresses to audible wheezing, chest tightness, a cough that produces thick mucus, and severe dyspnea. Other signs include accessory muscle use, cyanosis, diaphoresis, flaring nostrils, flushing, intercostal and supraclavicular retractions on inspiration, prolonged expirations, tachycardia, and tachypnea.

Interstitial lung disease
With interstitial lung disease, the patient has a nonproductive cough and progressive dyspnea. He or she may also be cyanotic and fatigued and have fine crackles, finger clubbing, chest pain, and recent weight loss.

Other causes
A nonproductive cough may stem from airway occlusion, atelectasis, the common cold, hypersensitivity pneumonitis,

pericardial effusion, pleural effusion, pulmonary embolism, *Hantavirus* infection, sinusitis, medications such as angiotensin-converting enzyme (ACE) inhibitors, and gastroesophageal reflux disease. Also, incentive spirometry, intermittent positive-pressure breathing, and suctioning can induce a nonproductive cough.

AGE ALERT

Acute otitis media, which commonly occurs in infants and young children because of their short eustachian tubes, also produces nonproductive coughing.

Cough (productive)

With productive coughing, the airway passages are cleared of accumulated secretions that normal mucociliary action does not remove. The sudden, forceful, noisy expulsion contains sputum, blood, or both.

Usually caused by a cardiopulmonary disorder, productive coughing typically stems from an acute or chronic infection that causes inflammation, edema, and increased production of mucus in the airways. Such coughing can also result from inhaling antigenic or irritating substances. The most common cause is cigarette smoking.

Health history

- When did the cough begin? How much sputum do you cough up daily? Is sputum production associated with the time of day, meals, activities, or the environment? Has it increased since coughing began? What are the color, odor, and consistency of the sputum? How does the cough sound and feel? Have you ever had a productive cough before?
- Have you noticed recent changes in your appetite or weight?
- Do you have a history of recent surgery or allergies? Do you smoke or drink alcohol? If so, how much? Do you work around chemicals or respiratory irritants?
- What medications are you taking?
- Do you currently or have you in the past lived with anyone diagnosed with tuberculosis?

Physical examination

As you examine the patient's mouth and nose for congestion, drainage, and inflammation, note his or her breath odor. Then inspect his or her neck for jugular vein distention. As he or she breathes, observe the chest for accessory muscle use, intercostal and supraclavicular retractions, and uneven expansion.

Palpate his or her neck for enlarged lymph nodes, masses, and tenderness. Next, percuss his or her chest, listening for dullness, flatness, and tympany. Finally, auscultate for abnormal breath sounds, crackles, pleural friction rubs, rhonchi, and wheezes.

Causes

Bacterial pneumonia

With bacterial pneumonia, an initially dry cough becomes productive. Rust-colored sputum appears in pneumococcal pneumonia, brick-red or currant-jelly sputum in *Klebsiella* pneumonia, salmon-colored sputum in staphylococcal pneumonia, and mucopurulent sputum in streptococcal pneumonia.

Lung abscess

The cardinal sign of a ruptured lung abscess is coughing that produces copious amounts of purulent, foul-smelling, and, possibly, blood-tinged sputum. A ruptured abscess can also cause anorexia, diaphoresis, dyspnea, fatigue, fever with chills, halitosis, headache, inspiratory crackles, pleuritic chest pain, tubular or amphoric breath sounds, and weight loss.

Other causes

A productive cough can result from acute bronchiolitis, aspiration and chemical pneumonitis, bronchiectasis, the common cold, cystic fibrosis, lung cancer, pertussis, pulmonary embolism, pulmonary edema, and tracheobronchitis. Also, expectorants, incentive spirometry, and intermittent positive-pressure breathing can cause a productive cough.

Diarrhea

Usually a chief sign of an intestinal disorder, diarrhea is an increase in the frequency or volume of stools compared with the patient's normal bowel habits. It varies in severity and may be acute, persistent, or chronic. Acute diarrhea may result from acute infection, stress, fecal impaction, or the effect of a drug. It is usually self-limiting and lasts 1 or 2 days. Persistent diarrhea may result from viral infection, antibiotics such as erythromycin, and antacids that contain magnesium. It usually lasts for 2 to 4 weeks. Chronic diarrhea may result from chronic infection, obstructive and inflammatory bowel disease, malabsorption syndrome, an endocrine disorder (such as thyrotoxicosis, diabetes, or Addison's disease), side effects of chemotherapy, antiarrhythmic or antihypertensive medications, defect of the anal sphincter, AIDS, Zollinger-Ellison's syndrome, or gastrointestinal (GI) surgery. Periodic diarrhea may result from food intolerance or from ingestion of caffeine or spicy or high-fiber foods.

Health history

- Do you have abdominal pain and cramps?
- Do you have difficulty breathing?
- Are you weak or fatigued?
- What medications do you take?
- Have you had GI surgery or radiation therapy recently?
- Describe your diet.
- Do you have any known food allergies?
- Have you been experiencing any unusual stress?

Physical examination

If the patient is not in shock, proceed with a brief physical examination. Evaluate hydration; check skin turgor and the mucous membranes; and take blood pressure with the patient lying, sitting, and standing. Inspect the abdomen for distention, auscultate for bowel sounds, and palpate for tenderness. Check for tympany over the abdomen. Take the patient's temperature and note chills or rash. Conduct a rectal examination and a pelvic examination if indicated.

Causes

Anthrax, GI

GI anthrax manifests after the patient has eaten contaminated meat from an animal infected with *Bacillus anthracis*. Early signs and symptoms include decreased appetite, nausea, vomiting, and fever. Later signs and symptoms include severe bloody diarrhea, abdominal pain, and hematemesis.

Carcinoid syndrome

With carcinoid syndrome, severe diarrhea occurs with flushing—usually of the head and neck—that is commonly caused by emotional stimuli or the ingestion of food, hot water, or alcohol. Associated signs and symptoms include abdominal cramps, dyspnea, weight loss, anorexia, weakness, palpitations, valvular heart disease, and depression.

Cholera

After ingesting water or food contaminated by the bacterium *Vibrio cholerae*, the patient experiences abrupt watery diarrhea and vomiting. Other signs and symptoms include thirst (caused by severe water and electrolyte loss), weakness, muscle cramps, decreased skin turgor, oliguria, tachycardia, and hypotension. Without treatment, death can occur within hours.

Clostridium difficile infection

The patient may be asymptomatic or may have soft, unformed stools or watery diarrhea that may be foul smelling or grossly bloody; abdominal pain, cramping, and tenderness; fever; and a white blood cell count as high as 20,000/µl. In severe cases, the patient may have toxic megacolon, colonic perforation, or peritonitis.

Crohn's disease

Crohn's disease is a recurring inflammatory disorder that produces diarrhea accompanied by abdominal pain with guarding, tenderness, and nausea. The patient may also have fever, chills, weakness, anorexia, and weight loss.

Escherichia coli 0157:H7

With *Escherichia coli* infection, the patient has watery or bloody diarrhea, nausea, vomiting, fever, and abdominal cramps after eating undercooked beef or other foods contaminated with this strain of bacteria. Hemolytic uremic syndrome, which causes red blood cell destruction and eventually acute renal failure, is a complication of *E. coli* 0157:H7 infection in children age 5 and younger and in elderly people.

Infections

Acute viral, bacterial, and protozoal infections (such as cryptosporidiosis) cause the sudden onset of watery diarrhea as well as abdominal pain, cramps, nausea, vomiting, and fever. Significant fluid and electrolyte loss may cause signs of dehydration and shock. Chronic tuberculosis and fungal and parasitic infections may produce less severe but more persistent diarrhea, accompanied by epigastric distress, vomiting, weight loss, and, possibly, passage of blood and mucus.

Intestinal obstruction

Partial intestinal obstruction increases intestinal motility, resulting in diarrhea, abdominal pain with tenderness and guarding, nausea, and, possibly, distention.

Irritable bowel syndrome

Diarrhea alternates with constipation or normal bowel function. The patient may have abdominal pain, tenderness, and distention; dyspepsia; and nausea.

Ischemic bowel disease

Ischemic bowel disease is a life-threatening disorder that causes bloody diarrhea with abdominal pain. If severe, shock may occur, requiring surgery.

Lactose intolerance

With lactose intolerance, diarrhea occurs within several hours of ingesting milk or milk products. It is accompanied by cramps, abdominal pain, borborygmi, bloating, nausea, and flatus.

Large-bowel cancer

With large-bowel cancer, bloody diarrhea is seen with partial obstruction. Other signs and symptoms include abdominal pain, anorexia, weight loss, weakness, fatigue, exertional dyspnea, and depression.

Ulcerative colitis

The hallmark of ulcerative colitis is recurrent bloody diarrhea with pus or mucus. Other signs and symptoms include tenesmus, hyperactive bowel sounds, cramping lower abdominal pain, low-grade fever, anorexia, and, at times, nausea and vomiting. Weight loss, anemia, and weakness are late findings.

Other causes

Many antibiotics—such as ampicillin, cephalosporins, tetracyclines, and clindamycin—cause diarrhea. Other drugs that may cause diarrhea include magnesium-containing antacids, colchicine, guanethidine, lactulose, dantrolene, ethacrynic acid, mefenamic acid, methotrexate, metyrosine, and, in high doses, cardiac glycosides and quinidine. Laxative abuse can cause acute or chronic diarrhea. Foods that contain certain oils may inhibit absorption of food, causing acute, uncontrollable diarrhea and rectal leakage. Gastrectomy, gastroenterostomy, and pyloroplasty may produce diarrhea. High-dose radiation therapy may produce enteritis and diarrhea.

AGE ALERT

Diarrhea in children commonly results from infection, although chronic diarrhea may result from malabsorption syndrome, an anatomic defect, or allergies. Because dehydration and electrolyte imbalance occur rapidly in children, diarrhea can be life-threatening. Diligently monitor all episodes of diarrhea, and immediately replace lost fluids.

Dizziness

A common symptom, dizziness is a sensation of imbalance or faintness that is sometimes associated with blurred or double vision, confusion, and weakness. Dizziness may be mild or severe and may be aggravated by standing up quickly and alleviated by lying down. Onset may be abrupt or gradual. Episodes are usually brief.

Dizziness typically results from inadequate blood flow and oxygen supply to the cerebrum and spinal cord. It may occur with anxiety, respiratory and cardiovascular disorders, and postconcussion syndrome. Dizziness is also a key symptom of certain serious disorders, such as hypertension and vertebrobasilar artery insufficiency.

Health history

- When did the dizziness start? How severe is it? How often does it occur, and how long does each episode last? Does the dizziness abate spontaneously? Is it triggered by standing up suddenly or bending over?
- Do you have blurred vision, chest pain, a chronic cough, diaphoresis, a headache, or shortness of breath?
- Have you ever had hypertension or another cardiovascular disorder? What about diabetes mellitus, anemia, respiratory or anxiety disorders, or head injury?
- What medications and supplements are you taking?

AGE ALERT

Many children have difficulty describing dizziness and instead complain of tiredness, stomachache, and feeling sick.

Physical examination

Assess the patient's level of consciousness (LOC), body temperature, pulse rate, respirations, and blood pressure. As you observe his or her breathing, look for accessory muscle use or barrel chest. Look also for finger clubbing, cyanosis, dry mucous membranes, and poor skin turgor. Evaluate the patient's motor and sensory functions and reflexes.

Palpate the extremities for peripheral edema and capillary refill. Auscultate the patient's heart rate and rhythm and his or her breath sounds. Take the patient's blood pressure while he or she is lying down, sitting, and standing. If the diastolic pressure exceeds 100 mm Hg, notify the physician immediately and instruct the patient to lie down.

Causes

Cardiac arrhythmias

With cardiac arrhythmias, dizziness lasts for several minutes or longer and may precede fainting. Other signs and symptoms include blurred vision; confusion; hypotension; palpitations; paresthesia; weakness; and an irregular, rapid, or thready pulse.

Hypertension

With hypertension, dizziness may precede fainting but may be relieved by rest. Other findings include blurred vision; elevated blood pressure; headache; and retinal changes, such as hemorrhage and papilledema.

Transient ischemic attack

Dizziness of varying severity occurs during a transient ischemic attack. Lasting from a few seconds to 24 hours, an attack may be triggered by turning the head to the side and may signal an impending stroke. During an attack, the patient may experience blindness or visual field deficits, diplopia, hearing loss, numbness, paresis, ptosis, and tinnitus.

Other causes

Dizziness may result from anemia, generalized anxiety disorder, orthostatic hypotension, panic disorder, or postconcussion syndrome. Also, dizziness may be an adverse reaction to certain drugs, such as anxiolytics, central nervous system depressants, narcotic analgesics, decongestants, antihistamines, antihypertensives, or vasodilators. Some herbal medications, such as St. John's wort, can cause dizziness.

Dysphagia

Difficulty swallowing, or dysphagia, is the most common—and sometimes the only—symptom of an esophageal disorder. This symptom may also result from oropharyngeal, respiratory, and neurologic disorders, or from exposure to toxins. Patients with dysphagia have an increased risk of aspiration and choking and of malnutrition and dehydration.

Health history

- When did your difficulty swallowing start? Is swallowing painful? If so, is the pain constant or intermittent? Can you point to the spot where you have the most trouble swallowing? Does eating alleviate or aggravate the problem? Do you have more trouble swallowing solids or liquids? Does the problem disappear after you try to swallow a few times? Is swallowing easier if you change position?
- Have you or has anyone in your family ever had an esophageal, oropharyngeal, respiratory, or neurologic disorder? Have you recently had a tracheotomy or been exposed to a toxin?

Physical examination

Evaluate the patient's swallowing and his or her cough and gag reflexes. As you listen to his or her speech, note signs of muscle, tongue, or facial weakness; aphasia; or dysarthria. Is his or her voice nasal or hoarse? Check his or her mouth for dry mucous membranes and thick secretions.

Causes

Airway obstruction

A life-threatening condition, upper-airway obstruction is marked by mild to severe wheezing and respiratory distress. Dysphagia occurs along with gagging and dysphonia.

Esophageal carcinoma

In the patient with esophageal carcinoma, painless dysphagia typically accompanies rapid weight loss. As the carcinoma advances, dysphagia becomes painful and constant.

The patient has a cough with hemoptysis, hoarseness, sore throat, and steady chest pain.

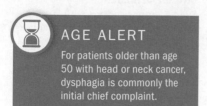

AGE ALERT

For patients older than age 50 with head or neck cancer, dysphagia is commonly the initial chief complaint.

Esophagitis

A patient with corrosive esophagitis has dysphagia accompanied by excessive salivation, fever, hematemesis, intense pain in the mouth and anterior chest, and tachypnea. *Candida* esophagitis produces dysphagia and sore throat. In reflux esophagitis, dysphagia is a late symptom that usually accompanies stricture.

Hiatal hernia

The patient with a hiatal hernia may complain of belching, dysphagia, dyspepsia, flatulence, heartburn, regurgitation, and retrosternal or substernal chest pain that is aggravated by lying down or bending over.

Other causes

Dysphagia results from botulism, esophageal diverticula or stricture, external esophageal compression, hypocalcemia, laryngeal nerve damage, and Parkinson's disease. Radiation therapy and tracheotomy may also cause dysphagia.

Dyspnea

Patients typically describe dyspnea as shortness of breath, but this symptom also refers to difficult or uncomfortable breathing. Its severity varies greatly and is generally unrelated to the seriousness of the underlying cause. Dyspnea may arise suddenly or slowly and may subside rapidly or persist for years.

Health history

- When did the dyspnea first occur? Did it begin suddenly or gradually? Is it constant or intermittent? Does it occur during activity or while you are resting? Does anything seem to trigger, worsen, or relieve it? Have you ever had dyspnea before?
- Do you have chest pain or a productive or nonproductive cough?
- Have you recently had an upper respiratory tract infection or experienced trauma? Do you smoke? If so, how much and for how long? Have you been exposed to any allergens? Do you have any known allergies?
- What medications and supplements are you taking?

Physical examination

Observe the patient's respirations, noting his or her rate and depth as well as breathing difficulties or abnormal respiratory patterns. Check for flaring nostrils, grunting respirations, inspiratory stridor, intercostal retractions during inspirations, and pursed-lip expirations.

Examine the patient for barrel chest, diaphoresis, jugular vein distention, finger clubbing, and peripheral edema. Note the color, consistency, and odor of sputum.

Palpate his or her chest for asymmetrical expansion, decreased diaphragmatic excursion, tactile fremitus, and subcutaneous crepitation. Also check the rate, rhythm, and intensity of his or her peripheral pulses.

As you percuss the lung fields, note dull, hyperresonant, or tympanic percussion sounds. Auscultate the lungs for bronchophony, crackles, decreased or absent unilateral breath sounds, egophony, pleural friction rubs, rhonchi, whispered pectoriloquy, and wheezing. Auscultate the heart for abnormal sounds or rhythms, such as ventricular or atrial gallop, and for pericardial friction rubs and tachycardia. Also monitor the patient's blood pressure and pulse pressure.

Causes

Acute respiratory distress syndrome

In acute respiratory distress syndrome (ARDS), acute dyspnea is followed by accessory muscle use, crackles, grunting respirations, progressive respiratory distress, rhonchi, and wheezes. In the late stages, anxiety, cyanosis, decreased mental acuity, and tachycardia occur. Severe ARDS can produce signs of shock, such as cool, clammy skin and hypotension. The typical patient has no history of underlying cardiac or pulmonary disease but has had a recent pulmonary or systemic insult.

Airway obstruction (partial)

Inspiratory stridor and acute dyspnea occur as the patient tries to overcome the obstruction. Related findings include accessory muscle use, anxiety, asymmetrical chest expansion, cyanosis, decreased or absent breath sounds, diaphoresis, hypotension, and tachypnea. The patient may have aspirated vomitus or a foreign body or may have been exposed to an allergen.

Asthma

Acute dyspneic attacks occur along with accessory muscle use, apprehension, dry cough, flushing or cyanosis, intercostal retractions, tachypnea, and tachycardia. On palpation, you will detect decreased tactile fremitus. Hyperresonance occurs on chest percussion. On auscultation, you will note wheezing and rhonchi or, during a severe episode, decreased breath sounds.

Heart failure

Dyspnea usually develops gradually or occurs as chronic paroxysmal nocturnal dyspnea. In ventricular failure, dyspnea occurs with basilar crackles, dependent peripheral edema, distended jugular veins, fatigue, orthopnea, tachycardia, ventricular or atrial gallop, and weight gain. The patient may have a history of cardiovascular disease, or he or she may be taking a drug—such as amiodarone (Cordarone), a beta-adrenergic blocker, or a corticosteroid—that can precipitate heart failure.

Myocardial infarction

Sudden dyspnea occurs with crushing substernal chest pain that may radiate to the back, neck, jaw, and arms. The patient's history may include heart disease, hypertension, hypercholesterolemia, or use of a drug—such as cocaine, dextrothyroxine sodium (Choloxin), estramustine phosphate sodium (Emcyt), or aldesleukin (Proleukin)—that can precipitate an MI.

Pneumonia

Dyspnea occurs suddenly and is usually accompanied by fever, pleuritic chest pain that worsens with deep inspiration, and shaking chills. The patient also has a dry or productive cough, depending on the stage and type of pneumonia. Sputum may be discolored and foul smelling. Crackles, decreased breath sounds, dullness on percussion, and rhonchi may also be present. The history may include exposure to a contagious organism, hazardous fumes, or air pollution.

Pulmonary edema

In pulmonary edema, severe dyspnea is commonly preceded by signs of heart failure, such as crackles in both lung fields, cyanosis, tachycardia, tachypnea, and marked anxiety. The patient may have a dry cough or one that produces copious amounts of pink, frothy sputum. The history may show cardiovascular disease, cyanosis, fatigue, and pallor.

Pulmonary embolism

Severe dyspnea occurs with intense angina-like or pleuritic pain that is aggravated by deep breathing and thoracic movement. Other findings include crackles, cyanosis, diffuse wheezing, dull percussion sounds, low-grade fever, nonproductive cough, pleural friction rubs, restlessness, tachypnea, and tachycardia. The patient's history may include acute MI, heart failure, a hip or leg fracture, recent abdominal surgery, hormonal contraceptive use, pregnancy, thrombophlebitis, immobility, or thrombophilias.

Other causes

Dyspnea may also result from anemia, anxiety, cardiac arrhythmias, cor pulmonale, inhalation injury, lung cancer, pleural effusion, and sepsis.

Eye pain

Eye pain, also known as *ophthalmalgia*, may be described as a burning, throbbing, aching, or stabbing sensation in or around the eye. It may also be characterized as a foreign-body sensation. This sign varies from mild to severe; its duration and exact location provide clues to the cause.

Eye pain usually results from corneal abrasion, but it may also be caused by glaucoma or other eye disorders, trauma, and neurologic or systemic disorders. Any of these may stimulate nerve endings in the cornea or external eye, producing pain.

Health history

- Can you rate the pain on a scale of 0 to 10, with 10 being the worst pain imaginable? Can you describe your pain? Is it an ache or a sharp pain? How long does it last? Is it accompanied by burning, itching, or discharge? When did the pain begin? Is it worse in the morning or in the evening?
- Have you had any recent trauma or surgery?
- Do you have headaches? If yes, how often and at what time of day do they occur?

Physical examination

During the physical examination, *do not* manipulate the eye if you suspect trauma. Carefully assess the lids and conjunctiva for redness, inflammation, and swelling. Then examine the eyes

for ptosis or exophthalmos. Finally, test visual acuity with and without correction, and assess extraocular movements. Characterize any discharge.

Causes

Acute angle-closure glaucoma

Blurred vision and sudden, excruciating pain in and around the eye characterize acute angle-closure glaucoma. The pain may be so severe that it causes nausea, vomiting, and abdominal pain. Other findings include halo vision; rapidly decreasing visual acuity; and a fixed, nonreactive, moderately dilated pupil.

Blepharitis

Blepharitis is a burning pain in both eyelids that is accompanied by itching, a sticky discharge, and conjunctival injection. Related findings include foreign-body sensation, lid ulcerations, and loss of eyelashes.

Burns

With chemical burns, sudden and severe eye pain may occur with erythema and blistering of the face and lids, photophobia, miosis, conjunctival injection, blurring, and inability to keep the eyelids open. With ultraviolet radiation burns, moderate to severe pain occurs about 12 hours after exposure along with photophobia and vision changes.

Chalazion

A chalazion causes localized tenderness and swelling on the upper or lower eyelid. Eversion of the lid shows conjunctival injection and a small red lump.

Conjunctivitis

Some degree of eye pain and excessive tearing occurs with four types of conjunctivitis. Allergic conjunctivitis causes bilateral mild burning pain accompanied by itching, conjunctival injection, and a characteristic ropy discharge.

Bacterial conjunctivitis causes pain only when it affects the cornea. Otherwise, it produces burning and a foreign-body sensation. A purulent discharge and conjunctival injection are also typical.

If the cornea is affected, fungal conjunctivitis may cause pain and photophobia. Even without corneal involvement, it causes itching; burning eyes; a thick, purulent discharge; and conjunctival injection.

Viral conjunctivitis produces itching, redness, a foreign-body sensation, visible conjunctival follicles, and eyelid edema.

Corneal abrasions

With corneal abrasions, eye pain is characterized by a foreign-body sensation. Excessive tearing, photophobia, conjunctival injection, and an inability to keep the eyelid open are also common.

Corneal ulcers

Both bacterial and fungal corneal ulcers cause severe eye pain. They may also cause a purulent eye discharge, sticky eyelids, photophobia, and impaired visual acuity. Bacterial corneal ulcers also produce a gray-white, irregularly shaped ulcer on the cornea; unilateral pupil constriction; and conjunctival injection. Fungal corneal ulcers produce conjunctival injection; eyelid edema and erythema; and a dense, cloudy, central ulcer surrounded by progressively clearer rings.

Foreign bodies in the cornea and conjunctiva

Sudden, severe pain is common with foreign bodies in the cornea and conjunctiva, but vision usually remains intact. Other findings include excessive tearing, photophobia, miosis, a foreign-body sensation, a dark speck on the cornea, and dramatic conjunctival injection.

Glaucoma

Open-angle glaucoma may cause mild aching in the eyes as well as loss of peripheral vision, halo vision, and reduced visual acuity that is not corrected by glasses. Angle-closure glaucoma may cause pain and pressure over the eye,

blurred vision, halo vision, decreased visual acuity, and nausea and vomiting.

Iritis (acute)

Acute iritis causes moderate to severe eye pain with severe photophobia, dramatic conjunctival injection, and blurred vision. The constricted pupil may respond poorly to light.

Migraine headache

Migraines can produce pain so severe that the eyes also ache. Additionally, the patient may have nausea, vomiting, blurred vision, and sensitivity to light and noise.

Ocular laceration and intraocular foreign bodies

Penetrating eye injuries usually cause mild to severe unilateral eye pain and impaired visual acuity. Eyelid edema, conjunctival injection, and an abnormal pupillary response may also occur.

Optic neuritis

With optic neuritis, the patient may have pain in and around the eye. Severe vision loss and tunnel vision develop but improve in 2 to 3 weeks. Pupils respond sluggishly to direct light but normally to consensual light.

Other causes

Contact lenses may cause eye pain and a foreign-body sensation. Ocular surgery may also produce eye pain that ranges from a mild ache to a severe pounding or stabbing sensation.

AGE ALERT

Glaucoma, which can cause eye pain, is usually a disease of older patients, becoming clinically significant after age 40. It usually occurs bilaterally and leads to slowly progressive vision loss, especially in the peripheral visual fields.

Fatigue

A common symptom, fatigue is a feeling of excessive tiredness, lack of energy, or exhaustion, accompanied by a strong desire to rest or sleep. Fatigue differs from weakness, which involves the muscles and may occur with fatigue.

Fatigue is a normal response to physical overexertion, emotional stress, and sleep deprivation. It can also result from psychological and physiologic disorders, especially viral infections and endocrine, cardiovascular, or neurologic disorders.

Health history

- When did the fatigue begin? Is it constant or intermittent? If it is intermittent, when does it occur? Does the fatigue worsen with activity and improve with rest, or vice versa? (The former usually signals a physiologic disorder; the latter, a psychological disorder.)
- Have you experienced any recent stressful changes at home or at work?
- Have you changed your eating habits? Have you recently lost or gained weight?
- Have you or has anyone in your family been diagnosed with any cardiovascular, endocrine, or neurologic disorders? What about viral infections or psychological disorders?
- What medications and supplements are you taking?

AGE ALERT

Always ask older patients about fatigue because this symptom may be insidious and mask a more serious underlying condition.

Physical examination

Observe the patient's general appearance for signs of depression or organic illness. Is he or she unkempt? Expressionless? Tired or unhealthy looking? Is he or she slumped over? Assess his or her mental status, noting especially agitation, attention deficits, mental clouding, or psychomotor impairment.

Causes

Anemia

Fatigue after mild activity is generally the first symptom of anemia. Other signs and symptoms typically include dyspnea, pallor, and tachycardia.

Cancer

Unexplained fatigue is commonly the earliest indication of cancer. Related signs and symptoms reflect the type, location, and stage of the tumor. They usually include abnormal bleeding, anorexia, nausea, pain, a palpable mass, vomiting, and weight loss.

Chronic infection

In a patient with a chronic infection, fatigue is usually the most prominent symptom—and sometimes the only one.

Depression

Chronic depression is usually accompanied by persistent fatigue unrelated to exertion. The patient may also have anorexia, constipation, headache, and sexual dysfunction.

Diabetes mellitus

The most common symptom of diabetes mellitus is fatigue, which may begin insidiously or abruptly. Related findings include polydipsia, polyphagia, polyuria, and weight loss.

Heart failure

Persistent fatigue and lethargy are characteristic symptoms of heart failure. Left-sided heart failure produces exertional and paroxysmal nocturnal dyspnea, orthopnea, and tachycardia. Right-sided heart failure causes jugular vein distention and, sometimes, a slight but persistent nonproductive cough.

Hypothyroidism

Fatigue occurs early in the course of hypothyroidism, along with forgetfulness, cold intolerance, weight gain, metrorrhagia, and constipation.

Myasthenia gravis

The cardinal symptoms of myasthenia gravis are easy fatigability and muscle weakness that worsen with exertion and abate with rest. These symptoms are related to the specific muscle groups affected.

Other causes

Anxiety, MI, rheumatoid arthritis, systemic lupus erythematosus, and malnutrition can cause fatigue, as can certain drugs—notably antihypertensives and sedatives—and most types of surgery.

Fever

An abnormal elevation of body temperature above 98.6° F (37° C), fever (or pyrexia) is a common sign arising from disorders that affect virtually every body system. As a result, fever alone has little diagnostic value. However, persistently high fever is a medical emergency.

Fever can be classified as low (oral reading of 99° to 100.4° F [37.2° to 38° C]), moderate (100.5° to 104° F [38° to 40° C]), or high (greater than 104° F [40° C]). Fever above 108° F (42.2° C) causes unconsciousness and, if prolonged, brain damage.

AGE ALERT

Infants and young children experience higher and more prolonged fevers, more rapid temperature increases, and greater temperature fluctuations than do older children or adults.

Health history

- When did the fever begin? How high did it reach? Is the fever constant, or does it disappear and then reappear later?
- Do you also have chills, fatigue, or pain?
- Have you had any immunodeficiency disorders, infections, recent trauma or surgery, or diagnostic tests? Have you traveled recently?
- What medications and supplements are you taking? Have you recently had anesthesia?

Causes

Infectious and inflammatory disorders

Fever may be low, as in Crohn's disease and ulcerative colitis, or extremely high, as in bacterial pneumonia. It may be remittent, as in infectious mononucleosis; sustained, as in meningitis; or relapsing, as in malaria. Fever may arise abruptly, as in Rocky Mountain spotted fever, or insidiously, as in mycoplasmal pneumonia. Typically, it accompanies a self-limiting disorder such as the common cold.

Medications

Fever and rash commonly result from hypersensitivity to such medications as quinidine, methyldopa (Aldomet), procainamide, phenytoin (Dilantin), anti-infectives, barbiturates, iodides, and some antitoxins. Fever can also result from the use of chemotherapeutic agents and medications that decrease sweating such as anticholinergics. Toxic doses of salicylates, amphetamines, and antidepressants can cause fever.

Other causes

Fever may also result from an injection of contrast media used in diagnostic tests or from surgery. Other causes include blood transfusion reactions, exercise, heat stroke, malignant hypothermia, or neuroleptic malignant syndrome.

Headache

Headache is the most common neurologic symptom. A headache may be mild to severe, localized or generalized, and constant or intermittent. About 90% of all headaches are benign and can be described as vascular, muscle contracting, or a combination of both.

Occasionally, this symptom indicates a severe neurologic disorder. A generalized, pathologic headache may result from disorders associated with intracranial inflammation, increased intracranial pressure (ICP), meningeal irritation, or vascular disturbance. A headache may also result from disorders of the eye or sinus and from the effects of drugs, tests, and treatments.

Health history

- When did the headache first occur? Describe your pain on a scale of 0 to 10, with 10 being the worst pain imaginable. Is the pain mild, moderate, or severe? Is it localized or generalized? If it is localized, where does it occur? Is it constant or intermittent? If it is intermittent, what is the duration? How would you describe the pain; for example, is it stabbing, dull, throbbing, or viselike? Does anything seem to trigger it, exacerbate it, or relieve it? Have you had this kind of headache before?
- Have you also experienced confusion, dizziness, drowsiness, eye pain, fever, muscle twitching, nausea, photophobia, seizures, difficulty speaking or walking, neck stiffness, visual disturbances, vomiting, or weakness?
- Have you been under unusual stress at home or at work? For family members: Have you noticed any changes in the patient's behavior or personality?
- Do you have a history of blood dyscrasia, cardiovascular disease, glaucoma, hemorrhagic disorders, hypertension, poor vision, seizures, migraine headaches, or smoking? Have you had a recent traumatic injury; dental work; or a sinus, ear, or systemic infection?
- What medications and supplements are you taking?

Physical examination

Observe the rate and depth of the patient's respirations, noting breathing difficulty or abnormal patterns. Inspect his or her head for bruising, swelling, and sinus bleeding. Check also for Battle's sign, neck stiffness, otorrhea, and rhinorrhea.

Assess the patient's LOC. Is he or she drowsy, lethargic, or comatosed? Examine his or her eyes, noting pupil size, equality, and response to light and accommodation. With the patient both at rest and active, note tremors.

Gently palpate the skull and sinuses for tenderness. Unless head trauma has occurred, slowly move the neck to check for nuchal rigidity or pain. Then assess the patient's motor strength. Palpate his or her peripheral pulses, noting their rate, rhythm, and intensity.

Check for Babinski's reflex. As you percuss for other reflexes, note hyperreflexia. Then auscultate over the temporal artery, listening for bruits. Also monitor the patient's blood pressure and pulse pressure.

Causes

Brain abscess

Headache caused by a brain abscess typically intensifies over a few days. It localizes to a particular spot and is aggravated by straining. The headache may be accompanied by a decreased LOC (drowsiness to deep stupor), focal or generalized seizures, nausea, and vomiting. Depending on the abscess site, the patient may also have aphasia, ataxia, impaired visual acuity, hemiparesis, personality changes, or tremors.

Signs of infection may or may not appear. The patient may have a history of systemic, chronic middle ear, mastoid, or sinus infection; osteomyelitis of the skull or a compound fracture; or a penetrating head wound.

Brain tumor

Headache caused by a brain tumor develops near the tumor site and becomes generalized as the tumor grows. Pain is usually intermittent, deep-seated, dull, and most intense in the morning. It is aggravated by coughing, stooping, Valsalva's maneuver, and changes in head position.

Cerebral aneurysm (ruptured)

Headache caused by a cerebral aneurysm is sudden and excruciating. It may be unilateral and usually peaks within minutes of the rupture. The headache may be accompanied by nausea, vomiting, and signs of meningeal irritation, and the patient may lose consciousness. His or her history may include hypertension or other cardiovascular disorders, a stressful lifestyle, or smoking.

Encephalitis

Headache caused by encephalitis is severe and generalized and is accompanied by a deteriorating LOC over a 48-hour period. Fever, focal neurologic deficits, irritability, nausea, nuchal rigidity, photophobia, seizures, and vomiting may also develop. The patient may have a history of exposure to the viruses that commonly cause encephalitis, such as mumps or herpes simplex.

Epidural hemorrhage (acute)

With acute epidural hemorrhage, a progressively severe headache immediately follows a brief loss of consciousness. Then the patient's LOC declines rapidly and steadily. Accompanying signs and symptoms include increasing ICP, ipsilateral pupil dilation, nausea, and vomiting. The patient's history usually shows head trauma within the last 24 hours.

Glaucoma (acute angle-closure)

Glaucoma is an ophthalmic emergency that may cause an excruciating headache. Other signs and symptoms include blurred vision, a cloudy cornea, halo vision, a moderately dilated and fixed pupil, photophobia, nausea, and vomiting.

Hypertension

Patients with hypertension may have a slightly throbbing occipital headache on awakening. During the day, the severity may decrease. However, if the patient's diastolic blood pressure exceeds 120 mm Hg and the headache remains constant, this situation is considered a medical emergency because of the potential for stroke.

Meningitis

With meningitis, the patient has a severe constant, generalized headache that starts suddenly and worsens with movement. He or she may also have chills, fever, hyperreflexia, nuchal rigidity, and positive Kernig's and Brudzinski's signs. His or her history may include recent systemic or sinus infection, dental work, or exposure to bacteria or viruses that commonly cause meningitis, such as *Haemophilus influenzae*, *Streptococcus pneumoniae*, enteroviruses, and mumps.

Migraine

A severe, throbbing headache, a migraine may follow a 5- to 15-minute prodrome of dizziness; tingling of the face, lips, or hands; unsteady gait; and visual disturbances. Other signs and symptoms include anorexia, nausea, photophobia, and vomiting.

Sinusitis (acute)

Patients with sinusitis have a dull, periorbital headache that is typically aggravated by bending over or touching the face. They may also have fever, malaise, nasal discharge, nasal turbinate edema, sinus tenderness, and sore throat. Sinus drainage relieves the sinusitis.

Subarachnoid hemorrhage

The hallmarks of subarachnoid hemorrhage are a sudden, violent headache and dizziness; hypertension; ipsilateral pupil dilation; nausea; nuchal rigidity; seizures; vomiting; and an altered LOC that may progress rapidly to coma. The patient's history may include congenital vascular defects, arteriovenous malformation, cardiovascular disease, smoking, hypertension, or excessive stress.

Subdural hematoma

A severe, localized headache usually follows head trauma that causes an immediate loss of consciousness, a latent period of drowsiness, confusion or personality changes, and agitation. Later, signs of increased ICP may develop. If the head trauma occurred within 3 days of the onset of signs and symptoms, the hematoma is acute. If it occurred within 3 weeks, it is subacute; after more than 3 weeks, chronic.

Other causes

Cervical traction; lumbar puncture; myelography; withdrawal from a vasopressor or a sympathomimetic; or the use of indomethacin (Indocin), digoxin (Lanoxin), nitroglycerin (Nitrostat), isosorbide (Isordil), or another vasodilator can cause headaches. Also, the use of certain herbal medicines—such as St. John's wort, ginseng, and ephedra—can cause headaches.

Heartburn

A substernal burning sensation that rises in the chest and may radiate to the neck or throat, heartburn (also known as *pyrosis*) results from the reflux of gastric contents into the esophagus. Usually, it is accompanied by regurgitation. Because increased intra-abdominal pressure contributes to reflux, heartburn commonly occurs with pregnancy, ascites, or obesity, but it may also be caused by GI disorders, connective tissue disease, and certain drugs.

In most cases, heartburn develops after meals or occurs when a person lies down, bends over, lifts heavy objects, or exercises vigorously. It usually worsens with swallowing and improves when the person sits upright or takes antacids. Some patients confuse heartburn with an MI, but a patient who is having an MI typically has other symptoms besides a burning sensation.

Health history

- When did the heartburn start? Do certain foods or beverages seem to trigger it? Does stress or fatigue seem to aggravate it? Do movement, certain body positions, or very hot or cold liquids worsen or relieve it? Where exactly is the burning sensation? Does it radiate to other areas? Does it cause you to regurgitate sour or bitter fluids? Have you ever had heartburn before? If so, what relieved it?
- Do you have a history of GI problems or connective tissue disease? For women of childbearing age: Are you pregnant?
- What medications are you taking?

Physical examination

Auscultate the heart and lungs to rule out a heart or lung disorder. Palpate the abdomen for abdominal pain.

Causes

Esophageal cancer

Heartburn may indicate esophageal cancer. The first symptom is usually painless dysphagia that progressively worsens. Eventually, partial obstruction and rapid weight loss occur. The patient may have a feeling of substernal fullness, hoarseness, nausea, sore throat, steady pain in the posterior and anterior chest, and vomiting.

Gastroesophageal reflux

Severe, chronic heartburn is the most common symptom of gastroesophageal reflux. Heartburn usually occurs within 1 hour after eating and may be triggered by certain foods or beverages. It worsens when the person lies down or bends over and abates when he or she sits, stands, or ingests antacids. Other findings include dull retrosternal pain that may radiate, hypersalivation, odynophagia, dysphagia, flatulent dyspepsia, and postural regurgitation.

Peptic ulcer

Heartburn and indigestion usually signal the onset of a peptic ulcer attack. Most patients have a gnawing, burning pain in the left epigastrium, although some report sharp pain. The pain typically occurs when the stomach is empty and is generally relieved by taking antacids. The pain may also occur after the patient drinks coffee, other caffeinated beverages, or alcohol or takes aspirin.

Scleroderma

A connective tissue disease, scleroderma may cause esophageal dysfunction resulting in heartburn, bloating after meals, odynophagia, the sensation of food sticking behind the sternum, and weight loss. Other GI effects include abdominal distention; constipation or diarrhea; and malodorous, floating stools.

Other causes

Heartburn may also be caused by esophageal diverticula; obesity; and the use of certain drugs, including aspirin, nonsteroidal anti-inflammatory drugs, anticholinergics, inhaled corticosteroids, inhaled beta-adrenergic blockers, and drugs that have anticholinergic effects.

Hematuria

A cardinal sign of renal and urinary tract disorders, hematuria is blood in the urine. Hematuria may be evident or may be confirmed by a urine test for occult blood.

Bleeding may be continuous or intermittent, is commonly accompanied by pain, and may be aggravated by prolonged standing or walking. Dark or brownish blood indicates renal or upper urinary tract bleeding; bright red blood, lower urinary tract bleeding.

Health history

- When did you first notice blood in your urine? Does it occur every time you urinate? Are you passing any clots? Have you ever had this problem before?
- Do you have any pain? If so, does the pain occur only when you urinate, or is it continuous? On a scale of 0 to 10, with 10 being the worst pain imaginable, rate the pain.
- Do you have bleeding hemorrhoids? Have you had any recent trauma or performed any strenuous exercise? Do you have a history of renal, urinary, prostatic, or coagulation disorders? For female patients: Are you menstruating?
- What medications are you taking?

Physical examination

Check the urinary meatus for bleeding or abnormalities. Palpate the abdomen and flanks, noting pain or tenderness. Finally, percuss the abdomen and flanks, especially the costovertebral angle, to elicit tenderness.

Causes

Bladder cancer

A primary cause of gross hematuria in men, bladder cancer may produce pain in the bladder, rectum, pelvis, flank, back, or legs. You may also note signs of urinary tract infection.

Calculi

Both bladder and renal calculi produce hematuria that may be accompanied by signs and symptoms of urinary tract infection. Bladder calculi usually produce gross hematuria, pain referred to the penile or vulvar areas, and, in some patients, bladder distention. Renal calculi may produce either microscopic or gross hematuria.

Glomerulonephritis

Usually, acute glomerulonephritis begins with gross hematuria. It may also produce anuria or oliguria, flank and abdominal pain, and increased blood pressure. Chronic glomerulonephritis typically causes microscopic hematuria accompanied by generalized edema, increased blood pressure, and proteinuria.

Nephritis

Acute nephritis causes fever, a maculopapular rash, and microscopic hematuria. In chronic interstitial nephritis, the patient may have dilute, almost colorless urine along with polyuria.

Pyelonephritis (acute)

A typical sign of pyelonephritis is microscopic or gross hematuria that progresses to grossly bloody hematuria. After the infection resolves, microscopic hematuria may persist for a few months. Other findings include flank pain, high fever, and signs and symptoms of a urinary tract infection.

Renal infarction

Patients with renal infarction usually have gross hematuria. Other symptoms include anorexia; costovertebral angle tenderness; and constant, severe flank and upper abdominal pain.

Other causes

Hematuria may result from benign prostatic hyperplasia, bladder trauma, obstructive nephropathy, polycystic kidney disease, renal trauma, and urethral trauma. It may result from a diagnostic test, such as cystoscopy or renal biopsy. It may also result from the use of a drug, such as an anticoagulant; a chemotherapeutic agent, such as cyclophosphamide, bacillus Calmette-Guérin intravesical (TheraCys), or leuprolide (Lupron); or thiabendazole (Mintezol). Also, certain herbal medicines, such as garlic and ginkgo biloba, may cause hematuria when taken with an anticoagulant.

Hemoptysis

The expectoration of blood or bloody sputum from the lungs or tracheobronchial tree is known as hemoptysis. Usually caused by an abnormality of the tracheobronchial tree, hemoptysis is associated with inflammatory conditions or lesions that cause erosion and necrosis of the bronchial tissues and blood vessels.

Hemoptysis is sometimes confused with bleeding from the mouth, throat, nasopharynx, or GI tract. Severe hemoptysis requires emergency endotracheal intubation and suctioning.

Health history

- When did you begin expectorating blood? How much blood or sputum are you expectorating? How often?
- Did you recently have a flulike syndrome? Have you had any recent invasive pulmonary procedures or chest trauma?
- Do you smoke? Did you ever smoke? If so, how much? Have you ever been diagnosed with a cardiac, respiratory, or bleeding disorder?
- What medications are you taking? Are you taking an anticoagulant?

Physical examination

After assessing the patient's LOC, examine his or her nose, mouth, and pharynx for sources of bleeding. Observe the rate and depth of his or her respirations, noting breathing difficulty or abnormal breathing patterns. Also, look for abnormal chest movement, accessory muscle use, and retractions. Inspect the skin for central and peripheral cyanosis, diaphoresis, lesions, and pallor.

Palpate the rate, rhythm, and intensity of the peripheral pulses. Then feel the chest, noting abnormal pulsations, diaphragmatic tenderness, and fremitus.

Check for respiratory excursion. If the patient has a history of trauma, carefully check the position of the trachea and note edema.

As you percuss over the lung fields, note dullness, flatness, hyperresonance, or tympany. Auscultate the lungs for crackles, rhonchi, and wheezes and the heart for bruits, gallops, murmurs, and pleural friction rubs. Also, monitor the patient's blood pressure and pulse pressure.

Causes

Bronchitis (chronic)

The patient with chronic bronchitis usually has a productive cough that lasts at least 3 months and leads to expectoration of blood-streaked sputum. Other respiratory signs include dyspnea, prolonged expiration, scattered rhonchi, and wheezing.

Lung abscess

A patient with a lung abscess expectorates copious amounts of bloody, purulent, foul-smelling sputum. He or she also has anorexia, chills, diaphoresis, fever, headache, and pleuritic or dull chest pain. Lung auscultation may show tubular breath sounds or crackles. Percussion shows dullness on the affected side. The patient may have a history of a recent pulmonary infection or evidence of poor oral hygiene, with dental or gingival disease.

Lung cancer

Ulceration of the bronchus commonly causes recurring hemoptysis (an early sign), which can vary from blood-streaked sputum to blood. Related findings include anorexia, chest pain, dyspnea, fever, a productive cough, weight loss, and wheezing.

Pulmonary edema

A patient with pulmonary edema may expectorate copious amounts of frothy, blood-tinged, pink sputum. He or she may also have dyspnea and orthopnea.

On examination, you may detect diffuse crackles in both lung fields and a ventricular gallop (S_3).

Tracheal trauma

With tracheal trauma, the bleeding appears to come from the back of the throat. Accompanying signs and symptoms include airway occlusion, dysphagia, hoarseness, neck pain, and respiratory distress.

Other causes

Hemoptysis may also result from bronchiectasis, coagulation disorders, cystic fibrosis, lung or airway injuries from diagnostic procedures, and primary pulmonary hypertension.

Hoarseness

A rough or harsh-sounding voice, hoarseness can be acute or chronic. It may result from infections or inflammatory lesions or exudates in the larynx, from laryngeal edema, from compression or disruption of the vocal cords or recurrent laryngeal nerve damage, or from irritating polyps on the vocal cords. Hoarseness can also occur with aging because the laryngeal muscles and mucosa atrophy, leading to diminished control of the vocal cords. Hoarseness may be exacerbated by excessive alcohol intake, smoking, inhalation of noxious fumes, excessive talking, and shouting.

Health history

- When did the hoarseness start? Is it constant or intermittent? Does anything relieve or exacerbate it? Have you been overusing your voice?
- Have you also had a cough, a dry mouth, difficulty swallowing dry food, shortness of breath, or a sore throat?
- Have you ever had cancer or other disorders? Have you had recent surgery?
- Do you regularly drink alcohol or smoke? If so, how much?

Physical examination

Inspect the patient's mouth and throat for redness or exudate, possibly indicating an upper respiratory tract infection. Ask the patient to stick out his or her tongue: If he or she cannot, the hypoglossal nerve (cranial nerve XII) may be impaired.

As the patient breathes, observe him or her for asymmetrical chest expansion, intercostal retractions, nasal flaring, stridor, and other signs of respiratory distress.

Palpate the patient's neck for masses and the cervical lymph nodes and thyroid gland for enlargement. Then palpate the trachea to check for deviation.

As you percuss the chest wall, note dullness. Auscultate the lungs for crackles, rhonchi, tubular sounds, or wheezes. To detect bradycardia, auscultate the heart.

Causes

Inhalation injury

Exposure to a fire or an explosion can cause an inhalation injury that produces coughing, hoarseness, orofacial burns, singed nasal hair, and soot-stained sputum. Subsequent signs and symptoms include crackles, rhonchi, wheezes, and respiratory distress.

Laryngitis

Persistent hoarseness may be the only sign of chronic laryngitis. In acute laryngitis, hoarseness or complete loss of the voice develops suddenly. Related findings include cough, fever, pain (especially during swallowing or speaking), profuse diaphoresis, rhinorrhea, and sore throat.

Vocal cord polyps

A patient with vocal cord polyps has raspy hoarseness and may also have a chronic cough and a crackling voice.

Other causes

Hoarseness may result from hypothyroidism, pulmonary tuberculosis, rheumatoid arthritis, and laryngeal cancer (most common in men ages 50 to 70).

Prolonged intubation, surgical severing of the recurrent laryngeal nerve, and a tracheostomy may also produce hoarseness.

AGE ALERT

In infants and young children, hoarseness commonly stems from acute laryngotracheo-bronchitis (croup).

Nausea

A profound feeling of revulsion to food or a signal of impending vomiting, nausea is usually accompanied by anorexia, diaphoresis, hypersalivation, pallor, tachycardia, tachypnea, and vomiting. A common symptom of GI disorders, nausea may also result from electrolyte imbalances; infections; metabolic, endocrine, and cardiac disorders; early pregnancy; drug therapy; surgery; and radiation therapy. Also, severe pain, anxiety, alcohol intoxication, overeating, and ingestion of something distasteful can trigger nausea.

Health history

- When did the nausea begin? Is it intermittent or constant? How severe is it?
- Do you have any other signs and symptoms, such as abdominal pain, loss of appetite, changes in bowel habits, excessive belching or gas, weight loss, or vomiting?
- For female patients: Are you pregnant, or could you be? Have you ever had a GI, endocrine, or metabolic disorder? Have you had any recent infections? Have you ever had cancer, radiation therapy, or chemotherapy?
- What medications and supplements are you taking? Do you drink alcohol, and, if so, how much?

Physical examination

Examine the patient's skin for bruises, jaundice, poor turgor, and spider angiomas. Inspect his or her abdomen for distention.

Because palpation and percussion can affect the frequency and intensity of bowel sounds, you should auscultate the abdomen first. Listen for bowel sounds in each quadrant. Then, using the bell of the stethoscope, listen for abdominal bruits.

As you palpate the abdomen, note rigidity, tenderness, or rebound tenderness. Next, palpate the size of the liver. Then percuss the abdomen and liver for abnormalities.

Causes

Appendicitis

A patient with appendicitis will feel nauseated and may vomit. He or she will also have vague epigastric or periumbilical discomfort that localizes to the right lower quadrant.

Cholecystitis (acute)

In acute cholecystitis, nausea commonly follows severe right upper quadrant pain that may radiate to the back or shoulders. Associated findings include abdominal tenderness; vomiting and, possibly, abdominal rigidity and distention; diaphoresis; and fever with chills.

Gastritis

Patients with gastritis commonly experience nausea, especially after ingestion of alcohol, aspirin, spicy foods, or caffeine. Belching, epigastric pain, fever, malaise, and vomiting of mucus or blood may also occur.

Other causes

Nausea may result from cirrhosis, an electrolyte imbalance, labyrinthitis, metabolic acidosis, MI, a renal or urologic disorder, or ulcerative colitis. Use of an anesthetic, an antibiotic, an antineoplastic, ferrous sulfate, oral potassium, or quinidine, or an overdose of a cardiac glycoside or theophylline may also trigger nausea, as may radiation therapy or surgery—especially abdominal surgery. Certain herbal medicines, such as ginkgo biloba and St. John's wort, may also cause nausea.

Pain (abdominal)

Usually, abdominal pain results from GI disorders, but it can also stem from reproductive, genitourinary, musculoskeletal, or vascular disorders; from drug use; or from the effect of toxins. Abdominal pain may originate in the abdominopelvic viscera; the parietal peritoneum; or the capsules of the liver, kidneys, or spleen. The pain may be acute or chronic and diffuse or localized.

Health history

- Can you rate the pain on a scale of 0 to 10, with 10 being the worst pain imaginable? When did the pain begin? What does it feel like? How long does it last? Where exactly is it? Does it radiate to other areas, such as the chest or back? Does it get better or worse when you change position, move, exert yourself, cough, eat, or have a bowel movement?
- Does fever occur during episodes of pain? Do you have appetite changes, constipation, diarrhea, nausea, pain with urination, pink or cloudy urine, vomiting, or urinary frequency or urgency?
- Do you have a history of adrenal disease, heart disease, recent infection, or recent blunt trauma to the abdomen, flank, or chest? Have you had any condition that could predispose you to emboli or that could narrow an arterial lumen? Have you recently had a urinary tract procedure or surgery? Have you traveled to a foreign country recently?
- For women of childbearing age: What was the date of your last

normal menses? Has your menstrual pattern changed? Could you be pregnant?

- Have you ever used I.V. drugs? Do you drink alcohol? If so, how much and how often? What medications and supplements do you take?

Physical examination

After assessing the patient's LOC, observe his or her skin for diaphoresis, jaundice, and turgor. Then check for coolness, discoloration, and edema of the arms and legs. Inspect the abdomen and chest for signs of trauma: A bluish discoloration around the umbilicus (Cullen's sign) and around the flank area (Turner's sign) can indicate blunt trauma. Obtain and record a baseline measurement of abdominal girth at the umbilicus.

After inspecting for jugular vein distention, observe the rate and depth of respirations, noting abnormal patterns. Observe the color and odor of the patient's urine.

Because palpation and percussion can affect the frequency and intensity of bowel sounds, you should auscultate the abdomen first. Listen for bowel sounds in each quadrant, noting whether the sounds are high pitched and tinkling, hyperactive, or absent.

Listen to the patient's heart and breath sounds for abnormalities. Also, monitor his or her blood pressure and pulse pressure.

As you systematically palpate the abdominal, pelvic, flank, and epigastric areas, note enlarged organs, masses, rigidity, tenderness, rebound tenderness, or tenderness with guarding. Check the patient's peripheral pulses for rate, rhythm, and intensity.

Percuss each abdominal quadrant, noting tenderness, increased pain, and percussion sounds. Dull percussion sounds indicate free fluid; hollow sounds, air.

Causes

Abdominal aortic aneurysm (dissecting)

Constant, dull upper abdominal pain radiating to the lower back typically accompanies rapid enlargement of the aneurysm and may indicate a rupture. On auscultation, you may detect a systolic bruit over the aneurysm. Palpation may show an epigastric mass that pulsates before rupture. You may also note abdominal rigidity, increasing abdominal girth, and signs of hypovolemic shock.

Abdominal trauma

The patient may have generalized or localized abdominal pain along with abdominal ecchymosis, abdominal tenderness, or vomiting. If he or she is hemorrhaging into the peritoneal cavity, you may note abdominal rigidity, dullness on percussion, and increasing abdominal girth. You may hear hollow bowel sounds if an abdominal organ has been perforated, or bowel sounds may be absent. Bowel sounds heard in the chest cavity usually signal a diaphragmatic tear.

Appendicitis

The patient with appendicitis may have sudden pain in the epigastric or umbilical region that increases over a few hours or days, along with flulike symptoms. Anorexia, constipation or diarrhea, nausea, and vomiting precede the pain, which may be dull or severe. Pain localizes at McBurney's point in the right lower quadrant. Abdominal rigidity and rebound tenderness may also occur.

Ectopic pregnancy

With ectopic pregnancy, lower abdominal pain may be sharp, dull, or cramping and either constant or intermittent. The pain may be accompanied by breast tenderness, nausea, vaginal bleeding, vomiting, and urinary frequency. The patient typically has a 1- to 2-month history of amenorrhea. Rupture of the fallopian tube produces sharp lower abdominal pain that may radiate to the shoulders and neck and become extreme on cervical or adnexal palpation.

Hepatitis

Liver enlargement from any type of hepatitis causes discomfort or dull pain and tenderness in the right upper quadrant.

Intestinal obstruction

Intestinal obstruction causes short episodes of intense, colicky, cramping pain. These episodes alternate with pain-free periods.

Pancreatitis

The characteristic symptom of pancreatitis is fulminating, continuous upper abdominal pain that may radiate to both flanks and to the back.

Renal calculi

Depending on the location of the calculi, the patient may have severe abdominal or back pain. However, the classic symptom of renal calculi is colicky pain that travels from the costovertebral angle to the flank, the suprapubic region, and the external genitalia.

Other causes

Abdominal pain may result from adrenal crisis, cholecystitis, heart failure, diabetic ketoacidosis, diverticulitis, hepatic abscess, mesenteric artery ischemia, MI, an ovarian cyst, a perforated ulcer, peritonitis, pneumonia, pneumothorax, pyelonephritis, renal infarction, or splenic infarction. Other causes include the use of salicylates and nonsteroidal anti-inflammatory drugs.

Pain (back)

Back pain may be acute, chronic, constant, or intermittent. It may also remain localized in the back or may radiate along the spine or down one or both legs. Pain may be exacerbated by activity (most commonly, stooping or lifting) and alleviated by rest or may be unaffected by either.

Intrinsic back pain results from muscle spasm, nerve root irritation, fracture, or a combination of these causes. It usually occurs in the lower back or lumbosacral area. Back pain may also be referred from the abdomen, possibly signaling a life-threatening disorder.

Health history

- When did the pain first occur? What does it feel like? Is it mild, moderate, or severe? Is it constant or intermittent? Where exactly is it? Is it associated with activity? What relieves or exacerbates it? For women of childbearing age: Does the pain occur before or during your menses?
- Have you had recent episodes of abdominal tenderness or rigidity, fever, nausea, or vomiting? Do you feel unusual sensations in your legs? Have you had urinary frequency or urgency or painful urination?
- Do you have a history of trauma; back surgery; or urinary tract surgery, procedures, obstructions, or infections?
- What medications and supplements are you taking?

Physical examination

Observe the rate and depth of respirations, noting breathing difficulty or abnormal breathing patterns. Check the skin for diaphoresis, discoloration, edema, mottling, and pallor. Then inspect the back, legs, and abdomen for signs of trauma. After you check for abdominal distention, take a baseline abdominal girth measurement.

Because palpation and percussion can affect the frequency and intensity of bowel sounds, you should auscultate the abdomen first. Listen for bowel sounds in each quadrant. Then listen over the abdominal aorta for bruits and over the lungs for crackles. Also monitor the patient's blood pressure and pulse pressure.

Palpate the abdominal, epigastric, and pelvic areas for abdominal rigidity, enlarged organs, masses, and tenderness. If you feel pulsations, do not palpate deeply. Check the peripheral pulses for rate, rhythm, and intensity. Gently palpate the painful area, noting contractions, excessive muscle tone, or spasm.

Finally, percuss each abdominal quadrant. Note abnormal sounds, increased pain, and tenderness.

Causes

Abdominal aortic aneurysm (dissecting)

Lower back pain and dull upper abdominal pain commonly accompany a rapidly enlarging aneurysm and may indicate the early stages of rupture. On palpation, you may detect tenderness over the area of the aneurysm as well as a pulsating epigastric mass. Other signs include absent femoral and pedal pulses, mottling of the skin below the waist, and signs of hypovolemic shock.

Pancreatitis

Fulminating, continuous abdominal pain that may radiate to the back and both flanks characterizes pancreatitis. You may also note abdominal tenderness, rigidity, and distention; fever; hypoactive bowel sounds; pallor; tachycardia; and vomiting. The history may include alcohol abuse, use of a thiazide diuretic, gallbladder disease, or trauma.

Pyelonephritis (acute)

The patient with acute pyelonephritis has progressive back pain or flank tenderness accompanied by costovertebral angle pain and abdominal pain in one or two quadrants. Associated signs and symptoms include dysuria, high fever,

hematuria, nocturia, shaking chills, vomiting, and urinary frequency and urgency. The history may show a recent urinary tract procedure, urinary tract infection or obstruction, compromised renal function, or a neurogenic bladder.

Other causes

Back pain may also result from appendicitis, cholecystitis, a herniated disk, lumbosacral sprain, osteoporosis, a perforated ulcer, renal calculi, a tumor, or vertebral osteomyelitis.

Pain (chest)

Patients describe chest pain in many ways. They may report a dull ache; a sensation of heaviness or fullness; a feeling of indigestion; or a sharp, shooting pain. The pain may be constant or intermittent, may radiate to other body parts, and may arise suddenly or gradually. Patients may say that stress, anxiety, exertion, deep breathing, or certain foods seem to trigger the pain.

Chest pain may indicate several acute and life-threatening cardiopulmonary and GI conditions. It can also result from musculoskeletal and hematologic disorders, anxiety, and the use of certain drugs.

Health history

- When did the chest pain begin? Did it develop suddenly or gradually? Can you rate the pain on a scale of 0 to 10, with 10 being the worst pain imaginable? Is the pain localized or diffuse? Does it radiate to the neck, jaw, arms, or back? Is the pain sharp and stabbing or dull and aching? Is it constant or intermittent? Does breathing, changing positions, or eating certain foods worsen or relieve the pain?
- Do you have other signs and symptoms, such as coughing, shortness of breath, headache, nausea, palpitations, vomiting, diaphoresis, or weakness?

- Have you ever had cardiac or respiratory disease, cardiac surgery, chest trauma, or intestinal disease? Do you have a family history of cardiac disease?
- Do you drink alcohol or use illicit drugs? What medications and supplements are you taking?

Physical examination

Assess the patient's skin temperature, color, and general appearance, noting coolness, cyanosis, diaphoresis, mottling below the waist, pallor, peripheral edema, and prolonged capillary refill time. Look for facial edema, jugular vein distention, and tracheal deviation. Note signs of altered LOC, anxiety, dizziness, or restlessness.

Observe the rate and depth of the patient's respirations, noting abnormal patterns or breathing difficulty. If the patient has a productive cough, examine the sputum.

Palpate the patient's neck, chest, and abdomen. Note asymmetrical chest expansion, masses, subcutaneous crepitation, tender areas, tracheal deviation, or tactile fremitus. Also palpate his or her peripheral pulses, and record their rate, rhythm, and intensity.

As you percuss over an affected lung, note dullness. Auscultate the lungs to identify crackles, diminished or absent breath sounds, pleural friction rubs, rhonchi, or wheezes. Auscultate the heart for clicks, gallops, murmurs, and a pericardial friction rub. To check for abdominal bruits, apply the bell of the stethoscope over the abdominal aorta. Also, monitor the patient's blood pressure closely.

Causes

Angina

Angina usually begins gradually, builds to a peak, and subsides slowly. The pain can last from 2 to 10 minutes. It occurs in the retrosternal region and radiates to the neck, jaw, and arms.

Associated signs and symptoms include diaphoresis, dyspnea, nausea, vomiting, palpitations, and tachycardia. On auscultation, you may detect an atrial gallop (or fourth heart sound [S_4]) or a murmur. Attacks may occur at rest or may be provoked by exertion, emotional stress, or a heavy meal.

Aortic aneurysm (dissecting)

A patient with a dissecting aortic aneurysm has sudden, excruciating, tearing pain in the chest and neck, radiating to the upper back, lower back, and abdomen. Other signs and symptoms include abdominal tenderness, heart murmurs, jugular vein distention, systolic bruits, tachycardia, syncope, and dyspnea.

Cholecystitis

The patient with cholecystitis has sudden epigastric or right upper quadrant pain. The pain may be steady or intermittent, may radiate to the back, and may be sharp or intense. Other signs and symptoms include chills, diaphoresis, nausea, and vomiting. Palpation of the right upper quadrant may show distention, rigidity, tenderness, and a mass.

Myocardial infarction

With MI, the patient has severe, crushing substernal pain that radiates to the left arm, jaw, or neck. The pain may be accompanied by anxiety, clammy skin, diaphoresis, dyspnea, a feeling of impending doom, nausea, vomiting, pallor, and restlessness. The patient may have an atrial gallop (or an S_4), crackles, hypotension or hypertension, murmurs, and a pericardial friction rub. A history of heart disease, hypertension, hypercholesterolemia, or cocaine abuse is common.

Peptic ulcer

A sharp, burning pain arising in the epigastric region, usually hours after eating, characterizes a peptic ulcer. Other signs and symptoms include epigastric tenderness, nausea, and vomiting. Food or antacids usually relieve the pain.

Pneumothorax

In pneumothorax, a collapsed lung produces sudden, sharp, severe chest pain that is commonly unilateral and increases with chest movement. You may detect decreased breath sounds, hyperresonant or tympanic percussion sounds, and subcutaneous crepitation. Other signs and symptoms include accessory muscle use, anxiety, asymmetrical chest expansion, nonproductive cough, tachycardia, and tachypnea. The history may include chronic obstructive pulmonary disease, lung cancer, diagnostic or therapeutic procedures involving the thorax, or thoracic trauma.

Pulmonary embolism

Typically, the patient with pulmonary embolism has sudden dyspnea with intense angina-like or pleuritic ischemic pain that is aggravated by deep breathing and thoracic movement. Other findings include anxiety, cough with blood-tinged sputum, dull percussion sounds, crackles, restlessness, and tachycardia. If the embolism is large, the cardiovascular, pulmonary, and neurologic systems may be compromised. The patient's history may include thrombophlebitis, hip or leg injury, abdominal surgery, acute MI, heart failure, pregnancy, the use of hormonal contraceptives, or immobility.

Other causes

Chest pain may also result from abrupt withdrawal of beta-adrenergic blockers, acute bronchitis, anxiety, esophageal spasm, esophageal reflux, lung abscess, muscle strain, pancreatitis, pneumonia, a rib fracture, or tuberculosis.

Palpitations

Defined as a person's conscious awareness of his or her own heartbeat, palpitations are usually felt over the precordium or in the throat or neck.

The patient may describe his or her heart as pounding, jumping, turning, fluttering, flopping, or missing or skipping beats. Palpitations may be regular or irregular, fast or slow, and paroxysmal or sustained. Besides cardiac causes, palpitations may stem from anxiety, drug reactions, hypertension, thyroid hormone deficiency, and several other problems.

Health history

- When did the palpitations start? Where do you feel them? How would you describe them? What were you doing when they started? How long did they last? Have you ever had palpitations before?
- Do you have chest pain, dizziness, or weakness along with the palpitations?
- Are you under unusual stress at home or at work? Have you recently had multiple blood transfusions or an infusion of phosphate?
- Have you ever had thyroid disease, calcium or vitamin D deficiency, malabsorption syndrome, bone cancer, renal disease, hypoglycemia, or cardiovascular or pulmonary disorders that may produce arrhythmias or hypertension?
- What medications and supplements are you taking? Are you taking an over-the-counter drug that contains caffeine or a sympathomimetic, such as a cough, cold, or allergy preparation? Do you smoke or drink alcohol? If so, how much?

Physical examination

Assess the patient's LOC, noting anxiety, confusion, or irrational behavior. Check his or her skin for pallor and diaphoresis, and observe the eyes for exophthalmos.

Note the rate and depth of his or her respirations, checking for abnormal patterns and breathing difficulty. Also inspect the fingertips for capillary nail bed pulsations.

To check for thyroid gland enlargement, gently palpate the patient's neck. Then palpate his or her muscles for weakness and twitching. Evaluate his or her peripheral pulses, noting the rate, rhythm, and intensity. Assess his or her reflexes for hyperreflexia.

Auscultate the heart for gallops and murmurs and the lungs for abnormal breath sounds. Also monitor blood pressure and pulse pressure.

Causes

Acute anxiety attack

During an acute anxiety attack, palpitations may be accompanied by diaphoresis, facial flushing, and trembling. The patient usually hyperventilates, which may lead to dizziness, syncope, and weakness.

Cardiac arrhythmias

With cardiac arrhythmias, paroxysmal or sustained palpitations may occur with dizziness, fatigue, and weakness. Other signs and symptoms include chest pain; confusion; decreased blood pressure; diaphoresis; pallor; and an irregular, rapid, or slow pulse rate. The patient may be taking a drug that can cause cardiac arrhythmias—for instance, an antihypertensive, a sympathomimetic, a ganglionic blocker, an anticholinergic, or a methylxanthine.

Thyrotoxicosis

In patients with thyrotoxicosis, sustained palpitations may accompany diaphoresis, diarrhea, dyspnea, heat intolerance, nervousness, tachycardia, tremors, and weight loss despite increased appetite. Exophthalmos and an enlarged thyroid gland may also develop.

Other causes

Palpitations may also arise from anemia, aortic insufficiency, hypocalcemia, hypertension, hypoglycemia, mitral valve stenosis or prolapse, and pheochromocytoma. Also, certain herbal medicines, such as ginseng and ephedra, may cause palpitations.

Paresthesia

Paresthesia is an abnormal sensation, commonly described as numbness, prickling, or tingling, that is felt along the peripheral nerve pathways. It may develop suddenly or gradually and may be transient or permanent. A common symptom of many neurologic disorders, paresthesia may also occur in certain systemic disorders and with the use of certain drugs.

Health history

- When did the paresthesia begin? What does it feel like? Where does it occur? Is it transient or constant?
- Have you had recent trauma, surgery, or an invasive procedure that may have injured the peripheral nerves? Have you been exposed to industrial solvents or heavy metals? Have you had long-term radiation therapy? Do you have neurologic, cardiovascular, metabolic, renal, or chronic inflammatory disorders, such as arthritis or lupus erythematosus?
- What medications and supplements are you taking?

Physical examination

Focus on the patient's neurologic status, assessing his or her LOC and cranial nerve function. Also note his or her skin color and temperature.

Test muscle strength and deep tendon reflexes in the extremities that are affected by paresthesia. Systematically evaluate light touch, pain, temperature, vibration, and position sensation. Then palpate the pulses.

Causes

Acute lower extremity, arterial occlusion

A patient with an arterial embolus may have sudden paresthesia and coldness in one or both legs. Severe pain at rest, intermittent claudication, and paresis are also characteristic. The leg becomes cyanotic, and a line of temperature and color demarcation develops at the level of the occlusion. Pulses are absent below the occlusion, and capillary refill time is prolonged.

Brain tumor
Tumors that affect the parietal lobe may cause progressive contralateral paresthesia accompanied by agnosia, anomia, agraphia, apraxia, homonymous hemianopsia, and loss of proprioception.

Herniated disk
Herniation of a lumbar or cervical disk may cause acute or gradual paresthesia along the distribution pathways of the affected spinal nerves. Other neuromuscular effects include muscle spasms, severe pain, and weakness.

Herpes zoster
Paresthesia, an early symptom of herpes zoster, occurs in the dermatome supplied by the affected spinal nerve. Within several days, this dermatome is marked by a pruritic, erythematous, vesicular rash accompanied by sharp, shooting pain.

Spinal cord injury
Paresthesia may occur after spinal shock resolves in a patient with partial spinal cord transection. The paresthesia may be unilateral or bilateral and may occur at or below in the level of the lesion.

Other disorders
Paresthesia may result from arthritis, stroke, migraine headache, multiple sclerosis, peripheral neuropathies, vitamin B_{12} deficiency, hypocalcemia, and heavy metal or solvent poisoning. Also, long-term radiation therapy, parenteral gold therapy, and certain drugs—such as chemotherapeutic agents, paclitaxel (Taxol), interferons, and isoniazid (Laniazid)—may cause paresthesia.

Rash (papular)
Consisting of small, raised, circumscribed, and, possibly, discolored lesions, a papular rash can erupt anywhere on the body and in various configurations. A characteristic sign of many cutaneous disorders, a papular rash may also result from allergies or from infectious, neoplastic, or systemic disorders.

AGE ALERT

In bedridden elderly patients, the first sign of a pressure ulcer is commonly an erythematous area, sometimes with firm papules.

Health history
- When and where did the rash erupt? What did it look like? Has it spread or changed in any way? If so, when and how did it spread?
- Does the rash itch or burn? Is it painful or tender?
- Have you had a fever, GI distress, or a headache? Do you have any allergies? Have you had any previous skin disorders, infections, sexually transmitted diseases, or tumors? What childhood diseases have you had?
- Have you recently been bitten by an insect or a rodent or exposed to anyone with an infectious disease?
- What medications and supplements are you taking? Have you applied any topical agents to the rash, and, if so, what was it and when was the last application?

Physical examination
Observe the color, configuration, and location of the rash.

Causes

Acne vulgaris

In acne vulgaris, the rupture of enlarged comedones produces inflamed and, possibly, painful and pruritic papules, pustules, nodules, or cysts. They may appear on the face, shoulders, chest, or back.

Insect bites

Venom from insect bites—especially those of ticks, lice, flies, and mosquitoes—may cause an allergic reaction that produces a papular, macular, or petechial rash. Associated findings include fever, headache, lymphadenopathy, myalgia, nausea, and vomiting.

Kaposi's sarcoma

Kaposi's sarcoma is a neoplastic disorder that is most commonly found in patients with AIDS. Kaposi's sarcoma produces purple or blue papules or macules on the extremities, ears, and nose. Firm pressure causes these lesions to decrease in size, but they return to their original size within 10 to 15 seconds. The lesions may become scaly, ulcerate, and bleed.

Psoriasis

Psoriasis causes small, erythematous, pruritic papules on the scalp, chest, elbows, knees, back, buttocks, and genitalia. The papules may be painful. They enlarge and coalesce, forming red, elevated plaques covered by silver scales, except in moist areas, such as the genitalia. The scales may flake off easily or may thicken, covering the plaque. Other common findings include pitted fingernails and arthralgia.

Other causes

Infectious mononucleosis or sarcoidosis may produce a papular rash. This type of rash may also be caused by nonsteroidal anti-inflammatory drugs, succimer (Chemet), and interferons.

Rash (pustular)

Crops of pustules (small, elevated, circumscribed lesions), vesicles (small blisters), and bullae (large blisters) filled with purulent exudate make up a pustular rash. The lesions vary in size and shape and may be generalized or localized (limited to the hair follicles or sweat glands).

Pustules may result from skin disorders, systemic disorders, ingestion of certain drugs, and exposure to skin irritants. Although many pustular lesions are sterile, a pustular rash usually indicates infection.

Health history

- When and where did the rash erupt? Did another type of skin lesion precede the pustules?
- What does the rash look like? Has it spread or changed in any way? If so, how and where did it spread?
- Have you or has a family member ever had a skin disorder or allergies?
- What medications are you taking? Have you applied topical medication to the rash, and, if so, what was it and when did you last apply it?

Physical examination

Examine the entire skin surface, noting if it is dry, oily, moist, or greasy. Record the exact location, distribution, color, shape, and size of the lesions.

Causes

Folliculitis

A bacterial infection of the hair follicles, folliculitis produces individual pustules, each pierced by a hair. The patient may also have pruritus. Hot-tub folliculitis is characterized by pustules on the areas normally covered by a bathing suit.

Scabies

Threadlike channels or burrows under the skin characterize scabies, a disorder that can also produce pustules, vesicles, and excoriations. The lesions are 1 to 10 cm long, with a swollen nodule or red papule containing the itch mite. In men, crusted lesions commonly develop on the glans and shaft of the penis and on the scrotum. In women, lesions may form on the nipples. Other common sites include the wrists, elbows, axillae, and waist.

Other causes

A pustular rash may result from acne vulgaris, blastomycosis, furunculosis, and pustular psoriasis. Also, certain drugs—such as bromides, iodides, corticotropin, corticosteroids, lithium (Eskalith), phenytoin (Dilantin), phenobarbital (Luminal), isoniazid (Laniazid), and hormonal contraceptives—can cause a pustular rash.

Rash (vesicular)

The lesions in a vesicular rash are scattered or linear vesicles that are sharply circumscribed and are usually less than 0.5 cm in diameter. They may be filled with clear, cloudy, or bloody fluid. Lesions larger than 0.5 cm in diameter are called bullae. A vesicular rash may be mild or severe and may be transient or permanent.

Health history

- When and where did the rash erupt? Did other skin lesions precede the vesicles?
- What does the rash look like? Has it spread or changed in any way? If so, how and where did it spread?
- Do you or does anyone in your family have a history of allergies or skin disorders?
- Have you recently had an infection or been bitten by an insect?

Physical examination

Examine the patient's skin and note the location, general distribution, color, shape, and size of the lesions. Check for crusts, macules, papules, scales, scars, and wheals. Note whether the outer layer of epidermis separates easily from the basal layer.

Palpate the vesicles or bullae to determine whether they are flaccid or tense.

Causes

Burns

Thermal burns that affect the epidermis and part of the dermis commonly cause vesicles and bullae, along with erythema, moistness, pain, and swelling.

Herpes zoster

In herpes zoster, fever and malaise occur first. Then the vesicular rash appears along a dermatome. This rash is accompanied by pruritus, deep pain, and paresthesia or hyperesthesia, usually of the trunk and sometimes of the arms and legs. The vesicles erupt, dry up, and form scabs in about 10 days. Occasionally, herpes zoster involves the cranial nerves; such involvement produces dizziness, eye pain, facial palsy, hearing loss, impaired vision, and loss of taste.

Other causes

Other causes of vesicular rashes include dermatitis, herpes simplex, insect bites, pemphigus, scabies, tinea pedis, and toxic epidermal necrolysis.

Vision loss

Vision loss can occur suddenly or gradually, may be temporary or permanent, and may range from a slight impairment to total blindness. It may result from eye, neurologic, and systemic disorders as well as from trauma and reactions to certain drugs.

Health history

- When did the loss first occur? Did it occur suddenly or gradually? Does it affect one eye or both eyes? Does it affect all or part of the visual field?
- Are you experiencing blurred vision, halo vision, nausea, pain, photosensitivity, or vomiting with the vision loss?

- Do you wear glasses? Have you had your eyes checked recently? If yes, what was the result?
- Have you had a recent facial or eye injury?
- Have you ever had a cardiovascular or endocrine disorder, an infection, or allergies? Does anyone in your family have a history of vision loss or other eye problems?
- What medications and supplements are you taking?

Physical examination

Check the patient's visual acuity. Observe the patient's eyes for conjunctival or scleral redness, drainage, edema, foreign bodies, and signs of trauma. With a flashlight, examine the cornea and iris. Observe the size, shape, and color of the pupils. Then test direct and consensual light reflexes and visual accommodation, and extraocular muscle function. Gently palpate each eye, noting hardness.

Causes

Glaucoma

Acute angle-closure glaucoma may cause rapid blindness. Findings include halo vision, nonreactive pupillary response, photophobia, rapid onset of unilateral inflammation and pain, and reduced visual acuity. In contrast, chronic open-angle glaucoma progresses slowly. Usually bilateral, it causes aching eyes, halo vision, peripheral vision loss, and reduced visual acuity.

Eye trauma

Sudden unilateral or bilateral vision loss may occur after eye injury. The loss may be total or partial and permanent or temporary. The eyelids may be reddened, edematous, and lacerated.

Other causes

Vision loss may also be caused by congenital rubella or syphilis; herpes zoster; Marfan's syndrome; pituitary tumor; retrolental fibroplasia; and

drugs, such as cardiac glycosides, indomethacin (Indocin), ethambutol (Myambutol), and methanol.

Visual floaters

Particles of blood or cellular debris that move about in the vitreous humor appear as spots or dots when they enter the visual field. Chronic floaters commonly occur in elderly or myopic patients. However, sudden onset of visual floaters commonly signals retinal detachment, an ocular emergency.

Health history

- When did the floaters first appear? What do they look like? Did they appear suddenly or gradually? If they appeared suddenly, did you also see flashing lights and have a curtain-like loss of vision?
- Are you nearsighted, and do you wear corrective lenses?
- Do you have a history of eye trauma or other eye disorders, allergies, granulomatous disease, diabetes mellitus, or hypertension?
- What medications and supplements are you taking?

Physical examination

Inspect the eyes for signs of injury, such as bruising or edema. Then assess the patient's visual acuity, using the Snellen's alphabet chart, or "E" chart.

Causes

Retinal detachment

Many floaters and light flashes appear suddenly in the portion of the visual field where the retina has detached. As retinal detachment progresses (a painless process), gradual vision loss occurs, with the patient seeing a "dark curtain" falling in front of his or her eyes. Ophthalmoscopic examination shows a gray, opaque, detached retina with an indefinite margin. The retinal vessels appear almost black.

Vitreous hemorrhage

Vitreous hemorrhage, or the rupture of the retinal vessels, produces a shower of red or black dots or a red haze across the visual field. Vision blurs suddenly in the affected eye, and visual acuity may be greatly reduced.

Other causes

Visual floaters may also result from posterior uveitis.

Weight gain

Weight gain occurs when ingested calories exceed body requirements for energy, causing increased adipose tissue storage. It can also occur when fluid retention causes edema. When weight gain results from overeating, emotional factors—most commonly anxiety, guilt, and depression—and social factors may be the primary causes.

Among elderly people, weight gain commonly reflects a sustained food intake in the presence of the normal, progressive decline in basal metabolic rate. Among women, progressive weight gain occurs with pregnancy, whereas periodic weight gain usually occurs with menstruation.

Weight gain, a primary sign of many endocrine disorders, also occurs with conditions that limit activity, especially cardiovascular and pulmonary disorders. It can also result from drug therapy that increases appetite or causes fluid retention or from cardiovascular, hepatic, and renal disorders that cause edema.

Health history

- Do you have any past patterns of weight gain and loss?
- Do you have a family history of obesity, thyroid disease, or diabetes mellitus?
- Describe your eating habits. Has your appetite increased?
- Do you exercise regularly or at all?
- Have you experienced visual disturbances, hoarseness, paresthesia, or increased urination and thirst?

- Have you had any episodes of impotence?
- If the patient is female: Have you had menstrual irregularities or experienced weight gain during menstruation?
- Have you felt anxious or depressed?
- Are you having any difficulties with your memory?
- What medications and supplements are you taking?

Physical examination

During your physical examination, measure skinfold thickness to estimate fat reserves. Note fat distribution, localized or generalized edema, and overall nutritional status. Also look for other abnormalities, such as abnormal body hair distribution or hair loss and dry skin. Take and record the patient's vital signs.

Causes

Acromegaly

Acromegaly causes moderate weight gain. Other findings include coarsened facial features, prognathism, enlarged hands and feet, increased sweating, oily skin, deep voice, back and joint pain, lethargy, sleepiness, and heat intolerance. Occasionally, hirsutism may occur.

Diabetes mellitus

The increased appetite associated with diabetes mellitus may lead to weight gain, although weight loss sometimes occurs instead. Other findings include fatigue, polydipsia, polyuria, nocturia, weakness, polyphagia, and somnolence.

Heart failure

In heart failure, weight gain may result from edema despite anorexia. Other typical findings include paroxysmal nocturnal dyspnea, orthopnea, and fatigue.

Hypercortisolism

Excessive weight gain, usually over the trunk and the back of the neck (buffalo hump), characteristically occurs in hypercortisolism. Other cushingoid features include slender extremities, moon face, weakness, purple striae, emotional lability, and increased susceptibility to infection. Men may have gynecomastia. Women may have hirsutism, acne, and menstrual irregularities.

Hyperinsulinism

Hyperinsulinism increases appetite, leading to weight gain. Emotional lability, indigestion, weakness, diaphoresis, tachycardia, visual disturbances, and syncope also occur.

Hypogonadism

Weight gain is common in hypogonadism. Prepubertal hypogonadism causes eunuchoid body proportions with relatively sparse facial and body hair and a high-pitched voice. Postpubertal hypogonadism causes loss of libido, impotence, and infertility.

Hypothalamic dysfunction

Conditions of hypothalamic dysfunction such as Laurence-Moon-Biedl's syndrome cause a voracious appetite with subsequent weight gain, along with altered body temperature and sleep rhythms.

Hypothyroidism

With hypothyroidism, weight gain occurs despite anorexia. Related signs and symptoms include fatigue; cold intolerance; constipation; menorrhagia; slowed intellectual and motor activity; dry, pale, cool skin; dry, sparse hair; and thick, brittle nails. Myalgia, hoarseness, hypoactive deep tendon reflexes, bradycardia, and abdominal distention may occur. Eventually, the face assumes a dull expression with periorbital edema.

Nephrotic syndrome

With nephrotic syndrome, weight gain results from edema. In severe cases, anasarca develops—increasing body weight up to 50%. Related effects include abdominal distention, orthostatic hypotension, and lethargy.

Pancreatic islet cell tumor

A pancreatic islet cell tumor causes excessive hunger that leads to weight gain. Other findings include emotional lability, weakness, malaise, fatigue, restlessness, diaphoresis, palpitations, tachycardia, visual disturbances, and syncope.

Preeclampsia

With preeclampsia, rapid weight gain (exceeding the normal weight gain of pregnancy) may accompany nausea and vomiting, epigastric pain, elevated blood pressure, and visual blurring or double vision.

Sheehan's syndrome

Sheehan's syndrome may cause weight gain and is most common in women who have severe obstetric hemorrhage.

Other causes

Corticosteroids, phenothiazines, and tricyclic antidepressants cause weight gain from fluid retention and increased appetite. Other drugs that can lead to weight gain include hormonal contraceptives, which cause fluid retention; cyproheptadine, which increases appetite; and lithium, which can induce hypothyroidism.

AGE ALERT

Weight gain in children can result from an endocrine disorder, such as hypercortisolism. Other causes include inactivity caused by Prader-Willi's syndrome, Down's syndrome, Werdnig-Hoffmann's disease, late stages of muscular dystrophy, severe cerebral palsy, and an adverse effect from atypical antipsychotic medications such as risperidone (Risperdal).

Nonpathologic causes include poor eating habits, sedentary recreation, and emotional problems, especially among adolescents. Regardless of the cause, discourage fad diets and provide the patient with a balanced weight loss program. The incidence of obesity is increasing among children.

Weight loss

Weight loss can reflect decreased food intake, increased metabolic requirements, or a combination of the two. Its causes include endocrine, neoplastic, GI, and psychological disorders; nutritional deficiencies; infections; and neurologic lesions that cause paralysis and dysphagia. Weight loss may also accompany conditions that prevent sufficient food intake, such as painful oral lesions, ill-fitting dentures, and tooth loss. Weight loss may stem from poverty, adherence to fad diets, excessive exercise, or drug use.

Health history

- When did you first notice that you were losing weight? How much weight have you lost? Was the loss intentional? If not, can you think of any reason for it?
- What do you usually eat in a day? Have your eating habits changed recently? Why?
- Have your stools changed recently? For instance, have you noticed bulky, floating stools, or have you had diarrhea? What about abdominal pain, excessive thirst, excessive urination, heat intolerance, nausea, or vomiting?
- Have you felt anxious or depressed? If so, why?
- What medications and supplements are you taking? Do you take diet pills or laxatives to lose weight?

Physical examination

Record the patient's height and weight. As you take the vital signs, note general appearance. Does he or she appear well nourished? Does his or her clothes fit? Is muscle wasting evident? Next, examine his or her skin for turgor and abnormal pigmentation, especially around the joints. Does he or she have jaundice or pallor? Examine his or her mouth, including the condition of his or her teeth or dentures. Also, check his or her eyes for exophthalmos and neck for swelling.

Finally, palpate the patient's abdomen for liver enlargement, masses, and tenderness.

Causes

Anorexia nervosa

A psychogenic disorder, anorexia nervosa is most common in young women and is characterized by severe, self-imposed weight loss. Weight loss may be accompanied by amenorrhea, blotchy or sallow skin, cold intolerance, constipation, frequent infections, loss of fatty tissue, loss of scalp hair, and skeletal muscle atrophy.

Cancer

Weight loss is a common sign of cancer. Associated signs and symptoms reflect the type, location, and stage of the tumor. They typically include abnormal bleeding, anorexia, fatigue, nausea, pain, a palpable mass, and vomiting.

Crohn's disease

Weight loss occurs with abdominal pain, anorexia, and chronic cramping. Other findings include abdominal distention, tenderness, and guarding; diarrhea; hyperactive bowel sounds; pain; and tachycardia.

Depression

Patients with severe depression may experience weight loss, anorexia, apathy, fatigue, feelings of worthlessness, and insomnia or hypersomnia. Other signs and symptoms include incoherence, indecisiveness, and suicidal thoughts or behavior.

Leukemia

Acute leukemia causes progressive weight loss accompanied by bleeding tendencies, high fever, and severe prostration. Chronic leukemia causes progressive weight loss with anemia, anorexia, bleeding tendencies, enlarged spleen, fatigue, fever, pallor, and skin eruptions.

Other causes

Weight loss may result from adrenal insufficiency, diabetes mellitus, gastroenteritis, cryptosporidiosis, lymphoma, ulcerative colitis, and thyrotoxicosis. Drugs, such as amphetamines, chemotherapeutic agents, laxatives, and thyroid preparations, can also cause weight loss.

Selected references

Bickley, L. S., & Szilagyi, P. G. (2017). *Bates' guide to physical examination and history taking* (12th ed.). Philadelphia, PA: Wolters Kluwer.

Good, V. S., & Kirkwood, P. L. (2018). *Advanced critical care nursing* (2nd ed.). St. Louis, MO: Elsevier.

Hinkle, J. L., & Cheever, K. H. (2018). *Brunner & Suddarth's textbook of medical-surgical nursing* (14th ed.). Philadelphia, PA: Wolters Kluwer.

Papadakis, M. A., & McPhee, S. J. (2019). *Current medical diagnosis & treatment* (58th ed.). New York, NY: McGraw-Hill Education.

3

ECGs

Interpreting them with ease and accuracy

Normal ECG

Analyzing the ECG waveform

An electrocardiogram (ECG) complex represents the electrical events occurring in one cardiac cycle. A complex consists of five waveforms labeled with the letters P, Q, R, S, and T. The letters Q, R, and S are referred to as a unit known as the *QRS complex*. The ECG tracing represents the conduction of electrical impulses from the atria to the ventricles. (See *Components of an ECG waveform.*)

- The P wave is the first component of the normal ECG waveform. It represents atrial depolarization.
- The PR interval tracks the atrial impulse from the atria through the atrioventricular (AV) node, the bundle of His, and the right and left bundle branches. It begins with atrial depolarization and ends with the beginning of ventricular depolarization.

- The QRS complex follows the P wave and represents ventricular depolarization.
- The ST segment represents the end of ventricular depolarization and the beginning of ventricular repolarization. The J point marks the end of the QRS complex and the beginning of the ST segment.
- The T wave represents ventricular repolarization.
- The QT interval measures the time needed for ventricular depolarization and repolarization.
- The U wave represents His-Purkinje repolarization.

How to read an ECG rhythm strip: The 8-step method

Analyzing a rhythm strip is a skill that is developed through practice. You can use several methods, as long as you are consistent. (See *The 8-step method of rhythm strip analysis*, pages 107 and 108.)

(Text continues on page 109.)

Components of an ECG waveform

This illustration shows the components of a normal ECG waveform.

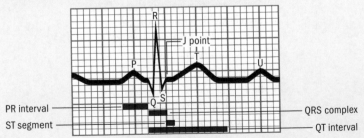

The 8-step method of rhythm strip analysis

Rhythm strip analysis requires a sequential and systematic approach. The following eight steps provide a good outline for you to follow.

Step 1: Determine rhythm

To determine the heart's atrial and ventricular rhythms, use either the pen-and-pencil method or the caliper method.

To determine the atrial rhythm, measure the P-P intervals, the intervals between consecutive P waves. These intervals should occur regularly, with only small variations associated with respirations. Then compare the P-P intervals in several cycles. Consistently similar P-P intervals indicate regular atrial rhythm; dissimilar P-P intervals indicate irregular atrial rhythm.

To determine the ventricular rhythm, measure the intervals between two consecutive R waves in the QRS complexes. If an R wave is not present, use either Q waves or S waves of consecutive QRS complexes. The R-R intervals should occur regularly. Then compare the R-R intervals in several cycles. As with atrial rhythms, consistently similar intervals mean a regular rhythm; dissimilar intervals point to an irregular rhythm.

After completing your measurements, ask yourself:

- Is the rhythm regular or irregular? Consider a rhythm with only slight variations (up to 0.04 second) to be regular.
- If the rhythm is irregular, is it slightly irregular or markedly irregular? Does the irregularity occur in a pattern (a regularly irregular pattern)?

Step 2: Calculate rate

You can use one of three methods to determine the atrial and ventricular heart rates from an electrocardiogram (ECG) waveform. Although these methods can provide accurate information, you should not rely solely on them when assessing your patient. Keep in mind that the ECG waveform represents electrical, not mechanical, activity. Therefore, although an ECG can show that ventricular depolarization has occurred, it does not mean that ventricular contraction has occurred. To determine this, you must assess the patient's pulse.

- *Times-ten method.* The simplest, quickest, and most common way to calculate rate is the times-ten method, especially if the rhythm is irregular. ECG paper is marked in increments of 3 seconds, or 15 large boxes. To calculate the atrial rate, obtain a 6-second strip, count the number of P waves that appear on it, and multiply this number by 10. Ten 6-second strips equal 1 minute. Calculate the ventricular rate the same way, using the R waves.

- *1,500 method.* If the heart rhythm is regular, use the 1,500 method, so named because 1,500 small squares equal 1 minute. Count the number of small squares between identical points on two consecutive P waves and then divide 1,500 by that number to determine the atrial rate. To obtain the ventricular rate, use the same method with two consecutive R waves.

- *Sequence method.* The third method of estimating heart rate is the sequence method, which requires memorizing a sequence of numbers. For the atrial rate, find a P wave that peaks on a heavy black line and assign the following numbers to the next six heavy black lines: 300, 150, 100, 75, 60, and 50. Then find the next P-wave peak and estimate the atrial rate, based on the number assigned to the nearest heavy black line. Estimate the ventricular rate the same way, using the R wave.

(continued)

The 8-step method of rhythm strip analysis *(continued)*

Step 3: Evaluate P waves

When examining a rhythm strip for P waves, ask yourself:

- Are P waves present?
- Do the P waves have a normal configuration?
- Do all of the P waves have a similar size and shape?
- Is there one P wave for every QRS complex?

Step 4: Determine PR interval duration

To measure the PR interval, count the small squares between the start of the P wave and the start of the QRS complex and then multiply the number of squares by 0.04 second. After you perform this calculation, ask yourself:

- Does the duration of the PR interval fall within normal limits, 0.12 to 0.20 second (or 3 to 5 small squares)?
- Is the PR interval constant?

Step 5: Determine QRS complex duration

When determining QRS complex duration, make sure to measure straight across from the end of the PR interval to the end of the S wave, not just to the peak. Remember, the QRS complex has no horizontal components. To calculate duration, count the number of small squares between the beginning and the end of the QRS complex and multiply this number by 0.04 second. Then ask yourself the following questions:

- Does the duration of the QRS complex fall within normal limits, 0.06 to 0.10 second?
- Are all QRS complexes the same size and shape? (If not, measure each one and describe them individually.)
- Does a QRS complex appear after every P wave?

Step 6: Evaluate T wave

Examine the T waves on the ECG strip. Then ask yourself:

- Are T waves present?
- Do all of the T waves have a normal shape?
- Could a P wave be hidden in a T wave?
- Do all of the T waves have a normal amplitude?
- Do the T waves have the same deflection as the QRS complexes?

Step 7: Determine QT interval duration

Count the number of small squares between the beginning of the QRS complex and the end of the T wave, where the T wave returns to the baseline. Multiply this number by 0.04 second. Ask yourself:

- Does the duration of the QT interval fall within normal limits, 0.36 to 0.44 second?

Step 8: Evaluate other components

Note the presence of ectopic or aberrantly conducted beats or other abnormalities. Also, check the ST segment for abnormalities and look for the presence of a U wave.

Next, interpret your findings by classifying the rhythm strip according to one or all of the following features:

- *Site of origin of the rhythm.* For example, sinus node, atria, atrioventricular node, or ventricles
- *Rate.* Normal (60 to 100 beats/minute), bradycardia (less than 60 beats/minute), or tachycardia (greater than 100 beats/minute)
- *Rhythm.* Normal or abnormal; for example, flutter, fibrillation, heart block, escape rhythm, or other arrhythmias

Normal sinus rhythm

When the heart functions normally, the sinoatrial (SA) node acts as the primary pacemaker, initiating the electrical impulses. The SA node assumes this role because its automatic firing rate exceeds that of the heart's other pacemakers, allowing cells to depolarize spontaneously.

Normal sinus rhythm records an impulse that starts with the sinus node and progresses to the ventricles through a normal conduction pathway—from the sinus node to the atria and AV node, through the bundle of His, to the bundle branches, and onto the Purkinje fibers. Normal sinus rhythm is the standard against which all other rhythms are compared; you must be able to recognize normal sinus rhythm before you can recognize an arrhythmia.

Based on the location of the electrical disturbance, arrhythmias can be classified as sinus, atrial, junctional, or ventricular arrhythmias, or as AV blocks. Functional disturbances in the SA node produce sinus arrhythmias. Enhanced automaticity of atrial tissue or reentry may produce atrial arrhythmias, the most common arrhythmias.

Junctional arrhythmias originate in the area around the AV node and bundle of His. These arrhythmias usually result from a suppressed higher pacemaker or from blocked impulses at the AV node.

Ventricular arrhythmias originate in ventricular tissue below the bifurcation of the bundle of His. These rhythms may result from reentry or enhanced automaticity or may occur after depolarization.

An AV block results from an abnormal interruption or delay of atrial impulse conduction to the ventricles. It may be partial or total and may occur in the AV node, bundle of His, or Purkinje system.

Characteristics of normal sinus rhythm

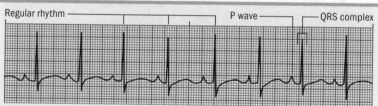

Lead II

Atrial rhythm: regular
Ventricular rhythm: regular
Atrial rate: 60 to 100 beats/minute (80 beats/minute shown)
Ventricular rate: 60 to 100 beats/minute (80 beats/minute shown)
P wave: normally shaped (All P waves have similar size and shape; a P wave precedes each QRS complex.)
PR interval: within normal limits (0.12 to 0.20 second) and constant (0.20-second duration shown)

QRS complex: within normal limits (0.06 to 0.10 second) (All QRS complexes have the same configuration. The duration shown here is 0.12 second.)
T wave: normally shaped; upright and rounded in lead II (Each QRS complex is followed by a T wave.)
QT interval: within normal limits (0.36 to 0.44 second) and constant (0.44-second duration shown)

Arrhythmias

Sinus arrhythmia

In sinus arrhythmia, the heart rate stays within normal limits, but the rhythm is irregular and corresponds to the respiratory cycle and to variations in vagal tone. During inspiration, an increased volume of blood returns to the heart, reducing vagal tone and increasing sinus rate. During expiration, venous return decreases, vagal tone increases, and sinus rate slows.

Conditions unrelated to respiration may also produce sinus arrhythmia. These conditions include inferior wall myocardial infarction (MI) and digoxin toxicity.

Sinus arrhythmia is easily recognized in elderly, pediatric, and sedated patients. The patient's pulse rate increases with inspiration and decreases with expiration. Usually, the patient is asymptomatic.

Intervention

Treatment is not necessary unless the patient is symptomatic or the sinus arrhythmia stems from an underlying cause. If symptoms are associated with symptomatic bradycardia, atropine may be administered.

Characteristics of sinus arrhythmia

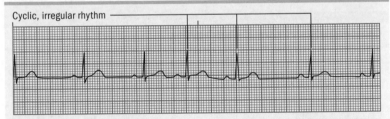

Cyclic, irregular rhythm

Lead II

Atrial rhythm: irregular, corresponding to the respiratory cycle
Ventricular rhythm: irregular, corresponding to the respiratory cycle
Atrial rate: within normal limits; varies with respiration (60 beats/minute shown)
Ventricular rate: within normal limits; varies with respiration (60 beats/minute shown)
P wave: normal size and configuration (One P wave precedes each QRS complex.)

PR interval: within normal limits (0.16-second, constant interval shown)
QRS complex: normal duration and configuration (0.06-second duration shown)
T wave: normal size and configuration
QT interval: within normal limits (0.36-second interval shown)
Other: phasic slowing and quickening of the rhythm

Sinus bradycardia

Characterized by a sinus rate of less than 60 beats/minute, sinus bradycardia usually occurs as the normal response to a reduced demand for blood flow. It is common among athletes, whose well-conditioned hearts can maintain stroke volume with reduced effort. It may also be caused by drugs, such as cardiac glycosides, calcium channel blockers, and beta-adrenergic blockers. Sinus bradycardia may occur after an inferior wall MI involving the right coronary artery, which supplies the blood to the SA node. This rhythm may develop during sleep and in patients with increased intracranial pressure. It may also result from vagal stimulation caused by vomiting or defecating. Pathologic sinus bradycardia may occur with sick sinus syndrome.

The patient with sinus bradycardia is asymptomatic if he or she can compensate for the decrease in heart rate by increasing stroke volume. If he or she cannot, he or she may have signs and symptoms of decreased cardiac output, such as hypotension, syncope, confusion, and blurred vision.

Intervention

If the patient is asymptomatic, treatment is not necessary. If he or she has signs and symptoms, the goal of treatment is to distinguish symptoms of poor perfusion and determine if those signs caused bradycardia. The initial treatment for symptomatic bradycardia is atropine. A temporary (transcutaneous or transvenous) or permanent pacemaker may be necessary if bradycardia persists. Patients with poor perfusion should be externally paced.

Characteristics of sinus bradycardia

Regular rhythm with rate
less than 60 beats/minute

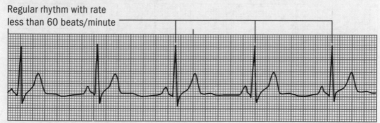

Lead II

Atrial rhythm: regular
Ventricular rhythm: regular
Atrial rate: less than 60 beats/minute (50 beats/minute shown)
Ventricular rate: less than 60 beats/minute (50 beats/minute shown)
P wave: normal size and configuration (One P wave precedes each QRS complex.)

PR interval: within normal limits and constant (0.14-second duration shown)
QRS complex: normal duration and configuration (0.08-second duration shown)
T wave: normal size and configuration
QT interval: within normal limits (0.40-second interval shown)

Sinus tachycardia

Sinus tachycardia is an acceleration of firing of the SA node beyond its normal discharge rate. In an adult, it is characterized by a sinus rate of more than 100 beats/minute. The rate rarely exceeds 180 beats/minute except during strenuous exercise. The maximum rate achieved with exercise decreases with age.

A normal response to cellular demands for increased oxygen delivery and blood flow commonly produces sinus tachycardia. Conditions that cause such a demand include heart failure, shock, anemia, exercise, fever, hypoxia, pain, and stress. Drugs that stimulate the beta receptors in the heart also cause sinus tachycardia.

They include aminophylline, epinephrine, dobutamine, and dopamine. Alcohol, caffeine, and nicotine may also produce sinus tachycardia.

An elevated heart rate increases myocardial oxygen demands. If the patient cannot meet these demands (for example, because of coronary artery disease), ischemia and further myocardial damage may occur.

Intervention

Treatment focuses on finding the primary cause. If it is high catecholamine levels, a beta-adrenergic blocker may slow the heart rate. After MI, persistent sinus tachycardia may precede heart failure or cardiogenic shock.

Characteristics of sinus tachycardia

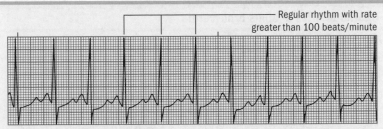

Regular rhythm with rate greater than 100 beats/minute

Lead II

Atrial rhythm: regular
Ventricular rhythm: regular
Atrial rate: 100 to 160 beats/minute (110 beats/minute shown)
Ventricular rate: 100 to 160 beats/minute (110 beats/minute shown)
P wave: normal size and configuration (One P wave precedes each QRS complex. As the sinus rate reaches about 150 beats/minute, the P wave merges with the preceding T wave and may be difficult to identify. Examine the descending slope of the preceding T wave closely for notches, indicating presence of the P wave. The P wave shown is normal.)
PR interval: within normal limits and constant (0.16-second duration shown)
QRS complex: normal duration and configuration (0.10-second duration shown)
T wave: normal size and configuration
QT interval: within normal limits and constant (0.36-second duration shown)
Other: gradual onset and cessation

Sinus arrest

In sinus arrest, the normal sinus rhythm is interrupted by an occasional, prolonged failure of the SA node to initiate an impulse. Therefore, sinus arrest is caused by episodes of failure in the automaticity of impulse formation of the SA node. The atria are not stimulated, and an entire PQRST complex is missing from the ECG strip. Except for the missing complex, or pause, the ECG usually remains normal.

During a sinus arrest, the sinus node resets itself so that when the impulse is initiated, the complex that occurs after the pause will be out of the cycle and the rate will usually be different from the rate before the pause.

Sinus arrest may result from an acute inferior wall MI, increased vagal tone, or the use of certain drugs, such as cardiac glycosides, calcium channel blockers, and beta-adrenergic blockers. The arrhythmia may also be linked to sick sinus syndrome. The patient has an irregular pulse rate associated with the pauses in sinus rhythm. If the pauses are infrequent, the patient is asymptomatic. If they occur frequently and last for several seconds, however, the patient may have signs of decreased cardiac output.

Intervention

For a symptomatic patient, treatment focuses on maintaining cardiac output and discovering the cause of sinus arrest. If indicated, atropine may be given or a temporary (transcutaneous or transvenous) or permanent pacemaker may be inserted.

Characteristics of sinus arrest

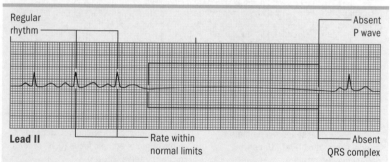

Atrial rhythm: regular, except for the missing PQRST complexes
Ventricular rhythm: regular, except for the missing complex
Atrial rate: within normal limits but varies because of pauses (94 beats/minute shown)
Ventricular rate: within normal limits but varies because of pauses (94 beats/minute shown)
P wave: normal size and configuration (One P wave precedes each QRS complex but is absent during a pause.)

PR interval: within normal limits and constant when the P wave is present; not measurable when the P wave is absent (0.20-second duration shown on all complexes surrounding the arrest)
QRS complex: normal duration and configuration; absent during pause (0.08-second duration shown)
T wave: normal size and configuration; absent during pause
QT interval: within normal limits; not measurable during pause (0.40-second, constant interval shown)

Premature atrial contractions

Premature atrial contractions (PACs) usually result from an irritable focus in the atrium that supersedes the SA node as the pacemaker for one or more beats.

Although PACs commonly occur in normal hearts, they are also associated with coronary and valvular heart disease. In an inferior wall MI, PACs may indicate a concomitant right atrial infarct. In an anterior wall MI, PACs are an early sign of left-sided heart failure. They may also warn of more severe atrial arrhythmia, such as atrial flutter or atrial fibrillation.

Possible causes include digoxin toxicity, hyperthyroidism, elevated catecholamine levels, acute respiratory failure, and chronic obstructive pulmonary disease. Alcohol, caffeine, or tobacco use can also trigger PACs. Patients who eliminate or control these factors can usually correct the arrhythmia.

Intervention

Symptomatic patients may be treated with beta-adrenergic blockers or calcium channel blockers.

Characteristics of premature atrial contractions

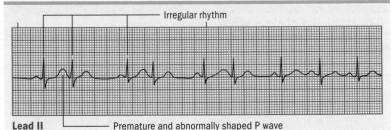

Irregular rhythm

Lead II — Premature and abnormally shaped P wave

Atrial rhythm: irregular (Incomplete compensatory pause follows premature arterial contraction [PAC]. Underlying rhythm may be regular.)
Ventricular rhythm: irregular (Incomplete compensatory pause follows PAC. Underlying rhythm may be regular.)
Atrial rate: varies with underlying rhythm (90 beats/minute shown)
Ventricular rate: varies with underlying rhythm (90 beats/minute shown)
P wave: premature and abnormally shaped; possibly lost in previous T wave (Varying configurations indicate multiform PACs.)

PR interval: usually normal but may be shortened or slightly prolonged, depending on the origin of ectopic focus (0.16-second, constant interval shown)
QRS complex: usually normal duration and configuration (0.08-second, constant duration shown)
T wave: usually normal configuration; may be distorted if the P wave is hidden in the previous T wave
QT interval: usually normal (0.36-second, constant interval shown)
Other: may occur in bigeminy or couplets

Atrial tachycardia

Atrial tachycardia is a supraventricular tachycardia, which means that the impulse originates above the ventricles. In this rhythm, the impulse originates in the atria. The rapid atrial rate shortens diastole, resulting in a loss of atrial kick, reduced cardiac output, reduced coronary perfusion, and ischemic myocardial changes.

Although atrial tachycardia can occur in healthy patients, it is usually associated with high catecholamine levels, digoxin toxicity, MI, cardiomyopathy, hyperthyroidism, hypertension, and valvular heart disease. Three types of atrial tachycardia exist: atrial tachycardia with block, multifocal atrial tachycardia, and paroxysmal atrial tachycardia.

Intervention

If the patient has atrial tachycardia or paroxysmal atrial tachycardia and is symptomatic, prepare for immediate synchronized cardioversion. If the patient is stable, the physician may perform carotid sinus massage (if no bruits are present), a Valsalva's maneuver, or order drug therapy, such as adenosine (Adenocard), a calcium channel blocker, a beta-adrenergic blocker, or digoxin (Lanoxin). If these treatments are ineffective in rhythm conversion, then procainamide, amiodarone, or sotalol may be needed. If these measures fail, cardioversion may be necessary.

Characteristics of atrial tachycardia

Regular rhythm — Rate between 160 and 250 beats/minute

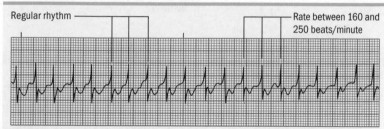

Lead II

Atrial rhythm: regular
Ventricular rhythm: regular
Atrial rate: three or more successive ectopic atrial beats at a rate of 160 to 250 beats/minute (210 beats/minute shown)
Ventricular rate: varies with atrioventricular conduction ratio (210 beats/minute shown)
P wave: 1:1 ratio with QRS complex, although commonly indiscernible because of rapid rate; may be hidden in previous ST segment or T wave
PR interval: may not be measurable if P wave cannot be distinguished from preceding T wave (If P wave is present,

PR interval is short when conduction through the atrioventricular (AV) node is 1:1. On this strip, the PR interval is not discernible.)
QRS complex: usually normal unless aberrant intraventricular conduction is present (0.10-second duration shown)
T wave: may be normal or inverted if ischemia is present (inverted T waves shown)
QT interval: usually normal but may be shorter because of rapid rate (0.20-second interval shown)
Other: appearance of ST-segment and T-wave changes if tachyarrhythmia persists longer than 30 minutes

Atrial flutter

Characterized by an atrial rate of 250 beats/minute or more, atrial flutter is caused by multiple reentry circuits within the atrial tissue. On the ECG, the P waves lose their normal appearance as a result of rapid atrial rate and blend together in a sawtooth configuration known as flutter waves. These waves are the hallmark of atrial flutter.

Causes of atrial flutter include conditions that enlarge atrial tissue and elevate atrial pressures. Atrial flutter is associated with MI, increased catecholamine levels, hyperthyroidism, and digoxin toxicity.

If the patient's pulse rate is normal, he or she usually has no symptoms. If his or her pulse rate is high, however, he or she will probably have signs and symptoms of decreased cardiac output, such as hypotension and syncope.

Intervention

If the patient is symptomatic, prepare for immediate cardioversion. The focus of treatment for stable patients with atrial flutter includes controlling the rate and converting the rhythm. Specific interventions depend on the patient's cardiac function, the presence of preexcitation syndromes, and the duration (less than or greater than 48 hours) of arrhythmia. For example, in patients with atrial flutter, normal cardiac function, and duration of rhythm less than 48 hours, cardioversion may be considered. When duration is greater than 48 hours, avoid nonemergent cardioversion unless adequate anticoagulation has been achieved.

Drugs that may be ordered to control atrial rate include beta blocker and nondihydropyridine calcium channel blockers such as diltiazem. Digoxin and amiodarone may also be used.

Characteristics of atrial flutter

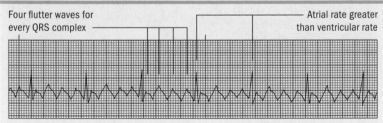

Four flutter waves for every QRS complex

Atrial rate greater than ventricular rate

Lead II

Atrial rhythm: regular
Ventricular rhythm: may be regular or irregular, depending on the conduction ratio (regular rhythm shown)
Atrial rate: 300 to 350 beats/minute (300 beats/minute shown)
Ventricular rate: variable (70 beats/minute shown)

P wave: atrial activity seen as flutter waves, with a classic sawtooth appearance
PR interval: not measurable
QRS complex: usually normal but can be distorted by the underlying flutter waves (0.10-second, normal duration shown)
T wave: unidentifiable
QT interval: not measurable

Atrial fibrillation

Atrial fibrillation is chaotic, asynchronous electrical activity in the atrial tissue. It results from impulses in many reentry pathways. These multiple and multidirectional impulses cause the atria to quiver instead of contracting regularly.

With this type of arrhythmia, blood may pool in the left atrial appendage and form thrombi that can be ejected into the systemic circulation. An associated rapid ventricular rate can decrease cardiac output.

Possible causes include valvular disorders, hypertension, coronary artery disease, MI, chronic lung disease, ischemia, thyroid disorders, and Wolff-Parkinson-White's syndrome. The disorder may also result from high adrenergic tone as a result of physical exertion, sepsis, alcohol withdrawal, or the use of drugs, such as

aminophylline (theophylline ethylenediamine) and cardiac glycosides.

Intervention

If the patient is symptomatic, synchronized cardioversion should be used immediately. Vagal stimulation may be used to slow the ventricular response, but it will not convert the arrhythmia. Drugs that may be ordered to slow AV conduction include calcium channel blockers and beta-adrenergic blockers. Digoxin may be ordered if the patient is stable. After the rate slows, if conversion to a normal sinus rhythm has not occurred, amiodarone (Cordarone), flecainide, or sotalol may be ordered. If atrial fibrillation is of several days' duration, anticoagulant therapy is recommended before pharmacologic or electrical conversion. If atrial fibrillation is of recent onset, ibutilide (Corvert) may be used to convert the rhythm.

Characteristics of atrial fibrillation

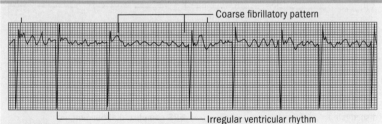

Lead MCL₁

Atrial rhythm: grossly irregular
Ventricular rhythm: grossly irregular
Atrial rate: greater than 400 beats/minute
Ventricular rate: varies from 40 to 250 beats/minute (80 beats/minute shown)
P wave: absent; appearance of erratic baseline fibrillatory waves (f waves) (When the f waves are pronounced, the arrhythmia is called coarse atrial fibrillation. When the

f waves are not pronounced, the arrhythmia is known as fine atrial fibrillation. On this strip, the f waves are pronounced.)
PR interval: indiscernible
QRS complex: duration usually within normal limits, with aberrant intraventricular conduction (0.08-second duration shown)
T wave: indiscernible
QT interval: not measurable

Junctional rhythm

Junctional rhythm, also known as *junctional escape rhythm*, occurs in the AV junctional tissue. It causes retrograde depolarization of the atrial tissue and antegrade depolarization of the ventricular tissue. It results from conditions that depress SA node function, such as an inferior wall MI, digoxin toxicity, and vagal stimulation. The arrhythmia may also stem from increased automaticity of the junctional tissue, which can be caused by digoxin toxicity or ischemia associated with an inferior wall MI.

Junctional rhythm is a regular rhythm with a ventricular rate of 40 to 60 beats/minute. A junctional rhythm with a ventricular rate of 60 to 100 beats/minute is known as an accelerated junctional rhythm. If the ventricular rate exceeds 100 beats/minute, the arrhythmia is called junctional tachycardia.

Intervention

Treatment aims to identify and manage the primary cause of arrhythmia. If the patient is symptomatic, treatment may include atropine to increase the sinus or junctional rate. Alternately, the physician may insert a pacemaker or use transcutaneous pacing to maintain an effective heart rate.

Characteristics of junctional rhythm

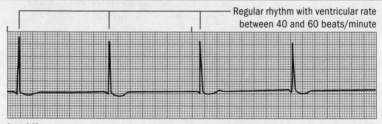

Regular rhythm with ventricular rate between 40 and 60 beats/minute

Lead II

Atrial rhythm: regular
Ventricular rhythm: regular
Atrial rate: if discernible, 40 to 60 beats/minute (On this strip, the rate is not discernible.)
Ventricular rate: 40 to 60 beats/minute (40 beats/minute shown)
P wave: usually inverted; may precede, follow, or fall within the QRS complex; may be absent (On this strip, the P wave is absent.)

PR interval: less than 0.12 second and constant if the P wave precedes the QRS complex; otherwise, not measurable (not measurable on this strip)
QRS complex: duration normal; configuration usually normal (0.08-second duration shown)
T wave: usually normal configuration
QT interval: usually normal (0.32-second duration shown)

Accelerated junctional rhythm

An accelerated junctional rhythm is an arrhythmia that originates in the AV junction and is usually caused by enhanced automaticity of the AV junctional tissue. It is called "accelerated" because it occurs at a rate of 60 to 100 beats/minute, exceeding the inherent junctional rate of 40 to 60 beats/minute.

Digoxin toxicity is a common cause of accelerated junctional rhythm.

Other causes include electrolyte disturbances, ventricular heart disease, heart failure, and inferior or posterior MI.

Intervention

Treatment aims to identify and manage the primary cause of arrhythmia. Assessing the patient for signs and symptoms of decreased cardiac output and hemodynamic instability is key, as is monitoring serum digoxin and electrolyte levels.

Characteristics of accelerated junctional rhythm

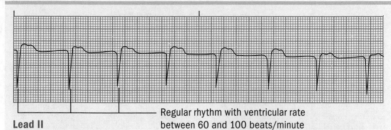

Lead II

Regular rhythm with ventricular rate between 60 and 100 beats/minute

Atrial rhythm: regular
Ventricular rhythm: regular
Atrial rate: if discernible, 60 to 100 beats/minute (On this strip, the rate is not discernible.)
Ventricular rate: 60 to 100 beats/minute (75 beats/minute shown)
P wave: usually inverted; may precede, follow, or fall within the QRS complex; may be absent (On this strip, the P wave is absent.)

PR interval: less than 0.12 second and constant if the P wave precedes the QRS complex; otherwise, not measurable (not measurable on this strip)
QRS complex: duration normal; configuration usually normal (0.10-second duration shown)
T wave: usually normal configuration
QT interval: usually normal (0.32-second duration shown)

Junctional tachycardia

In junctional tachycardia, three or more premature junctional contractions (PJCs) occur in a row. This supraventricular tachycardia generally occurs as a result of enhanced automaticity of the AV junction, which causes the AV junction to override the SA node.

Digoxin toxicity is the most common cause of junctional tachycardia. Other causes include inferior or posterior MI, heart failure, and electrolyte imbalances.

Intervention

The goal of treatment is to identify and manage the primary cause of arrhythmia. If the cause is digoxin toxicity, the drug should be discontinued. Drugs such as the calcium channel blocker verapamil may slow the heart rate in symptomatic patients.

Characteristics of junctional tachycardia

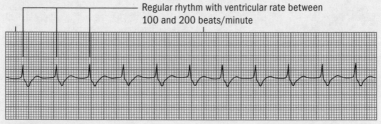

Regular rhythm with ventricular rate between 100 and 200 beats/minute

Lead II

Atrial rhythm: regular
Ventricular rhythm: regular
Atrial rate: if discernible, 100 to 200 beats/minute (On this strip, the rate is not discernible.)
Ventricular rate: 100 to 200 beats/minute (115 beats/minute shown)
P wave: usually inverted; may precede, follow, or fall within the QRS complex; may be absent (On this strip, the P wave is absent.)

PR interval: less than 0.12 second and constant if the P wave precedes the QRS complex; otherwise, not measurable (not measurable on this strip)
QRS complex: duration normal; configuration usually normal (0.08-second duration shown)
T wave: usually normal configuration
QT interval: usually normal (0.36-second duration shown)

Premature junctional contractions

In PJCs, a junctional beat occurs before the next normal sinus beat. Ectopic beats and PJCs commonly result from increased automaticity in the bundle of His or the surrounding junctional tissue, which interrupts the underlying rhythm.

Digoxin toxicity is the most common cause of PJCs. Other causes include ischemia associated with inferior wall MI, excessive caffeine ingestion, and excessive levels of amphetamines.

Intervention

In most cases, treatment is directed at the underlying cause.

Characteristics of premature junctional contractions

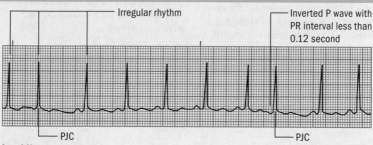

Lead II

Atrial rhythm: irregular with premature junctional contractions (PJCs), but underlying rhythm may be regular
Ventricular rhythm: irregular with PJCs, but underlying rhythm may be regular
Atrial rate: follows the underlying rhythm (100 beats/minute shown)
Ventricular rate: follows the underlying rhythm (100 beats/minute shown)
P wave: usually inverted; may precede, follow, or fall within the QRS complex; may be absent (shown preceding the QRS complex)

PR interval: less than 0.12 second on the PJC if P wave precedes the QRS complex; otherwise, not measurable (On this strip, the PR interval is 0.14 second and constant on the underlying rhythm and 0.06 second on the PJC.)
QRS complex: normal duration and configuration (0.06-second duration shown)
T wave: usually normal configuration
QT interval: usually within normal limits (0.30-second interval shown)

Premature ventricular contractions

Premature ventricular contractions (PVCs) occur singly or in bigeminy, trigeminy, quadrigeminy, or clusters. PVCs may be caused by certain drugs, electrolyte imbalance, or stress.

Paired PVCs can produce ventricular tachycardia (VT) because the second PVC usually meets refractory tissue. Three or more PVCs in a row are a run of VT. Multiform PVCs do not look alike and may arise from different ventricular sites or be abnormally conducted. In the R-on-T phenomenon, the PVC occurs so early that it falls on the downslope of the previous T wave. Because the cells have not depolarized, VT or fibrillation can result.

The earlier the PVC, the shorter the diastolic filling time and the lower the stroke volume. Frequent PVCs may cause palpitations.

Intervention

If the PVCs are believed to result from a serious cardiac problem, antiarrhythmics, such as lidocaine, procainamide, or amiodarone, may be given to suppress ventricular irritability. When the PVCs are believed to result from a noncardiac problem, treatment aims at correcting the underlying cause—an acid-base or electrolyte imbalance, antiarrhythmic therapy, hypothermia, high catecholamine levels, or hypoxia.

Characteristics of premature ventricular contractions

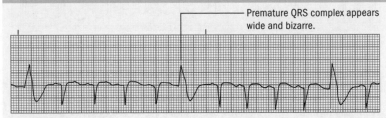

Premature QRS complex appears wide and bizarre.

Lead MCL₁

Atrial rhythm: irregular during premature ventricular contractions (PVCs); underlying rhythm may be regular.
Ventricular rhythm: irregular during PVCs; underlying rhythm may be regular.
Atrial rate: follows underlying rhythm (120 beats/minute shown)
Ventricular rate: follows underlying rhythm (120 beats/minute shown)
P wave: atrial activity independent of the PVC (If retrograde atrial depolarization exists, a retrograde P wave will distort the ST segment of the PVC. On this strip, no P wave appears before the PVC, but one occurs with each QRS complex.)
PR interval: determined by underlying rhythm; not associated with the

PVC (0.12-second, constant interval shown)
QRS complex: occurs earlier than expected; duration exceeds 0.12 second and complex has a bizarre configuration; may be normal in the underlying rhythm (On this strip, it is 0.08 second in the normal beats; it is bizarre and 0.14 second in the PVC.)
T wave: occurs in the direction opposite that of the QRS complex; normal in the underlying complexes
QT interval: not usually measured in the PVC but may be within normal limits in the underlying rhythm (On this strip, the QT interval is 0.28 second in the underlying rhythm.)

Ventricular tachycardia

The life-threatening arrhythmia VT develops when three or more PVCs occur in a row and the ventricular rate exceeds 100 beats/minute. VT may result from enhanced automaticity or reentry within the Purkinje system. The rapid ventricular rate reduces ventricular filling time, and because atrial kick is lost, cardiac output drops, putting the patient at risk for ventricular fibrillation.

VT usually results from acute MI, coronary artery disease, valvular heart disease, heart failure, or cardiomyopathy. The arrhythmia can also stem from an electrolyte imbalance or from toxic levels of a drug, such as digoxin, procainamide, or quinidine. You may detect two variations of this arrhythmia: ventricular flutter and torsades de pointes.

Intervention

Treatment depends on the patient's clinical status. This rhythm commonly degenerates into ventricular fibrillation and cardiovascular collapse, requiring immediate cardiopulmonary resuscitation and defibrillation. Patients with pulseless VT are treated the same as those with ventricular fibrillation and require immediate defibrillation. If the patient is unstable and has a pulse, prepare for immediate synchronized cardioversion followed by antiarrhythmic therapy. Drug therapy may include amiodarone, lidocaine, magnesium, or procainamide. Patients with chronic, recurrent episodes of VT that are unresponsive to drug therapy may need an implantable cardioverter-defibrillator.

Characteristics of ventricular tachycardia

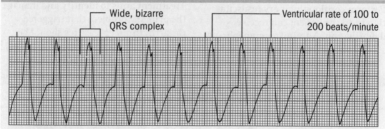

Wide, bizarre QRS complex

Ventricular rate of 100 to 200 beats/minute

Lead MCL₁

Atrial rhythm: independent P waves possibly discernible with slower ventricular rates (On this strip, the P waves are not visible.)
Ventricular rhythm: usually regular but may be slightly irregular (On this strip, it is regular.)
Atrial rate: cannot be determined
Ventricular rate: usually 100 to 200 beats/minute (120 beats/minute shown)

P wave: usually absent; possibly obscured by the QRS complex; retrograde P waves may be present.
PR interval: not measurable
QRS complex: duration greater than 0.12 second; bizarre appearance, usually with increased amplitude (0.16-second duration shown)
T wave: opposite direction of the QRS complex
QT interval: not measurable

Ventricular fibrillation

Defined as chaotic, asynchronous electrical activity within the ventricular tissue, ventricular fibrillation is a life-threatening arrhythmia that results in death if the rhythm is not stopped immediately. Conditions that lead to ventricular fibrillation include myocardial ischemia, hypokalemia, cocaine toxicity, hypoxia, hypothermia, severe acidosis, and severe alkalosis.

Patients with MI are at greatest risk for ventricular fibrillation during the first 2 hours after the onset of chest pain.

In ventricular fibrillation, lack of cardiac output results in loss of consciousness, pulselessness, and respiratory arrest. Initially, you may see coarse fibrillatory waves on the ECG strip. As acidosis develops, the waves become fine and progress to asystole unless defibrillation restores cardiac rhythm.

Intervention

Perform cardiopulmonary resuscitation until the patient can receive defibrillation. Administer epinephrine, amiodarone, or lidocaine if the initial defibrillation series is unsuccessful.

Idioventricular rhythm

Idioventricular rhythm, also referred to as ventricular escape rhythm, originates in an escape pacemaker site in the ventricles. The inherent firing rate of this ectopic pacemaker is less than 40 beats/minute. The rhythm acts as a safety mechanism when all potential pacemakers above the ventricles do not discharge or when a block prevents supraventricular impulses from reaching the ventricles.

The slow ventricular rate and loss of atrial kick associated with this arrhythmia markedly reduce cardiac output. In turn, reduced cardiac output causes hypotension, confusion, vertigo, and syncope. If it is not identified rapidly and managed appropriately, idioventricular rhythm may cause death.

Intervention

Treatment aims to identify and manage the primary problem that triggered the arrhythmia. Measures should be

Characteristics of ventricular fibrillation

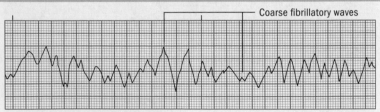

Coarse fibrillatory waves

Lead MCL$_1$

Atrial rhythm: cannot be determined
Ventricular rhythm: irregular
Atrial rate: cannot be determined
Ventricular rate: cannot be determined
P wave: indiscernible

PR interval: not measurable
QRS complex: replaced with fibrillatory waves; duration not discernible
T wave: cannot be determined
QT interval: not measurable

initiated to increase the patient's heart rate, improve cardiac output, and establish a normal rhythm. Atropine may be administered to increase the heart rate.

ALERT

If atropine is not effective or if hypotension or other signs of clinical instability develop, a pacemaker (transcutaneous or transvenous) may be needed to reestablish a heart rate that provides enough cardiac output to perfuse the organs properly.

ALERT

The goal of treating idioventricular rhythm does not include suppressing the rhythm because it acts as a safety mechanism to protect the heart from ventricular standstill. Idioventricular rhythm should never be treated with antiarrhythmics such as lidocaine because these drugs would suppress the escape beats.

Characteristics of idioventricular rhythm

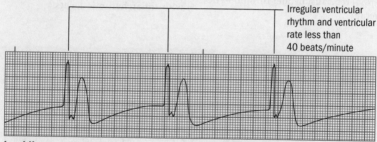

Irregular ventricular rhythm and ventricular rate less than 40 beats/minute

Lead II

Atrial rhythm: cannot be determined
Ventricular rhythm: usually regular, except with isolated escape beats (irregular rhythm shown)
Atrial rate: cannot be determined
Ventricular rate: less than 40 beats/minute (30 beats/minute shown)
P wave: absent
PR interval: usually not measurable

QRS complex: duration greater than 0.12 second; complex is wide and has a bizarre configuration (On this strip, the complex is 0.20 second and bizarre.)
T wave: directed opposite the terminal forces of the QRS complex
QT interval: usually greater than 0.44 second (0.46-second interval shown)

Accelerated idioventricular rhythm

When the pacemaker cells above the ventricles do not generate an impulse or when a block prevents supraventricular impulses from reaching the ventricles, idioventricular rhythms result. When the rate of an idioventricular rhythm ranges from 40 to 100 beats/minute, it is considered accelerated idioventricular rhythm, denoting a rate greater than that of the inherent pacemaker.

In this life-threatening arrhythmia, the cells of the His-Purkinje system operate as pacemaker cells. The characteristic waveform results from an area of enhanced automaticity within the ventricles, which may be associated with MI, digoxin toxicity, or metabolic imbalances. In addition, the arrhythmia commonly occurs during myocardial reperfusion after thrombolytic therapy.

The patient may be symptomatic, depending on his or her heart rate and ability to compensate for the loss of the atrial kick. A symptomatic patient may have signs and symptoms of decreased cardiac output, including hypotension, confusion, syncope, and loss of consciousness.

Intervention

An asymptomatic patient needs no treatment. For a symptomatic patient, treatment focuses on maintaining cardiac output and identifying the cause of arrhythmia. The patient may require a transcutaneous or transvenous temporary pacemaker to enhance cardiac output and may need a permanent pacemaker for long-term therapy. Remember, this rhythm protects the heart from ventricular standstill and should not be treated with antiarrhythmic agents.

Characteristics of accelerated idioventricular rhythm

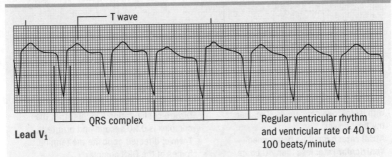

Lead V$_1$

T wave

QRS complex

Regular ventricular rhythm and ventricular rate of 40 to 100 beats/minute

Atrial rhythm: cannot be determined
Ventricular rhythm: usually regular
Atrial rate: cannot be determined
Ventricular rate: 40 to 100 beats/minute
P wave: absent
PR interval: not measurable

QRS complex: duration greater than 0.12 second; wide and bizarre configuration
T wave: deflection usually opposite that of the QRS complex
QT interval: may be within normal limits or prolonged

First-degree atrioventricular block

First-degree AV block occurs when there is a delay in the conduction of electrical impulses from the atria to the ventricles. This delay usually occurs at the level of the AV node but may also be infranodal.

First-degree AV block is characterized by a constant PR interval greater than 0.20 second. It may result from myocardial ischemia, MI, myocarditis, or degenerative changes in the heart associated with aging. Certain drugs, such as digoxin, calcium channel blockers, and beta-adrenergic blockers, may also cause this condition.

Most patients with first-degree AV block are asymptomatic.

Intervention

Management of first-degree AV block includes identifying and treating the underlying cause and monitoring the patient for signs of progressive AV block.

Characteristics of first-degree atrioventricular block

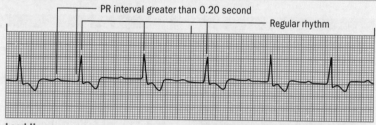

PR interval greater than 0.20 second

Regular rhythm

Lead II

Atrial rhythm: regular
Ventricular rhythm: regular
Atrial rate: usually within normal limits (60 beats/minute shown)
Ventricular rate: usually within normal limits (60 beats/minute shown)
P wave: normal size and configuration (One P wave precedes each QRS complex.)

PR interval: greater than 0.20 second and constant (0.32-second duration shown)
QRS complex: usually normal duration and configuration (0.08-second duration and normal configuration shown)
T wave: normal size and configuration
QT interval: usually within normal limits (0.32-second interval shown)

Second-degree atrioventricular block, type I

Type I (Wenckebach or Mobitz I) second-degree AV block occurs when each successive impulse from the SA node is delayed in the AV node slightly longer than the previous impulse. This pattern of progressive prolongation of the PR interval continues until an impulse is not conducted to the ventricles.

Type I block most commonly occurs at the level of the AV node and is caused by inferior wall MI, vagal stimulation, or digoxin toxicity. The arrhythmia usually does not cause symptoms; however, a patient may have signs and symptoms of decreased cardiac output, such as hypotension, confusion, and syncope. These effects occur especially if the patient's ventricular rate is slow.

Intervention

If the patient is asymptomatic, no intervention is required other than monitoring the ECG frequently to see if a more serious form of AV block develops.

If the patient is symptomatic, atropine may be ordered to increase the ventricular rate. Treatment may also include a temporary pacemaker (transcutaneous or transvenous) to maintain an effective cardiac output.

Characteristics of second-degree atrioventricular block, type I

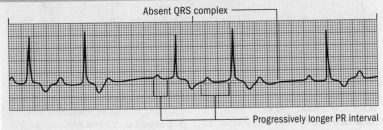

Absent QRS complex

Progressively longer PR interval

Lead II

Atrial rhythm: regular
Ventricular rhythm: irregular
Atrial rate: determined by the underlying rhythm (80 beats/minute shown)
Ventricular rate: slower than the atrial rate (50 beats/minute shown)
P wave: normal size and configuration
PR interval: progressively prolonged with each beat until a P wave appears without a QRS complex

QRS complex: normal duration and configuration; periodically absent (0.08-second duration shown)
T wave: normal size and configuration
QT interval: usually within normal limits (0.46-second, constant interval shown)
Other: usually distinguished by a pattern of group beating, referred to as the footprints of Wenckebach

Second-degree atrioventricular block, type II

Produced by a conduction disturbance in the His-Purkinje system, a type II (Mobitz II) second-degree AV block causes intermittent absence of conduction. In type II block, two or more atrial impulses are conducted to the ventricles with constant PR intervals, when suddenly, without warning, the atrial impulse is blocked. This type of block occurs in an anterior wall MI, severe coronary artery disease, and chronic degeneration of the conduction system.

Type II second-degree AV block is more serious than type I second-degree AV block and can be a life-threatening arrhythmia. It requires prompt intervention.

Intervention

If the patient is hypotensive, treatment aims at increasing his or her heart rate to improve cardiac output. Because the conduction block occurs in the His-Purkinje system, drugs that act directly on the myocardium usually prove more effective than those that increase the atrial rate. As a result, dopamine or epinephrine instead of atropine may be ordered to increase the ventricular rate.

If the patient has an anterior wall MI, the physician will immediately insert a temporary pacemaker to prevent ventricular asystole. A transcutaneous pacemaker should be used until a transvenous pacemaker is placed. For long-term management, the patient may need a permanent pacemaker.

Characteristics of second-degree atrioventricular block, type II

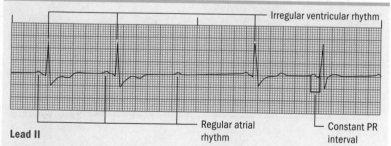

Irregular ventricular rhythm

Regular atrial rhythm

Constant PR interval

Lead II

Atrial rhythm: regular
Ventricular rhythm: regular or irregular
Atrial rate: usually within normal limits (60 beats/minute shown)
Ventricular rate: may be within normal limits but less than the atrial rate (40 beats/minute shown)
P wave: normal size and configuration (Not all P waves are followed by a QRS complex.)

PR interval: constant and frequently within normal limits for all conducted beats
QRS complex: duration within normal limits if the block occurs at the bundle of His; greater than 0.16 second if the block occurs at the bundle branches (0.12-second complex shown)
T wave: usually normal size and configuration
QT interval: usually within normal limits (0.44-second interval shown)

Third-degree atrioventricular block

Also called complete heart block, third-degree AV block indicates the complete absence of impulse conduction between the atria and ventricles. The atrial rate is generally equal to or faster than the ventricular rate. Third-degree AV block may occur at the level of the AV node, the bundle of His, or the bundle branches. Treatment and prognosis vary depending on the anatomic level of the block.

If this type of block originates at the AV node, a junctional escape rhythm occurs; if it originates below the AV node, an idioventricular escape rhythm occurs.

Third-degree AV block involving the AV node may result from inferior wall MI or drug toxicity (cardiac glycosides, beta-adrenergic blockers, calcium channel blockers). Third-degree AV block below the AV node may result from anterior wall MI or chronic degeneration of the conduction system.

Some patients with complete heart block are relatively free from symptoms, complaining only that they cannot tolerate exercise or increased activity. However, most patients have significant signs and symptoms, including severe fatigue, dyspnea, chest pain, light-headedness, and changes in mental status. The severity of the symptoms depends on the ventricular rate and the patient's ability to compensate for decreased cardiac output.

Characteristics of third-degree atrioventricular block

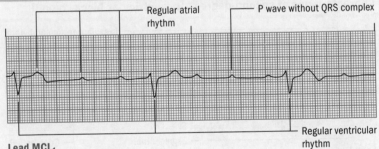

Regular atrial rhythm — P wave without QRS complex

Lead MCL₁ — Regular ventricular rhythm

Atrial rhythm: usually regular
Ventricular rhythm: usually regular
Atrial rate: usually within normal limits (90 beats/minute shown)
Ventricular rate: slow (30 beats/minute shown)
P wave: normal size and configuration
PR interval: not measurable because the atria and ventricles beat independently of each other

QRS complex: determined by the site of the escape rhythm (With a junctional escape rhythm, the duration and configuration are normal; with an idioventricular escape rhythm, the duration is greater than 0.12 second and the complex is distorted. In the complex shown, the duration is 0.16 second, the configuration is abnormal, and the complex is distorted.)
T wave: normal size and configuration
QT interval: may or may not be within normal limits (0.56-second interval shown)

Intervention

Third-degree AV block can be a life-threatening arrhythmia; it requires prompt intervention. If the patient has serious signs and symptoms and cardiac output is not adequate, interventions may include transcutaneous or transvenous pacing or I.V. atropine, dopamine, or epinephrine. Patients with third-degree AV block at the infranodal level associated with an extensive anterior MI usually require a permanent pacemaker.

 ALERT

Atropine is not indicated for third-degree atrioventricular (AV) block with new wide QRS complexes. In such cases, a pacemaker is indicated because atropine rarely increases sinus rate and AV node conduction when AV block occurs at the His-Purkinje level.

12-Lead ECGs

Basic components and principles

Whereas rhythm strips are used to detect arrhythmias, the 12-lead or standard ECG has a different purpose. The most common procedure for evaluating cardiac status, this diagnostic test helps to identify various pathologic conditions—most commonly, acute MI.

The 12-lead ECG provides 12 views of the electrical activity of the heart. (See *12 views of the heart*, page 132.) The 12 leads include:

- three bipolar limb leads (I, II, and III)
- three unipolar augmented limb leads (aV_R, aV_L, and aV_F)
- six unipolar precordial, or chest, leads (V_1, V_2, V_3, V_4, V_5, and V_6).

Leads

The six limb leads record electrical potential from the frontal plane, and the six precordial leads record electrical potential from the horizontal plane. Each waveform reflects the orientation of a lead to the wave of depolarization passing through the myocardium. Normally, this wave moves through the heart from right to left and from top to bottom.

Bipolar leads

Bipolar leads record the difference in electrical potential between two points on the patient's body where you place electrodes.

- Lead I goes from the right arm (−) to the left arm (+).
- Lead II goes from the right arm (−) to the left leg (+).
- Lead III goes from the left arm (−) to the left leg (+).

Because of the orientation of these leads to the wave of depolarization, QRS complexes typically appear upright. In lead II, these complexes are usually the tallest because this lead parallels the wave of depolarization.

Unipolar leads

Unipolar leads (the augmented limb leads and the precordial leads) have only one electrode, which represents the positive pole. The negative pole is computed by the ECG. Lead aV_R typically records negative QRS complex deflections because the wave of depolarization moves away from it. In the aV_F lead, QRS complexes are positive; in the aV_L lead, they are biphasic.

Unipolar precordial leads V_1 and V_2 usually have a small R wave because the direction of ventricular activation is left to right initially. That is because conduction time is normally faster down the left bundle branch than it is down the right. The wave of depolarization, however, moves toward the left ventricle and away from these leads, causing a low S wave.

12 views of the heart

Each of the leads on a 12-lead electrocardiogram (ECG) views the heart from a different angle. These illustrations show the direction of electrical activity (depolarization) monitored by each lead and the 12 views of the heart.

Views reflected on a 12-lead ECG

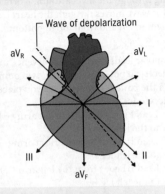

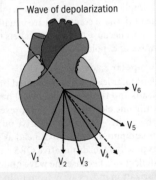

Lead	View of heart
Standard limb leads (bipolar)	
I	Lateral wall
II	Inferior wall
III	Inferior wall
Augmented limb leads (unipolar)	
aV_R	No specific view
aV_L	Lateral wall
aV_F	Inferior wall
Precordial, or chest, leads (unipolar)	
V_1	Septal wall
V_2	Septal wall
V_3	Anterior wall
V_4	Anterior wall
V_5	Lateral wall
V_6	Lateral wall

In leads V_3 and V_4, the R and S waves may have the same amplitude, and you will not see a Q wave. In leads V_5 and V_6, the initial ventricular activation appears as a small Q wave; the following tall R wave represents the strong wave of depolarization moving toward the left ventricle. These leads record a small or absent S wave.

Determining electrical axis

As electrical impulses travel through the heart, they generate small electrical forces called instant-to-instant vectors. The mean of these vectors represents the direction and force of the wave of depolarization, also known as the electrical axis of the heart.

In a healthy heart, the wave of depolarization originates in the SA node and travels through the atria and the AV node and on to the ventricles. The normal movement is downward and to the left—the direction of a normal electrical axis.

In an unhealthy heart, the wave of depolarization (or the direction of the electrical axis) varies. That is because the direction of electrical activity swings away from areas of damage or necrosis.

A simple method to determine the direction of your patient's electrical axis is the quadrant method. Before you use this method, you must understand the hexaxial reference system—a schematic view of the heart that uses the six limb leads.

As discussed earlier, these leads include the three standard limb leads (I, II, and III), which are bipolar, and the three augmented limb leads (aV$_R$, aV$_L$, and aV$_F$), which are unipolar. Combined, these leads give a view of the wave of depolarization in the frontal plane, including the right, left, inferior, and superior portions of the heart.

Hexaxial reference system

The axes of the six limb leads also make up the hexaxial reference system, which divides the heart into six equal areas. To use the hexaxial reference system, picture the position of each lead: Lead I connects the right arm (negative pole) with the left arm (positive pole); lead II connects the right arm (negative pole) with the left leg (positive pole); and lead III connects the left arm (negative pole) with the left leg (positive pole). The augmented limb leads have only one electrode, which represents the positive pole. As a result, lead aV$_R$ goes from the heart toward the right arm (positive pole), aV$_L$ goes from the heart toward the left arm (positive pole),

and aV$_F$ goes from the heart to the left leg or leg foot (positive pole).

Now, take this mental picture one step further and draw an imaginary line to illustrate the axis of each lead. For example, for lead I, you would draw a horizontal line between the right and left arms; for lead II, between the right arm and left leg; and so on. All of the lines should intersect near the center, somewhere over the heart. If you draw a circle to represent the heart, you would end up with a rough pie shape, with each wedge representing a portion of the heart monitored by each lead. (See *Understanding the hexaxial reference system*, page 134.)

This schematic representation of the heart allows you to plot your patient's electrical axis. If his or her axis falls in the right lower quadrant, between 0 degrees and +90 degrees, it is considered normal. An axis between +90 degrees and +180 degrees indicates right axis deviation; one between 0 degrees and −90 degrees, left axis deviation; and one between −180 degrees and −90 degrees, extreme axis deviation (sometimes called the no-man's-land axis or northwest axis).

Quadrant method

A simple, rapid method for determining the heart's axis is the quadrant method. With this method, you observe the main deflection of the QRS complex in leads I and aV$_F$. The QRS complex serves as the traditional marker for determining the electrical axis because the ventricles produce the greatest amount of electrical force when they contract. Lead I indicates whether impulses are moving to the right or left; lead aV$_F$ indicates whether they are moving up or down.

On the waveform for lead I, a positive main deflection of the QRS complex indicates that the electrical impulses are

Understanding the hexaxial reference system

The hexaxial reference system consists of six bisecting lines, each representing one of the six limb leads, and a circle representing the heart. The intersection of these lines divides the circle into equal 30-degree segments.

Note that 0 degrees appears at the 3 o'clock position. Moving counterclockwise, the degrees become increasingly negative until they reach ±180 degrees at the 9 o'clock position. The bottom half of the circle contains the corresponding positive degrees. It is important to remember that a positive-degree designation does not necessarily mean that the pole is positive.

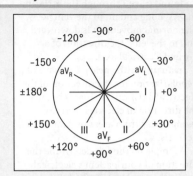

moving to the right, toward the positive pole of the lead, which is at the 0-degree position on the hexaxial reference system. Conversely, a negative deflection indicates that the impulses are moving to the left, toward the negative pole of the lead, which is at the ±180-degree position on the hexaxial reference system. On the waveform for lead aV_F, a positive deflection of the QRS complex indicates that the electrical impulses are traveling downward, toward the positive pole of the lead, which is at the +90-degree position of the hexaxial reference system. A negative deflection indicates that impulses are traveling upward, toward the negative pole of the lead, which is at the −90-degree position of the hexaxial reference system.

Plotting this information on the hexaxial reference system (with the horizontal axis representing lead I and the vertical axis representing lead aV_F) shows the patient's electrical axis. For example, if lead I shows a positive deflection of the QRS complex, darken the horizontal axis between the center

of the hexaxial reference system and the 0-degree position. If lead aV_F also shows a positive deflection of the QRS complex, darken the vertical axis between the center of the reference system and the +90-degree position. The quadrant between the two axes you have darkened indicates the patient's electrical axis. In this case, it is the left lower quadrant, which indicates a normal electrical axis. (See *Using the quadrant method.*)

Causes of axis deviation

Determining a patient's electrical axis can help to confirm a diagnosis or narrow the range of clinical possibilities. Many factors influence the electrical axis, including the position of the heart within the chest, the size of the heart, the conduction pathways, and the force of electrical generation.

Cardiac electrical activity swings away from areas of damage or necrosis. More specifically, electrical forces in the healthy portion of the heart take over for weak or absent electrical forces

Using the quadrant method

This chart will help you to determine quickly the direction of a patient's electrical axis. Observe the deflections of the QRS complexes in leads I and aV$_F$. Then check the chart to determine whether the patient's axis is normal or has a left, right, or extreme axis deviation.

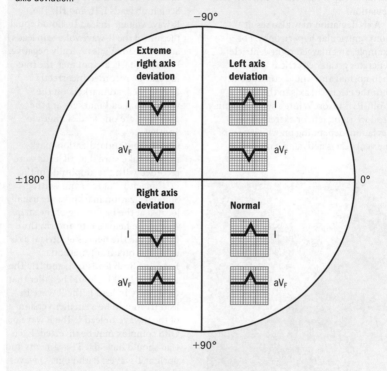

in the damaged portion. For instance, after an inferior wall MI, portions of the inferior wall can no longer conduct electricity. As a result, the major electrical vectors shift to the left, resulting in left axis deviation.

Typically, the damaged portion of the heart is the last area to be depolarized. For example, in a left anterior hemiblock, the left anterior fascicle of the left bundle branch can no longer conduct electricity. Therefore, the portion

normally served by the left bundle branch is the last portion of the heart to be depolarized. This shifts electrical forces to the left; consequently, the ECG shows left axis deviation.

An opposite shift occurs with right bundle-branch block. In this condition, the wave of impulse travels quickly down the normal left side but much more slowly down the damaged right side. This shifts the electrical forces to the right, causing right axis deviation.

An axis shift also takes place when the right or left ventricle is being paced artificially. Likewise, it takes place when the ventricles are depolarizing abnormally, such as occurs in VT. Both of these conditions can cause left axis deviation or, occasionally, extreme axis deviation.

Axis deviation may also result from ventricular hypertrophy. For example, an enlarged right ventricle generates greater electrical forces than normal and would consequently shift the electrical axis to the right. Wolff-Parkinson-White's syndrome may produce right, left, or extreme axis deviation, depending on which part of the ventricle is activated early.

AGE ALERT

Sometimes, axis deviation may be a normal variation, as in infants and children who normally experience right axis deviation. It may also stem from noncardiac causes. For example, if the heart is shifted in the chest cavity because of a high diaphragm as a result of pregnancy, expect to find left axis deviation.

If a patient's heart is situated on the right side of his or her chest instead of the left (a condition called dextrocardia), expect to find right axis deviation.

How to interpret a 12-lead ECG

To interpret a 12-lead ECG, use a systematic approach. Compare the patient's previous ECG, if available, with the current one. This will help you to identify changes. You can use various methods to interpret a 12-lead ECG.

Here is a logical, easy-to-follow method that will help to ensure that you are interpreting it accurately:

- Check the ECG tracing to see if it is technically correct. Make sure that the baseline is free from electrical interference and drift.
- Scan limb leads I, II, and III. The R-wave voltage in lead II should equal the sum of the R-wave voltage in leads I and III. Lead aV_R is typically negative. If these criteria are not met, the tracing may be recorded incorrectly.
- Locate the lead markers on the waveform. Lead markers are the points where one lead changes to another.
- Check the standardization markings to make sure that all leads were recorded with the amplitude of the ECG machine at the same setting. Standardization markings are usually located at the beginning of the strip.
- Assess the heart's rate and rhythm.
- Determine the heart's electrical axis using the quadrant method.
- Examine limb leads I, II, and III. The R wave in lead II should be taller than the R wave in lead I. The R wave in lead III should be a smaller version of the R wave in lead I. The P wave or QRS complex may be inverted. Each lead should have flat ST segments and upright T waves. Pathologic Q waves should be absent.
- Examine limb leads aV_L, aV_F, and aV_R. The tracings from leads aV_L and aV_F should be similar, but lead aV_F should have taller P and R waves. Lead aV_R has little diagnostic value. Its P wave, QRS complex, and T wave should be deflected downward.
- Examine the R wave in the precordial leads. Normally, the R wave— the first positive deflection of the QRS complex—gets progressively taller from lead V_1 to V_5. It gets slightly smaller in lead V_6.

(Text continues on page 139.)

Normal findings

Lead I

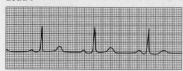

P wave: upright
Q wave: small or none
R wave: large
S wave: none or smaller than R wave
T wave: upright
U wave: none
ST segment: may vary from +1 to −0.5 mm

Lead II

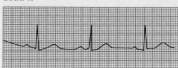

P wave: upright
Q wave: small or none
R wave: largest
S wave: none or smaller than R wave
T wave: upright
U wave: none
ST segment: may vary from +1 to −0.5 mm

Lead III

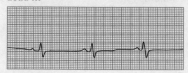

P wave: upright, diphasic, or inverted
Q wave: usually small or none (A Q wave must also be present in lead aV$_F$ to be considered diagnostic.)
R wave: none to large
S wave: none to large, indicating horizontal heart
T wave: upright, diphasic, or inverted
U wave: none
ST segment: may vary from +1 to −0.5 mm

Lead aV$_R$

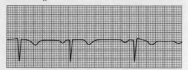

P wave: inverted
Q wave: none, small, or large
R wave: none or small
S wave: large (may be QS)
T wave: inverted
U wave: none
ST segment: may vary from +1 to −0.5 mm

Lead aV$_L$

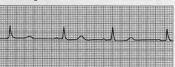

P wave: upright, diphasic, or inverted
Q wave: none, small, or large
(A Q wave must also be present in lead I or the precordial leads to be considered diagnostic.)
R wave: none, small, or large (A large wave indicates a horizontal heart.)
S wave: none to large (A large wave indicates a vertical heart.)
T wave: upright, diphasic, or inverted
U wave: none
ST segment: may vary from +1 to −0.5 mm

(continued)

Normal findings *(continued)*

Lead aV$_F$

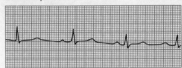

P wave: upright
Q wave: none or small
R wave: none, small, or large (A large wave suggests a vertical heart.)
S wave: none to large (A large wave suggests a horizontal heart.)
T wave: upright, diphasic, or inverted
U wave: none
ST segment: may vary from +1 to −0.5 mm

Lead V$_1$

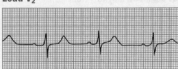

P wave: upright, diphasic, or inverted
Q wave: Deep QS pattern may be present.
R wave: none or less than S wave
S wave: large (part of the QS pattern)
T wave: usually inverted but may be upright and diphasic
U wave: none
ST segment: may vary from 0 to +1 mm

Lead V$_2$

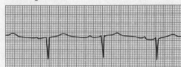

P wave: upright
Q wave: Deep QS pattern may be present.
R wave: none or less than S wave (Wave may become progressively larger.)
S wave: large (part of the QS pattern)
T wave: upright

U wave: upright; lower amplitude than T wave
ST segment: may vary from 0 to +1 mm

Lead V$_3$

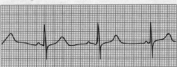

P wave: upright
Q wave: none or small
R wave: less than, greater than, or equal to S wave (Wave may become progressively larger.)
S wave: large (greater than, less than, or equal to R wave)
T wave: upright
U wave: upright; lower amplitude than T wave
ST segment: may vary from 0 to +1 mm

Lead V$_4$

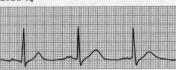

P wave: upright
Q wave: none or small
R wave: progressively larger; greater than S wave
S wave: progressively smaller; less than R wave
T wave: upright
U wave: upright; lower amplitude than T wave
ST segment: may vary from +1 to −0.5 mm

Normal findings *(continued)*

Lead V₅

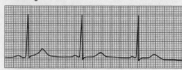

P wave: upright
Q wave: small
R wave: progressively larger but less than 26 mm
S wave: progressively smaller; less than the S wave in V₄
T wave: upright
U wave: none
ST segment: may vary from +1 to −0.5 mm

Lead V₆

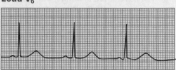

P wave: upright
Q wave: small
R wave: largest wave but less than 26 mm
S wave: smallest; less than S wave in V₅
T wave: upright
U wave: none
ST segment: may vary from +1 to −0.5 mm

- Examine the S wave (the negative deflection after an R wave) in the precordial leads. It should appear extremely deep in lead V₁ and become progressively more shallow, usually disappearing by lead V₅.
- If you suspect MI, start with lead I and continue through to lead V₆, observing the waveforms for changes in ECG characteristics that can indicate acute MI, such as T-wave inversion, ST-segment elevation, and pathologic Q waves. Note the leads in which you see such changes, and describe the changes. When you are first learning to interpret the 12-lead ECG, ignore lead aV_R because it will not provide clues to left ventricular infarction or injury.
- Determine the site and extent of myocardial damage. (See *Locating myocardial damage*, page 140.) Then follow these steps:
  - Identify the leads that record pathologic Q waves. Look at the second column of the chart to identify those leads. Then look at the first column to find the corresponding myocardial wall, where infarction has occurred. Keep in mind that this chart serves as a guideline only. Actual areas of infarction may overlap or may be larger or smaller than listed.
  - Identify the leads that record ST-segment elevation (or depression for reciprocal leads). Use the chart to locate the corresponding areas of myocardial injury.
  - Identify the leads that record T-wave inversion and locate the corresponding areas of ischemia.

Acute myocardial infarction

Acute MI can arise from any condition in which the myocardial oxygen supply cannot meet oxygen demand. Starved of oxygen, the myocardium suffers progressive ischemia, leading to injury and eventually to infarction.

In most cases, an acute MI involves the left ventricle, although it can also involve the right ventricle or the atria. Acute MIs are classified as ST-segment elevation MI or non–ST-segment elevation MI.

Locating myocardial damage

After you have noted characteristic lead changes in an acute myocardial infarction, use this chart to identify the areas of damage. Match the lead changes (ST elevation, abnormal Q waves) in the second column with the affected wall in the first column and the involved artery in the third column. The fourth column shows reciprocal lead changes.

Affected wall	Leads	Artery involved	Reciprocal changes
Anterior	V_2, V_3, V_4	Left coronary artery (LCA) and left anterior descending (LAD) artery	II, III, aV_F
Anterolateral	I, aV_L, V_3, V_4, V_5, V_6	LAD and diagonal branches; circumflex and marginal branches	II, III, aV_F
Anteroseptal	V_1, V_2, V_3, V_4	LAD	None
Inferior	II, III, aV_F	Right coronary artery (RCA)	I, aV_L
Lateral	I, aV_L, V_5, V_6	Circumflex branch of the LCA	II, III, aV_F
Posterior	V_8, V_9	RCA or circumflex	V_1, V_2, V_3, V_4 (R greater than S in V_1 and V_2, ST-segment depression, and elevated T wave)
Right ventricular	V_{4R}, V_{5R}, V_{6R}	RCA	None

In an acute MI, the characteristic ECG changes result from the three *I*'s: ischemia, injury, and infarction.

- Ischemia results from a temporary interruption of the myocardial blood supply. Its characteristic ECG change is T-wave inversion, a result of altered tissue repolarization. ST-segment depression may also occur.

Ischemia

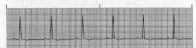

Ischemia produces T-wave inversion.

- Injury to myocardial cells results from prolonged interruption of blood flow. Its characteristic ECG change, ST-segment elevation, reflects altered depolarization. Usually, an elevation greater than 0.1 mV is considered significant.

Injury

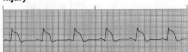

Injury produces ST-segment elevation.

- Infarction results from an absence of blood flow to myocardial tissue, leading to necrosis. The ECG shows pathologic Q waves, reflecting abnormal depolarization in damaged tissue or absent depolarization in scar tissue. The characteristic of a pathologic Q wave is a duration of 0.04 second or an amplitude that is at least one-third the height of the entire QRS complex.

Infarction

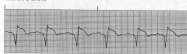

Infarction produces pathologic Q waves.

- In addition to these three characteristic ECG changes, you may see reciprocal (or mirror image) changes. Reciprocal changes—most commonly ST-segment depression or tall R waves—occur in the leads opposite those that reflect the area of ischemia, injury, or infarction.

Acute MI phases

To detect an acute MI, look for ST-segment elevation first, followed by T-wave inversion and pathologic Q waves.

Serial ECG recordings yield the best evidence of an MI. Normally, an acute MI progresses through the following phases.

Hyperacute phase

The hyperacute phase begins a few hours after the onset of acute MI. You will see ST-segment elevation and upright (usually peaked) T waves.

Fully evolved phase

The fully evolved phase starts several hours after the onset of MI. You will see deep T-wave inversion and pathologic Q waves.

Resolution phase

The resolution phase appears within a few weeks of acute MI. You will see normal T waves.

Stabilized chronic phase

After the resolution phase, you will see permanent pathologic Q waves that show an old infarction.

With an acute non–Q-wave MI, you may see persistent ST-segment depression, T-wave inversion, or both; however, pathologic Q waves may not appear. To differentiate an acute non–Q-wave MI from myocardial ischemia, cardiac enzyme tests must be performed.

For a true clinical diagnosis of acute MI, a patient must have symptoms, ECG changes, and elevated cardiac biomarker levels. If the patient shows such signs and symptoms as chest pain, left arm pain, diaphoresis, and nausea, proceed as if he or she has had an acute MI until this possibility has been ruled out.

Right-sided ECG, leads V_{1R} to V_{6R}

A right-sided ECG provides information about the extent of damage to the right ventricle, especially during the first 12 hours of MI. Right-sided ECG leads, placed over the right side of the chest in similar but reversed positions from the left precordial leads, are called unipolar right-sided chest leads.

Placing electrodes

Right-sided ECG leads are precordial leads designated by the letter V, a number representing the electrode position, and the letter R, indicating placement on the right side of the chest. Lead positions are:
- V_{1R}: in the fourth intercostal space at the left sternal border
- V_{2R}: in the fourth intercostal space at the right sternal border
- V_{3R}: midway between V_{1R} and V_{4R}, on a line joining these two locations
- V_{4R}: in the fifth intercostal space at the right midclavicular line
- V_{5R}: in the fifth intercostal space at the right anterior axillary line
- V_{6R}: in the fifth intercostal space at the right midaxillary line.

Right-sided ECG

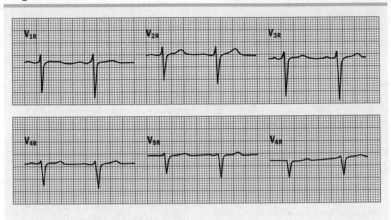

Viewing the heart

Chest leads, whether on the left or the right side of the chest, view the horizontal plane of the heart. The placement of left precordial leads gives a good picture of the electrical activity within the left ventricle. Because the right ventricle lies behind the left ventricle, the ability to evaluate right ventricular electrical activity when using only left precordial leads is limited. Right-sided ECG leads better visualize the right ventricular wall. This may be especially useful when evaluating a patient for a right ventricular MI.

Posterior-lead ECG, leads V_7 to V_9

Because of lung and muscle barriers, the usual chest leads cannot "see" the posterior portion of the heart to record myocardial damage there. To compensate, some practitioners add three posterior leads to the 12-lead ECG: leads V_7, V_8, and V_9. The addition of the posterior leads to the 12-lead ECG increases the sensitivity of the ECG in identifying posterior wall infarction so that appropriate treatment can begin.

Placing electrodes

To ensure an accurate ECG reading, make sure that the posterior electrodes V_7, V_8, and V_9 are placed at the same level horizontally as lead V_6 at the fifth intercostal space. Lead positions are:
- V_7: at the posterior axillary line
- V_8: halfway between V_7 and V_9
- V_9: at the paraspinal line.

Left bundle-branch block

In left bundle-branch block, a conduction delay or block occurs in both the left posterior and left anterior fascicles of the left bundle. This delay or block disrupts the normal left-to-right direction of depolarization. As a result, normal septal Q waves are absent. Because of the block, the wave of depolarization must move down the right bundle first and then spread from right to left.

This arrhythmia may indicate underlying heart disease such as coronary artery disease. It carries a more serious prognosis than right bundle-branch block because of its close correlation with organic heart disease, and it

Posterior-lead ECG

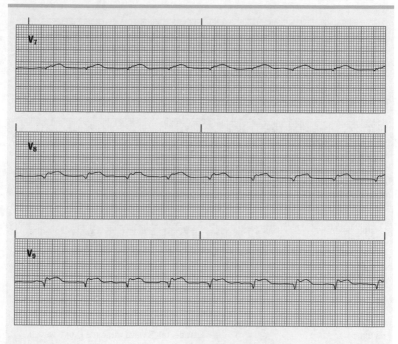

requires a large lesion to block the thick, broad left bundle branch.

Intervention

When left bundle-branch block occurs with an anterior wall MI, it usually signals complete heart block, which requires insertion of a pacemaker.

Right bundle-branch block

In the conduction delay or block associated with right bundle-branch block, the initial left-to-right direction of depolarization is not affected. The left ventricle depolarizes on time, so the intrinsic deflection in leads V_5 and V_6 (the left precordial leads) occurs on time as well. However, the right ventricle depolarizes late, causing a late intrinsic deflection in leads V_1 and V_2 (the right precordial leads). This late depolarization also causes the axis to deviate to the right.

Intervention

One potential complication of an MI is a bundle-branch block. Some blocks require treatment with a temporary pacemaker. Others are monitored only to detect progression to a more complete block.

Pericarditis

Pericarditis is the inflammation of the pericardium—the fibroserous sac that envelops the heart. It can be acute or chronic. The acute form may be fibrinous or effusive, with a purulent serous

(Text continues on page 146.)

Characteristics of left bundle-branch block

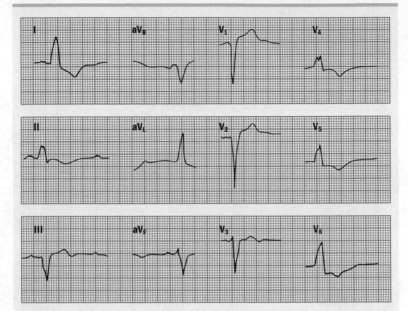

Rhythm: regular atrial and ventricular rhythms

Rate: atrial and ventricular rates within normal limits

P wave: normal size and configuration

PR interval: within normal limits

QRS complex: duration that varies from 0.10 to 0.12 second in incomplete left bundle-branch block (It is at least 0.12 second in complete block. Lead V_1 shows a wide, entirely negative rS or QS complex. Leads I, aV_L, and V_6 show a wide, tall R wave without a Q or S wave.)

T wave: deflection opposite that of the QRS complex in most leads

QT interval: may be prolonged or within normal limits

Other: magnitude of changes paralleling the magnitude of the QRS complex aberration, with normal axis or left axis deviation; delayed intrinsicoid deflection over the left ventricle (lead V_6)

Characteristics of right bundle-branch block

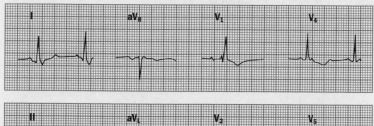

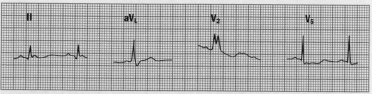

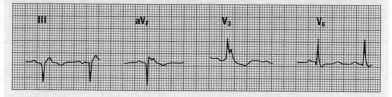

Rhythm: regular atrial and ventricular rhythms

Rate: atrial and ventricular rates within normal limits

PR interval: within normal limits

QRS complex: Duration is at least 0.12 seconds in complete block and 0.10 to 0.12 seconds in incomplete block. (In lead V_1, the QRS complex is wide and can appear in one of several patterns: an rSR′ complex with a wide S and R′ wave; an rsR′ complex with a wide R wave; and a wide R wave with an M-shaped pattern.

The complex is mainly positive, with the R wave occurring late. In leads I, aV_L, and V_6, a broad S wave can be seen.)

T wave: in most leads, deflection opposite that of the QRS deflection

QT interval: may be prolonged or within normal limits

Other: in the precordial leads, occurrence of triphasic complexes because the right ventricle continues to depolarize after the left ventricle depolarizes, thereby producing a third phase of ventricular stimulation

or hemorrhagic exudate. Chronic constrictive pericarditis causes dense fibrous pericardial thickening. Regardless of the type, pericarditis can cause cardiac tamponade if fluid accumulates too quickly. It can also cause heart failure if constriction occurs.

In pericarditis, ECG changes occur in four stages. Stage 1 coincides with the onset of chest pain. Stage 2 begins within several days. Stage 3 starts several days after stage 2. Stage 4 occurs weeks later.

Intervention

Pericarditis is usually treated with aspirin or nonsteroidal anti-inflammatory drugs or colchicine. A last resort is corticosteroid therapy, quickly tapered over 3 days.

Characteristics of pericarditis

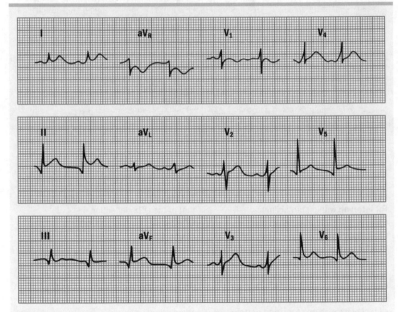

Rhythm: usually regular atrial and ventricular rhythms
Rate: atrial and ventricular rates usually within normal limits
P wave: normal size and configuration
PR interval: usually depressed in all leads except V_1 and aV_R in which it may be elevated
QRS complex: within normal limits, with a possible decrease in amplitude

ST segment: in stage 1, elevated 1 to 2 mm in a concave pattern in leads I, II, and III and the precordial leads
T wave: flattened in stage 2, inverted in stage 3 (lasting for weeks or months), and returning to normal in stage 4 (although sometimes becoming deeply inverted)
QT interval: within normal limits
Other: possible atrial fibrillation or tachycardia from sinoatrial node irritation

Selected references

American Heart Association. (2015a). *Part 7: Adult advanced cardiovascular life support. Web-based integrated guidelines for cardiopulmonary resuscitation and emergency cardiovascular care.* Retrieved from https://eccguidelines.heart.org/index .php/circulation/cpr-ecc-guidelines-2 /part-7-adult-advanced-cardiovascular -life-support/

American Heart Association. (2015b). *Part 10: Special circumstances of resuscitation: Web-based integrated guidelines for cardiopulmonary resuscitation and emergency cardiovascular care.* Retrieved from https:// eccguidelines.heart.org/index.php /circulation/cpr-ecc-guidelines-2/part-10 -special-circumstances-of-resuscitation/

Galluzzo, A., & Imazio, M. (2018). Advances in medical therapy for pericardial diseases. *Expert Review Cardiovascular Therapy, 16*(9), 635–643. doi:10.1080 /14779072.2018.1510315

4

Common
Laboratory Tests

Giving care and interpreting results

Alanine aminotransferase

The alanine aminotransferase (ALT) test is used to measure serum levels of ALT, one of two enzymes that catalyze a reversible amino group transfer reaction in the Krebs cycle. ALT is necessary for energy production in tissues. It is found primarily in the liver, with lesser amounts in the kidneys, heart, and skeletal muscles. ALT is a sensitive indicator of acute hepatocellular disease.

Purpose

- To detect acute hepatic disease, especially hepatitis and cirrhosis without jaundice, and evaluate its treatment
- To distinguish between myocardial and hepatic tissue damage (used with aspartate aminotransferase [AST])
- To assess the hepatotoxicity of some drugs

Patient preparation

- Explain to the patient that this test is used to assess liver function.

• Explain that the test requires a blood sample, and tell the patient when and where it will be taken.
• Inform the patient that there is no food or fluid restriction.

Reference values

Serum ALT levels range from 10 to 40 U/L (SI, 0.17 to 0.68 μkat/L) in males and 7 to 35 U/L (SI, 0.12 to 0.60 μkat/L) in females. The values may be a little higher among African Americans and men. Check the laboratory's reference range for normal values because they vary according to the testing method that the laboratory uses.

Abnormal findings

Very high ALT levels (up to 50 times normal) suggest viral or severe drug-induced hepatitis or other hepatic disease with extensive necrosis. Moderate to high levels may indicate infectious mononucleosis, chronic hepatitis, intrahepatic cholestasis or cholecystitis, early or improving acute viral hepatitis, or severe hepatic congestion as a result of heart failure.

Slight to moderate elevations of ALT may appear in any condition that produces acute hepatocellular injury, such as active cirrhosis and drug-induced or alcoholic hepatitis. Marginal elevations occasionally occur in acute myocardial infarction (MI), reflecting secondary hepatic congestion or the release of small amounts of ALT from myocardial tissue.

Aldosterone, serum

The aldosterone test measures serum aldosterone levels by quantitative analysis and radioimmunoassay. Aldosterone regulates ion transport across cell membranes to promote reabsorption of sodium and chloride in exchange for potassium and hydrogen ions. Consequently, it helps to maintain blood pressure and volume and regulate fluid and electrolyte balance.

This test identifies aldosteronism and, when supported by plasma renin levels, distinguishes between the primary and secondary forms of this disorder.

Purpose

• To aid in the diagnosis of primary and secondary aldosteronism, adrenal hyperplasia, hypoaldosteronism, and salt-losing syndrome

Patient preparation

• Explain to the patient that this test helps determine if symptoms are caused by improper hormonal secretion.
• Explain that the test requires a blood sample, and tell the patient when and where it will be taken.
• Instruct him or her to maintain a low-carbohydrate, normal-sodium diet (135 mEq or 3 g/day) for at least 2 weeks or, preferably, for 30 days before the test.
• Withhold all drugs that alter fluid, sodium, and potassium balance—especially diuretics, antihypertensives, steroids, hormonal contraceptives, and estrogens—for at least 2 weeks or, preferably, for 30 days before the test, as ordered.
• Withhold all renin inhibitors for 1 week before the test, as ordered. If they must be continued, note this information on the laboratory request.
• Tell the patient to avoid licorice for at least 2 weeks before the test because it produces an aldosterone-like effect.

Reference values

Laboratory values vary with the time of day and with the patient's posture—values are higher when patients are in an upright position. In upright individuals, a normal value is 7 to 30 ng/dl (SI, 0.19 to 0.83 nmol/L). In supine individuals, values are 3 to 16 ng/dl (SI, 0.08 to 0.44 nmol/L).

Abnormal findings

Excessive aldosterone secretion may indicate a primary or secondary disease. Primary aldosteronism (Conn's syndrome) may result from adrenocortical adenoma or carcinoma or from bilateral adrenal hyperplasia. Secondary aldosteronism can result from renovascular hypertension, heart failure, cirrhosis of the liver, nephrotic syndrome, idiopathic cyclic edema, and the third trimester of pregnancy.

Low serum aldosterone levels may indicate primary hypoaldosteronism, salt-losing syndrome, eclampsia, or Addison's disease.

Alkaline phosphatase

The alkaline phosphatase (ALP) test is used to measure serum levels of ALP, an enzyme that affects bone calcification as well as lipid and metabolite transport. ALP measurements reflect the combined activity of several ALP isoenzymes that are found in the liver, bones, kidneys, intestinal lining, and placenta. Bone and liver ALP is always present in adult serum, with liver ALP the most prominent except during the third trimester of pregnancy, when about half of all ALP originates in the placenta. The intestinal variant of ALP can be a normal component (found in less than 10% of normal patterns and almost exclusively in the sera of patients with blood groups B and O) or it can be an abnormal finding associated with hepatic disease.

Purpose

- To detect and identify skeletal diseases that are primarily characterized by marked osteoblastic activity

- To detect focal hepatic lesions that cause biliary obstruction, such as a tumor or abscess
- To assess the patient's response to vitamin D in the treatment of rickets
- To supplement information from other liver function studies and gastrointestinal (GI) enzyme tests

Patient preparation

- Explain to the patient that this test is used to assess liver and bone function.
- Instruct the patient to fast for at least 8 hours before the test because fat intake stimulates intestinal secretion of ALP.
- Explain that this test requires a blood sample, and tell the patient when and where it will be taken.

Reference values

Total ALP levels normally range from 25 to 100 U/L (SI, 0.43 to 1.70 μkat/L) in females older than 15 years and males older than 20 years.

Abnormal findings

Although significant elevations may occur with diseases that affect many organs, an elevated ALP level usually indicates skeletal disease or extrahepatic or intrahepatic biliary obstruction causing cholestasis. Many acute hepatic diseases cause elevated ALP levels before they affect serum bilirubin levels.

Moderate increases in ALP levels may reflect acute biliary obstruction as a result of hepatocellular inflammation in active cirrhosis, mononucleosis, and viral hepatitis. Moderate increases also occur in osteomalacia and deficiency-induced rickets.

Sharp elevations in ALP levels may indicate complete biliary obstruction by malignant or infectious infiltrations or fibrosis. These are most common in Paget's disease and occasionally occur in biliary obstruction, extensive bone metastasis, and hyperparathyroidism. Metastatic bone tumors caused by pancreatic cancer increase ALP levels without a concomitant rise in serum ALT levels.

Isoenzyme fractionation and additional enzyme tests (gamma glutamyl transferase, lactate dehydrogenase [LD], 5'-nucleotidase, and leucine aminopeptidase) are sometimes performed when the cause of ALP elevation is in doubt.

Rarely, low levels of serum ALP are associated with hypophosphatasia, hypothyroidism, malnutrition, and protein or magnesium deficiency.

Amylase, serum

An enzyme that is synthesized primarily in the pancreas and salivary glands, amylase (alpha-amylase, or AML) helps to digest starch and glycogen in the mouth, stomach, and intestine. In cases of suspected acute pancreatic disease, measurement of serum or urinary AML is the most important laboratory test.

Purpose

- To diagnose acute pancreatitis
- To distinguish between acute pancreatitis and other causes of abdominal pain that require immediate surgery
- To evaluate possible pancreatic injury caused by abdominal trauma or surgery

Patient preparation

- Explain to the patient that this test is used to assess pancreatic function.
- Inform the patient that he or she need not fast before the test but must abstain from alcohol.
- Explain that this test requires a blood sample, and tell the patient when and where it will be taken.

Reference values

Normal serum AML levels range from 25 to 125 U/L (SI, 0.4 to 2.1 μkat/L) for adults age 18 and older, 24 to 151 U/L (SI, 0.4 to 2.5 μkat/L) for adults 60 and older, and 6 to 65 U/L (SI, 0.1 to 1.1 μkat/L) for newborns . Check the laboratory's reference range for normal values because they vary according to the testing method that the laboratory uses. Amylase levels tend to be low up to 2 months of age.

Abnormal findings

After the onset of acute pancreatitis, AML levels begin to rise within 2 hours, peak within 12 to 48 hours, and return to normal within 3 to 4 days. Urine levels of AML should be measured after normal serum AML results are obtained to rule out pancreatitis. Moderate serum elevations may accompany obstruction of the common bile duct, pancreatic duct, or ampulla of Vater; pancreatic injury from a perforated peptic ulcer; pancreatic cancer; and acute salivary gland disease. Impaired kidney function may increase serum levels.

Levels may be slightly elevated in a patient who is asymptomatic or responds unusually to therapy.

Decreased levels can occur in chronic pancreatitis, pancreatic cancer, cirrhosis, hepatitis, and toxemia of pregnancy.

Antinuclear antibodies

In conditions such as systemic lupus erythematosus (SLE), scleroderma, and certain infections, the body's immune system may perceive parts of its own cell nuclei as foreign and may produce antinuclear antibodies (ANAs). Specific ANAs include antibodies to DNA, nucleoprotein, histones, nuclear ribonucleoprotein, and other nuclear constituents.

Because they do not penetrate living cells, ANAs are harmless, but they sometimes form antigen-antibody complexes that cause tissue damage (as in SLE). Because several organs may be involved, test results are not diagnostic and can only partially confirm clinical evidence.

Purpose

- To screen for SLE (The absence of ANAs essentially rules out active SLE.)
- To monitor the effectiveness of immunosuppressive therapy for SLE

Patient preparation

- Explain to the patient that this test evaluates the immune system and that further testing is usually required for diagnosis.
- Inform the patient that the test will be repeated to monitor his or her response to therapy, if appropriate.
- Inform the patient that he or she need not restrict food or fluids.
- Explain that the test requires a blood sample, and tell the patient when and where it will be taken.
- Check the patient's history for drugs that may affect test results, such as isoniazid and procainamide. Note the findings on the laboratory request.

Reference values

Test results are reported as positive (with pattern and serum titer noted) or negative.

Abnormal findings

Although this test is a sensitive indicator of ANAs, it is not specific for SLE. Low titers may occur in patients with viral diseases, chronic hepatic disease, collagen vascular disease, and autoimmune diseases and in some healthy adults; the incidence increases with age. The higher the titer, the more specific the test is for SLE. The titer commonly exceeds 1:256.

The pattern of nuclear fluorescence helps identify the type of immune disease present. A peripheral pattern is almost exclusively associated with SLE because it indicates anti-DNA antibodies; sometimes anti-DNA antibodies are measured by radioimmunoassay if ANA titers are high or if a peripheral pattern is observed. A homogeneous, or diffuse, pattern is also associated with SLE and related connective tissue disorders. A nucleolar pattern is associated with scleroderma, and a speckled, irregular pattern is associated with infectious mononucleosis and mixed connective tissue disorders (for example, SLE).

A single serum sample, especially one collected from a patient with collagen vascular disease, may contain antibodies to several parts of the nucleus of the cell. In addition, as serum dilution increases, the fluorescent pattern may change because different antibodies are reactive at different titers.

Arterial blood gas analysis

Arterial blood gas (ABG) analysis is used to measure the partial pressure of arterial oxygen (PaO_2), the partial pressure of arterial carbon dioxide ($PaCO_2$), and the pH of an arterial sample. It also measures the oxygen content (O_2CT), arterial oxygen saturation (SaO_2), and bicarbonate (HCO_3-) level. A blood sample for ABG analysis may be drawn by percutaneous arterial puncture or with an arterial line.

Purpose

- To evaluate the efficiency of pulmonary gas exchange
- To assess the integrity of the ventilatory control system
- To determine the acid-base level of the blood
- To monitor respiratory therapy

Patient preparation

- Explain to the patient that this test is used to evaluate how well the lungs are delivering oxygen to the blood and eliminating carbon dioxide.
- Tell the patient that the test requires a blood sample. Explain when and where the test will be performed and tell the patient which site, that is, radial, brachial, or femoral artery from an arterial line or arterial stick.
- Inform the patient that he or she need not restrict food or fluids.
- Instruct the patient to breathe normally during the test and that brief cramping or throbbing pain at the puncture site may occur.

Reference values

Check the laboratory's reference range for normal values because they vary according to the laboratory. Normal ABG values fall within the following ranges:

- Pao_2: 80 to 100 mm Hg (SI, 10.6 to 13.3 kPa)
- $Paco_2$: 35 to 45 mm Hg (SI, 4.7 to 5.9 kPa)
- pH: 7.35 to 7.45 (SI, 7.35 to 7.45)
- O_2CT: 15% to 23% (SI, 0.15 to 0.23)
- Sao_2: 95% to 100% (SI, 0.95 to 1.00)
- HCO_3^-: 22 to 26 mEq/L (SI, 22 to 26 mmol/L)

Abnormal findings

Low Pao_2, O_2CT, and Sao_2 levels and a high $Paco_2$ may result from conditions that impair respiratory function, such as respiratory muscle weakness or paralysis, respiratory center inhibition (from head injury, brain tumor, or drug abuse), and airway obstruction (possibly from mucus plugs or a tumor). Similarly, low readings may result from obstruction of the bronchioles as a result of asthma or emphysema, from an abnormal ventilation-perfusion ratio caused by partially blocked alveoli or pulmonary capillaries, or from alveoli that are damaged or filled with fluid because of disease, hemorrhage, or near drowning.

When inspired air contains insufficient oxygen, Pao_2, O_2CT, and Sao_2 decrease, but $Paco_2$ may be normal. Such findings are common in pneumothorax, in patients with impaired diffusion between the alveoli and blood (as a result of interstitial fibrosis, for example), and in patients who have an arteriovenous shunt that permits blood to bypass the lungs.

Low O_2CT—with normal Pao_2, Sao_2, and, possibly, $Paco_2$ values—may result from severe anemia, decreased blood volume, and reduced capacity to carry hemoglobin (Hb) oxygen.

In addition to clarifying blood oxygen disorders, ABG values can give considerable information about acid-base disorders. (See *Recognizing acid-base disorders.*)

Aspartate aminotransferase

AST is one of two enzymes that catalyze the conversion of the nitrogenous portion of an amino acid to an amino acid residue. It is essential to energy production in the Krebs cycle. AST is found in the cytoplasm and mitochondria of many cells, primarily in the liver, heart, skeletal muscles, kidneys, pancreas, and red blood cells (RBCs). It is released into serum in proportion to cellular damage.

Purpose

- To aid in the detection and differential diagnosis of acute hepatic disease
- To monitor the progress and prognosis of patients with cardiac and hepatic diseases
- To aid in the diagnosis of MI in correlation with creatine kinase (CK), LD, and troponin levels

Recognizing acid-base disorders

Disorder	ABG findings	Possible causes
Respiratory acidosis (excess CO_2 retention)	• pH <7.35 • HCO_3- >26 mEq/L (if compensating) • $Paco_2$ >45 mm Hg	• Central nervous system depression from drugs, injury, or disease • Hypoventilation from respiratory, cardiac, musculoskeletal, or neuromuscular disease
Respiratory alkalosis (excess CO_2 loss)	• pH >7.45 • HCO_3- <22 mEq/L (if compensating) • $Paco_2$ <35 mm Hg	• Hyperventilation as a result of anxiety, pain, or improper ventilator settings • Respiratory stimulation from drugs, disease, hypoxia, fever, or high room temperature • Gram-negative bacteremia
Metabolic acidosis (HCO_3- loss or acid retention)	• pH <7.35 • HCO_3- <22 mEq/L • $Paco_2$ <35 mm Hg (if compensating)	• Depletion of HCO_3- from renal disease, diarrhea, or small-bowel fistulas • Excessive production of organic acids from hepatic disease, endocrine disorders such as diabetes ketoacidosis, hypoxia, shock, or drug toxicity • Inadequate excretion of acids as a result of renal disease
Metabolic alkalosis (HCO_3- retention or acid loss)	• pH >7.45 • HCO_3- >26 mEq/L • $Paco_2$ >45 mm Hg (if compensating)	• Loss of hydrochloric acid from prolonged vomiting or gastric suctioning • Loss of potassium from increased renal excretion (as in diuretic therapy) or corticosteroid overdose • Excessive ingestion of alkali

Patient preparation

- Explain to the patient that this test is used to assess heart and liver function.
- Inform the patient that the test usually requires three venipunctures (one on admission and one each day for the next 2 days).
- Tell the patient that he or she need not restrict food or fluids.

Reference values

AST levels range from 14 to 20 U/L (SI, 0.23 to 0.33 μkat/L) in males and from 10 to 36 U/L (SI, 0.17 to 0.60 μkat/L) in females. In newborns, levels are 47 to 150 U/L (SI, 0.78 to 2.5 μkat/L). In children, they are 9 to 80 U/L (SI, 0.15 to 1.3 μkat/L). Check the laboratory's reference range for normal values because they vary according to the laboratory.

Abnormal findings

AST levels fluctuate in response to the extent of cellular necrosis. They are transiently and minimally increased early in the disease process and extremely increased during the most acute phase. Depending on when the initial sample is drawn, AST levels may increase, indicating increasing severity of disease and tissue damage, or they may decrease, indicating resolution of disease and tissue repair.

Maximum elevations (more than 20 times normal) may indicate acute viral hepatitis, severe skeletal muscle trauma, extensive surgery, drug-induced hepatic injury, or severe passive liver congestion.

High levels (10 to 20 times normal) may indicate severe MI, severe infectious mononucleosis, or alcoholic cirrhosis. High levels may also occur during the prodromal and resolving stages of conditions that cause maximum elevations.

Moderate to high levels (5 to 10 times normal) may indicate dermatomyositis, Duchenne muscular dystrophy, or chronic hepatitis. Moderate to high levels also occur during the prodromal and resolving stages of diseases that cause high elevations.

Low to moderate levels (2 to 5 times normal) occur at some time during the course of the conditions or diseases discussed earlier or may indicate hemolytic anemia, metastatic hepatic tumors, acute pancreatitis, pulmonary emboli, delirium tremens, or fatty liver. AST levels increase slightly after the first few days of biliary duct obstruction.

Bilirubin, serum

The bilirubin test is used to measure serum levels of bilirubin, the predominant pigment in bile. Bilirubin is the major product of Hb catabolism. There are two forms of bilirubin in the body: the conjugated (direct reacting) and the unconjugated (indirect reacting). Serum bilirubin measurements are especially significant in neonates because elevated unconjugated bilirubin can accumulate in the brain, causing irreparable damage.

Purpose

- To evaluate liver function
- To aid in the differential diagnosis of jaundice and monitor its progress
- To aid in the diagnosis of biliary obstruction and hemolytic anemia
- To determine whether a neonate requires an exchange transfusion or phototherapy because of dangerously high levels of unconjugated bilirubin

Patient preparation

- Explain to the patient that this test is used to evaluate liver function and the condition of RBCs.
- Explain that the test requires a blood sample, and tell the patient when and where it will be taken.
- Inform the adult patient not to restrict fluids, but he or she should fast for at least 4 hours before the test. (Fasting is not necessary for neonates.)
- If the patient is an infant, tell the parents that a small amount of blood will be drawn from his or her heel. Tell them who will be performing the heel stick and when it will be performed.

Reference values

In adults, the normal indirect serum bilirubin level is 1 mg/dl (SI, 17 μmol/L) and the direct serum bilirubin level is less than 0.5 mg/dl (SI, <6.8 μmol/L). In neonates, the total serum bilirubin level is 2 to 12 mg/dl (SI, 34 to 205 μmol/L).

Abnormal findings

Elevated indirect serum bilirubin levels usually indicate hepatic damage. High levels of indirect bilirubin are also likely in severe hemolytic anemia. If hemolysis continues, levels of both direct and indirect bilirubin may rise. Other causes of elevated indirect bilirubin levels include congenital enzyme deficiencies such as Gilbert's disease.

Elevated direct serum bilirubin levels usually indicate biliary obstruction. If the obstruction continues, both direct and indirect bilirubin levels may rise. In severe chronic hepatic damage, direct bilirubin concentrations may return to normal or near-normal levels, but indirect bilirubin levels remain elevated.

In neonates, total bilirubin levels of 15 mg/dl (SI, 257 μmol/L) or more indicate the need for an exchange transfusion.

Blood urea nitrogen

The blood urea nitrogen (BUN) test is used to measure the nitrogen fraction of urea, the chief end product of protein metabolism. Formed in the liver from ammonia and excreted by the kidneys, urea constitutes 40% to 50% of the nonprotein nitrogen in the blood. The BUN level reflects protein intake and renal excretory capacity but is a less reliable indicator of uremia than the serum creatinine level.

Purpose

- To evaluate kidney function and aid in the diagnosis of renal disease
- To aid in the assessment of hydration

Patient preparation

- Tell the patient that this test is used to evaluate kidney function.
- Inform the patient that he or she need not restrict food or fluids but should avoid a diet high in meat.
- Explain that the test requires a blood sample, and tell the patient when and where it will be taken.

Reference values

BUN values normally range from 6 to 20 mg/dl (SI, 2.1 to 7.1 mmol/L),

with slightly higher values in elderly patients. In adults 60 years and older, the range is 8 to 23 mg/dl (SI, 2.9 to 8.2 mmol/L) and in children, 5 to 18 mg/dl (SI, 1.8 to 6.4 mmol/L).

Abnormal findings

Elevated BUN levels occur in renal disease, reduced renal blood flow (as a result of dehydration or congestive heart failure, for example), urinary tract obstruction, and increased protein catabolism (such as, burn injuries or cancer).

Low BUN levels occur in severe hepatic damage, malnutrition, impaired absorption (such as celiac disease), and overhydration.

Calcium, serum

About 99% of the calcium in the body is found in the teeth. Approximately 1% of total calcium in the body circulates in the blood. Of this, about 50% is bound to plasma proteins and 40% is ionized, or free. Evaluation of serum calcium levels measures the total amount of calcium in the blood, and ionized calcium measures the fraction of serum calcium that is in the ionized form.

Purpose

- To evaluate endocrine function, calcium metabolism, and acid-base balance
- To guide therapy in patients with renal failure, renal transplant, endocrine disorders, malignancies, cardiac disease, and skeletal disorders

Patient preparation

- Explain to the patient that this test is used to determine blood calcium levels.
- Explain that the test requires a blood sample, and tell the patient when and where it will be taken.
- Inform the patient that he or she need not restrict food or fluids.

Reference values

Normally, total calcium levels range from 8.8 to 10.4 mg/dl (SI, 2.2 to 2.6 mmol/L) in adults and from 7.6 to 10.7 mg/dl (SI, 1.90 to 2.67 mmol/L) in children. Ionized calcium levels in adults are 4.65 to 5.28 mg/dl (SI, 1.16 to 1.32 mmol/L), 4.80 to 5.52 mg/dl (SI, 1.20 to 1.38 mmol/L) in children, and 4.40 to 5.48 mg/dl (SI, 1.10 to 1.37 mmol/L) in newborns. Check the laboratory's reference range for normal values because they vary according to the laboratory.

Abnormal findings

Abnormally high serum calcium levels (hypercalcemia) may occur in hyperparathyroidism and parathyroid tumors, Paget's disease of the bone, multiple myeloma, metastatic carcinoma, multiple fractures, and prolonged immobilization. Elevated levels may also result from inadequate excretion of calcium, such as in adrenal insufficiency and renal disease; from excessive ingestion of calcium; and from overuse of antacids such as calcium carbonate.

Low calcium levels (hypocalcemia) may result from hypoparathyroidism, total parathyroidectomy, and malabsorption. Decreased serum calcium levels may also occur with Cushing's syndrome, renal failure, acute pancreatitis, peritonitis, malnutrition with hypoalbuminemia, renal failure, and blood transfusions (as a result of citrate).

In the patient with hypocalcemia, be alert for circumoral and peripheral numbness and tingling, muscle twitching, Chvostek's sign (facial muscle spasm), tetany, muscle cramping, Trousseau's sign (carpopedal spasm), seizures, arrhythmias, laryngeal spasm, decreased cardiac output, prolonged bleeding time, fractures, and prolonged Q interval.

Carcinoembryonic antigen

Carcinoembryonic antigen (CEA) is a protein that is normally found in embryonic entodermal epithelium and fetal GI tissue. Production of CEA stops before birth, but it may begin again later if a neoplasm develops. Because biliary obstruction, alcoholic hepatitis, chronic heavy smoking, and other conditions also increase CEA levels, this test cannot be used as a general indicator of cancer. The measurement of enzyme CEA levels by immunoassay is useful for staging and monitoring the treatment of certain cancers.

Purpose

- To monitor the effectiveness of colon or pancreatic cancer therapy
- To assist in the preoperative staging of colorectal cancers, assess the adequacy of surgical resection, and test for recurrence of colorectal cancers
- To compare with other laboratory tests for diagnosing an inflammatory condition, cancer of the GI tract, or pancreatic cancer

Patient preparation

- Explain to the patient that this test detects and measures a special protein that is not normally present in adults.
- Inform the patient that the test will be repeated to monitor the effectiveness of therapy, if appropriate.
- Inform the patient that he or she need not restrict food, fluids, or medications.
- Explain that the test requires a blood sample, and tell the patient when and where it will be taken.

Reference values

Normal serum CEA values are less than 5 ng/ml (SI, <5 mg/L).

Abnormal findings

Persistent elevation of CEA levels suggests residual or recurrent tumor.

If levels exceed normal before surgical resection, chemotherapy, or radiation therapy, a return to normal within 6 weeks suggests successful treatment.

High CEA levels are characteristic of various malignant conditions, particularly entodermally derived neoplasms of the GI organs and lungs, and of certain nonmalignant conditions, such as benign hepatic disease, hepatic cirrhosis, alcoholic pancreatitis, and inflammatory bowel disease.

Elevated CEA concentrations may occur in nonendodermal carcinomas, such as breast and ovarian cancers.

Cerebrospinal fluid analysis

For qualitative analysis, cerebrospinal fluid (CSF) is most commonly obtained by lumbar puncture (spinal tap), performed in the lumbar sac at L3–L4 or at L4–L5 and, rarely, by cisternal or ventricular puncture. A CSF specimen may also be obtained during other neurologic tests such as myelography.

Purpose

- To measure CSF pressure as an aid in detecting obstruction of CSF circulation
- To aid in the diagnosis of viral or bacterial meningitis, subarachnoid or intracranial hemorrhage, tumors, and brain abscesses
- To aid in the diagnosis of neurosyphilis and chronic central nervous system infections
- To aid in the diagnosis of dementia

Patient preparation

- Describe the procedure to the patient, and explain that this test analyzes the fluid around the spinal cord.
- Inform the patient that he or she need not restrict food or fluids.

- Tell him or her who will perform the procedure and where it will be performed.
- Advise the patient that a headache is the most common adverse effect of a lumbar puncture and that his or her cooperation during the test helps to minimize this effect.
- Make sure that the patient or legal guardian signed the appropriate consent form.
- If the patient is unusually anxious, assess him or her and report his or her vital signs.

Normal findings

For a summary of normal and abnormal findings, see *Findings in cerebrospinal fluid analysis*, page 160.

Normally, CSF pressure is recorded and the appearance of the specimen is checked. Three tubes of CSF are collected routinely and are sent to the laboratory for analysis of protein, sugar, and cells as well as for serologic testing, such as the Venereal Disease Research Laboratory test for neurosyphilis. A separate specimen is sent to the laboratory for culture and sensitivity testing. Electrolyte analysis and Gram stain may be ordered as supplementary tests. CSF electrolyte levels are of special interest in patients with abnormal serum electrolyte levels or CSF infection and in those receiving hyperosmolar agents.

Chloride, serum

The chloride test is used to measure serum levels of chloride, the major extracellular fluid anion. Chloride helps maintain the osmotic pressure of blood and, therefore, helps regulate blood volume and arterial pressure. Chloride levels also affect the acid-base balance. Chloride is absorbed from the intestines and excreted primarily by the kidneys.

Findings in cerebrospinal fluid analysis

Test	Normal	Abnormal	Implications
Pressure	50 to 180 mm H_2O	Increase	• Increased intracranial pressure
		Decrease	• Spinal subarachnoid obstruction above puncture site • Hypovolemia
Appearance	Clear, colorless	Cloudy	• Infection
		Xanthochromic (yellow) or bloody	• Subarachnoid, intracerebral, or intraventricular hemorrhage; spinal cord obstruction; traumatic tap (usually noted only in initial specimen)
		Brown, orange, or yellow	• Elevated protein levels, red blood cell (RBC) breakdown (blood present for at least 3 days)
Protein	15 to 45 mg/dl (SI, 150 to 450 mg/L)	Marked increase	• Tumors, trauma, hemorrhage, diabetes mellitus, polyneuritis, blood in cerebrospinal fluid (CSF)
		Marked decrease	• Rapid production of CSF
Gamma globulin	3% to 12% of total protein	Increase	• Demyelinating disease, neurosyphilis, Guillain-Barré syndrome
Glucose	40 to 70 mg/dl (SI, 2.2 to 3.9 mmol/L)	Increase	• Systemic hyperglycemia
		Decrease	• Systemic hypoglycemia, bacterial or fungal infection, meningitis, mumps, postsubarachnoid hemorrhage
Cell count	0 to 5 white blood cells	Increase	• Active disease: meningitis, acute infection, onset of chronic illness, tumor, abscess, infarction, demyelinating disease

Findings in cerebrospinal fluid analysis (continued)

Test	Normal	Abnormal	Implications
	No RBCs	RBCs	• Hemorrhage or traumatic lumbar puncture
Venereal Disease Research Laboratory test for syphilis and other serologic tests	Nonreactive	Positive	• Neurosyphilis
Chloride	118 to 130 mEq/L (SI, 118 to 130 mmol/L)	Decrease	• Infected meninges
Gram stain	No organisms	Gram-positive or gram-negative organisms	• Bacterial meningitis

Purpose

- To detect an acid-base imbalance (acidosis or alkalosis) and to aid in the evaluation of fluid status and extracellular cation-anion balance

Patient preparation

- Explain to the patient that this test is used to evaluate the chloride content of blood.
- Explain that the test requires a blood sample, and tell the patient when it will be taken.
- Inform the patient that he or she need not restrict food or fluids.

Reference values

Normally, serum chloride levels range from 96 to 106 mEq/L (SI, 96 to 106 mmol/L) in adults and 96 to 113 in newborns mEq/L (SI, 96 to 113 mmol/L).

Abnormal findings

Chloride levels are inversely related to bicarbonate levels, reflecting the acid-base balance. Excessive loss of gastric juices or other secretions that contain chloride may cause hypochloremic metabolic alkalosis; excessive retention or ingestion of chloride may lead to hyperchloremic metabolic acidosis.

Increased blood chloride levels occur in patients with severe dehydration, complete renal shutdown, head injury (producing neurogenic hyperventilation), and primary aldosteronism.

Decreased blood chloride levels occur in patients with low sodium and potassium levels as a result of prolonged vomiting, gastric suctioning, intestinal fistula, chronic renal failure, and Addison's disease. Heart failure or edema resulting in excess extracellular fluid can cause dilutional hypochloremia.

Cholesterol, total

The total cholesterol test, the quantitative analysis of serum cholesterol, is used to measure the circulating levels of free cholesterol and cholesterol esters. It reflects the level of the two forms in which this biochemical compound appears in the body. High serum cholesterol levels may be associated with an increased risk of coronary artery disease (CAD) and atherosclerosis.

Purpose

- To assess the risk for CAD and atherosclerosis
- To evaluate fat metabolism
- To aid in the diagnosis of nephrotic syndrome, pancreatitis, hepatic disease, hypothyroidism, and hyperthyroidism
- To assess the efficacy of lipid-lowering drug therapy, dietary and lifestyle changes, and the management of stress

Patient preparation

- Explain to the patient that this test is used to assess the body's fat metabolism.
- Explain that the test requires a blood sample, and tell the patient when and where it will be taken.
- Instruct the patient not to eat or drink for 12 hours before the test, but it is okay to have water.

Reference values

Total cholesterol concentrations vary with age and sex. Total cholesterol values are:

- adults: desirable, less than 200 mg/dl (SI, <5.18 mmol/L)
- children ages 12 to 18: desirable, less than 170 mg/dl (SI, <4.40 mmol/L).

Abnormal findings

Elevated serum cholesterol levels (hypercholesterolemia) may indicate a risk for CAD and atherosclerosis as well as incipient hepatitis, lipid disorders, bile duct blockage, nephrotic syndrome, obstructive jaundice, pancreatitis, and hypothyroidism.

Low serum cholesterol levels (hypocholesterolemia) are commonly associated with malnutrition, cellular necrosis of the liver, and hyperthyroidism. Patients who have abnormal cholesterol levels typically must undergo further testing to pinpoint the cause.

Creatine kinase

CK is an enzyme that catalyzes the creatine-creatinine metabolic pathway in muscle cells and brain tissue. The enzyme is highly concentrated in the heart and skeletal muscles, with a low concentration in brain tissue. Because of its intimate role in energy production, CK reflects normal tissue catabolism. Increased serum levels indicate trauma to cells.

Fractionation and measurement of three distinct CK isoenzymes—CK-BB (CK$_1$), CK-MB (CK$_2$), and CK-MM (CK$_3$)—have replaced the use of total CK levels to localize the site of increased tissue destruction. CK-BB is most commonly found in brain tissue, genitourinary track, and GI system. CK-MM is primarily found in skeletal muscle. CK-MM and CK-MB are found primarily in heart muscle. In addition, subunits of CK-MB and CK-MM, called isoforms or isoenzymes, can be assayed to increase the sensitivity of the test.

Purpose

- To detect and diagnose acute MI and reinfarction (CK-MB is primarily used.)
- To evaluate possible causes of chest pain and to monitor the severity of myocardial ischemia after cardiac surgery, cardiac catheterization, and cardioversion (CK-MB is primarily used.)
- To detect early dermatomyositis and musculoskeletal disorders that are not neurogenic in origin such

as Duchenne muscular dystrophy (Total CK is primarily used.)

Patient preparation

- Explain to the patient that this test is used to assess myocardial and musculoskeletal function and that multiple blood samples are required to detect fluctuations in serum levels.
- Tell the patient when and where the blood samples will be taken.
- If the patient is being evaluated for musculoskeletal disorders, advise him or her to avoid exercising for 24 hours before the test.
- Inform the patient that there is no food or fluid restrictions.

Reference values

Total CK values determined by ultraviolet or kinetic measurement range from 38 to 174 U/L (SI, 0.63 to 2.90 μkat/L) for men and from 26 to 140 U/L (SI, 0.46 to 2.38 μkat/L) for women. CK levels may be significantly higher in muscular people. Infants up to age 1 have levels two to three times higher than adult levels, possibly reflecting birth trauma and striated muscle development. Normal ranges for isoenzyme levels are as follows: CK-BB, undetectable; CK-MB, less than 6% (SI, <0.06); CK-MM, 90% to 100% (SI, 0.90 to 1.00). Check the laboratory about the values because they may vary depending on the testing method and the temperature of the reaction. The CK levels tend to be higher among African Americans who are healthy compared to Caucasians and Hispanics.

Abnormal findings

CK-MM makes up 99% of the total CK that is normally present in serum. Detectable CK-BB isoenzyme may indicate, but does not confirm, a diagnosis of brain tissue injury, widespread malignant tumors, severe shock, or renal failure.

CK-MB levels greater than 6% of the total CK level indicate MI, especially if the LD isoenzyme ratio is greater than 1 (flipped LD). In acute MI and after cardiac surgery, CK-MB begins to increase within 2 to 4 hours, peaks within 12 to 24 hours, and usually returns to normal within 24 to 48 hours. Persistent elevations and increasing levels indicate ongoing myocardial damage. The total CK level follows roughly the same pattern but increases slightly later. CK-MB levels may not increase in heart failure or during angina pectoris that is not accompanied by myocardial cell necrosis. Serious skeletal muscle injury that occurs in certain muscular dystrophies, polymyositis, and severe myoglobinuria may cause a mild increase in CK-MB because a small amount of this isoenzyme is present in some skeletal muscles.

CK-MM values increase after skeletal muscle damage as a result of trauma, such as surgery and I.M. injections, and from diseases, such as dermatomyositis and muscular dystrophy (values may be 50 to 100 times normal). CK-MM levels increase moderately in patients with hypothyroidism; sharp increases occur with muscle activity caused by agitation, such as during an acute psychotic episode.

Total CK levels may be increased in patients with severe hypokalemia, carbon monoxide poisoning, malignant hyperthermia, and alcoholic cardiomyopathy. They may also be increased after seizures and, occasionally, in patients who have had pulmonary or cerebral infarctions. Troponin I and cardiac troponin C are present in the contractile cells of cardiac myocardial tissue and are released when myocardial tissue is injured. Troponin levels increase within 1 hour of infarction and may remain elevated for as long as 14 days. (See *Serum protein and isoenzyme levels after MI*, page 164.)

Serum protein and isoenzyme levels after MI

Because they are released by damaged tissue, serum proteins and isoenzymes (catalytic proteins that vary in concentration in specific organs) can help identify the compromised organ and assess the extent of damage after myocardial infarction (MI). The serum protein and isoenzyme determinations listed below are most significant after MI.

Isoenzymes

- Creatine kinase-MB (CK-MB): in heart muscle and a small amount in skeletal muscle

Proteins

- Troponin I and troponin T (the cardiac contractile proteins) have greater sensitivity than CK-MB in detecting myocardial injury

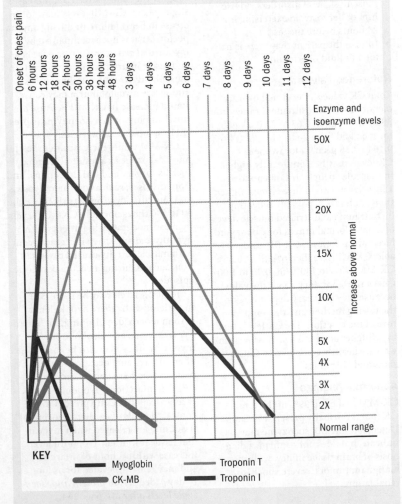

KEY
- Myoglobin
- CK-MB
- Troponin T
- Troponin I

Creatinine, serum

Analysis of serum creatinine levels provides a more sensitive measure of renal damage than BUN levels. Creatinine is a nonprotein end product of creatine metabolism that appears in serum in amounts proportional to muscle mass.

Purpose

- To assess glomerular filtration
- To screen for renal damage

Patient preparation

- Explain to the patient that this test is used to evaluate kidney function.
- Explain that the test requires a blood sample, and tell the patient when and where it will be taken.
- Instruct the patient that he or she need not restrict food or fluids.

Reference values

Creatinine concentrations normally range from 0.6 to 1.2 mg/dl (SI, 71 to 106 μmol/L) in men and 0.4 to 1.0 mg/dl (SI, 36 to 90 μmol/L) in women.

Abnormal findings

Elevated serum creatinine levels usually indicate renal disease that has seriously damaged 50% or more of the nephrons. Elevated levels may also be associated with gigantism and acromegaly.

Creatinine clearance (urine)

An anhydride of creatine, creatinine is formed and excreted in constant amounts by an irreversible reaction. It functions solely as the main end product of creatine. Creatinine production is proportional to total muscle mass and is relatively unaffected by urine volume, normal physical activity, or diet.

Creatinine clearance is an excellent diagnostic indicator of renal function.

The test determines how efficiently the kidneys are clearing creatinine from the blood. The rate of clearance is expressed in terms of the volume of blood (in milliliters) that can be cleared of creatinine in 1 minute. Creatinine levels become abnormal when more than 50% of the nephrons have been damaged.

Purpose

- To assess renal function (primarily glomerular filtration)
- To monitor the progression of renal insufficiency

Patient preparation

- Explain to the patient that this test assesses kidney function.
- Inform the patient that he or she may need to avoid meat, poultry, fish, tea, or coffee for 6 hours before the test.
- Advise the patient to avoid strenuous physical exercise during the collection period.
- Tell the patient that the test requires a timed 12- or 24-hour urine specimen and at least one blood sample.
- Tell the patient how the urine specimen will be collected, and inform him or her when and where the blood sample will be taken.

Reference values

Normal creatinine clearance varies with age: in men, it ranges from 14 to 26 mg/kg/24 hours (124 to 230 μmol/kg/day); in women, 11 to 20 mg/kg/24 hours (97 to 177 μmol/kg/day).

Abnormal findings

Low creatinine clearance may result from reduced renal blood flow (associated with shock or renal artery obstruction), acute tubular necrosis, acute or chronic glomerulonephritis, advanced bilateral chronic pyelonephritis, advanced bilateral renal lesions (which may occur in polycystic kidney disease, renal tuberculosis, and cancer), nephrosclerosis, congestive heart failure, hyperthyroidism, or severe dehydration.

High creatinine clearance can suggest hypothyroidism, hypertension (renovascular), or exercise.

Erythrocyte sedimentation rate

The erythrocyte sedimentation rate (ESR) measures the degree of erythrocyte settling that occurs in a blood sample during a specified amount of time. The ESR is a sensitive but nonspecific test that is commonly the earliest indicator of disease when other chemical or physical signs are normal. The ESR usually increases significantly in widespread inflammatory disorders; elevations may be prolonged in localized inflammation and malignant disease.

Purpose
- To monitor inflammatory or malignant disease
- To aid in the detection and diagnosis of occult disease, such as tuberculosis, tissue necrosis, rheumatoid, or connective tissue disease

Patient preparation
- Explain to the patient that this test is used to evaluate the condition of RBCs.
- Explain that a blood sample will be needed, and tell the patient when and where it will be taken.
- Inform the patient that he or she need not restrict food or fluids.

Reference values
The ESR normally ranges from 0 to 15 mm/hour (SI, 0 to 15 mm/hour) in men and 0 to 20 mm/hour (SI, 0 to 20 mm/hour) in women. Rates gradually increase with age.

Abnormal findings
The ESR increases in pregnancy, anemia, acute or chronic inflammation, tuberculosis, paraproteinemias (especially multiple myeloma and Waldenström's macroglobulinemia), rheumatic fever, rheumatoid arthritis, and some cancers.

Polycythemia, sickle cell anemia, hyperviscosity, and low plasma fibrinogen or globulin levels tend to depress the ESR.

Estrogens

Estrogens (and progesterone) are secreted by the ovaries, adrenal cortex, and testes. These hormones are responsible for the development of secondary female sexual characteristics and for normal menstruation. Levels are usually undetectable in children. These hormones are secreted by the ovarian follicular cells during the first half of the menstrual cycle and by the corpus luteum during the luteal phase and during pregnancy. In menopause, estrogen secretion drops to a constant, low level.

This radioimmunoassay measures serum levels of estradiol, estrone, and estriol (the only estrogens that appear in serum in measurable amounts) and has diagnostic significance in evaluating female gonadal dysfunction. (See *Predicting premature labor.*) Tests of hypothalamic-pituitary function may be required to confirm the diagnosis.

Purpose
- To determine sexual maturation and fertility
- To aid in the diagnosis of gonadal dysfunction, such as precocious or delayed puberty, menstrual disorders (especially amenorrhea), and infertility

Predicting premature labor

A simple salivary test can help determine whether a pregnant woman is at risk for premature labor, a complication that is detrimental to the health of the premature infant. The test, known as the SalEst test, measures salivary levels of estriol, an estrogen that increases a thousand fold during pregnancy. For women determined to be at risk, the SalEst test is 98% accurate in ruling out premature labor and delivery.

The test is performed on women between 22 and 36 weeks' gestation. The level of estriol has been found to increase 2 to 3 weeks before the spontaneous onset of labor and delivery. A positive result indicates that the patient is at risk for premature labor. With this knowledge and evaluation by a physician, precautions can be instituted to decrease the risk of preterm labor and maintain fetal viability.

- To determine fetal well-being
- To aid in the diagnosis of tumors that are known to secrete estrogen

Patient preparation

- Tell the patient that this test helps determine if the secretion of female hormones is normal, and explain that the test may be repeated during the various phases of the menstrual cycle.
- Tell the patient that there is no food or fluid restriction.
- Explain that the test requires a blood sample, and tell the patient when and where it will be taken.
- Withhold all steroid and pituitary-based hormones, as ordered. If they must be continued, note this on the laboratory request.

Reference values

Normal serum estrogen levels for premenopausal women vary widely during the menstrual cycle, ranging from 26 to 149 pg/ml (SI, 90 to 550 pmol/L). The range for postmenopausal women is 0 to 34 pg/ml (SI, 0 to 125 pmol/L).

Serum estrogen levels in men range from 12 to 34 pg/ml (SI, 40 to 125 pmol/L). In children younger than age 6, the normal level of serum estrogen is 3 to 10 pg/ml (SI, 10 to 36 pmol/L).

During pregnancy, the placenta secretes large amounts of estriol. Levels range from 2 ng/ml (SI, 7 nmol/L) by week 30 to 30 ng/ml (SI, 105 nmol/L) by week 40.

Abnormal findings

Decreased estrogen levels may indicate primary hypogonadism, or ovarian failure, as in Turner's syndrome or ovarian agenesis; secondary hypogonadism, such as in hypopituitarism; anorexia nervosa; or menopause.

Abnormally high estrogen levels may occur with estrogen-producing tumors, in precocious puberty, and in severe hepatic disease (such as cirrhosis) that prevents the clearance of plasma estrogens. High levels may also result from congenital adrenal hyperplasia (increased conversion of androgens to estrogen) and testicular cancer.

Glucose, fasting plasma

The fasting plasma glucose (or fasting blood sugar) test is used to measure plasma glucose levels after a 12- to 14-hour fast. This test is commonly used to screen for diabetes mellitus, in which absence or deficiency of insulin allows persistently high glucose levels.

Purpose

- To screen for prediabetic state and diabetes mellitus
- To monitor drug or diet therapy in patients with diabetes mellitus

Patient preparation

- Explain to the patient that this test is used to detect disorders of glucose metabolism and aids in the diagnosis of diabetes.
- Explain that the test requires a blood sample, and tell the patient when and where it will be taken.
- Instruct the patient to fast for 12 to 14 hours before the test.
- Alert the patient to the symptoms of hypoglycemia (weakness, restlessness, nervousness, hunger, and sweating), and tell the patient to report such symptoms immediately.

Reference values

The normal range for fasting plasma glucose level varies according to the laboratory procedure. Usually, a normal true glucose value after a fast of at least 8 hours is 70 to 110 mg/dl (SI, 3.9 to 6.1 mmol/L) of blood.

Abnormal findings

Confirmation of diabetes mellitus requires fasting plasma glucose levels of 126 mg/dl (SI, 7 mmol/L) or more obtained on two or more occasions. In patients with borderline or transient elevated levels, a 2-hour postprandial plasma glucose test or an oral glucose tolerance test may be performed to confirm the diagnosis.

Increased fasting plasma glucose levels can also result from diabetic acidosis, pancreatitis, recent acute illness (such as MI), Cushing's syndrome, acromegaly, burns, renal failure, and pheochromocytoma. Hyperglycemia may also stem from hyperlipoproteinemia (especially type III, IV, or V), chronic hepatic disease, nephrotic syndrome, brain tumor, sepsis, or gastrectomy with dumping syndrome. It is also typical in eclampsia, anoxia, and seizure disorder.

Low plasma glucose levels can result from hyperinsulinism, insulinoma, von Gierke's disease, functional and reactive hypoglycemia, myxedema, adrenal insufficiency, congenital adrenal hyperplasia, hypopituitarism, malabsorption syndrome, and some cases of hepatic insufficiency.

Glucose, 2-hour postprandial plasma

Also called the 2-hour postprandial blood sugar test, the 2-hour postprandial plasma glucose test is a valuable screening tool for detecting diabetes mellitus. The test is performed when the patient shows symptoms of diabetes (polydipsia and polyuria) or when the results of the fasting plasma glucose test suggest diabetes.

Purpose

- To aid in the diagnosis of diabetes mellitus
- To monitor drug or diet therapy in patients with diabetes mellitus

Patient preparation

- Explain to the patient that this test is used to evaluate glucose metabolism and to detect diabetes.
- Explain that the test requires a blood sample, and tell the patient when and where it will be taken.
- Tell the patient to eat a balanced meal or one containing 100 g of carbohydrates before the test and then to fast for 2 hours. Instruct him or her to avoid smoking and strenuous exercise after the meal.

Reference values

In a patient who does not have diabetes, postprandial glucose values are less than 145 mg/dl (SI, <8 mmol/L) by the glucose oxidase or hexokinase method; levels are slightly elevated in people older than age 50.

Abnormal findings

Two 2-hour postprandial blood glucose values of 200 mg/dl (SI, 11.1 mmol/L) or above indicate diabetes mellitus. High levels may also occur with pancreatitis, Cushing's syndrome, acromegaly, and pheochromocytoma. Hyperglycemia may also be caused by hyperlipoproteinemia (especially type III, IV, or V), chronic hepatic disease, nephrotic syndrome, brain tumor, sepsis, gastrectomy with dumping syndrome, eclampsia, anoxia, and seizure disorders.

Low glucose levels occur in hyperinsulinism, insulinoma, von Gierke's disease, functional and reactive hypoglycemia, myxedema, adrenal insufficiency, congenital adrenal hyperplasia, hypopituitarism, malabsorption syndrome, and some cases of hepatic insufficiency.

Glucose tolerance test, oral

The oral glucose tolerance test is the most sensitive method of evaluating borderline cases of diabetes mellitus. Plasma and urine glucose levels are monitored for 3 hours after the patient ingests a challenge dose of glucose. This test is performed to assess insulin secretion and the ability to metabolize glucose.

The oral glucose tolerance test is not normally used in patients with fasting plasma glucose values greater than 140 mg/dl (SI, >7.7 mmol/L) or postprandial plasma glucose values greater than 200 mg/dl (SI, >11 mmol/L).

Purpose

- To confirm the diagnosis of diabetes mellitus in selected patients, such as patients with a family history of diabetes mellitus

- To aid in the diagnosis of hypoglycemia and malabsorption syndrome

Patient preparation

- Explain to the patient that this test is used to evaluate glucose metabolism.
- Instruct the patient to maintain a high-carbohydrate diet of >150 g for 3 days and then fast for 12 to 16 hours before the test.
- Tell the patient not to smoke, drink coffee or alcohol, or exercise strenuously for 8 hours before or during the test.
- Tell the patient that this test requires five blood samples and usually five urine samples.
- Suggest to the patient that he or she bring a book or another quiet diversion with him or her to the test. The procedure usually takes 3 hours but can last as long as 6 hours.
- Alert the patient to the symptoms of hypoglycemia (weakness, restlessness, nervousness, hunger, and sweating), and tell him or her to report such symptoms immediately.

Reference values

Normal plasma glucose levels peak at 160 to 170 mg/dl (SI, 8.8 to 9.4 mmol/L) within 30 minutes to 1 hour after the administration of an oral glucose test dose. They return to fasting levels or lower within 2 to 3 hours. Urine glucose test results remain negative throughout.

Abnormal findings

Decreased glucose tolerance, in which levels peak sharply before falling slowly to fasting levels, may confirm diabetes mellitus or may result from Cushing's disease, hemochromatosis, protein malnutrition, pheochromocytoma, or central nervous system lesions.

Increased glucose tolerance, in which levels may peak at less than normal, may indicate insulinoma, malabsorption syndrome, adrenocortical insufficiency (Addison's disease), pancreatic cancer, alcoholism, eclampsia, hypothyroidism, or hypopituitarism.

Hematocrit

A hematocrit (HCT) test may be done separately or as part of a complete blood count. It measures the percentage of packed RBCs by volume in a sample of whole blood; for example, an HCT of 40% indicates that a 100-ml (1 dl) sample of blood contains 40 ml (0.40 dl) of packed RBCs. Packing is achieved by centrifuging anticoagulated whole blood in a capillary tube so that RBCs are packed tightly without hemolysis.

Purpose

- To aid in the diagnosis of polycythemia, anemia, or abnormal states of hydration
- To aid in the calculation of RBC indices

Patient preparation

- Explain to the patient that HCT is tested to detect anemia and other abnormal blood conditions.
- Explain that the test requires a blood sample, and tell the patient when and where it will be taken.
- If the patient is a child, explain to him or her (if patient is old enough) and his or her parents that a small amount of blood will be taken from the finger or earlobe.
- Inform the patient that he or she need not restrict food or fluids.

Reference values

HCT is usually measured electronically. The results are 3% lower than those obtained with manual measurements, which trap plasma in the column of packed RBCs.

Reference values vary, depending on the type of sample, the laboratory performing the test, and the patient's age and sex, as follows:
- Neonates age 2 weeks: 44% to 64% (SI, 0.44 to 0.64)
- Infants age 1 month: 37% to 49% (SI, 0.37 to 0.49)
- Infants age 3 months: 30% to 36% (SI, 0.3 to 0.36)
- Infants age 1 year: 29% to 41% (SI, 0.29 to 0.41)
- Children ages 1 to 6 years: 30% to 40% (SI, 0.3 to 0.4)
- Children ages 6 to 16 years: 32% to 42% (SI, 0.32 to 0.42)
- Children ages 16 to 18 years: 34% to 44% (SI, 0.34 to 0.44)
- Men: 42% to 52% (SI, 0.42 to 0.52)
- Women: 36% to 48% (SI, 0.36 to 0.48)

Abnormal findings

Low HCT suggests anemia, hemodilution, or massive blood loss. High HCT indicates polycythemia or hemoconcentration as a result of blood loss and dehydration.

Hemoglobin, glycosylated

Also called total fasting Hb, the glycosylated Hb test is used to screen for diabetes and monitor diabetes therapy. Measurement of glycosylated Hb levels provides information about the average blood glucose level during the preceding 2 to 3 months. This test requires only one venipuncture every 6 to 8 weeks. Therefore, it can be used to evaluate the long-term effectiveness of diabetes therapy.

Purpose

- To test for prediabetes and diabetes
- To assess control of diabetes mellitus

Patient preparation

- Explain to the patient that this test is used to evaluate diabetes therapy.
- Explain that the test requires a blood sample, and tell the patient when and where it will be taken.

- Inform the patient that he or she need not restrict food or fluids, and instruct the patient to maintain his or her prescribed medication and diet regimens.

Reference values

Glycosylated Hb values are reported as a percentage of the total Hb within an RBC. Glycosylated Hb accounts for 4% to 7%.

Abnormal findings

A patient with diabetes has good control of blood glucose concentrations when the glycosylated Hb value is less than 8%. A glycosylated Hb value greater than 8% indicates poor control.

Hemoglobin, total

Total Hb is used to measure the amount of Hb found in a deciliter (dl, or 100 ml) of whole blood. It is usually part of a complete blood count. Hb concentration correlates closely with the RBC count and affects the Hb-RBC ratio (mean corpuscular Hb [MCH] and mean corpuscular Hb concentration [MCHC]).

Purpose

- To measure the severity of anemia or polycythemia and monitor the response to therapy
- To obtain data to calculate MCH and MCHC

Patient preparation

- Explain to the patient that this test is used to detect anemia or polycythemia or to assess his or her response to treatment.
- Explain that a blood sample will be needed, and tell the patient when and where it will be taken.
- If the patient is an infant or a child, explain to the parents that a small amount of blood will be taken from the finger or earlobe.
- Inform the patient that he or she need not restrict food or fluids.

Reference values

Hb concentration varies depending on the type of sample drawn and the patient's age and sex:

- Neonates ages 0 to 2 weeks: 14.5 to 24.5 g/dl (SI, 145 to 245 g/L)
- Infants ages 2 to 8 weeks: 12.5 to 20.5 g/dl (SI, 125 to 205 g/L)
- Infants ages 2 to 6 months: 10.7 to 17.3 g/dl (SI, 107 to 173 g/L)
- Infants ages 6 months to 1 year: 9.9 to 14.5 g/dl (SI, 99 to 145 g/L)
- Children ages 1 to 6 years: 9.5 to 14.1 g/dl (SI, 95 to 141 g/L)
- Children ages 6 to 16 years: 10.3 to 14.9 g/dl (SI, 103 to 149 g/L)
- Adolescents ages 16 to 18 years: 11.1 to 15.7 g/dl (SI, 111 to 157 g/L)
- Men: 14 to 17.4 g/dl (SI, 140 to 174 g/L)
- Women: 12 to 16 g/dl (SI, 120 to 160 g/L)

Those who are more physically active or who live in high altitudes may have higher values.

Abnormal findings

Low Hb concentration may indicate anemia, recent hemorrhage, or fluid retention, causing hemodilution. It may also indicate liver cirrhosis and leukemias.

Elevated Hb suggests hemoconcentration from polycythemia or dehydration.

Hepatitis B surface antigen

Hepatitis B surface antigen (HBsAg), also called hepatitis-associated antigen or Australia antigen, appears in the sera of patients with hepatitis B virus. It can be detected by radioimmunoassay or, less commonly, by reverse passive hemagglutination during the extended incubation period and usually during the first 3 weeks of acute infection or if the patient is a carrier.

Because the transmission of hepatitis is one of the gravest complications associated with blood transfusion, all donors must be screened for hepatitis B before their blood is stored. This screening, which is required by the U.S. Food and Drug Administration Center for Biologics Evaluation and Research, has helped reduce the incidence of hepatitis. This test does not screen for hepatitis A virus (infectious hepatitis).

Purpose

- To screen blood donors for hepatitis B infection
- To screen people at high risk for contracting hepatitis B such as hemodialysis nurses
- To aid in the differential diagnosis of viral hepatitis

Patient preparation

- Explain to the patient that this test helps identify a type of viral hepatitis.
- Explain that the test requires a blood sample, and tell the patient when and where it will be taken.
- Inform the patient that he or she need not restrict food or fluids.
- Check the patient's history for administration of hepatitis B vaccine.

Normal findings

Normal serum is negative for HBsAg.

Abnormal findings

The presence of HBsAg in a patient with hepatitis confirms the diagnosis of hepatitis B. In chronic carriers and in people with chronic active hepatitis, HBsAg may be present in the serum several months after the onset of acute infection. It may also occur in more than 5% of patients with certain diseases other than hepatitis, such as hemophilia, Hodgkin's disease, and leukemia. If HBsAg is found in donor blood, that blood must be discarded because it carries a risk of transmitting hepatitis. Blood samples with positive results should be retested, however, because inaccurate results occur.

Human chorionic gonadotropin, serum

Human chorionic gonadotropin (hCG) is a glycoprotein hormone that is produced in the placenta. If conception occurs, a specific assay for hCG—commonly called the beta-subunit assay—may detect this hormone in the blood 9 days after ovulation occurs. This interval coincides with the implantation of the fertilized ovum into the uterine wall. Although the precise function of hCG is unclear, it appears that hCG, with progesterone, maintains the corpus luteum during early pregnancy.

The production of hCG increases steadily during the first trimester, peaking around 8 to 10 weeks' gestation. During the remainder of the pregnancy, levels decrease to less than 10% of the first trimester peak levels. About 3 to 4 weeks after delivery, the hormone may no longer be detectable.

This serum immunoassay, a quantitative analysis of hCG beta-subunit level, is both more sensitive and more expensive than the routine pregnancy test that is performed with a urine sample.

Purpose

- To detect early pregnancy
- To determine the adequacy of hormone production in high-risk pregnancies (for example, in a patient with habitual abortion)
- To aid in the diagnosis of trophoblastic tumors, such as hydatidiform moles and choriocarcinoma, and tumors that secrete hCG ectopically
- To monitor treatment for the induction of ovulation and conception

Patient preparation

- Explain to the patient that this test determines if she is pregnant. If detection of pregnancy is not the diagnostic objective, explain why the test is being done.
- Explain that the test requires a blood sample, and tell the patient when and where it will be taken.
- Inform her that she need not restrict food or fluids.
- Inform the patient to have the test done 2 weeks (no earlier than 5 days) after the first missed menstrual period.

Reference values

Normally, hCG levels are less than 4 IU/L. During pregnancy, hCG levels vary widely, depending in part on the number of days since the patient's last normal menstrual period.

Abnormal findings

Elevated hCG beta-subunit levels indicate pregnancy; significantly higher concentrations are present in a multiple pregnancy. Increased levels may also suggest hydatidiform mole, trophoblastic neoplasms of the placenta, and non-trophoblastic carcinomas that secrete hCG (including gastric, pancreatic, and ovarian adenocarcinomas). Low hCG beta-subunit levels can occur in ectopic pregnancy or pregnancy of less than 9 days. The beta-subunit level cannot differentiate between pregnancy and tumor recurrence because levels are high in both conditions.

Human chorionic gonadotropin, urine

Qualitative analysis of urine levels of hCG allows for the detection of pregnancy as early as 14 days after ovulation. The production of hCG, a glycoprotein that prevents degeneration of the corpus luteum at the end of the normal menstrual cycle, begins after conception. During the first trimester, hCG levels increase steadily and rapidly, peaking around the 10th week of gestation, and subsequently tapering off to less than 10% of peak levels.

The most common method of evaluating hCG in urine is hemagglutination inhibition. This laboratory procedure can provide both qualitative and quantitative information. The qualitative urine test is easier and less expensive than the serum hCG test (beta-subunit assay); therefore, it is used more commonly to detect pregnancy.

Purpose

- To detect and confirm pregnancy
- To aid in the diagnosis of hydatidiform mole or hCG-secreting tumors, threatened abortion, or dead fetus

Patient preparation

- If appropriate, explain to the patient that this test determines whether she is pregnant or determines the status of her pregnancy. Alternatively, explain how the test is used to screen for some types of cancer.
- Tell the patient that she need not restrict food but should restrict fluids for 8 hours before the test.
- Inform the patient that the test requires a first-voided morning specimen or urine collection over a 24-hour period, depending on whether a qualitative or quantitative test is done.

Normal findings

In a qualitative immunoassay analysis, results are reported as negative (nonpregnant) or positive (pregnant) for hCG. In a quantitative analysis, urine hCG levels in the first trimester of a normal pregnancy may be as high as 500,000 IU/24 hours; in the second trimester, they range from 10,000 to 25,000 IU/24 hours; and in the third trimester, from 5,000 to 15,000 IU/24 hours.

Measurable levels of hCG do not normally appear in the urine of men or nonpregnant women.

Abnormal findings

During pregnancy, elevated urine hCG levels may indicate multiple pregnancy or erythroblastosis fetalis; depressed urine hCG levels may indicate threatened abortion or ectopic pregnancy.

Measurable levels of hCG in men and nonpregnant women may indicate choriocarcinoma; ovarian or testicular tumors; melanoma; multiple myeloma; or gastric, hepatic, pancreatic, or breast cancer.

Human immunodeficiency virus (HIV) antibodies

The HIV antibody test detects antibodies to HIV in the serum. HIV is the virus that causes AIDS.

HIV testing

Test type	Specimen (mode of collection)	Sensitivity/specificity
Fourth-generation HIV-1/HIV-2 combination test*	Serum or plasma (phlebotomy)	High
Standard HIV antibody test[†]	Serum or plasma (phlebotomy)	High
Rapid test	Serum, plasma, or whole blood (phlebotomy) or finger stick	High for patients with chronic infection
Home sample collection test[‡]	Dried blood spot (finger stick)	Moderate
Oral fluid test	Oral mucosal transudate (oral fluid collection device)	Less sensitive for oral samples (can get false-negative results)

*Preferred approach to testing due to its ability to detect acute/early infections in up to 80% of patients with HIV who would otherwise be undetected with the standard HIV tests. (Data from UpToDate: https://www.uptodate.com/contents/screening-and-diagnostic-testing-for-hiv-infection.)
[†]ELISAs and Western blot can detect HIV-1. A confirmatory HIV-1 Western blot is performed if an ELISA test is positive to exclude the possibility of a false-positive result. If HIV-2 is being considered,

Transmission occurs by direct exposure of the blood to body fluids that contain the virus. The virus may be transmitted from one person to another through exchange of contaminated blood and blood products, during sexual intercourse with an infected partner, when needles used to inject I.V. drugs are shared, and from an infected mother to her child during pregnancy or breastfeeding.

Initial identification of HIV is usually achieved through enzyme-linked immunosorbent assay. Positive findings are confirmed by Western blot test and immunofluorescence. Other tests may also be performed to detect antibodies. (See *HIV testing*.)

Purpose

- To screen for HIV infection in high-risk patients
- To screen donated blood for HIV
- To monitor HIV status during drug therapy

Screening; confirmation	Strains detected[†]	Results
HIV-1/HIV-2 immunoassay	HIV-1, HIV-2, and HIV P24 antigen	HIV negative: no further testing needed HIV positive: An HIV-1/HIV-2 antibody differentiation test is performed: confirmed results at next visit
Enzyme-linked immunosorbent assays (ELISAs), HIV-1/HIV-2 differentiation assays, Western blot	HIV-1 and HIV-2	HIV negative: test result at return visit (typically a few days to 1 to 2 weeks) HIV positive: confirmed result at return visit
ELISA	HIV-1	HIV negative: test result at time of testing (<20 minutes) HIV positive: Preliminary positive test result at time of testing will need follow-up test: confirmed result at return visit
ELISA	HIV-1	HIV negative: test result when patient calls (typically 3 to 7 days) HIV positive: confirmed result when patient calls
ELISA	HIV-1	HIV negative: test result at return visit (typically 1 to 2 weeks) HIV positive: will need follow-up test: confirmed result at return visit

a special HIV-2 Western blot must be performed. (Data from UpToDate: https://www.uptodate.com/contents/screening-and-diagnostic-testing-for-hiv-infection.)
[‡]The tests performed on blood samples collected at home reveal infection later than most lab-based tests using blood from a vein but earlier than tests obtained from an oral swab. (Data from Centers for Disease Control and Prevention: https://www.cdc.gov/hiv/testing/hometests.html.)

Patient preparation

- Explain to the patient that this test detects HIV infection.
- Provide adequate counseling about the reasons for performing the test, which is usually requested by the patient's physician.
- If the patient has questions about his or her condition, provide full and accurate information.
- Explain that the test requires a blood sample. Tell the patient who will perform the venipuncture and when and where it will be performed.
- Inform the patient that there is no food or fluid restriction.

Normal findings

Test results are normally negative.

Abnormal findings

The test detects previous exposure to the virus. However, it does not identify patients who have been exposed to the virus but have not yet made antibodies. Most patients with AIDS have antibodies to HIV. A positive result on a test for the HIV antibody cannot determine whether a patient harbors an actively replicating virus or when the patient will show the signs and symptoms of AIDS.

Many apparently healthy people have been exposed to HIV and have circulating antibodies. The test results for such people are not false-positive findings. Furthermore, patients with late stages of AIDS may show no detectable antibody in their sera because they can no longer mount an antibody response.

Human leukocyte antigen test

The human leukocyte antigen (HLA) test identifies a group of antigens present on the surface of all nucleated cells but that is most easily detected on lymphocytes. There are four types of HLA: HLA-A, HLA-B, HLA-C, and HLA-D. These antigens are essential to immunity and determine the degree of histocompatibility between transplant recipients and donors. Many antigenic determinants (>60, for instance, at the HLA-B locus) are present for each site; one set of each antigen is inherited from each parent.

A high incidence of specific HLA types has been linked to specific diseases, such as rheumatoid arthritis and multiple sclerosis, but these findings have little diagnostic significance.

Purpose

- To provide histocompatibility typing of transplant recipients and donors
- To aid genetic counseling
- To aid paternity testing

Patient preparation

- Explain to the patient that this test detects antigens on white blood cells (WBCs).
- Explain that the test requires a blood sample, and tell the patient when and where it will be taken.
- Inform the patient that he or she need not restrict food or fluids.
- Check the patient's history for recent blood transfusions. HLA testing may need to be postponed if he or she has recently undergone a transfusion.

Normal findings

In HLA-A, HLA-B, and HLA-C testing, lymphocytes that react with the test antiserum undergo lysis; they are detected by phase microscopy. In HLA-D testing, leukocyte incompatibility is marked by blast formation, DNA synthesis, and proliferation.

Abnormal findings

Incompatible HLA-A, HLA-B, HLA-C, and HLA-D groups may cause unsuccessful tissue transplantation.

Many diseases have a strong association with certain types of HLA.

For example, HLA-DR5 is associated with Hashimoto's thyroiditis. HLA-B8 and HLA-Dw3 are associated with Graves' disease, whereas HLA-B8 alone is associated with chronic autoimmune hepatitis, celiac disease, and myasthenia gravis. HLA-Dw3 alone is associated with Addison's disease, Sjögren's syndrome, dermatitis herpetiformis, and SLE.

In paternity testing, a putative father who has a phenotype (two haplotypes: one from the father and one from the mother) with no haplotype or antigen pair identical to one of the child's is excluded as the father. A putative father with one haplotype identical to one of the child's may be the father; the probability varies with the incidence of the haplotype in the population.

International Normalized Ratio

The International Normalized Ratio (INR) system is considered the best method for standardizing the measurement of prothrombin time (PT) to monitor oral anticoagulant therapy. It is not used as a screening test for coagulopathies.

Purpose
- To evaluate the effectiveness of oral anticoagulant therapy

Patient preparation
- Explain to the patient that this test is used to determine the effectiveness of oral anticoagulant therapy.
- Explain that a blood sample will be needed, and tell the patient when and where it will be taken.

Reference values
A normal INR for patients receiving warfarin therapy is 2.0 to 3.0 (SI, 2.0 to 3.0). For those with mechanical prosthetic heart valves, an INR of 2.5 to 3.5 (SI, 2.5 to 3.5) is suggested.

Abnormal findings
An increased INR may indicate disseminated intravascular coagulation, cirrhosis, hepatitis, vitamin K deficiency, salicylate intoxication, or uncontrolled oral anticoagulation, or massive blood transfusion.

Lactate dehydrogenase

LD catalyzes the reversible conversion of muscle lactic acid into pyruvic acid, an essential step in the metabolic processes that ultimately produce cellular energy. Because LD is present in almost all body tissues, cellular damage increases the total serum LD level, limiting the diagnostic usefulness of LD.

Five tissue-specific isoenzymes can be identified and measured: LD_1 and LD_2 appear primarily in the heart, RBCs, and kidneys; LD_3 is found primarily in the lungs, spleen, placenta, and the pancreas; and LD_4 and LD_5 occur in the liver, skin, and skeletal muscles.

Purpose
- To aid in the differential diagnosis of MI, skeletal damage, pulmonary infarction, anemias, and hepatic disease
- To support the results of CK isoenzyme tests in diagnosing MI or to provide a diagnosis when CK-MB samples are obtained too late to show an increase
- To monitor patient response to some forms of chemotherapy

Patient preparation
- Explain to the patient that this test is used primarily to detect tissue alterations.
- Explain that the test requires a blood sample, and tell the patient when and where it will be taken.
- Inform the patient that he or she need not restrict food or fluids.

- If MI is suspected, tell the patient that the test will be repeated on the next two mornings to monitor progressive changes.

Reference values

Total LD levels normally range from 71 to 207 U/L (SI, 1.2 to 3.52 μkat/L). Normal distribution is as follows:

- LD_1: 17% to 27% (SI, 0.17 to 0.27) of total
- LD_2: 29% to 39% (SI, 0.29 to 0.39) of total
- LD_3: 19% to 27% (SI, 0.19 to 0.27) of total
- LD_4: 8% to 16% (SI, 0.08 to 0.16) of total
- LD_5: 6% to 16% (SI, 0.06 to 0.16) of total

Abnormal findings

Because many common diseases increase total LD levels, isoenzyme electrophoresis is usually necessary for diagnosis. In some disorders, the total LD level may be within normal limits, but abnormal proportions of each enzyme indicate tissue damage to specific organs. For instance, in acute MI, the concentration of LD_1 is greater than that of LD_2 within 12 to 48 hours after the onset of symptoms; therefore, the LD_1/LD_2 ratio is greater than 1. This reversal of the normal isoenzyme pattern is typical of myocardial damage and is known as flipped LD.

Midzone fractions (LD_2, LD_3, LD_4) can be increased in granulocytic leukemia, lymphomas, and platelet disorders.

Lipoprotein-cholesterol fractionation

Cholesterol fractionation tests are used to isolate and measure the types of cholesterol in serum. The types of cholesterol are low-density lipoproteins (LDLs) and high-density lipoproteins (HDLs). The HDL level is inversely related to the risk of CAD and atherosclerosis; the higher the HDL level, the lower the incidence of CAD and atherosclerosis. In contrast, the higher the LDL level, the higher the incidence of CAD and atherosclerosis.

Purpose

- To assess the risk of CAD and atherosclerosis
- To assess the efficacy of lipid-lowering drug therapy

Patient preparation

- Tell the patient that this test is used to determine the risk of CAD and atherosclerosis.
- Explain that the test requires a blood sample, and tell the patient when and where it will be taken.
- Instruct the patient to maintain his or her normal diet for 2 weeks before the test, to abstain from alcohol for 24 hours before the test, and to fast and avoid exercise for 12 to 14 hours before the test.

Reference values

Normal lipoprotein values vary by age, sex, geographic area, and ethnic group; check the laboratory for reference values. HDL levels range from 37 to 70 mg/dl (SI, 0.96 to 1.8 mmol/L) for men and from 40 to 85 mg/dl for women (SI, 1.03 to 2.2 mmol/L). LDL levels are less than 130 mg/dl (SI, <3.36 mmol/L) in people who do not have CAD. Borderline high levels are greater than 160 mg/dl (SI, >4.1 mmol/L).

The American College of Cardiology recommends an HDL level of 40 mg/dl or greater, with women maintaining an HDL cholesterol level of at least 45 mg/dl. An HDL level greater than 60 mg/dl is considered the heart is healthy. Optimally, the LDL level should be less than 100 mg/dl, with levels of 130 mg/dl or greater considered high.

Abnormal findings

High LDL levels increase the risk of CAD. Elevated HDL levels usually indicate a healthy state but can also indicate chronic hepatitis, early-stage primary biliary cirrhosis, and alcohol consumption. Increased HDL levels can occur as a result of long-term aerobic and vigorous exercise. Rarely, a sharp increase (to as high as 100 mg/dl [SI, 2.58 mmol/L]) in a second type of HDL (alpha2-HDL) signals CAD.

Lyme disease serology

Lyme disease is a multisystem disorder that is characterized by dermatologic, neurologic, cardiac, and rheumatic manifestations in various stages. Epidemiologic and serologic studies implicate a common tick-borne spirochete, *Borrelia burgdorferi*, as the causative agent. Serologic tests for Lyme disease, both indirect immunofluorescent and enzyme-linked immunosorbent assays, measure antibody response to this spirochete and indicate current infection or previous exposure. Serologic tests can identify 50% of patients with early-stage Lyme disease and all patients with later complications of carditis, neuritis, and arthritis as well as patients in remission.

Purpose

- To confirm the diagnosis of Lyme disease

Patient preparation

- Explain to the patient that this test helps determine whether his or her symptoms are caused by Lyme disease.
- Explain that the test requires a blood sample, and tell the patient when and where it will be taken.
- Inform the patient that there is no food or fluid restriction.

Reference values

Normal serum values are nonreactive.

Abnormal findings

A positive test result can help confirm the diagnosis, but it is not definitive. Other treponemal diseases and high rheumatoid factor titers can cause false-positive results. More than 15% of patients with Lyme disease do not have antibodies.

Magnesium, serum

The magnesium test is used to measure serum levels of magnesium, an electrolyte that is vital to neuromuscular function. It also helps in intracellular metabolism, activates many essential enzymes, and affects the metabolism of nucleic acids and proteins. Magnesium also helps to transport sodium and potassium across cell membranes and influences intracellular calcium levels. Most magnesium is found in bone and intracellular fluid; a small amount is found in extracellular fluid. Magnesium is absorbed by the small intestine and excreted in urine and stools.

Purpose

- To evaluate electrolyte status
- To assess neuromuscular and renal function

Patient preparation

- Explain to the patient that this test is used to determine the magnesium content of the blood.
- Explain that the test requires a blood sample, and tell the patient when and where it will be taken.
- Instruct the patient not to use magnesium salts (such as milk of magnesia or Epsom salt) for at least 3 days before the test, but tell him or her that he or she need not restrict food or fluids.

Reference values

Serum magnesium levels for adults range from 1.8 to 2.6 mg/dl (SI, 0.74 to 1.07 mmol/L); for children, 1.7 to 2.1 mg/dl (SI, 0.70 to 0.86 mmol/L); and for newborns, 1.5 to 2.2 mg/dl (SI, 0.62 to 0.91 mmol/L).

Abnormal findings

Elevated serum magnesium levels (hypermagnesemia) most commonly occur in renal failure, when the kidneys excrete inadequate amounts of magnesium, and also with the administration or ingestion of magnesium. Adrenal insufficiency (Addison's disease) can also increase serum magnesium levels.

In suspected or confirmed hypermagnesemia, observe the patient for lethargy; flushing; diaphoresis; decreased blood pressure; slow, weak pulse; muscle weakness; diminished deep tendon reflexes; slow, shallow respiration; and electrocardiogram (ECG) changes (prolonged PR interval, wide QRS complex, elevated T waves, atrioventricular block, premature ventricular contractions).

Decreased serum magnesium levels (hypomagnesemia) most commonly result from chronic alcoholism. Other causes include malabsorption syndrome, diarrhea, faulty absorption after bowel resection, prolonged bowel or gastric aspiration, acute pancreatitis, primary aldosteronism, severe burns, hypercalcemic conditions (including hyperparathyroidism), malnutrition, and certain diuretic therapy.

In hypomagnesemia, watch for leg and foot cramps, hyperactive deep tendon reflexes, arrhythmias, muscle weakness, seizures, twitching, tetany, tremors, and ECG changes (premature ventricular contractions and ventricular fibrillation).

Myoglobin

Myoglobin, which is usually found in skeletal and cardiac muscle, functions as an oxygen-binding muscle protein. It is released into the bloodstream in ischemia, trauma, and muscle inflammation.

Purpose

- As a nonspecific test, to estimate damage to skeletal or cardiac muscle tissue
- To predict flare-ups of polymyositis
- Specifically, to determine if MI has occurred

Patient preparation

- Explain the purpose of the test to the patient.
- Explain that a blood sample is required, and tell the patient when and where it will be obtained.
- Obtain a patient history, including disorders that may be associated with increased myoglobin levels.
- Inform the patient that the results must be correlated with the results of other tests such as cardiac enzymes to obtain a definitive diagnosis.

Reference values

Normal myoglobin values are 5 to 70 ng/ml (SI, 5 to 70 μg/L).

Abnormal findings

Besides MI, increased myoglobin levels may occur in acute alcohol intoxication, dermatomyositis, hypothermia (with prolonged shivering), muscular dystrophy, polymyositis, rhabdomyolysis, severe burn injuries, trauma, severe renal failure, and SLE.

Occult blood, fecal

Fecal occult blood is detected by microscopic analysis or by chemical tests for Hb, such as the guaiac test.

Normally, stools contain small amounts of blood (2 to 2.5 ml/day); therefore, tests for occult blood detect larger quantities. Testing is indicated when clinical symptoms and preliminary blood studies suggest GI bleeding. Additional tests are required to pinpoint the origin of the bleeding.

Purpose

- To detect GI bleeding
- To aid in the early diagnosis of colorectal cancer

Patient preparation

- Explain to the patient that this test helps detect abnormal GI bleeding.
- Tell him or her that the test requires collection of three stool specimens. Occasionally, only a random specimen is collected.
- Instruct the patient to maintain a high-fiber diet and to refrain from eating red meat, turnips, and horseradish for 48 to 72 hours before the test and throughout the collection period.

Normal findings

Zero to <2.5 ml of blood should be present in stools, resulting in a green reaction.

Abnormal findings

A positive test result indicates GI bleeding, which may result from many disorders, such as gastritis, varices, peptic ulcer, carcinoma, ulcerative colitis, dysentery, or hemorrhagic disease. This test is particularly important for the early diagnosis of colorectal cancer. Further tests, such as barium swallow, analysis of gastric contents, and endoscopic procedures, are necessary to define the site and extent of bleeding.

Partial thromboplastin time

The partial thromboplastin time (PTT) is used to evaluate the clotting factors of the intrinsic pathway—except platelets—by measuring the time required for a fibrin clot to form after a calcium and phospholipid emulsion is added to a plasma sample. An activator such as kaolin is used to shorten clotting time.

Purpose

- To screen for deficiencies of the clotting factors in the intrinsic pathways
- To monitor the response to heparin therapy

Patient preparation

- Explain to the patient that this test is used to determine if his or her blood clots normally.
- Explain that a blood sample will be needed, and tell the patient when and where it will be taken.
- When appropriate, tell the patient who is receiving heparin therapy that this test may be repeated at regular intervals to assess the response to treatment.
- Inform the patient that he or she need not restrict food or fluids.

Reference values

Normally, a fibrin clot forms 21 to 35 seconds (SI, 21 to 35 s) after reagents are added. If the patient is receiving anticoagulant therapy, ask the attending physician to specify the reference values for the therapy that is being delivered.

Abnormal findings

Prolonged PTT may indicate a deficiency of certain plasma clotting factors; vitamin K deficiency; the presence of heparin; or the presence of fibrin split products, fibrinolysins, or circulating anticoagulants that are antibodies to specific clotting factors.

Phosphate, serum

The phosphate test is used to measure serum levels of phosphate, which is the primary anion in intracellular fluid. Phosphates are essential in energy storage and use; calcium regulation; RBC function; acid-base balance; bone formation; and carbohydrate, protein, and fat metabolism. The intestines absorb most phosphates from dietary sources; the kidneys excrete phosphates and serve as a regulatory mechanism. Abnormal concentrations of serum phosphates usually result from improper excretion rather than faulty ingestion or absorption from dietary sources.

Normally, calcium and phosphate levels have an inverse relationship; if one is increased, the other is decreased.

Purpose

- To aid in the diagnosis of renal insufficiency or failure and acid-base imbalance
- To detect endocrine, skeletal, and calcium disorders

Patient preparation

- Explain to the patient that this test is used to measure phosphate levels in the blood.
- Explain that the test requires a blood sample, and tell the patient when and where it will be taken.
- Inform the patient that he or she need not restrict food or fluids.

Reference values

Normally, serum phosphate levels in adults range from 2.7 to 4.5 mg/dl (SI, 0.87 to 1.45 mmol/L). In children, the normal range is 4.5 to 5.5 mg/dl (SI, 1.45 to 1.78 mmol/L).

Abnormal findings

Decreased phosphate levels (hypophosphatemia) may result from malnutrition, malabsorption syndromes, vitamin D deficiency, hyperparathyroidism, renal tubular acidosis, and treatment of diabetic ketoacidosis. In children, hypophosphatemia can suppress normal growth. Symptoms of hypophosphatemia include anemia, prolonged bleeding, bone demineralization, decreased WBC count, and anorexia.

Increased levels (hyperphosphatemia) may result from skeletal disease, healing fractures, hypoparathyroidism, acromegaly, diabetic ketoacidosis, high intestinal obstruction, lactic acidosis (as a result of hepatic impairment), and renal insufficiency, or renal failure. Hyperphosphatemia is seldom clinically significant, but it can alter bone metabolism if it is prolonged. Symptoms of hyperphosphatemia include tachycardia, muscular weakness, diarrhea, cramping, and hyperreflexia.

Platelet count

Platelets, or thrombocytes, are the smallest formed elements in blood. They promote coagulation and the formation of a hemostatic plug in vascular injury.

Platelet count is one of the most important screening tests of platelet function. Accurate counts are vital.

Purpose

- To evaluate platelet production
- To assess the effects of chemotherapy or radiation therapy on platelet production
- To diagnose and monitor severe thrombocytosis or thrombocytopenia
- To confirm a visual estimate of the number and morphologic features of platelets from a stained blood film

Patient preparation

- Explain to the patient that this test is used to determine if his or her blood clots normally.

- Explain that a blood sample will be needed and tell the patient when and where it will be taken.
- Inform the patient that there is no food or fluid restriction.

Reference values

Normal platelet counts range from 140,000 to 400,000/mm³ (SI, 140 to 400 × 10⁹/L) in adults and from 150,000 to 450,000/mm³ (SI, 150 to 450 × 10⁹/L) in children.

Abnormal findings

A decreased platelet count (thrombocytopenia) can result from aplastic or hypoplastic bone marrow; infiltrative bone marrow disease, such as leukemia or disseminated infection; megakaryocytic hypoplasia; ineffective thrombopoiesis as a result of folic acid or vitamin B₁₂ deficiency; pooling of platelets in an enlarged spleen; increased platelet destruction as a result of drugs or immune disorders; disseminated intravascular coagulation; Bernard-Soulier syndrome; or mechanical injury to platelets.

An increased platelet count (thrombocytosis) can result from hemorrhage, fractures, infectious disorders, iron deficiency anemia, recent surgery, pregnancy, splenectomy, or inflammatory disorders. In such cases, the platelet count returns to normal after the patient recovers from the primary disorder. However, the count remains elevated in primary thrombocythemia, myelofibrosis with myeloid metaplasia, polycythemia vera, and chronic myelogenous leukemia.

When the platelet count is abnormal, the diagnosis usually requires further studies, such as a complete blood count, bone marrow biopsy, direct antiglobulin test (direct Coombs test), and serum protein electrophoresis.

Potassium, serum

The potassium test is used to measure serum levels of potassium, the major intracellular cation. Potassium helps maintain osmotic equilibrium in the cells as well as to regulate muscle activity, enzyme activity, and acid-base balance. It also affects renal function.

The body has no efficient method for conserving potassium; the kidneys excrete nearly all ingested potassium, even when the body's supply is depleted. Potassium deficiency can develop rapidly and is quite common. The average daily dietary potassium requirement that is necessary to maintain balance in adults is 80 to 200 mEq.

Purpose

- To evaluate the clinical signs of potassium excess (hyperkalemia) or potassium depletion (hypokalemia)
- To monitor renal function, acid-base balance, and glucose metabolism
- To evaluate neuromuscular and endocrine disorders
- To detect the origin of arrhythmias

Patient preparation

- Explain to the patient that this test is used to determine the potassium content of blood.
- Explain that the test requires a blood sample, and tell the patient when and where it will be taken.
- Inform the patient that there is no food or fluid restriction.

Reference values

Normally, serum potassium levels range from 3.5 to 5.2 mEq/L (SI, 3.5 to 5.2 mmol/L) for adults, 3.4 to 4.7 mEq/L (SI, 3.4 to 4.7 mmol/L) for children 1 year old to 18 years old, 4.1 to 5.3 mEq/L (SI, 4.1 to 5.3 mmol/L) in infants who are 7 days to 1 year old, and 3.7 to 5.9 mEq/L (SI, 3.7 to 5.9 mmol/L) in neonates who are 0 to 7 days old.

Abnormal findings

Abnormally high serum potassium levels are common in conditions in which excess cellular potassium enters the blood, such as burn injuries, crush injuries, diabetic ketoacidosis, transfusions of large amounts of blood, and MI. Hyperkalemia may also indicate reduced sodium excretion, possibly from acute renal failure (preventing normal exchange of sodium and potassium) or Addison's disease (as a result of potassium buildup and sodium depletion).

The patient with hyperkalemia may have weakness, malaise, nausea, diarrhea, colicky pain, and muscle irritability that progresses to flaccid paralysis, oliguria, anuria, and bradycardia. The ECG shows flattened P waves; a prolonged PR interval; a wide QRS complex; a tall, tented T wave; and ST-segment depression. Cardiac arrest may occur without warning.

Decreased potassium levels commonly result from aldosteronism or Cushing's syndrome, loss of body fluids (such as long-term diuretic therapy, vomiting, or diarrhea), and excessive ingestion of licorice. Although serum values and clinical symptoms can indicate a potassium imbalance, an ECG allows a definitive diagnosis.

A patient with hypokalemia may show decreased reflexes; a rapid, weak, irregular pulse; mental confusion; hypotension; anorexia; muscle weakness; and paresthesia. An ECG shows a flattened T wave, ST-segment depression, and U-wave elevation. In severe cases, ventricular fibrillation, respiratory paralysis, and cardiac arrest can develop.

Prostate-specific antigen

Prostate-specific antigen (PSA) is a glycoprotein found in prostatic tissues and is increased in both benign prostatic hyperplasia/hypertrophy (BPH) and prostate cancer; however, it is greatly increased in prostate cancer. Serum PSA levels are used to monitor the spread or recurrence of prostate cancer and to evaluate the patient's response to treatment. Measurement of serum PSA levels, along with a digital rectal examination, is now recommended as a screening test for prostate cancer in men older than age 50. African American males and males with a familial history of prostate cancer should start screening at age 40 years. It is also useful in assessing response to treatment in patients with stage B3 to D1 prostate cancer as well as in detecting tumor spread or recurrence.

Purpose

- To screen for prostate cancer in men older than age 50 and African American males at the age of 40
- To monitor the course of prostate cancer and aid in the evaluation of treatment

Patient preparation

- Explain to the patient that this test is used to screen for prostate cancer or, if appropriate, to monitor the course of treatment.
- Explain that the test requires a blood sample, and tell the patient when and where it will be taken.
- Inform the patient that he or she need not restrict food or fluids.

Reference values

Normal values are as follows:
- Ages 40 to 49: 0 to 2.5 ng/ml (SI, 0 to 2.5 mcg/L)
- Ages 50 to 59: 0 to 3.5 ng/ml (SI, 0 to 3.5 mcg/L)
- Ages 60 to 69: 0 to 4.5 ng/ml (SI, 0 to 4.5 mcg/L)
- Ages 70 and older: 0 to 6.5 ng/ml (SI, 0 to 6.5 mcg/L)

Abnormal findings

About 80% of patients with prostate cancer have pretreatment PSA values greater than 4.0 mcg/L. However, PSA results alone do not confirm a diagnosis of prostate cancer. About 20% of patients with benign prostatic hyperplasia/hypertrophy also have levels greater than 4.0 mcg/L. Further assessment and testing, including tissue biopsy, are needed to confirm the diagnosis of prostate cancer.

Protein, urine

A protein test is a quantitative test for proteinuria. Normally, the glomerular membrane allows only proteins of low molecular weight to enter the filtrate. The renal tubules reabsorb most of these proteins and normally excrete a small amount that is undetectable by a screening test. A damaged glomerular capillary membrane and impaired tubular reabsorption allow excretion of proteins in the urine.

A qualitative screening usually precedes this test. A positive result requires quantitative analysis of a 24-hour urine specimen by acid precipitation tests. Electrophoresis can detect Bence Jones protein, Hb, myoglobin, or albumin.

Purpose

- To aid in the diagnosis of pathologic states characterized by proteinuria, primarily renal disease

Patient preparation

- Explain to the patient that this test detects proteins in the urine.
- Tell the patient that the test usually requires urine collection over a 24-hour period; random collection can be done.
- Inform the patient that there is no food or fluid restriction.

Normal findings

At rest, normal urine protein values range from 10 to 140 mg/L (SI, 1 to 14 mg/dl) in a 24-hour urine sample for adult males, 30 to 100 mg/L (SI, 3 to 10 mg/dl) in a 24-hour urine sample for adult females, and 10 to 100 mg/L (SI, 1 to 10 mg/dl) in a 24-hour urine sample for children who are younger than 10 years old.

Abnormal findings

Proteinuria is a chief characteristic of renal disease. When proteinuria is present in a single/random specimen, a 24-hour urine collection is required to identify specific renal abnormalities.

Proteinuria can result from glomerular leakage of plasma proteins (a major cause of protein excretion), from overflow of filtered proteins of low molecular weight (when these are present in excessive concentrations), from impaired tubular reabsorption of filtered proteins, and from the presence of renal proteins derived from the breakdown of kidney tissue.

Persistent proteinuria indicates renal disease as a result of increased glomerular permeability. Minimal proteinuria (<0.5 g/24 hours), however, is commonly associated with renal diseases in which glomerular involvement is not a major factor, as in chronic pyelonephritis.

Moderate proteinuria (0.5 to 4 g/24 hours) occurs in several types of renal disease—acute or chronic glomerulonephritis, amyloidosis, and toxic nephropathies—or in diseases in which renal failure usually develops as a late complication (diabetes or heart failure, for example). Heavy proteinuria (>4 g/24 hours) is commonly associated with nephrotic syndrome.

When accompanied by an elevated WBC count, proteinuria indicates urinary tract infection. When accompanied by hematuria, proteinuria indicates local or diffuse urinary tract disorders. Other pathologic states (infections and lesions of the central nervous system, for example) can also result in detectable amounts of protein in the urine.

Many drugs (such as amphotericin B, gold preparations, aminoglycosides, polymyxins, and trimethadione) cause renal damage that leads to true proteinuria. For this reason, routine evaluation of urine protein is essential during such treatment. In all forms of proteinuria, fractionation results obtained by electrophoresis provide more precise information than the screening test. For example, excessive Hb in the urine indicates intravascular hemolysis; an elevated myoglobin level suggests muscle damage; an increased albumin level, increased glomerular permeability; and a high level of Bence Jones protein, multiple myeloma.

Not all forms of proteinuria have pathologic significance. Benign proteinuria can result from changes in body position. Functional proteinuria, which is associated with exercise and emotional or physiologic stress, is usually transient.

Protein electrophoresis, serum

Protein electrophoresis is used to measure the levels of serum albumin and globulins, which are the major blood proteins. This test separates the proteins into five distinct fractions: albumin, $alpha_1$, $alpha_2$, beta, and gamma globulin proteins.

The gamma globulins contribute to the body's immunity.

Purpose

- To aid in the diagnosis of hepatic disease, protein deficiency, renal disorders, and GI and neoplastic diseases

Patient preparation

- Explain to the patient that this test is used to determine the protein content of blood.
- Explain that the test requires a blood sample, and tell the patient when and where it will be taken.
- Inform the patient that there is no food or fluid restriction.

Reference values

Normally, total serum protein levels range from 6.4 to 8.3 g/dl (SI, 64 to 83 g/L), and the albumin fraction ranges from 3.5 to 5 g/dl (SI, 35 to 50 g/L). The $alpha_1$-globulin fraction ranges from 0.1 to 0.3 g/dl (SI, 1 to 3 g/L); $alpha_2$-globulin ranges from 0.6 to 1 g/dl (SI, 6 to 10 g/L). Beta-globulin ranges from 0.7 to 1.1 g/dl (SI, 7 to 11 g/L); gamma-globulin ranges from 0.8 to 1.6 g/dl (SI, 8 to 16 g/L).

Abnormal findings

For common abnormal findings, see *Clinical implications of abnormal protein levels.*

Prothrombin time

PT measures the time required for a fibrin clot to form in a citrated plasma sample after the addition of calcium ions and tissue thromboplastin (factor III).

Purpose

- To evaluate the extrinsic coagulation system (factors V, VII, and X and prothrombin and fibrinogen)
- To monitor the response to oral anticoagulant therapy

Patient preparation

- Explain to the patient that this test is used to determine whether the patient's blood clots normally.
- When appropriate, explain that this test is used to monitor the effects of oral anticoagulants; the test will be performed daily when therapy begins

and will be repeated at longer intervals when medication levels stabilize.

- Explain that a blood sample will be needed, and tell the patient when and where it will be taken.
- Inform the patient that there is no food or fluid restriction.

Reference values

Normally, PT values range from 10 to 14 seconds (SI, 10 to 14 s). Values vary, however, depending on the source of tissue thromboplastin and the method and type of reagents used to measure

clot formation. In a patient who is receiving oral anticoagulants, PT is usually maintained between 1 and 2.5 times the normal control value.

Abnormal findings

Prolonged PT may indicate deficiencies in fibrinogen; prothrombin; factor V, VII, or X (specific assays can pinpoint such deficiencies); or vitamin K. It may also result from ongoing oral anticoagulant therapy. Prolonged PT that exceeds 2.5 times the control value is commonly associated with abnormal bleeding.

Clinical implications of abnormal protein levels

Protein fractions	Decreased level	Increased level
Albumin	Chronic liver disease Chronic renal failure Severe burns Heart failure Leukemia	Dehydration Exercise
Alpha$_1$	Emphysema	Acute and chronic infection Tissue necrosis Neoplasm
Alpha$_2$	Hemolytic anemia Severe liver disease	Acute infection Trauma Severe burns Rheumatic fever
Beta	Hypocholesterolemia	Biliary cirrhosis Hypothyroidism Diabetes mellitus Malignant hypertension
Gamma	Nephrotic syndrome Lymphosarcoma	Collagen disease Rheumatoid arthritis Hodgkin's disease Liver disease

Adapted from LeFever, K. J. (2014). *Laboratory and diagnostic tests with nursing implications* (9th ed.). London, United Kingdom: Pearson.

(continued)

Clinical implications of abnormal protein levels *(continued)*

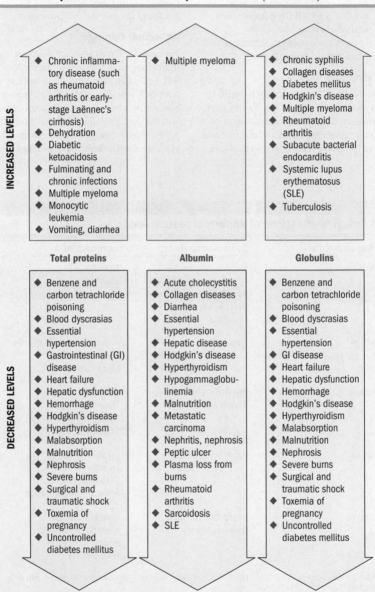

INCREASED LEVELS

Total proteins
- Chronic inflammatory disease (such as rheumatoid arthritis or early-stage Laënnec's cirrhosis)
- Dehydration
- Diabetic ketoacidosis
- Fulminating and chronic infections
- Multiple myeloma
- Monocytic leukemia
- Vomiting, diarrhea

Albumin
- Multiple myeloma

Globulins
- Chronic syphilis
- Collagen diseases
- Diabetes mellitus
- Hodgkin's disease
- Multiple myeloma
- Rheumatoid arthritis
- Subacute bacterial endocarditis
- Systemic lupus erythematosus (SLE)
- Tuberculosis

DECREASED LEVELS

Total proteins
- Benzene and carbon tetrachloride poisoning
- Blood dyscrasias
- Essential hypertension
- Gastrointestinal (GI) disease
- Heart failure
- Hepatic dysfunction
- Hemorrhage
- Hodgkin's disease
- Hyperthyroidism
- Malabsorption
- Malnutrition
- Nephrosis
- Severe burns
- Surgical and traumatic shock
- Toxemia of pregnancy
- Uncontrolled diabetes mellitus

Albumin
- Acute cholecystitis
- Collagen diseases
- Diarrhea
- Essential hypertension
- Hepatic disease
- Hodgkin's disease
- Hyperthyroidism
- Hypogammaglobulinemia
- Malnutrition
- Metastatic carcinoma
- Nephritis, nephrosis
- Peptic ulcer
- Plasma loss from burns
- Rheumatoid arthritis
- Sarcoidosis
- SLE

Globulins
- Benzene and carbon tetrachloride poisoning
- Blood dyscrasias
- Essential hypertension
- GI disease
- Heart failure
- Hepatic dysfunction
- Hemorrhage
- Hodgkin's disease
- Hyperthyroidism
- Malabsorption
- Malnutrition
- Nephrosis
- Severe burns
- Surgical and traumatic shock
- Toxemia of pregnancy
- Uncontrolled diabetes mellitus

Red blood cell count

The RBC count, also called erythro-cyte count, is part of a complete blood count. It is used to detect the number of RBCs in a microliter, or cubic millimeter, of whole blood.

Purpose

- To provide data for calculating mean corpuscular volume (MCV), MCH, and MCHC which show RBC size, weight, and Hb concentration
- To support other hematologic tests that are used to diagnose anemia or polycythemia

Patient preparation

- Explain to the patient that this test is used to evaluate the number of RBCs and to detect possible blood disorders.
- Explain that a blood sample will be needed, and tell the patient when and where it will be taken.
- If the patient is a child, explain to the patient (if he or she is old enough) and the parents that a small amount of blood will be taken from his or her finger or earlobe.
- Inform the patient that there is no food or fluid restriction.

Reference values

Normal RBC values vary, depending on the type of sample and the patient's age and sex, as follows:

- Men: 4.5 to 5.5 million RBCs/μl (SI, 4.5 to 5.5 $\times$ 10^{12}/L) of venous blood
- Women: 4 to 5 million RBCs/μl (SI, 4 to 5 $\times$ 10^{12}/L) of venous blood
- Children: 4.6 to 4.8 million/μl (SI, 4.6 to 4.8 $\times$ 10^{12}/L) of venous blood
- Full-term neonates: 4.4 to 5.8 million/μl (SI, 4.4 to 5.8 $\times$ 10^{12}/L) of capillary blood at birth, decreasing to 3 to 3.8 million/μl (SI, 3 to 3.8 $\times$ 10^{12}/L) at age 2 months, and increasing slowly thereafter

Normal values may exceed these levels in patients who live at high altitudes or are very active.

Abnormal findings

An elevated RBC count may indicate absolute or relative polycythemia. A depressed count may indicate anemia, fluid overload, or hemorrhage more than 24 hours ago. Further tests, such as stained cell examination, HCT, Hb, RBC indices, and WBC studies, are needed to confirm the diagnosis.

Red blood cell indices

Using the results of the RBC count, HCT, and total Hb tests, RBC indices (eryth-rocyte indices) provide important information about the size, Hb concentration, and Hb weight of an average RBC.

Purpose

- To aid in the diagnosis and classifi-cation of anemias

Patient preparation

- Explain to the patient that this test helps determine if he or she has anemia.
- Explain that a blood sample will be needed, and tell the patient when and where it will be taken.

Reference values

The indices tested include MCV, MCH, and MCHC.

MCV, the ratio of HCT (packed cell volume) to the RBC count, expresses the average size of the erythrocytes and indi-cates whether they are undersized (micro-cytic), oversized (macrocytic), or normal (normocytic). MCH, the Hb-RBC ratio, gives the weight of Hb in an average RBC. MCHC, the ratio of Hb weight to HCT, defines the concentration of Hb in 100 ml of packed RBCs. It helps distinguish normally colored (normochromic) RBCs from paler (hypochromic) RBCs.

Comparative red cell indices in anemias

	Normal findings (normocytic, normochromic)	Iron deficiency anemia (microcytic, hypochromic)	Pernicious anemia (macrocytic, normochromic)
MCV	82 to 98 μm^3	60 to 80 μm^3	96 to 150 μm^3
MCH	26 to 34 pg/cell	5 to 25 pg/cell	33 to 53 pg/cell
MCHC	32 to 36 g/dl	20 to 30 g/dl	33 to 38 g/dl

MCV, mean corpuscular volume; MCH, mean corpuscular hemoglobin; MCHC, mean corpuscular hemoglobin concentration.

The range of normal RBC indices is as follows:

- MCV: 82 to 98 μm^3
- MCH: 26 to 34 pg/cell
- MCHC: 32 to 36 g/dl

Abnormal findings

Low MCV and MCHC indicate microcytic, hypochromic anemias caused by iron deficiency anemia, pyridoxine-responsive anemia, or thalassemia. A high MCV suggests macrocytic anemia caused by megaloblastic anemia, folic acid or vitamin B_{12} deficiency, inherited disorders of DNA synthesis, or reticulocytosis. Because MCV reflects the average volume of many cells, a value within the normal range can encompass RBCs of varying size, from microcytic to macrocytic. (See *Comparative red cell indices in anemias*.)

Sodium, serum

The sodium test is used to measure serum levels of sodium in relation to the amount of water in the body. Sodium, the major extracellular cation, affects the distribution of water in the body, maintains the osmotic pressure of extracellular fluid, and helps promote neuromuscular function. It also helps maintain the acid-base balance and influences chloride and potassium levels.

Purpose

- To evaluate the fluid-electrolyte balance and the acid-base balance and related neuromuscular, renal, and adrenal functions

Patient preparation

- Explain to the patient that this test is used to determine the sodium content of blood.
- Explain that the test requires a blood sample, and tell the patient when and where it will be taken.
- Inform the patient that there is no food or fluid restriction.

Reference values

Normally, serum sodium levels range from 136 to 145 mEq/L (SI, 136 to 145 mmol/L).

Abnormal findings

Sodium imbalance can result from a loss or gain of sodium or from a change in the patient's state of hydration. Increased serum sodium levels (hypernatremia) may be caused by inadequate water intake, water loss in excess of sodium loss (such as diabetes insipidus, impaired renal function, prolonged hyperventilation, and, occasionally, severe vomiting or diarrhea), and sodium retention (such as aldosteronism). Hypernatremia can also result from excessive sodium intake. If a patient has hypernatremia and associated loss of water, observe him or her for signs of thirst, restlessness, dry and sticky mucous membranes, flushed skin, oliguria, and diminished reflexes. If increased total body sodium causes water retention, observe the patient for hypertension, dyspnea, edema, and heart failure.

Abnormally low serum sodium levels (hyponatremia) may result from inadequate sodium intake or from excessive sodium loss as a result of profuse sweating, GI suctioning, diuretic therapy, diarrhea, vomiting, adrenal insufficiency, burns, and chronic renal insufficiency with acidosis. Urine sodium measurements are usually more sensitive to early changes in sodium balance and should be evaluated simultaneously with serum sodium levels.

If a patient has hyponatremia, watch him or her for apprehension, lassitude, headache, decreased skin turgor, abdominal cramps, and tremors that may progress to seizures.

Thyroid-stimulating immunoglobulin

Thyroid-stimulating immunoglobulin (TSI), formerly called long-acting thyroid stimulator, appears in the blood of most patients with Graves' disease. It stimulates the thyroid gland to produce and excrete excessive amounts of thyroid hormone.

Reportedly, 90% of people with Graves' disease have elevated TSI levels. Positive test results strongly suggest Graves' disease, despite normal results on routine thyroid tests, in patients who are still suspected of having Graves' disease or progressive exophthalmos.

Purpose

- To aid in the evaluation of suspected thyroid disease
- To aid in the diagnosis of suspected thyrotoxicosis, especially in patients with exophthalmos
- To monitor the treatment of thyrotoxicosis

Patient preparation

- Explain to the patient that this test evaluates thyroid function, as appropriate.
- Explain that the test requires a blood sample, and tell the patient when and where it will be taken.

Reference values

TSI does not normally appear in serum. However, it is considered normal at levels equal to or greater than the 1.3 index.

Abnormal findings

Increased TSI levels are associated with exophthalmos, Graves' disease (thyrotoxicosis), and recurrence of hyperthyroidism.

Thyroxine

Thyroxine (T_4) is an amine that is secreted by the thyroid gland in response to thyroid-stimulating hormone (TSH) and, indirectly, thyrotropin-releasing hormone. It is the major hormone secreted by the thyroid gland. The rate of secretion is normally regulated by a complex system of negative and positive feedback mechanisms.

Only a fraction of T_4 (about 0.05%) circulates freely in the blood; the rest binds strongly to plasma proteins, primarily T_4-binding globulin (TBG).

This minute fraction is responsible for the clinical effects of thyroid hormone. TBG binds so tenaciously that T_4 survives in the plasma for a relatively long time, with a half-life of about 6 days. This immunoassay, one of the most common thyroid diagnostic tools, measures the total circulating T_4 level when TBG is normal. An alternative test is the Murphy-Pattee test, or T_4 (D) test, which is based on competitive protein binding.

Purpose

- To evaluate thyroid function
- To aid in the diagnosis of hyperthyroidism and hypothyroidism
- To monitor the response to antithyroid medication in hyperthyroidism or to thyroid replacement therapy in hypothyroidism (TSH estimates are needed to confirm hypothyroidism.)

Patient preparation

- Explain to the patient that this test helps evaluate the function of the thyroid gland.
- Explain that the test requires a blood sample, and tell the patient when and where it will be taken.
- Inform him or her that there is no need to fast or restrict activity.

Reference values

Normally, total T_4 levels range from 5.4 to 11.5 mcg/dl (SI, 57 to 148 nmol/L).

Abnormal findings

Abnormally elevated T_4 levels are consistent with primary and secondary hyperthyroidism, including excessive T_4 (levothyroxine) replacement therapy (factitious or iatrogenic hyperthyroidism). Low levels suggest primary or secondary hypothyroidism or may be caused by T_4 suppression by normal, elevated, or replacement levels of triiodothyronine (T_3). If the diagnosis of hypothyroidism is in doubt, TSH levels may be obtained.

Normal T_4 levels do not guarantee euthyroidism; for example, normal readings occur in T_3 toxicosis. Overt signs of hyperthyroidism require further testing.

Thyroxine, free and triiodothyronine, free

The free thyroxine (FT_4) and free triiodothyronine (FT_3) tests, which are commonly performed simultaneously, measure serum levels of FT_4 and FT_3, the minute portions of T_4 and T_3 that are not bound to TBG and other serum proteins. These unbound hormones are responsible for the thyroid's effects on cellular metabolism. Measurement of free hormone levels is the best indicator of thyroid function.

Because of disagreement as to whether FT_4 or FT_3 is the better indicator, laboratories commonly measure both. Disadvantages of these tests include a cumbersome and difficult laboratory method, inaccessibility, and cost. This test may be useful in the 5% of patients in whom standard T_3 or T_4 tests do not produce diagnostic results.

Purpose

- To measure the metabolically active form of the thyroid hormones
- To aid in the diagnosis of hyperthyroidism and hypothyroidism when TBG levels are abnormal

Patient preparation

- Explain to the patient that this test helps evaluate thyroid function.
- Explain that the test requires a blood sample, and tell the patient when and where it will be taken.

Reference values

The normal range for FT_4 is 0.9 to 2.3 ng/dl (SI, 10 to 30 pmol/L); for FT_3, it is 260 to 480 pg/dl (SI, 4.0 to 7.4 pmol/L). Values vary, depending on the laboratory.

Abnormal findings

Elevated FT_4 and FT_3 levels indicate hyperthyroidism, unless peripheral resistance to thyroid hormone is present. T_3 toxicosis, a distinct form of hyperthyroidism, yields high FT_3 levels with normal or low FT_4 values. Low FT_4 levels usually indicate hypothyroidism, except in patients who are receiving T_3 replacement therapy. Patients who are receiving thyroid therapy may have varying levels of FT_4 and FT_3, depending on the preparation used and the time of sample collection.

Triglycerides

Serum triglyceride analysis provides a quantitative analysis of triglycerides—the main storage form of lipids—which constitute about 95% of fatty tissue. Although not in itself diagnostic, the triglyceride test permits early identification of hyperlipidemia and helps determine the risk of CAD.

Purpose

- To screen for hyperlipidemia or pancreatitis
- To help identify nephrotic syndrome and patients with poorly controlled diabetes mellitus
- To determine the risk of CAD
- To calculate the LDL cholesterol level using the Friedewald equation

Patient preparation

- Explain to the patient that this test is used to detect disorders of fat metabolism.
- Explain that the test requires a blood sample, and tell the patient when and where it will be taken.
- Instruct the patient to fast for at least 12 hours before the test and to abstain from alcohol for 24 hours. Tell the patient that water is not restricted.

Reference values

Triglyceride values vary with age and sex. There is some controversy about the most appropriate normal ranges, but values of 0.30 to 148 mg/dl (SI, 0.34 to 1.67 mmol/L) for men and 32 to 131 mg/dl (SI, 0.36 to 1.48 mmol/L) for women are widely accepted.

Abnormal findings

Increased or decreased serum triglyceride levels suggest a clinical abnormality; additional tests are required for a definitive diagnosis.

A mild to moderate increase in serum triglyceride levels indicates biliary obstruction, diabetes mellitus, nephrotic syndrome, endocrinopathies, or overconsumption of alcohol. Markedly increased levels without an identifiable cause reflect congenital hyperlipoproteinemia and necessitate lipoprotein phenotyping to confirm the diagnosis.

Decreased serum triglyceride levels are rare and occur mainly in malnutrition and abetalipoproteinemia.

Triiodothyronine

The T_3 test is a highly specific radioimmunoassay that measures total (bound and free) serum content of T_3 to investigate clinical indications of thyroid dysfunction. Like T_4 secretion, T_3 secretion occurs in response to TSH and, secondarily, thyrotropin-releasing hormone.

Although T_3 is present in the bloodstream in minute quantities and is metabolically active for only a short time, its effect on body metabolism dominates that of T_4. Another significant difference between the two major thyroid hormones is that T_3 binds less firmly to TBG. Consequently, T_3 persists in the bloodstream for a short time. Half of T_3 disappears in about 1 day, whereas half of T_4 disappears in 6 days.

Purpose

- To aid in the diagnosis of T_3 toxicosis
- To aid in the diagnosis of hypothyroidism and hyperthyroidism
- To monitor the clinical response to thyroid replacement therapy in hypothyroidism

Patient preparation

- Explain to the patient that this test helps evaluate the function of the thyroid gland and determine the cause of his or her symptoms.
- Explain that the test requires a blood sample, and tell the patient when and where it will be taken.
- Withhold medications, such as steroids, propranolol, and cholestyramine, which may affect thyroid function, as ordered. If they must be continued, record this information on the laboratory request.

Reference values

Normal serum T_3 levels range from 80 to 200 ng/dl (SI, 1.2 to 3.0 nmol/L).

Abnormal findings

Serum T_3 and T_4 levels usually rise and fall in tandem. However, in T_3 toxicosis, T_3 levels rise, whereas total and free T_4 levels remain normal. T_3 toxicosis occurs in patients with Graves' disease, toxic adenoma, or toxic nodular goiter. T_3 levels also surpass T_4 levels in patients who are receiving thyroid replacement therapy containing more T_3 than T_4. In iodine-deficient areas, the thyroid may produce larger amounts of the more cellularly active T_3 than of T_4 in an effort to maintain the euthyroid state.

Usually, T_3 levels appear to be a more accurate diagnostic indicator of hyperthyroidism. Although T_3 and T_4 levels are increased in about 90% of patients with hyperthyroidism, there is a disproportionate increase in T_3. In some patients with hypothyroidism, T_3 levels may fall within the normal range and may not be diagnostically significant.

A rise in serum T_3 levels normally occurs during pregnancy. Low T_3 levels may appear in euthyroid patients who have a systemic illness (especially hepatic or renal disease), during severe acute illness, and after trauma or major surgery. In such patients, TSH levels are within normal limits. Low serum T_3 levels are found in some euthyroid patients with malnutrition.

Triiodothyronine uptake

The T_3 uptake test measures FT_4 levels indirectly by showing the availability of serum protein-binding sites for T_4. The results of T_3 uptake are usually combined with a T_4 radioimmunoassay or a T_4 (D) test (competitive protein-binding test) to determine the FT_4 index, which is a mathematical calculation that is believed to reflect FT_4 by correcting for TBG abnormalities.

The T_3 uptake test has become less popular recently because rapid tests for T_3, T_4, and TSH are readily available.

Purpose

- To aid in the diagnosis of hypothyroidism and hyperthyroidism when the TBG level is normal
- To aid in the diagnosis of primary disorders of TBG levels

Patient preparation

- Explain to the patient that this test helps evaluate thyroid function.
- Explain that the test requires a blood sample, and tell the patient when and where it will be taken.
- Tell him or her that the laboratory requires several days to complete the analysis.
- Withhold medications, such as estrogens, androgens, phenytoin, salicylates, and thyroid preparations, that may interfere with test results, as ordered. If they must be continued, note this information on the laboratory request.

Reference values

Normal T_3 uptake values are 25% to 35%.

Abnormal findings

A high T_3 uptake percentage in the presence of elevated T_4 levels indicates hyperthyroidism (implying few TBG free binding sites and high FT_4 levels). A low uptake percentage, together with low T_4 levels, indicates hypothyroidism (implying more TBG free binding sites and low FT_4 levels). Thus, in primary thyroid disease, T_4 and T_3 uptake vary in the same direction; the availability of binding sites varies inversely.

Discordant variance in T_4 and T_3 uptake suggests a TBG abnormality. For example, the finding of a high T_3 uptake percentage and a low or normal FT_4 level suggests decreased TBG levels. Such decreased levels may result from protein loss (as in nephrotic syndrome), decreased production (as a result of excess androgen or genetic or idiopathic causes), or competition for T_4 binding sites by certain drugs (salicylates, phenylbutazone, and phenytoin). Conversely, the finding of a low T_3 uptake percentage and a high or normal FT_4 level suggests increased TBG levels. Such increased levels may be caused by exogenous or endogenous estrogen (pregnancy) or may result from idiopathic causes. Thus, in primary disorders of TBG levels, values of measured T_4 and free sites change in the same direction.

Troponin

Cardiac troponin I (cTnI) and cardiac troponin T (cTnT) are proteins in the striated cells that are specific markers of cardiac damage. When the myocardial tissue is injured, these proteins are released into the bloodstream. Elevations in troponin levels can be seen within 1 hour of MI and persist for a week or longer.

Purpose

- To detect and diagnose acute MI and reinfarction
- To evaluate possible causes of chest pain

Patient preparation

- Explain to the patient that this test helps assess myocardial injury and that multiple samples may be drawn to detect fluctuations in serum levels.
- Explain that a blood sample will be needed, and tell the patient when and where it will be taken.
- Inform the patient that there is no food or fluid restriction.

Reference values

Laboratory results may vary. Some laboratories may consider a test result positive if detectable levels are found; others may give a range for abnormal results. Normally, cTnI levels are less than 0.35 ng/ml (SI, <0.35 mcg/L); cTnT levels are less than 0.1 ng/ml (SI, <0.1 mcg/L). A cTnI level greater than 2.0 ng/ml (SI, >2.0 mcg/L) suggests cardiac injury. Results of a qualitative cTnT rapid immunoassay that are greater than 0.1 ng/ml (SI, >0.1 mcg/L) are considered positive for cardiac injury. As long as tissue injury continues, the troponin levels will remain high.

Abnormal findings

- Troponin levels increase rapidly and are detectable within 1 hour of injury to the myocardial cells. Levels of cTnI are not detectable in people who do not have cardiac injury.

Uric acid, serum

The uric acid test is used to measure serum levels of uric acid, the major end metabolite of purine. Disorders of purine metabolism, rapid destruction of nucleic acids, and conditions that cause impaired renal excretion characteristically increase serum uric acid levels.

Purpose

- To confirm the diagnosis of gout
- To monitor serum uric acid during the treatment of gout
- To help detect renal dysfunction

Patient preparation

- Explain to the patient that this test is used to detect gout and kidney dysfunction.
- Explain that the test requires a blood sample, and tell the patient when and where it will be taken.
- There is no food or fluid restriction; however, in some cases, high-purine foods are restricted for 24 hours before the test.

Reference values

Uric acid concentrations in men normally range from 3.4 to 7 mg/dl (SI, 202 to 416 μmol/L); in women, normal levels range from 2.3 to 6 mg/dl (SI, 143 to 357 μmol/L).

Abnormal findings

Increased uric acid levels may indicate gout or impaired kidney function. Levels may also increase in heart failure, glycogen storage disease (type I, von Gierke's disease), infections, hemolytic and sickle cell anemia, polycythemia, neoplasms, and psoriasis.

Low uric acid levels may indicate defective tubular absorption (such as Fanconi syndrome) or acute hepatic atrophy.

Urinalysis, routine

A routine urinalysis is done to evaluate urinary and systemic disorders. This test evaluates the physical characteristics (color, odor, turbidity, and opacity) of urine; determines its specific gravity and pH; detects and measures protein, glucose, and ketone bodies; and examines the sediment for blood cells, casts, and crystals.

Diagnostic laboratory methods include visual examination, reagent strip screening, refractometry for specific gravity, and microscopic inspection of centrifuged sediment.

Purpose

- To screen the patient's urine for renal or urinary tract disease
- To help detect metabolic or systemic disease unrelated to renal disorders
- To detect substance (drug) use

Patient preparation

- Explain to the patient that this test aids in the diagnosis of renal or urinary tract disease and help evaluate overall body function.
- Inform the patient that food or fluids need not be restricted before the test.

Normal findings

See *Normal findings in routine urinalysis.*

Abnormal findings

Nonpathologic variations in normal values may result from diet, nonpathologic conditions, the time of specimen collection, and other factors.

Urine pH, which is greatly affected by diet and medications, affects the appearance of urine and the composition of crystals. An alkaline pH (>7.0)—characteristic of a vegetarian diet—causes turbidity and the formation of phosphate, carbonate, and amorphous crystals. An acid pH (<7.0)—typical of a high-protein diet—produces turbidity and the formation of oxalate, cystine, leucine, tyrosine, amorphous urate, and uric acid crystals.

Protein, which is normally absent from the urine, may be present in a benign condition known as orthostatic (postural) proteinuria. Most common in patients ages 10 to 20, this condition is intermittent, appears after prolonged standing, and disappears after the patient assumes a recumbent position.

Normal findings in routine urinalysis

Element	Findings
Macroscopic	
Color	• Straw to dark yellow
Odor	• Slightly aromatic
Appearance	• Clear
Specific gravity	• 1.005 to 1.035
pH	• 4.5 to 8
Protein	• None
Glucose	• None
Ketone bodies	• None
Bilirubin	• None
Urobilinogen	• Normal
Hemoglobin	• None
Erythrocytes (RBCs)	• None
Nitrites (bacteria)	• None
Leukocytes (WBCs)	• None
Microscopic	
RBCs	• 0 to 2/high-power field
WBCs	• 0 to 5/high-power field
Epithelial cells	• 0 to 5/high-power field
Casts	• None, except 1 to 2 hyaline casts/low-power field
Crystals	• Present
Bacteria	• None
Yeast cells	• None
Parasites	• None

RBCs, red blood cells; WBCs, white blood cells.

Transient benign proteinuria can also occur with fever, exposure to cold, emotional stress, or strenuous exercise. Systemic diseases that may cause proteinuria include lymphoma, hepatitis, diabetes mellitus, toxemia, hypertension, lupus erythematosus, and febrile illnesses.

Sugars, which are usually absent from the urine, may appear under normal conditions. The most common sugar found in urine is glucose. Transient nonpathologic glycosuria may result from emotional stress or pregnancy and may follow ingestion of a high-carbohydrate meal.

Centrifuged urine sediment contains cells, casts, crystals, bacteria, yeast, and parasites. RBCs do not usually appear in urine without pathologic significance; however, strenuous exercise can cause hematuria.

The following abnormal findings suggest pathologic conditions:
• *Color*: Color change can result from diet, drugs, and many diseases.
• *Odor*: In diabetes mellitus, starvation, and dehydration, a fruity odor

accompanies the formation of ketone bodies. In urinary tract infections, a foul or putrid odor commonly is associated with *Escherichia coli*. Maple syrup urine disease and phenylketonuria also cause distinctive odors. Other abnormal odors include those similar to a brewery, sweaty feet, cabbage, fish, and sulfur.

- *Turbidity*: Turbid urine may contain RBCs or WBCs, bacteria, fat, or chyle and may reflect renal infection.
- *Specific gravity*: Low specific gravity (<1.005) is characteristic of diabetes insipidus, nephrogenic diabetes insipidus, acute tubular necrosis, and pyelonephritis. Fixed specific gravity, in which the value remains 1.010 regardless of fluid intake, occurs in chronic glomerulonephritis with severe renal damage. High specific gravity (>1.035) occurs in nephrotic syndrome, dehydration, acute glomerulonephritis, heart failure, liver failure, diabetes mellitus, and shock.
- *pH*: Alkaline urine pH may result from Fanconi syndrome, urinary tract infection, and metabolic or respiratory alkalosis. Acid urine pH is associated with renal tuberculosis, pyrexia, phenylketonuria, alkaptonuria, and acidosis.
- *Protein*: Proteinuria suggests renal failure or disease (including nephrosis, glomerulosclerosis, glomerulonephritis, nephrolithiasis, nephrotic syndrome, and polycystic kidney disease) or, possibly, multiple myeloma.
- *Sugars*: Glycosuria usually indicates diabetes mellitus but may result from pheochromocytoma, Cushing's syndrome, impaired tubular reabsorption, advanced renal disease, and increased intracranial pressure. I.V. solutions containing glucose and total parenteral nutrition containing 10% to 50% glucose can cause glucose to spill over the renal threshold, leading to glycosuria. Fructosuria, galactosuria, and pentosuria usually suggest rare hereditary metabolic disorders (except for lactosuria during pregnancy and breastfeeding). However, an alimentary form of pentosuria and fructosuria may occur after excessive ingestion of pentose or fructose. When the liver does not metabolize these sugars, they spill into the urine because the renal tubules do not reabsorb them.

- *Ketone bodies*: Ketonuria occurs in diabetes mellitus when cellular energy needs exceed available cellular glucose. In the absence of glucose, cells metabolize fat for energy. Ketone bodies—the end products of incomplete fat metabolism— accumulate in the plasma and are excreted in the urine. Ketonuria may also occur in starvation states, low- or no-carbohydrate diets, and after diarrhea or vomiting.
- *Bilirubin*: Bilirubin in urine may occur in liver disease resulting from obstructive jaundice or hepatotoxic drugs or toxins or from fibrosis of the biliary canaliculi (which may occur in cirrhosis).
- *Urobilinogen*: Intestinal bacteria in the duodenum change bilirubin into urobilinogen. The liver reprocesses the remainder into bile. Increased urobilinogen in the urine may indicate liver damage, hemolytic disease, or severe infection. Decreased levels may occur with biliary obstruction, inflammatory disease, antimicrobial therapy, severe diarrhea, or renal insufficiency.
- *Cells*: Hematuria indicates bleeding within the genitourinary tract and may result from infection, obstruction, inflammation, trauma, tumors, glomerulonephritis, renal hypertension, lupus nephritis, renal tuberculosis, renal vein thrombosis, renal calculi, hydronephrosis,

pyelonephritis, scurvy, malaria, parasitic infection of the bladder, subacute bacterial endocarditis, polyarteritis nodosa, and hemorrhagic disorders. Strenuous exercise or exposure to toxic chemicals may also cause hematuria. An excess of WBCs in the urine usually implies urinary tract inflammation, especially cystitis or pyelonephritis. The finding of WBC and WBC casts in the urine suggests renal infection or noninfective inflammatory disease. Numerous epithelial cells suggest renal tubular degeneration, such as heavy metal poisoning, eclampsia, and kidney transplant rejection.

- *Casts (plugs of gelled proteinaceous material [high-molecular-weight mucoprotein])*: Casts form in the renal tubules and collecting ducts by agglutination of protein cells or cellular debris and are flushed loose by urine flow. Excessive numbers of casts indicate renal disease. Hyaline casts are associated with renal parenchymal disease, inflammation, trauma to the glomerular capillary membrane, and some physiologic states (such as after exercise); epithelial casts, with renal tubular damage, nephrosis, eclampsia, amyloidosis, and heavy metal poisoning; coarse and fine granular casts, with acute or chronic renal failure, pyelonephritis, and chronic lead intoxication; fatty and waxy casts, with nephrotic syndrome, chronic renal disease, and diabetes mellitus; RBC casts, with renal parenchymal disease (especially glomerulonephritis), renal infarction, subacute bacterial endocarditis, vascular disorders, sickle cell anemia, scurvy, blood dyscrasias, malignant hypertension, collagen disease, and acute inflammation; and WBC casts, with acute pyelonephritis and glomerulonephritis, nephrotic syndrome, pyogenic infection, and lupus nephritis.

- *Crystals*: Some crystals normally appear in urine, but numerous calcium oxalate crystals suggest hypercalcemia or ingestion of ethylene glycol. Cystine crystals (cystinuria) reflect an inborn error of metabolism.
- *Other components*: Bacteria, yeast cells, and parasites in urine sediment reflect genitourinary tract infection or contamination of external genitalia. Yeast cells, which may be mistaken for RBCs, are identifiable by their ovoid shape, lack of color, variable size, and, commonly, signs of budding. The most common parasite in sediment is *Trichomonas vaginalis*, which causes vaginitis, urethritis, and prostatovesiculitis.

White blood cell count

A WBC count, also called a leukocyte count, is part of a complete blood count. It indicates the number of white cells in a microliter, or cubic millimeter, of whole blood.

WBC counts may vary by as much as 2,000 cells/μl (SI, 2×10^9/L) on any given day as a result of strenuous exercise, stress, or digestion. The WBC count may increase or decrease significantly in certain diseases but is diagnostically useful only when the patient's WBC differential and clinical status are considered.

Purpose

- To identify infection or inflammation
- To determine the need for further tests, such as WBC differential or bone marrow biopsy
- To monitor the response to chemotherapy or radiation therapy

Patient preparation

- Explain to the patient that the test is used to detect an infection or inflammation.

- Explain that a blood sample will be needed, and tell the patient when and where it will be taken.
- Inform the patient that he or she should avoid strenuous exercise for 24 hours before the test. Also tell the patient that he or she should avoid eating a heavy meal before the test.
- If the patient is being treated for an infection, advise him or her that this test will be repeated to monitor his or her progress.
- Notify the laboratory and physician of medications that the patient is taking that may affect test results; they may need to be restricted.

Reference values

WBC count ranges from 4,000 to 10,000/μl (SI, 4 to 10 × 10^9/L).

Abnormal findings

An elevated WBC count (leukocytosis) commonly signals infection, such as an abscess, meningitis, appendicitis, or tonsillitis. A high count may also result from leukemia and tissue necrosis from burns, MI, or gangrene.

A low WBC count (leukopenia) indicates bone marrow depression that may result from viral infection or from a toxic reaction, such as those that occur after treatment with antineoplastics, ingestion of mercury or other heavy metals, or exposure to benzene or arsenicals. Leukopenia characteristically accompanies influenza, typhoid fever, measles, infectious hepatitis, mononucleosis, and rubella.

White blood cell differential

The WBC differential is used to evaluate the distribution and morphologic features of WBCs, providing more specific information about a patient's immune system than the WBC count alone.

WBCs are classified as one of five major types—neutrophils, eosinophils, basophils, lymphocytes, and monocytes—and the percentage of each type is determined. The differential count is the percentage of each type of WBC in the blood. The total number of each type of WBC is obtained by multiplying the percentage of each type by the total WBC count.

High levels of these leukocytes are associated with various allergic diseases and reactions to parasites. An eosinophil count is sometimes ordered as a follow-up test when the eosinophil level is elevated or depressed.

Purpose

- To evaluate the body's capacity to resist and overcome infection
- To detect and identify various types of leukemia
- To determine the stage and severity of an infection
- To detect allergic reactions and parasitic infections and assess their severity (eosinophil count)
- To distinguish viral infections from bacterial infections
- To monitor the effects of chemotherapeutic agents on the immune system

Patient preparation

- Explain to the patient that this test is used to evaluate the immune system.
- Explain that this test requires a blood sample, and tell the patient when and where it will be taken.
- Notify the laboratory and physician of medications the patient is taking that may affect test results; they may need to be restricted.
- Inform the patient that there is no food or fluid restriction but should refrain from strenuous exercise for 24 hours before the test.

Interpreting WBC differential values

The differential count measures the types of white blood cells (WBCs) as a percentage of the total WBC count (relative value). The absolute value is obtained by multiplying the relative value of each cell type by the total WBC count. The relative and absolute values must be considered to obtain an accurate diagnosis.

For example, consider a patient whose WBC count is 6,000/μl (SI, 6×10^9/L) and whose differential shows 30% (SI, 0.30) neutrophils and 70% (SI, 0.70) lymphocytes. His or her relative lymphocyte count seems high (lymphocytosis), but when this figure is multiplied by his or her WBC count (6,000 × 70% = 4,200 lymphocytes/μl) (SI, 6×10^9/L × 9.79 = 4.2×10^9/L lymphocytes), it is well within the normal range.

However, this patient's neutrophil count (30%) (SI, 0.30) is low; when this figure is multiplied by the WBC count (6,000 × 30% = 1,800 neutrophils/ml) (SI, 6×10^9/L × 0.30 = 1.8×10^9/L neutrophils), the result is a low absolute number, which may mean depressed bone marrow.

The normal percentages of WBC type in adults are:

Neutrophils: 54% to 75% (SI, 0.54 to 0.75)
Eosinophils: 1% to 4% (SI, 0.01 to 0.04)
Basophils: 0% to 1% (SI, 0 to 0.01)
Monocytes: 2% to 8% (SI, 0.02 to 0.08)
Lymphocytes: 25% to 40% (SI, 0.25 to 0.40)

Reference values

For normal values for the five types of WBCs classified in the differential for adults and children, see *Interpreting WBC differential values.* For an accurate diagnosis, differential test results must always be interpreted in relation to the total WBC count.

Abnormal findings

Abnormal differential patterns provide evidence of a wide range of disease states and other conditions.

Selected reference

Fischbach, F. T., & Fischbach, M. A. (2018). *Fischbach's manual of laboratory and diagnostic tests* (10th ed.). Philadelphia, PA: Wolters Kluwer.

5 > Common Disorders

Treating and preventing diseases

Alzheimer's disease

Overview

- Degenerative disorder of the cerebral cortex (especially the frontal lobe). Alzheimer's disease accounts for more than 50% of all cases of dementia.
- Poor prognosis
- No cure or definitive treatment
- May be a late onset
- Stages are:
  - pre-Alzheimer's (stage 1)—often not recognized and individual recognition is variable
  - mild (stage 2)—endures for 2 to 4 years
  - moderate (stage 3)—endures for about 2 years
  - severe (stage 4) endures for about 1.5 years.

Causes

- Unknown

Risk factors

Neurochemical

- Deficiencies of the neurotransmitters
- Genetics
  - Mutation on chromosome 21 causes amyloid plaques, which are considered the hallmark of Alzheimer's

- Health (lifestyle)
  - Heart disease; early-age hypertension; diabetes; smoking; overweight; no physical exercises daily; excessive alcohol; unhealthy diet that is related to too many carbohydrates, high cholesterol, sugar, and soft drinks; acute infections; medications taken for treatment of other medical illnesses side effects

Environmental

- Manganese, lead, and other heavy metal
- Repeated head trauma
- Slow-growing central nervous system (CNS) viruses

Assessment

History

- Obtained from a family member or caregiver
- Insidious onset
- Initial changes almost imperceptible
- Forgetfulness and subtle memory loss
- Recent memory loss
- Difficulty learning and remembering new information
- General deterioration in personal hygiene
- Inability to concentrate
- Tendency to perform repetitive actions and experience restlessness

- Negative personality changes (irritability, depression, paranoia, hostility)
- Nocturnal awakening
- Disorientation
- Suspicious and fearful of imaginary people and situations
- Misperceives own environment
- Misidentifies objects and people
- Complains of stolen or misplaced objects
- Labile emotions
- Mood swings, sudden angry outbursts, and sleep disturbances
- An expression of stare-blank face (Facial expression is like a mask.)
- Withdrawn
- Does not communicate
- Appetite declines significantly to no appetite.
- Inability to chew food or swallow
- Weight loss
- Decreased mobility that declines to immobility

Physical findings
- Impaired sense of smell (usually an early symptom)
- Impaired stereognosis
- Gait disorders
- Tremors
- Loss of recent memory
- Positive snout reflex
- Organic brain disease in adults
- Urinary or fecal incontinence
- Seizures

Diagnostic tests
- Diagnosis is made by exclusion.
- Tests are performed to rule out diseases such as Lewy bodies—a type of dementia similar to Alzheimer's dementia, vitamin or mineral deficiencies.
- Positive diagnosis is made on autopsy.

Imaging
- Positron emission tomography (PET) shows metabolic activity of the cerebral cortex.
- Computed tomography (CT) scan shows excessive and progressive brain atrophy.
- Magnetic resonance imaging (MRI) rules out intracranial lesions.
- Cerebral blood flow studies show abnormalities in blood flow to the brain.

Diagnostic procedures
- Cerebrospinal fluid analysis shows chronic neurologic infection.
- Electroencephalogram evaluates the brain's electrical activity and may show slowing of brain waves in late stages of the disease.

Other
- Neuropsychological tests may show impaired cognitive ability and reasoning.

Treatment
General
- Behavioral interventions (patient-centered or caregiver training) focused on managing cognitive and behavioral changes
- Physical therapy, exercise
- Well-balanced diet (may need to be monitored)
- Safe activities, as tolerated (may need to be monitored)

Medications
- N-methyl-D-aspartate antagonist
- Cerebral vasodilators
- Psychostimulators
- Antidepressants
- Anxiolytics
- Neurolytics
- Anticonvulsants (experimental)
- Anti-inflammatories (experimental)
- Anticholinesterase agents
- Omega-3 fatty acids
- Vitamin E

Nursing interventions

- Check vital signs and note any major changes such as a very low and/or high pulse, respirations, blood pressure—report to health care provider.
- Provide an effective communication system.
- Use soft tones and a slow, calm manner when speaking to the patient.
- Allow the patient sufficient time to answer questions.
- Encourage social activities, as indicated.
- Protect the patient from injury.
- Provide rest periods.
- Provide an exercise program.
- Encourage independence.
- Offer frequent toileting and reinforce the location of the bathroom.
- Assist with hygiene and dressing.
- Observe the skin for bruises, wounds, erythema, or cyanosis.
- Give prescribed drugs.
- Monitor for medication side effects.
- Provide familiar objects to help with orientation and behavior control.
- Monitor fluid intake, nutritional status, and safety.
- Assist with feeding, as needed.

Patient teaching

- Be sure to cover:
  - the disease processes
  - the exercise regimen
  - the importance of cutting food and providing finger foods, if indicated
  - the need to use plates with rim guards, built-up utensils, and cups with lids
  - promotion of independence.
- Refer the patient (and his or her family or caregivers) to the Alzheimer's Association.
- Refer the patient (and his or her family or caregivers) to a local support group.
- Refer the patient (and his or her family or caregivers) to social services for additional support.

Arterial occlusive disease (peripheral artery disease)

Overview

- Obstruction or narrowing of the lumen of arteries
- May affect any artery; commonly affects the aortic, iliac, carotid, vertebral, femoral, popliteal, anterior tibial, posterior tibial, renal, mesenteric, and celiac
- Arterial insufficiency is observed in individuals 50 years and older.
- Prognosis depends on the location of the occlusion and the development of collateral circulation that counteracts reduced blood flow.
- Ninety percent of acute peripheral arterial occlusions occur in the lower extremities.
- More common in men than women and current smokers

Causes

- Atherosclerosis
- Aneurysm
- Immune arteritis
- Embolism
- Dissection of an artery
- Thrombosis
- Thrombophilia
- Thromboangiitis obliterans
- Raynaud's disease
- Fibromuscular disease
- Atheromatous debris (plaques)
- Indwelling arterial catheter
- Direct blunt or penetrating trauma

Risk factors

- Smoking
- Hypertension
- Dyslipidemia
- Diabetes mellitus
- Advanced age
- Sedentary lifestyle
- Metabolic syndrome

Assessment

History

- One or more risk factors
- Intermittent claudication
- Family history of vascular disease
- Pain on resting
- Poor healing of wounds or ulcers
- Toe nails grow poorly
- Poor extremity hair growth
- Impotence
- Dizziness or near syncope
- Nausea
- Fatigue, weakness
- Palpitations
- Symptoms that are seen in a heart attack
- Symptoms of transient ischemic attack

Physical findings

- Trophic changes of the involved arm or leg
- Diminished or absent pulses in the carotid artery, arm, or leg
- Ischemic ulcers
- Pallor with elevation of the arm or leg
- Dependent rubor
- Arterial bruit
- Hypertension
- Pain cramping
- Pallor pale or bluish
- Pulselessness distal to the occlusion
- Paralysis (numbness)
- Paresthesia—prickly/burning/stinging
- Poikilothermy—one extremity is cooler than the other

Diagnostic tests

Imaging

- Arteriography shows the type, location, and degree of obstruction and the establishment of collateral circulation and evaluates arterial anatomy.
- Duplex Doppler ultrasonography shows decreased blood flow distal to the obstruction.
- Magnetic resonance angiography and CT angiography may show arterial abnormalities.

Other

- Segmental limb pressures and pulse volume measurements show the location and severity of the obstruction.
- Ophthalmodynamometry indirectly helps determine the degree of obstruction in the internal carotid artery.
- Electrocardiogram (ECG) and echocardiogram may show cardiovascular disease.

Treatment

General

- Smoking cessation
- Control of hypertension, diabetes, and dyslipidemia
- Foot and leg care
- Weight control
- Low-fat, low-cholesterol, high-fiber diet
- Regular walking program

Medications

- Antiplatelets
- Lipid-lowering agents
- Hypoglycemic agents
- Antihypertensives
- Thrombolytics
- Anticoagulation
- Niacin or vitamin B complex

Surgery

- Embolectomy
- Endarterectomy
- Atherectomy
- Laser angioplasty
- Endovascular stent placement
- Endovascular stent graft
- Percutaneous transluminal angioplasty
- Laser surgery
- Patch arterioplasty
- Bypass graft
- Amputation
- Bowel resection

Nursing interventions

For chronic arterial occlusive disease

- Monitor vital signs.
- Monitor intake and output to check kidney function.
- Use preventive measures, such as minimal pressure mattresses, heel protectors, a foot cradle, or a footboard.
- Avoid restrictive clothing such as antiembolism stockings.
- Give prescribed drugs.
- Allow the patient to express fears and concerns.

For preoperative care during an acute episode

- Assess the patient's circulatory status—distal pulses, skin color, temperature.
- Give prescribed analgesics.
- Give prescribed heparin or thrombolytics.
- Wrap the patient's affected foot in soft cotton batting, and reposition it frequently to prevent pressure on any one area.
- Strictly avoid elevating or applying heat to the affected leg.

For postoperative care

- Watch the patient closely for signs of hemorrhage.
- If the patient has mesenteric artery occlusion, connect a nasogastric (NG) tube to low-intermittent suction.
- Give prescribed analgesics.
- Monitor intake and output (low urine output indicates renal artery damage).
- Assist with early ambulation, but do not allow the patient to sit for an extended period.
- If amputation has occurred, check the stump carefully for drainage and note and record the color and amount of drainage as well as the time.
- Elevate the stump, as ordered.
- Perform neurovascular checks, as ordered.

Patient teaching

- Be sure to cover:
  - the disorder, diagnosis, and treatment
  - medications and potential adverse reactions
  - when to notify the health care provider
  - dietary restrictions
  - the regular exercise programs
  - foot care
  - signs and symptoms of graft occlusion
  - signs and symptoms of arterial insufficiency and occlusion—pain, pallor, pulselessness distal to the occlusion, paralysis, paresthesia, poikilothermy
  - the need to avoid crossing the legs and wearing constrictive clothing or garters
  - modification of risk factors
  - the need to avoid temperature extremes.
- Instruct to keep follow-up appointments with the health care provider
- Refer the patient to a physical and occupational therapist, as indicated.
- Refer the patient to a podiatrist for foot care, as needed.
- Refer the patient to an endocrinologist for glucose control, as indicated.
- Refer the patient to a smoking-cessation program, as indicated.

Asthma

Overview

- A chronic reactive airway disorder that involves episodic, reversible airway obstruction caused by bronchospasms, increased secretion of mucus, and mucosal edema
- Signs and symptoms that range from mild wheezing and dyspnea to life-threatening respiratory failure
- Signs and symptoms of bronchial airway obstruction that may persist between acute episodes

Causes
- Sensitivity to specific external allergens
- Internal, nonallergenic factors

Extrinsic asthma (atopic asthma)
- Pollen
- Animal dander
- House dust or mold
- Kapok or feather pillows
- Food additives that contain sulfites or other sensitizing substances

Intrinsic asthma (nonatopic asthma)
- Emotional stress
- Genetic factors

Bronchoconstriction
- Hereditary predisposition
- Sensitivity to allergens or irritants such as pollutants
- Viral infections
- Drugs, such as aspirin, beta-adrenergic blockers, and nonsteroidal anti-inflammatory drugs (NSAIDs)
- Tartrazine
- Psychological stress
- Cold air
- Exercise

Eosinophilic asthma
- Unusual type
- Inflammation results from eosinophils.
- The initial attack occurs in adult ages 30 to 50 years.

Intermittent asthma
- Mildest asthma
- May have episode zero to twice a week

Persistent asthma
- May be mild, moderate, or severe
- Episodes occur often.

Mild persistent asthma
- Episodes may occur more than twice a week.
- May awaken in the morning with symptoms three or four times a month

Moderate persistent asthma
- Episodes may occur every day.
- Often is awaken several nights in a week with symptoms
- There may be limitations to daily activities.

Severe persistent asthma
- Episodes occur throughout the day, every day, and every night with symptoms.
- May have to be hospitalized due to uncontrolled coughing
- Daily activities are very limited.

Risk/precipitating factors
- Allergens such as cockroaches, dust mites, indoor mold, sprays, perfume
- Smoke from cigarette, fireplace, and smoking products
- Pollution from grass, weeds
- Foods such as shrimp, dried fruits, and beverages that contain sulfites (beer, wine)
- Genetics
- Stress

Assessment
History
- Asthma is commonly preceded by severe respiratory tract infections, especially in adults.
- Irritants, emotional stress, fatigue, endocrine changes, temperature and humidity variations, and exposure to noxious fumes may aggravate asthma attacks.
- An asthma attack may begin dramatically, with simultaneous onset of severe, multiple symptoms, or insidiously, with gradually increasing respiratory distress.

Physical findings
- Visible dyspnea
- Ability to speak only a few words before pausing for breath
- Use of accessory respiratory muscles
- Diaphoresis

- Increased anteroposterior thoracic diameter
- Hyperresonance
- Tachycardia, tachypnea, and mild systolic hypertension
- Inspiratory and expiratory wheezes
- Prolonged expiratory phase of respiration
- Diminished breath sounds
- Cyanosis, confusion, and lethargy, which indicate onset of life-threatening status asthmaticus and respiratory failure

Diagnostic tests

Laboratory

- Arterial blood gas analysis shows hypoxemia.
- Increased serum immunoglobulin (Ig) E levels are caused by an allergic reaction.
- A complete blood count (CBC) with differential shows an increased eosinophil count.
- A peripheral blood test for eosinophil count in patients with eosinophilic asthma

Imaging

- Chest X-rays may show hyperinflation, with areas of focal atelectasis.

Diagnostic procedures

- Pulmonary function tests may show decreased peak flow and forced expiratory volume in 1 second, low-normal or decreased vital capacity, and increased total lung and residual capacities.
- Skin testing may identify specific allergens.
- Bronchial challenge testing shows the clinical significance of allergens that are identified by skin testing.
- Sputum eosinophilic test, fractional exhaled nitric oxide breath test, and serum IgE may identify eosinophilic asthma.

Other

- Pulse oximetry measurements may show decreased oxygen saturation.

Treatment

General

- Identification and avoidance of precipitating factors
- Desensitization to specific antigens
- Establishment and maintenance of a patent airway
- Fluid replacement
- Activity, as tolerated
- In patients who are unresponsive to drug therapy, possible admission for further treatment, which may include intubation or mechanical ventilation

Medications

- Bronchodilators
- Corticosteroids
- Histamine antagonists
- Leukotriene antagonists
- Anticholinergic bronchodilators
- Low-flow oxygen
- Antibiotics
- Trial of heliox (helium-oxygen mixture) before intubation
- I.V. magnesium sulfate (controversial)
- Biologic therapy—made from the products of living organisms or the living organism is used in eosinophilic asthma and is extending to use in all types of asthma.
  - Omalizumab (Xolair)
  - Mepolizumab (Nucala)
  - Reslizumab (Cinqair)
  - Benralizumab (Fasenra)

Nursing interventions

- Monitor vital signs.
- Give prescribed drugs.
- Place the patient in high Fowler's position.
- Encourage pursed-lip and diaphragmatic breathing.

- Administer prescribed humidified oxygen.
- Adjust oxygen administration according to the patient's vital signs, pulse oximetry, and arterial blood gas values.
- Assist with intubation and mechanical ventilation, if appropriate.
- Perform postural drainage and chest percussion, if tolerated.
- Suction an intubated patient, as needed.
- Treat the patient's dehydration with I.V. or oral fluids, as tolerated.
- Anticipate bronchoscopy or bronchial lavage.
- Keep the room temperature comfortable.
- Use an air conditioner or a fan in hot, humid weather.

Patient teaching

- Be sure to cover:
  - the disorder, diagnosis, and treatment
  - medications and potential adverse reactions
  - when to notify the health care provider
  - keeping of follow-up visits with health care provider
  - the importance of avoiding known allergens and irritants
  - the use of a metered-dose inhaler or dry powder inhaler
  - pursed-lip and diaphragmatic breathing
  - the use of a peak flow meter
  - effective coughing techniques
  - the importance of maintaining adequate hydration.
  - importance of getting annual flu vaccine
- Refer the patient to a local asthma support group.

Breast cancer

Overview

- Malignant proliferation of the epithelial cells that line the ducts or lobules of the breast
- Invasive or noninvasive
- Prognosis considerably affected by early detection and treatment
- Refer to the American Cancer Society, American College of Obstetricians and Gynecologists, and/or the U.S. Preventive Services Task Force's (USPSTF) recommendation regarding when to begin screening and frequency.

Causes

- Unknown

Risk factors

- Family history of breast cancer, particularly in first-degree relatives, including the patient's parents and siblings
- Positive results on tests for genetic mutations (BRCA 1 and BRCA 2)
- Older than age 45 and premenopausal
- Long menstrual cycles
- Early onset of menses, late menopause
- Nulliparous or first pregnancy after age 30
- High-fat diet
- History of endometrial or ovarian cancer
- History of unilateral breast cancer
- Radiation exposure
- Estrogen therapy
- Antihypertensive therapy
- Alcohol or tobacco use
- Preexisting fibrocystic disease
- Dense breast tissue
- Breast implants—textured surface implants or smooth surfaces
- Obesity

Men

- Klinefelter syndrome—small testicles and infertile
- Higher levels of estrogen and a decrease in androgen levels
- Gynecomastia
- Radiation exposure
- Estrogen treatment in transgender and transsexual individuals
- Undescended testicle
- Bilateral orchiectomy
- Mumps during the adult years
- Female family members with a history of breast cancer
- Positive results on tests for genetic mutations of (BRCA 2) than with (BRCA 1)

 ALERT

- Breast cancer is the leading cause of cancer deaths among women ages 35 to 54.
- Breast cancer is rare in men, but when it occurs, it is often diagnosed between ages 60 and 70.

Note: Findings, diagnostic tests, and treatment are the same in females and males.

Assessment

History

- Detection of a painless lump or mass in the breast
- Edematous breast
- Detection of lump in the axilla
- Change in breast tissue
- History of risk factors

Physical findings

- Clear, milky, or bloody nipple discharge; nipple retraction; scaly skin around the nipple; and skin changes, such as dimpling (peau d'orange) or inflammation
- Change in size or shape of breast
- Edema of the arm

- Hard lump, mass, or thickening of breast tissue
- Lymphadenopathy

Diagnostic tests

Laboratory

- Elevated alkaline phosphatase levels and liver function test results may indicate distant metastases.
- A hormonal receptor assay determines whether the tumor is estrogen dependent or progesterone dependent and guides decisions to use therapy that blocks the action of the hormone estrogen that supports tumor growth.
- Cytologic examination—nipple discharge test

Imaging

- Mammography can show a tumor that is too small to palpate.
- Ultrasonography can distinguish between a fluid-filled cyst and a solid mass.
- MRI can show very small tumors.
- Chest X-rays can show metastases to the lung.
- Scans of the bone, brain, liver, and other organs can detect distant metastases.

Diagnostic procedures

- Fine-needle aspiration and excisional biopsy of the breasts and/lymph node provide cells for histologic examination that may confirm the diagnosis.

Treatment

General

- The choice of treatment usually depends on the stage and type of disease, the woman's age and menopausal status, and the disfiguring effects of surgery.
- Therapy may include any combination of surgery, radiation therapy, chemotherapy, and hormone therapy, and targeted therapy.
- Some patients benefit from preoperative breast irradiation.

- The patient may require arm-stretching exercises after surgery.
- The patient may need primary radiation therapy.

Medications

- Chemotherapy such as a combination of drugs, including cyclophosphamide, fluorouracil, methotrexate, doxorubicin, vincristine, paclitaxel, and prednisone
- Antiestrogen therapy, such as tamoxifen or anastrozole
- Hormonal therapy, including estrogen, progesterone, androgen, or antiandrogen aminoglutethimide therapy
- Biologic or targeting treatment, such as trastuzumab, lapatinib, bevacizumab

Surgery

- Lumpectomy
- Partial, total, or modified radical mastectomy
- Sentinel node biopsy or axillary node dissection
- Reconstruction

Nursing interventions

- Provide information about the disease process, diagnostic tests, and treatment.
- Give prescribed drugs.
- Provide emotional support.
- Monitor for fatigue, infection, and adverse effects of drugs.

Patient teaching

- Be sure to cover:
  – all procedures and treatments
  – activities or exercises that promote healing
  – breast self-examination
  – the risks and the signs and symptoms of recurrence
  – the need to avoid venipuncture or blood pressure monitoring on the affected arm.
- Refer the patient to local and national support groups.

Bronchitis, chronic

Overview

- Inflammation of the lining of the bronchial tubes
- A form of chronic obstructive pulmonary disease
- Characterized by excessive production of tracheobronchial mucus with a cough for at least 3 months each year for 2 consecutive years
- Severity linked to the amount of cigarette smoke or other pollutants inhaled and the duration of inhalation
- Exacerbation of the cough and related symptoms by respiratory tract infections
- Development of significant airway obstruction in few patients with chronic bronchitis

Causes

- Cigarette smoking is the main cause.
- Possible genetic predisposition
- Environmental pollution
- Exposure to organic or inorganic dusts and noxious gas

Assessment

History

- Longtime smoker
- Frequent upper respiratory tract infections
- Productive cough
- Exertional dyspnea
- Cough, initially prevalent in winter, but gradually becoming year-round
- Increasingly severe coughing episodes
- Worsening dyspnea

Physical findings

- Cough that produces copious gray, white, or yellow sputum
- Cyanosis, also called a blue bloater
- Use of accessory respiratory muscles
- Tachypnea

- Substantial weight gain
- Pedal edema
- Jugular vein distention
- Wheezing
- Prolonged expiratory time
- Rhonchi

Diagnostic tests

Laboratory

- Arterial blood gas analysis shows decreased partial pressure of oxygen and normal or increased partial pressure of carbon dioxide.
- Sputum culture shows many micro-organisms and neutrophils.

Imaging

- Chest X-ray may show hyperinflation and increased bronchovascular markings.

Diagnostic procedures

- Pulmonary function test results show increased residual volume, decreased vital capacity and forced expiratory flow, and normal static compliance and diffusing capacity.
- Spirometry for the amount of air inhaled and exhaled

Other

- ECG may show atrial arrhythmias; peaked P waves in leads II, III, and aV_F; and right ventricular hypertrophy.

Treatment

General

- Smoking cessation
- Avoidance of air pollutants
- Chest physiotherapy
- Ultrasonic or mechanical nebulizer treatments
- Adequate fluid intake
- High-calorie, protein-rich diet
- Rest, fluids, cough
- Activity, as tolerated, with frequent rest periods

Medications

- Oxygen
- Antibiotics, if fever occurs
- Bronchodilators
- Corticosteroids
- Diuretics

Surgery

- Tracheostomy in advanced disease

Nursing interventions

- Monitor vital signs.
- Give prescribed drugs.
- Encourage the patient to express his or her fears and concerns.
- Include the patient and his or her family in care decisions.
- Perform chest physiotherapy.
- Provide a high-calorie, protein-rich diet.
- Offer small, frequent meals.
- Encourage energy-conservation techniques.
- Ensure adequate oral fluid intake.
- Provide frequent mouth care.
- Encourage daily activity.
- Provide diversional activities, as appropriate.
- Provide frequent rest periods.

Patient teaching

- Be sure to cover:
  - the disorder, diagnosis, and treatment
  - medications and possible adverse reactions
  - when to notify the health care provider
  - infection control practices
  - the importance of influenza and pneumococcus immunizations
  - the importance of home oxygen therapy, if required, including a demonstration, if needed
  - postural drainage and chest percussion
  - coughing and deep-breathing exercises
  - inhaler use
  - high-calorie, protein-rich meals

– adequate hydration
– avoidance of inhaled irritants
– prevention of bronchospasm
– exercise, as indicated.
- Refer the patient to a smoking-cessation program, if indicated.
- Refer the patient to the American Lung Association for information and support.

Colorectal cancer

Overview

- Malignant tumors of the colon or rectum are almost always adeno-carcinomas (about half are sessile lesions of the rectosigmoid area; all others are polypoid lesions).
- Slow progression
- Five-year survival rate of 50%; potentially curable in 75% of patients if early diagnosis allows resection before involvement of nodes
- Third most common type of cancer in Europe and North America

Causes

- Unknown

Risk factors

- Excessive intake of saturated animal fat
- Smoking
- Older than age 50
- Obesity
- History of ulcerative colitis
- History of Crohn's disease
- History of familial adenomatous polyposis, or Lynch syndrome (hereditary nonpolyposis colon cancer)
- Family history of colon cancer, rectal cancer
- High-protein, low-fiber diet
- Excessive alcohol intake
- Diabetes mellitus type 2
- Lack of physical activity

- Cooking meats at high temperatures (frying, grilling, broiling)
- Previous radiation to the abdomen or pelvis to treat prior cancer

Assessment

History

- Tumors of the right side of the colon: No signs and symptoms in the early stages because stool is liquid in that part of the colon.
- Black, tarry stools
- Manifested as weakness, fatigue
- Abdominal pain, aching, pressure, or dull cramps
- Weakness, chronic fatigue
- Diarrhea, constipation, or obstipation (change in bowel pattern)
- Anorexia (due to early satiety
- Weight loss that is unintentional, nausea, and vomiting
- Rectal bleeding
- Intermittent abdominal fullness
- Rectal pressure
- Urgent need to defecate on arising

Physical findings

- Abdominal distention or visible masses
- Enlarged abdominal veins
- Enlarged inguinal and supraclavicular nodes
- Abnormal bowel sounds
- Abdominal masses (Tumors on the right side usually feel bulky; tumors of the transverse portion are more easily detected.)
- Generalized abdominal tenderness

Diagnostic tests

Laboratory

- Stool DNA test is a multitargeted test that looks for DNA mutations.
- Fecal immunochemical test that looks for blood not readily visible, if positive for blood may indicate precancer

- A fecal occult blood test may show blood in the stools, a warning sign of rectal cancer.
- The carcinoembryonic antigen test permits patient monitoring before and after treatment to detect metastasis or recurrence.

Imaging

- Excretory urography verifies bilateral renal function and allows inspection to detect displacement of the kidneys, ureters, or bladder by a tumor pressing against these structures.
- Barium enema studies use dual contrast of barium and air to show the location of lesions that are not detectable manually or visually. This test should not precede colonoscopy or excretory urography because barium sulfate interferes with these tests.
- A CT scan allows better visualization if a barium enema test yields inconclusive results or if metastasis to the pelvic lymph nodes is suspected.

Diagnostic procedures

- Proctoscopy or sigmoidoscopy permits visualization of the lower gastrointestinal (GI) tract. It can detect up to 76% of colorectal cancers.
- Colonoscopy permits visual inspection and photography of the colon up to the ileocecal valve and provides access for polypectomy and biopsy of suspected lesions.

Other

- Digital rectal examination can be used to detect one-third of malignant tumors of the distal colon and rectum; specifically, it can be used to detect suspicious rectal and perianal lesions.
- *Note*: Refer to American Cancer Society and/or USPSTF recommendation regarding when to begin screening and frequency.

Treatment
General

- Radiation preoperatively and postoperatively to induce tumor regression
- High-fiber diet
- After surgery, avoidance of heavy lifting and contact sports

Medications

- Chemotherapy for metastasis, residual disease, or recurrent inoperable tumor
- Analgesics

Surgery

- Resection or right hemicolectomy for advanced disease (Surgery may include resection of the terminal segment of the ileum, cecum, ascending colon, and right half of the transverse colon with corresponding mesentery.)
- Right colectomy that includes the transverse colon and mesentery corresponding to the midcolic vessels or segmental resection of the transverse colon and associated midcolic vessels
- Resection usually limited to the sigmoid colon and mesentery
- Anterior or low anterior resection (A newer method that uses a stapler allows for much lower resections than were possible in the past.)
- Abdominoperineal resection and permanent sigmoid colostomy required

Nursing interventions

- Provide support and encourage the patient to express his or her concerns.
- Give prescribed drugs.

Postoperative

- Vital signs
- Intake and output
- Hydration and nutritional status
- Monitor for hemorrhage.

- Electrolyte levels
- Wound site
- Postoperative complications
- Bowel function
- Pain control
- Psychological status

Patient teaching

- Be sure to cover:
  - the disease process, treatment, and postoperative course
  - stoma care
  - the need to avoid heavy lifting
  - the need to keep follow-up appointments
  - risk factors and signs of reoccurrence.
- Refer the patient to resource and support services.

Coronary artery disease

Overview

- Heart disease that results from narrowing and hardening of the coronary arteries over time as a result of atherosclerosis
- Primary effect: loss of oxygen and nutrients to myocardial tissue because of decreased coronary blood flow

Causes

- Atherosclerosis
- Dissecting aneurysm
- Infectious vasculitis
- Syphilis
- Congenital defects
- Coronary artery spasm

Risk factors

- Family history
- Increasing age
- Gender
- Race
- High cholesterol level
- Smoking
- Insulin resistance
- Prediabetes
- Diabetes
- Hypertension
- Hormonal contraceptives
- Obesity
- Sedentary lifestyle
- Stress
- Increased homocysteine levels
- Increased levels of C-reactive protein (CRP)
- Poor diet
- Sleep apnea
- Preeclampsia
- Postmenopause

Assessment

History

- Angina that may radiate to the left arm, neck, jaw, or shoulder blade
- Angina that commonly occurs after physical exertion but may also follow emotional excitement, exposure to cold, or a large meal
- May develop during sleep (Symptoms wake the patient.)
- Nausea
- Vomiting
- Fainting
- Sweating
- Fatigue
- Shortness of breath
- Palpitations
- Stable angina (predictable and relieved by rest or nitrates)
- Unstable angina (increased frequency and duration, more easily induced, generally indicates extensive or worsening disease and, untreated, may progress to myocardial infarction [MI])
- Crescendo angina (effort-induced pain that occurs with increasing frequency and with decreasing provocation)
- Prinzmetal's angina or variant angina pectoris (severe, noneffort-produced pain that occurs at rest without provocation)

Physical findings

- Cool extremities
- Xanthoma
- Arteriovenous nicking of the eye
- Obesity
- Hypertension
- Positive Levine's sign (holding the fist to the chest)
- Decreased or absent peripheral pulses

Diagnostic tests

Laboratory

- CBC
- Comprehensive metabolic panel (CMP)
- Lipid panel

Imaging

- Chest X-ray shows heart failure signs.
- Myocardial perfusion imaging with thallium 201 during treadmill exercise shows ischemic areas of the myocardium. These are visualized as "cold spots."
- Pharmacologic myocardial perfusion imaging in arteries with stenosis shows a decrease in blood flow that is proportional to the percentage of occlusion.
- Multiple-gated acquisition scanning shows cardiac wall motion and reflects injury to cardiac tissue.

Diagnostic procedures

- Electrocardiographic findings may be normal between anginal episodes. During angina, the findings may show ischemic changes.
- Exercise testing may be performed to detect ST-segment changes during exercise, which indicate ischemia, and to determine a safe exercise prescription.
- Coronary angiography shows the location and degree of coronary artery stenosis or obstruction, the collateral circulation, and the condition of the artery beyond the narrowing.

- Stress echocardiography may show abnormal wall motion.
- Cardiac catheterization shows blood flow passage in the heart and blood vessels and if there is coronary artery disease (CAD), heat valve disease, or disease of the aorta.

Treatment

General

- Stress reduction techniques are essential, especially if known stressors precipitate pain.
- Lifestyle modifications, such as smoking cessation and maintaining ideal body weight
- Low-fat, low-sodium diet
- Possible restrictions on the patient's activity
- Regular exercise
- Enhanced external counter pulsation whereby inflation and deflation of cuffs on the legs enhance blood flow to the coronary arteries.
- Angiogenesis which refers to the use of stem cells in damage heart tissue

Medications

- Aspirin
- Nitrates
- Beta blockers
- Calcium channel blockers
- Antiplatelets
- Antilipemics
- Antihypertensives
- Angiotensin-converting enzyme inhibitors
- Vitamins

Surgery

- Coronary artery bypass graft
- "Keyhole," or minimally invasive surgery
- Angioplasty
- Placement of an endovascular stent
- Laser angioplasty
- Atherectomy

Nursing interventions

- Monitor vital signs.
- Ask the patient to grade the severity of his or her pain on a scale of 1 to 10, with 10 being the most severe.
- Keep nitroglycerin available for immediate use. Instruct the patient to call the nurse immediately whenever he or she feels pain and before he or she takes nitroglycerin.
- Monitor the patient's ECG for ST-T segment changes.
- Observe the patient for signs and symptoms that may signify worsening of his or her condition.
- Perform vigorous chest physiotherapy and guide the patient in pulmonary self-care.
- Monitor abnormal bleeding and distal pulses after interventions or procedures.
- Monitor drainage of the chest tube after surgery.

Patient teaching

- Be sure to cover:
  - risk factors for CAD
  - the need to avoid activities that precipitate episodes of pain
  - effective coping mechanisms for dealing with stress
  - the need to follow the prescribed drug regimen and side effects
  - the importance of following a low-sodium, low-calorie, and low-cholesterol diet, as indicated
  - the importance of regular, moderate exercise, as indicated
  - age-specific immunizations, such as flu and pneumonia.
- Refer the patient to a weight-loss program, if needed.
- Refer the patient to a smoking-cessation program, if needed.
- Refer the patient to a cardiac rehabilitation program, if indicated.

Diabetes mellitus

Overview

- Chronic disease of absolute or relative insulin deficiency or resistance
- Characterized by disturbances in the metabolism of carbohydrates, proteins, and fats
- Two primary forms
  - Type 1, which is characterized by absolute insufficiency of insulin
  - Type 2, which is characterized by insulin resistance with varying degrees of insulin secretory defects
- Other forms
  - Gestational diabetes: an increase in blood sugar levels during pregnancy
  - Secondary diabetes: an increase in blood sugar levels due to damage to the pancreas or by increased resistance to the effects of insulin by medications such as corticosteroids

Causes

- Genetic factors
- Hormonal disturbances: an increase in blood sugar levels by hormones such as growth hormone and cortisol
- Autoimmune disease (type 1)
- Beta cells continuous decline (type 2) as a result of a reduction in insulin secretion per pancreas islet as well as a reduction in the total number of pancreas islets

Risk factors (type 2)

- Family history of diabetes
- Race
- Sedentary lifestyle
- Obesity (body mass index [BMI] $\geq$25 kg/m^2)

- History of gestational diabetes, glucose intolerance, or delivery of a >9-lb (4.1 kg) baby
- High-density lipoprotein (HDL) ≤35 mg/dl (≥0.91 mmol/L) or triglyceride level ≤130 mg/dl (≤3.4mmol/L)
- Hypertension
- Insulin resistance
- Polycystic ovary syndrome
- Diet high in sugar (examples: soft drinks, snacks, desserts, other sweets), carbohydrates
- Age ≥45 years

AGE ALERT

Unless a diabetic woman's glucose levels are well controlled before conception and during pregnancy, her neonate has two to three times the risk of congenital malformations and fetal distress.

Assessment

History

- Polyuria, nocturia
- Dehydration
- Polydipsia
- Dry mucous membranes
- Poor skin turgor
- Weight loss and hunger
- Weakness and fatigue
- Vision changes
- Frequent skin and urinary tract infections
- Frequent vaginal infections
- Dry, itchy skin
- Sexual problems
- Numbness or pain in the hands or feet
- Postprandial feeling of nausea or fullness
- Nocturnal diarrhea
- Nausea and vomiting
- Slow healing wounds

Type 1
- Rapidly developing symptoms
  - Frequent urination
  - Extreme hunger
  - Blurred vision
  - Increased thirst
  - Fatigue and weakness
  - Mood changes and irritability
  - Unintended weight loss

Type 2
- Vague, long-standing symptoms that develop gradually
- Family history of diabetes mellitus
- Pregnancy
- Severe viral infection
- Other endocrine diseases
- Recent stress or trauma
- Use of drugs that increase blood glucose levels

Physical findings

- Retinopathy or cataract formation
- Acanthosis nigricans
- Skin changes, especially on the legs and feet
- Muscle wasting and loss of subcutaneous fat (type 1)
- Obesity, particularly in the abdominal area (type 2)
- Poor skin turgor
- Dry mucous membranes
- Decreased peripheral pulses
- Cool skin temperature
- Diminished deep tendon reflexes
- Orthostatic hypotension
- Characteristic "fruity" breath odor in ketoacidosis
- Possible hypovolemia and shock in ketoacidosis and hyperosmolar hyperglycemic state

Diagnostic tests

Laboratory
- Fasting plasma glucose level is 126 mg/dl or greater on at least two occasions.
- Random blood glucose level is 200 mg/dl or greater along with symptoms of diabetes.

- Two-hour postprandial blood glucose level is 200 mg/dl or greater.
- Glycosylated hemoglobin (hemoglobin A_{1c}) value is increased above 6.5%.
  - Result is inaccurate in patients with sickle cell disease or anemia.

Diagnostic procedures
- Ophthalmologic examination may show diabetic retinopathy.

Treatment
General
- Exercise and diet control
- Tight glycemic control for prevention of complications
- Modest calorie restriction for weight loss or maintenance
- American Diabetes Association recommendations to reach target glucose, hemoglobin A_{1c} lipid, and blood pressure levels
- Regular aerobic exercise
- Management of hypertension

Medications
- Exogenous insulin (type 1 or possibly type 2)
  - Insulin pump
    - Releases a programmed dose of insulin either continuously in small doses (basal) or a bolus dose close to a meal to control the increase level of blood glucose after a meal
  - Inhaled insulin
    - Used in patients with type 1 or type 2 diabetes; not to be used if there are lung disorders such as asthma, chronic obstructive pulmonary disorder, emphysema, is a current smoker or has not stopped smoking in the previous 6 or more months before use of insulin inhalation
- Oral antihyperglycemic drugs (type 2)
  - Alpha-glucosidase inhibitors
  - Biguanides
  - Dipeptidyl peptidase 4 (DPP-4) inhibitors
  - Glucagon-like peptides
  - Meglitinides
  - Sodium-glucose cotransporter 2 inhibitor
  - Sulfonylureas
  - Thiazolidinediones

Surgery
- Bariatric surgery is an alternate treatment option for type 2 diabetics not adequately controlled.
- Pancreas transplantation

Nursing interventions
- Give prescribed medications.
- Give rapidly absorbed carbohydrates for hypoglycemia or, if the patient is unconscious, give glucagon or I.V. dextrose, as ordered.
- Administer I.V. fluids and insulin replacement for hyperglycemic crisis, as ordered.
- Monitor electrolytes and administer replacements, as ordered.
- Provide meticulous skin care, especially to the feet and legs.
- Treat all injuries, cuts, and blisters immediately.
- Avoid constricting hose, slippers, or bed linens.
- Encourage adequate fluid intake.
- Encourage the patient to express his or her feelings.
- Offer emotional support.
- Help the patient to develop effective coping strategies.

Patient teaching
- Be sure to cover:
  - the disorder, diagnosis, and treatment
  - medication and potential adverse reactions
  - when to notify the health care provider
  - the prescribed meal plans
  - the prescribed exercise program

– signs and symptoms of infection, hypoglycemia, hyperglycemia, and diabetic neuropathy
– self-monitoring of blood glucose level
– complications of hyperglycemia
– daily foot care
– the importance of annual regular ophthalmologic examinations
– safety precautions, such as not walking barefoot at any time, including in the home
– management of diabetes during illness.
• Refer the patient to a dietitian.
• Refer the patient to a podiatrist if indicated.
• Refer the patient to an ophthalmologist.
• Refer adult diabetic patients who are planning families for preconception counseling.
• Refer the patient to the Juvenile Diabetes Research Foundation, the American Association of Diabetes Educators, and the American Diabetes Association, as appropriate, to obtain additional information.

Emphysema

Overview

• Chronic lung disease characterized by permanent enlargement of air spaces distal to the terminal bronchioles and by exertional dyspnea
• One of several diseases usually labeled collectively as chronic obstructive pulmonary disease or chronic obstructive lung disease

Causes

• Genetic deficiency of alpha$_1$-antitrypsin
• Cigarette smoking
• Air pollution

Assessment

History

• Smoking
• Shortness of breath
• Chronic cough
• Anorexia and weight loss
• Malaise

Physical findings

• Barrel chest
• Pursed-lip breathing—hallmark sign
• Use of accessory muscles
• Cyanosis
• Clubbed fingers and toes
• Tachypnea
• Decreased tactile fremitus
• Decreased chest expansion
• Hyperresonance
• Decreased breath sounds
• Crackles
• Inspiratory wheeze
• Prolonged expiratory phase with grunting respirations
• Distant heart sounds

Diagnostic tests

Laboratory

• Arterial blood gas analysis shows decreased partial pressure of oxygen; the partial pressure of carbon dioxide is normal until late in the course of disease.
• The red blood cell (RBC) count shows an increased hemoglobin level late in the course of disease.
• White blood cell count is needed for recognition of possible infection.

Imaging

• Chest X-ray may show:
– a flattened diaphragm
– reduced vascular markings at the lung periphery
– over aeration of the lungs
– a vertical heart
– enlarged anteroposterior chest diameter
– a large retrosternal air space.

Diagnostic procedures
- Pulmonary function tests typically show:
  – increased residual volume and total lung capacity
  – reduced diffusing capacity
  – increased inspiratory flow.
- ECG may show tall, symmetrical P waves in leads II, III, and aV_F; a vertical QRS axis; and signs of right ventricular hypertrophy late in the course of disease.

Treatment
General
- Chest physiotherapy
- Possible transtracheal catheterization and home oxygen therapy
- Adequate hydration
- High-protein, high-calorie diet
- Activity, as tolerated
- Smoking cessation

Medications
- Bronchodilators
- Anticholinergics
- Mucolytics
- Corticosteroids
- Antibiotics
- Oxygen

Surgery
- Insertion of a chest tube for pneumothorax
- Lung volume reduction surgery for patients who meet criteria
- Lung transplant

Nursing interventions
- Monitor vital signs.
- Monitor oxygen saturation.
- Give prescribed drugs.
- Provide supportive care.
- Help the patient adjust to lifestyle changes that are necessitated by a chronic illness.
- Encourage the patient to express his or her fears and concerns.
- Perform chest physiotherapy.

- Provide a high-calorie, protein-rich diet.
- Give small, frequent meals.
- Encourage daily activity and diversional activities.
- Provide frequent rest periods.

Patient teaching
- Be sure to cover:
  – the disorder, diagnosis, and treatment
  – medication and potential adverse reactions
  – when to notify the health care provider
  – the importance of avoiding smoking and areas where smoking is permitted
  – the need to avoid crowds and people with known infections
  – home oxygen therapy, if indicated
  – transtracheal catheter care, if needed
  – coughing and deep-breathing exercises
  – the proper use of handheld inhalers
  – the importance of a high-calorie, protein-rich diet
  – adequate oral fluid intake
  – avoidance of respiratory irritants
  – signs and symptoms of pneumothorax.

 ALERT

Urge the patient to notify the health care provider if he or she has sudden onset of worsening dyspnea or sharp pleuritic chest pain that is exacerbated by chest movement, breathing, or coughing.

- Refer the patient to a smoking-cessation program, if indicated.
- Refer the patient for influenza and pneumococcal pneumonia immunizations, as needed.
- Refer the family of a patient with familial emphysema for screening for alpha$_1$-antitrypsin deficiency.

Gastroenteritis

Overview

- Self-limiting inflammation of the stomach and small or large intestine
- Intestinal flu, traveler's diarrhea, viral enteritis, and food poisoning
- Eosinophilic allergy

Causes

- Bacteria, such as *Staphylococcus aureus*, *Salmonella*, *Shigella*, *Clostridium botulinum*, *Clostridium perfringens*, and *Escherichia coli*
- Amoebae, especially *Entamoeba histolytica*
- Parasites, such as *Ascaris*, *Enterobius*, and *Trichinella spiralis*
- Viruses, such as noroviruses, echoviruses, and coxsackieviruses
- Ingestion of toxins, such as poisonous plants and toadstools
- Drug reactions from antibiotics
- A high concentration of eosinophils in the mucosal lining of the stomach, esophagus, and small intestine causing food allergy response
- Food allergens—shellfish, wheat, egg, cow's milk
- Enzyme deficiencies
- Contact with an infected individual

Assessment

History

- Acute onset of diarrhea
- Abdominal pain and discomfort
- Nausea and vomiting
- Exposure to contaminated food
- Recent travel
- Malaise and fatigue
- Dysphagia, heartburn, anorexia, and weight loss if eosinophilic origin

Physical findings

- Slight abdominal distention
- Poor skin turgor (with dehydration)
- Hyperactive bowel sounds
- Decreased blood pressure

Diagnostic tests

Laboratory

- Gram stain, stool culture (by direct rectal swab), or blood culture shows the causative agent.

Treatment

General

- Supportive treatment for headaches, nausea, vomiting, and diarrhea
- Rehydration
- Initially, clear liquids, as tolerated
- Electrolyte solutions
- Avoidance of milk products, citrus fruit, alcohol, sodas, and spicy foods
- Activity, as tolerated (Encourage mobilization.)

Medications

- Antidiarrheal therapy
- Antiemetics
- Antibiotics
- I.V. fluids

Nursing interventions

- Monitor vital signs.
- Hand-washing technique
- Allow uninterrupted rest periods.
- Replace lost fluids and electrolytes through diet or I.V. fluids.
- Give prescribed drugs.
- Dietary restrictions, as indicated

Patient teaching

- Be sure to cover:
  - the disorder, diagnosis, and treatment
  - dietary modifications
  - all prescribed drugs, including administration and possible adverse effects
  - preventive measures
  - how to perform warm sitz baths three times per day to relieve anal irritation.

Gastroesophageal reflux disease

Overview

- Backflow of gastric or duodenal contents, or both, into the esophagus and past the lower esophageal sphincter (LES), without associated belching or vomiting
- Reflux of gastric acid, causing acute epigastric pain, usually after a meal
- Commonly called heartburn
- Also called GERD

Causes

- Pyloric surgery (alteration or removal of the pylorus), which allows reflux of bile or pancreatic juice
- Hiatal hernia with an incompetent sphincter
- Any condition or position that increases intra-abdominal pressure

Risk factors

- Any agent that lowers LES pressure: acidic and fatty food, alcohol, cigarettes, anticholinergics (atropine, belladonna, propantheline) or other drugs (morphine, diazepam, calcium channel blockers, meperidine)
- NG intubation for more than 4 days
- Obesity
- Pregnancy

Assessment

History

- Minimal or no symptoms in one-third of patients
- Heartburn that typically occurs 1½ to 2 hours after eating
- Heartburn that worsens with vigorous exercise, bending, lying down, wearing tight clothing, coughing, constipation, or obesity
- Relief obtained by using antacids or sitting upright

- Regurgitation without associated nausea or belching
- Sensation of accumulation of fluid in the throat without a sour or bitter taste
- Chronic pain radiating to the neck, jaws, and arms that may mimic angina pectoris
- Nocturnal hypersalivation and wheezing
- Cough
- Dysphagia
- Hiccups

Physical findings

- Odynophagia (sharp substernal pain on swallowing), possibly followed by a dull substernal ache
- Bright red or dark brown blood in the vomitus
- Laryngitis and morning hoarseness
- Chronic cough

Diagnostic tests

Imaging

- Upper endoscopy to examine the lining of the esophagus, stomach, duodenum
- Barium swallow with fluoroscopy shows evidence of recurrent reflux.

Diagnostic procedures

- An esophageal acidity test shows the degree of gastroesophageal reflux.
- Gastroesophageal scintillation testing shows reflux.
- Esophageal manometry shows abnormal LES pressure and sphincter incompetence.
- The result of an acid perfusion (Bernstein) test confirms esophagitis.
- The results of esophagoscopy and biopsy confirm pathologic changes in the mucosa.

Treatment

General

- Modification of lifestyle
- Positional therapy

Factors affecting LES pressure

Various dietary and lifestyle factors can increase or decrease lower esophageal sphincter (LES) pressure. Take these factors into account when you plan the patient's treatment program.

Factors that increase LES pressure	Factors that decrease LES pressure
• Protein	• Fat
• Carbohydrates	• Whole milk
• Nonfat milk	• Orange juice
• Low-dose ethanol	• Tomatoes
	• Antiflatulent (simethicone)
	• Chocolate
	• High-dose ethanol
	• Cigarette smoking
	• Lying on the right or left side
	• Sitting

- Removal of the cause
- Weight reduction, if appropriate
- Avoidance of dietary causes
- Avoidance of eating 2 hours before sleep (See *Factors affecting LES pressure*.)
- Parenteral nutrition or tube feedings
- No activity restrictions for medical treatment
- Lifting restrictions for surgical treatment

Medications

- Antacids
- Cholinergics
- Histamine-2 receptor antagonists
- Proton pump inhibitors (PPIs)

Surgery

- Hiatal hernia repair
- Vagotomy or pyloroplasty
- Esophagectomy

Nursing interventions

- Monitor vital signs.
- Offer emotional and psychological support.

- Upright position for 2 hours after all meals
- Assist with diet modification.
- Perform chest physiotherapy.
- Use semi-Fowler's position for the patient with an NG tube.

Patient teaching

- Be sure to cover:
  - the disorder, diagnosis, and treatment
  - the causes of GERD
  - the prescribed antireflux regimen of medication, diet, and positional therapy
  - development of a dietary plan
  - the time of the last meal of the day before going to sleep
  - wearing loose fitting cloths
  - no smoking
  - the need to identify situations or activities that increase intra-abdominal pressure
  - the need to avoid substances that reduce sphincter control
  - signs and symptoms to watch for and report.

Heart failure

Overview

- Buildup of fluid in the heart that occurs when the myocardium cannot provide sufficient cardiac output
- Usually occurs in a damaged left ventricle but may occur in the right ventricle primarily or secondary to left-sided heart failure

Causes

- Mitral stenosis secondary to rheumatic heart disease, constrictive pericarditis, or atrial fibrillation
- Mitral or aortic insufficiency
- Arrhythmias
- Hypertension
- Atherosclerosis with MI
- Myocarditis
- Ventricular and atrial septal defects
- Constrictive pericarditis
- Pregnancy
- Thyrotoxicosis
- Pulmonary embolism
- Infections
- Anemia
- Emotional stress
- Increased intake of salt or water
- Diabetes
- Smoking
- Alcohol abuse
- Illegal drugs use and abuse such as cocaine
- HIV/AIDS
- Too much vitamin E
- Radiation therapy/chemotherapy

Assessment

History

- A disorder or condition that can precipitate heart failure
- Dyspnea or paroxysmal nocturnal dyspnea
- Peripheral edema
- Fatigue
- Weakness
- Insomnia
- Anorexia
- Nausea
- Sense of abdominal fullness (particularly in right-sided heart failure)
- Substance abuse (alcohol, illegal drugs, tobacco of any type/method)
- Obesity
- Congenital heart defects
- Common in 65-year-olds and older
- Family history

Physical findings

- Cough that produces pink, frothy sputum, worse at night or when lying down
- Cyanosis of the lips and nail beds
- Pale, cool, clammy skin
- Diaphoresis
- Distention of the jugular veins
- Ascites
- Tachycardia
- Pulsus alternans
- Hepatomegaly and, possibly, splenomegaly
- Decreased pulse pressure
- S_3 and S_4 heart sounds
- Moist, bibasilar crackles, rhonchi, and expiratory wheezing
- Decreased pulse oximetry
- Fatigue
- Peripheral edema
- Decreased urinary output

Diagnostic tests

Laboratory

- B-type natriuretic peptide (BNP) immunoassay value is elevated.

Imaging

- Chest X-rays show increased pulmonary vascular markings, interstitial edema, or pleural effusion, and cardiomegaly.

Diagnostic procedures

- ECG shows heart strain, enlargement, or ischemia. It may also show atrial enlargement or fibrillation, tachycardia, or extrasystole.

- Pulmonary artery pressure monitoring typically shows elevated pulmonary artery and pulmonary artery wedge pressures, left ventricular end-diastolic pressure in left-sided heart failure, and elevated right atrial or central venous pressure in right-sided heart failure.
- Nuclear heart scan—use of radioactive tracer substance to show healthy and damaged parts of the heart
- PET scan shows chemistry activity in all areas of the heart to determine adequacy of blood flow to all areas of the heart.
- Cardiac catheterization shows the intended function of the coronary arteries.
- Stress test assesses, with exercise, how hard the heart is working and the rate and the rhythm of the heart during exercise.
- Cardiac MRI shows the function of the heart and damaged major blood vessels.

Treatment

General

- Antiembolism stockings
- Elevation of the legs
- Sodium-restricted diet
- Fluid restriction
- Calorie restriction, if indicated
- Low-fat diet, if indicated
- Decrease added sugar
- Walking program
- Activity, as tolerated
- Limit alcohol intake, if applicable
- Tobacco cessation, if applicable

Medications

- Diuretics
- Oxygen
- Inotropic drugs
- Vasodilators
- Angiotensin-converting enzyme inhibitors
- Angiotensin receptor blockers
- Cardiac glycosides
- Potassium supplements
- Beta-adrenergic blockers
- Anticoagulants
- Statins
- Angiotensin-receptor neprilysin inhibitors
- Calcium channel blockers

Surgery

- For valvular dysfunction with recurrent acute heart failure, surgical replacement
- Heart transplantation
- Placement of a ventricular assist device
- Placement of a stent
- Cardiac resynchronization therapy device (pace maker) allows both sides of the heart to pump at the same time.

Nursing interventions

- Monitor vital signs.
- Monitor intake and output.
- Monitor laboratory values.
- Place the patient in Fowler's position, and give supplemental oxygen.
- Provide continuous cardiac monitoring during the acute and advanced stages of disease.
- Assist the patient with range-of-motion exercises.
- Apply antiembolism stockings. Check for calf pain and tenderness.
- Monitor the patient's weight daily to detect peripheral edema and other signs and symptoms of fluid overload.

Patient teaching

- Be sure to cover:
  - the disorder, diagnosis, and treatment
  - signs and symptoms of worsening heart failure
  - when to notify the health care provider
  - importance of keeping appointments with the health care provider

– the maintenance of a current list of medications including vitamins and minerals, indicate date added and change in frequency, dosage, and/or route
– the need to avoid high-sodium foods
– the need to avoid fatigue
– instructions about fluid restrictions
– the need for the patient to weigh himself or herself every morning at the same time, before eating and after urinating; to keep a record of his or her weight; and to report a weight gain of 3 to 5 lb (1.4 to 2.3 kg) in 1 week
– the importance of smoking cessation, if appropriate
– weight reduction, as needed
– annual flu vaccine and pneumonia vaccine, as indicated
– medication dosage, administration, potential adverse effects, and monitoring needs.
• Encourage follow-up care.
• Refer the patient to a smoking-cessation program, if appropriate.

Hepatitis, viral

Overview

• Infection and inflammation of the liver caused by a virus
• Types recognized: A, B, C
• Marked by hepatic cell destruction, necrosis, and autolysis, leading to anorexia, jaundice, and hepatomegaly
• In most patients, eventual regeneration of hepatic cells, with little or no residual damage, allowing recovery
• Complications more likely with advanced age and serious underlying disorders
• Poor prognosis if edema and hepatic encephalopathy develop

Causes

• Infection with the causative virus for each of the six major forms

Type A

• Transmission by the fecal-oral or parenteral route or touching contaminated objects
• Ingestion of contaminated food, milk, or water

Type B

• Transmission by contact with contaminated human blood via percutaneous or mucosal contact, secretions, and stools and poor infection control in health care facilities; sexual contact; blood transfusion; tattooing; body piercing; the sharing of personal items such as tooth brushes, razors, needles and/or syringes, needle sticks; at birth of infected mother

Type C

• Transmission primarily by sharing of syringes, needles by I.V. drug users, through blood transfusions, hemodialysis, needle sticks, sexual contact, or through tattoo needles, poor infection control in health care facilities, at birth of infected mother

Assessment

History

• Many people do not have symptoms.
• Individuals who do have symptoms experience a low-grade fever, loss of appetite, sudden nausea and vomiting, fatigue, abdominal pain most often in the upper left quadrant with hepatitis A.
• No signs or symptoms of disease in 50% to 60% of people with hepatitis B
• No signs or symptoms of disease in 80% of people with hepatitis C
• Revelation of a source of transmission
• Clinical characteristics are the same for all types of acute viral hepatitis.

Prodromal stage

- Fatigue and generalized malaise
- Anorexia and mild weight loss
- Depression
- Headache and photophobia
- Weakness
- Arthralgia and myalgia (hepatitis B)
- Nausea and vomiting
- Changes in the senses of taste and smell

Clinical jaundice stage

- Pruritus
- Abdominal pain or tenderness
- Indigestion
- Anorexia
- Possible jaundice of the sclerae, mucous membranes, and skin
- Diarrhea

Posticteric stage

- Most symptoms decreasing

Physical findings

Prodromal stage

- Fever (100° to 102° F [37.8° to 38.9° C])
- Dark urine
- Clay-colored stools

Clinical jaundice stage

- Rashes, erythematous patches, or hives
- Abdominal tenderness in the right upper quadrant
- Tender, enlarged liver
- Splenomegaly
- Cervical adenopathy

Posticteric stage

- Decrease in liver enlargement

Diagnostic tests

Laboratory

- In patients with suspected viral hepatitis, a hepatitis profile is routinely performed. The result identifies antibodies specific to the causative virus and establishes the type of hepatitis:
  - Type A: an antibody to hepatitis A confirms the diagnosis; positive IgM antibody

  - Type B: Hepatitis B surface antigens and hepatitis B antibodies confirm the diagnosis.
  - Type C: The diagnosis depends on serologic testing for the specific antibody 1 or more months after the onset of acute illness. Until then, the diagnosis is established principally by obtaining negative test results for hepatitis A and B.

- Additional findings from liver function studies support the diagnosis:
  - Serum aspartate aminotransferase and serum alanine aminotransferase levels are increased in the prodromal stage of acute viral hepatitis.
  - Serum alkaline phosphatase levels are slightly increased.
  - Serum bilirubin levels are elevated and may remain elevated late in the course of disease, especially in patients with severe disease.
  - Prothrombin time (PT) is prolonged (>3 seconds longer than normal, indicating severe liver damage).
  - White blood cell counts commonly show transient neutropenia and lymphopenia, followed by lymphocytosis.

Diagnostic procedures

- Liver biopsy shows chronic hepatitis.

Treatment

General

Hepatitis A

- There is no treatment—the body clears the hepatitis A virus on its own; management of signs and symptoms

Hepatitis B

- No specific treatment; provide supportive treatment of signs and symptoms

Hepatitis C

- Aimed at clearing hepatitis C virus from the body, stopping or slowing hepatic damage, and providing symptomatic relief
- Symptomatic treatment
- Small, high-calorie, high-protein meals (Protein intake is reduced if signs of precoma—lethargy, confusion, and mental changes—develop.)
- Parenteral feeding, if appropriate
- Alcohol cessation
- Frequent rest periods, as needed
- Avoidance of contact sports and strenuous activity

Medications

- Standard Ig
- Vaccine
- Interferon alfa-2b (hepatitis B and C)
- Antiemetics
- Cholestyramine
- Lamivudine (hepatitis B)
- Adefovir dipivoxil (hepatitis B)
- Ribavirin and Peginterferon (hepatitis C)

Surgery

- Possible liver transplantation (hepatitis C)

Nursing interventions

- Monitor intake and output.
- Monitor PT and for signs of bleeding.
- Observe standard precautions to prevent transmission of the disease.
- Provide rest periods throughout the day.
- Give prescribed drugs.
- Encourage oral fluid intake.

Patient teaching

- Be sure to cover:
  - the disorder, diagnosis, and treatment
  - measures to prevent the spread of disease to close relatives, friends, public
  - the importance of rest and a proper diet that includes a variety of healthy foods
  - the need to abstain from alcohol
  - medication administration, dosage, and possible adverse effects
  - the need to avoid over-the-counter medications unless approved by the health care provider
  - the need for age-appropriate vaccinations
  - the need for follow-up care.
- Refer the patient to Alcoholics Anonymous, if indicated.

HIV and AIDS

Overview

- HIV type 1; retrovirus causing AIDS
- HIV type 2; related to HIV type 1; also found to cause AIDS
- Increases susceptibility to opportunistic infections, unusual cancers, and other abnormalities
- Marked by progressive failure of the immune system
- Transmitted by contact with infected blood or body fluids and associated with identifiable high-risk behaviors
- Stage 1: primary—body's natural response to HIV infection
- Stage 2: latency—HIV virus is multiplying without symptoms.
- Stage 3: AIDS—late stage—CD4 count is less than 200 cells/mm^3.

Causes

- Infection with HIV, a retrovirus

Risk factors

- Sharing of needles or syringes by I.V. drug users
- Unprotected sexual intercourse
- Placental transmission
- History of sexually transmitted disease
- Homosexual lifestyle

- Bisexual lifestyle
- Transgender women
- Contact with infected blood

Assessment

History

- A mononucleosis-like syndrome occurring after a high-risk exposure; may be followed by an asymptomatic period that may last for years
- A latent stage in which the only sign of HIV infection is laboratory evidence of seroconversion.
- Exposure to HIV in the last 6 months
- Stages
  - Stage 1: acute—fever, chills, rash, night sweats, muscle aches, sore throat, fatigue, swollen lymph glands, mouth ulcers
  - Stage 2: latency—often no symptoms or mild symptoms while the HIV virus is reproducing/multiplying at very low levels
  - Stage 3: AIDS—late stage—rapid weight loss, recurring fever or profuse night sweats, extreme fatigue, diarrhea that lasts more than a week, lymphadenopathy in groin, armpits, neck, mouth lesions, pneumonia, blotches of skin including eyelids and nose (red, brown, pink, or purplish), depression, memory loss

Physical findings

- Persistent generalized adenopathy
- Nonspecific symptoms (weight loss, fatigue, night sweats, fever)
- Neurologic symptoms resulting from HIV encephalopathy
- Opportunistic infection or cancer (Kaposi's sarcoma)

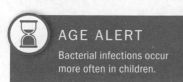

AGE ALERT

Bacterial infections occur more often in children.

Diagnostic tests

Laboratory

- A $CD4^+$ T-cell count of at least 200 cells/ml confirms HIV infection.
- A screening test (enzyme-linked immunosorbent assay) and a confirmatory test (Western blot) show HIV antibodies, which indicate HIV infection.

Treatment

General

- Variety of therapeutic options available for opportunistic infections (the leading cause of morbidity and mortality in patients infected with HIV)
- Disease-specific therapy for a variety of neoplastic and premalignant diseases and organ-specific syndromes
- Symptom management (fatigue and anemia)
- Well-balanced diet
- Regular exercise, as tolerated, with adequate rest periods

Medications

- Immunomodulatory agents
- Anti-infective agents
- Antineoplastic agents
- Highly active antiretroviral therapy
- HIV postexposure prophylaxis (PEP)
- Preexposure prophylaxis (PrEP)
- An integrase strand transfer inhibitor

Primary therapy

- Protease inhibitors
- Nucleoside reverse transcriptase inhibitors
- Nonnucleoside reverse transcriptase inhibitors

Nursing interventions

- Help the patient cope with an altered body image, the emotional burden of serious illness, and the threat of death.
- Avoid using glycerin swabs on the mucous membranes. Use normal saline or bicarbonate mouthwash for daily oral rinsing.

- Ensure adequate fluid intake during episodes of diarrhea.
- Provide meticulous skin care, especially in the debilitated patient.
- Encourage the patient to maintain as much physical activity as he or she can tolerate. Make sure his or her schedule includes time for exercise and rest.
- Monitor for progression of lesions in Kaposi's sarcoma.
- Monitor for opportunistic infections or signs of disease progression.

Patient teaching

- Be sure to cover:
  - medication regimens
  - the importance of informing potential sexual partners, caregivers, and health care workers of HIV infection
  - the signs of impending infection and the importance of seeking immediate medical attention
  - seeking information if traveling out of the country
  - the symptoms of AIDS dementia and its stages and progression
  - update/updating vaccinations, age appropriate.
- Refer the patient to a local support group.
- Refer the patient to hospice care, as indicated.

Hypertension

Overview

- Intermittent or sustained elevation of systolic blood pressure greater than 140 mm Hg and diastolic blood pressure greater than 90 mm Hg
- Disease usually benign initially, progressing slowly to accelerated or malignant state

- Two major types: essential (also called primary or idiopathic) hypertension and secondary hypertension, which results from renal disease thyroid dysfunction or another identifiable cause
- A severe, fulminant form commonly arising from both types—malignant hypertension—which is a medical emergency

Causes

- Unknown

Risk factors

- Family history
- Black race (in the United States)
- Stress
- Obesity
- Diet high in sodium and saturated fat
- Use of tobacco
- Use of hormonal contraceptives
- Excess alcohol intake
- Sedentary lifestyle
- Aging
- Chronic conditions, such as diabetes and sleep apnea

Assessment

History

- In many cases, no symptoms, with disorder detected incidentally during evaluation for another disorder or during routine blood pressure screening
- Symptoms that show the effect of hypertension on the organ systems
- Awakening with a headache in the occipital region that subsides spontaneously after a few hours
- Dizziness, fatigue, and confusion
- Palpitations, chest pain, and dyspnea
- Epistaxis
- Hematuria
- Blurred vision

Physical findings
- Bounding pulse
- Shortness of breath
- S_4 heart sound
- Peripheral edema in the late stages of disease
- Hemorrhages, exudates, and papilledema of the eye in the late stages of disease, if hypertensive retinopathy is present
- A pulsating abdominal mass, suggesting an abdominal aneurysm
- Elevated blood pressure on at least two consecutive occasions after initial screenings
- Bruits over the abdominal aorta and femoral arteries or the carotids

Diagnostic tests
Laboratory
- Urinalysis may show protein, RBC, white blood cells (suggesting renal disease), or glucose (suggesting diabetes mellitus).
- Serum potassium levels are less than 3.5 mEq/L, possibly indicating adrenal dysfunction (primary hyperaldosteronism).
- Blood urea nitrogen levels are normal or elevated to more than 20 mg/dl, and serum creatinine levels are normal or elevated to more than 1.5 mg/dl, suggesting renal disease.

Imaging
- Excretory urography may show renal atrophy, indicating chronic renal disease; one kidney more than $\frac{5}{8}''$ (1.6 cm) shorter than the other suggests unilateral renal disease.
- Chest X-rays may show cardiomegaly.
- Renal arteriography may show renal artery stenosis.

Diagnostic procedures
- ECG may show left ventricular hypertrophy or ischemia.
- Echocardiogram to detect enlarged heart and heart valve abnormalities

- An oral captopril challenge may be done to test for renovascular hypertension.
- Ophthalmoscopy shows arteriovenous nicking and, in hypertensive encephalopathy, edema.

Treatment
General
- Lifestyle modification, such as weight control, limiting alcohol use, regular exercise, and smoking cessation
- For a patient with secondary hypertension, correction of the underlying cause and control of hypertensive effects
- A diet that is low in sodium and saturated fat
- Adequate calcium, magnesium, and potassium in diet
- A regular exercise program

Medications
- Diuretics
- Beta-adrenergic blockers
- Calcium channel blockers
- Angiotensin-converting enzyme inhibitors
- Alpha blockers
- Alpha-receptor antagonists
- Vasodilators
- Angiotensin receptor blockers
- Aldosterone antagonist
- Central acting agents

Nursing interventions
- Promote rest.
- Administer medications, as ordered.
- Encourage dietary changes, as appropriate.
- Monitor intake and output.
- Help the patient identify risk factors and modify his or her lifestyle, as appropriate.
- Monitor vital signs, especially blood pressure.
- Monitor for signs of a stroke.

Patient teaching

- Be sure to cover:
  - the disorder, diagnosis, and treatment
  - how to use a self-monitoring blood pressure cuff and record the reading in a journal for review by the health care provider
  - the importance of complying with antihypertensive therapy and establishing a daily routine for taking medications
  - the need to report adverse effects of drugs
  - the need to avoid high-sodium antacids and over-the-counter cold and sinus medications that contain potentially harmful vasoconstrictors
  - the need for the patient to examine and modify his or her lifestyle, including diet
  - the need for a routine exercise program, particularly aerobic walking
  - dietary restrictions
  - the importance of follow-up care.
- Refer the patient to stress-reduction therapy or support groups, as needed.

Influenza

Overview

- Acute, highly contagious infection of the respiratory tract
- Capacity for antigenic variation (ability to mutate into different strains so that no immunologic resistance is present in those at risk)
- Antigenic variation characterized as antigenic drift (minor changes that occur yearly or every few years) and antigenic shift (major changes that lead to pandemics)
- Also called the grippe or the flu

Causes

- Type A: most prevalent; strikes annually, with new serotypes causing epidemics every 3 years
- Type B: occurs annually but causes epidemics only every 4 to 6 years
- Type C: endemic and causes only sporadic cases
- Infection transmitted by inhaling a respiratory droplet from an infected person or by indirect contact, such as drinking from a contaminated glass
- Transfer of virus to eyes, nose, mouth by putting infected hands after touching viral infected objects such as a keyboard, door knobs, counters, water faucets, cabinets, walls and others

Risk factors

- Age
- Living and/or work environment
- Weakened immune system
- Chronic illness—asthma, diabetes, heart conditions
- Pregnancy
- Obesity

Assessment

History

- Usually, recent exposure (typically within 48 hours) to a person with influenza
- No influenza vaccine received during the past season
- Headache
- Malaise
- Myalgia
- Fatigue, listlessness, and weakness

Physical findings

- Fever (usually higher in children)
- Signs of croup or dry persistent cough
- Red, watery eyes; clear nasal discharge
- Erythema of the nose and throat without exudate

- Tachypnea, shortness of breath, and cyanosis
- With bacterial pneumonia, purulent or bloody sputum
- Cervical adenopathy and tenderness
- Diminished breath sounds in areas of consolidation

Diagnostic tests

- After an epidemic is confirmed, diagnosis requires only observation of the clinical signs and symptoms.

Laboratory

- Inoculation of chicken embryos with nasal secretions from an infected patient shows the influenza virus.
- Throat swabs, nasopharyngeal washes, or sputum cultures show isolation of the influenza virus.
- Immunodiagnostic techniques show viral antigens in tissue culture or in exfoliated nasopharyngeal cells obtained by washings.
- White blood cell counts are elevated in secondary bacterial infection.
- White blood cell counts are decreased in overwhelming viral or bacterial infection.

Treatment

General

- Fluid and electrolyte replacement
- Oxygen and assisted ventilation, if indicated
- Increased fluid intake
- Rest periods, as needed

Medications

- Acetaminophen or aspirin (no aspirin for children or teens due to Reye's syndrome)
- NSAIDs
- Guaifenesin or an expectorant
- Oseltamivir (Tamiflu pills)—antiviral
- Zanamivir (Relenza inhaler)—antiviral
- Amantadine—an older antiviral
- Antibiotics

Nursing interventions

- Monitor vital signs.
- Place in a semi-Fowler's position for maximum lung expansion.
- Administer medications, as ordered.
- Follow standard precautions.
- Administer oxygen therapy, if warranted.
- Monitor for signs and symptoms of dehydration.

Patient teaching

- Be sure to cover:
  - the disorder, diagnosis, and treatment
  - the use of mouthwash or warm saline gargles to ease sore throat
  - the importance of increasing fluid intake to prevent dehydration
  - the use of a warm bath or a heating pad to relieve myalgia
  - the importance of covering coughs, following proper hand-washing technique, and properly disposing of tissues to prevent the virus from spreading
  - smoking cessation, as applicable
  - the need for influenza immunization annually.

Metabolic syndrome

Overview

- A cluster of conditions triggered by insulin resistance
- Confirmed if a patient has three or more of the following traits: increased abdominal fat with or without obesity, high blood pressure, high blood glucose levels, low serum HDL, and high triglyceride levels
- Associated with increased risk of diabetes, heart disease, and stroke
- Also known as metabolic X syndrome, insulin resistance syndrome, dysmetabolic syndrome, and multiple metabolic syndrome
- Currently affects approximately 25% of adults in the United States

Causes

- Insulin resistance, which results in cells being unable to respond to insulin, elevating both blood glucose and insulin levels
- High levels of circulating insulin, which raise triglyceride levels, affect renal function, and elevate blood pressure

Risk factors

- Genetic predisposition to hyper-insulinemia and impaired glucose tolerance
- Women more than men are at risk.
- Hispanic or Asian ethnicity
- Family history of type 2 diabetes
- Diabetes
- Gestational diabetes
- Aging
- Polycystic ovary syndrome
- Erectile dysfunction or decreased total testosterone
- High-fat, high-carbohydrate diet
- Insufficient physical activity
- Obesity
- Smoking

Assessment

History

- Family history of metabolic syndrome
- History of gestational diabetes
- Hypertension
- High low-density lipoprotein (LDL) levels
- Elevated triglyceride levels

- Low HDL levels
- Abdominal obesity
- Sedentary lifestyle
- Poor diet
- Smoking

Physical findings

- Obesity
- Large abdominal girth (See *Why abdominal obesity is dangerous.*)
- Waist circumference greater than 35″ (88.9 cm) in women and 40″ (102 cm) in men
- BMI greater than 25 kg/m^2
- Systolic blood pressure greater than 130 mm Hg or diastolic blood pressure greater than 85 mm Hg

Diagnostic tests

Laboratory

- Fasting serum glucose level is equal to or greater than 100 mg/dl.
- LDL level is equal to or greater than 130 mg/dl.
- HDL level is less than 40 mg/dl for men and less than 50 mg/dl for women.
- Triglyceride level is equal to or greater than 150 mg/dl.
- High-sensitivity CRP is equal to or greater than 1 mg/L.
- Insulin tolerance test (not widely used) measures glucose and insulin levels after a standard I.V. infusion of insulin; it may be helpful in obese patients and those with polycystic ovarian syndrome.

Why abdominal obesity is dangerous

People with excess weight around the waist have a greater risk of developing metabolic syndrome than people with excess weight around the hips. That is because intra-abdominal fat tends to be more resistant to insulin than fat in other areas of the body. Insulin resistance increases the release of free fatty acid into the portal system, leading to increased apolipoprotein B, increased low-density lipoprotein, decreased high-density lipoprotein, and increased triglyceride levels. As a result, the risk of cardiovascular disease increases.

Treatment

General

- Weight-reduction program
- Managing stress
- Low alcohol intake
- Low-cholesterol diet high in complex carbohydrates (grains, beans, vegetables, fruit) and low in refined carbohydrates (soft drinks, table sugar, high-fructose corn syrup)
- Moderately intense physical activity for at least 20 minutes a day, preferably for 30 to 60 minutes a day
- Smoking cessation

Medications

- Oral glucose-lowering drugs
- Insulin
- Antihypertensive drugs
- Cholesterol-lowering drugs
- Weight-loss drugs (orlistat, sibutramine)
- Vitamin supplements
- Low-dose aspirin

Surgery

- Possible gastric bypass procedure for patients with BMI greater than 40 kg/m^2 or, for patients with other obesity-related conditions, BMI greater than 35 kg/m^2

Nursing interventions

- Promote an exercise program for 30 to 60 minutes per day.
- Monitor laboratory values for laboratory markers and report abnormal results.
- Recommend smoking cessation; refer the patient to a smoking-cessation program, as needed.
- Alcohol cessation, as indicated because alcohol can affect weight gain
- Assist the patient with dietary choices, and answer all questions related to necessary dietary and weight changes.
- Monitor the patient's blood pressure and blood glucose, cholesterol, and triglyceride levels.

Patient teaching

- Be sure to cover:
  - the disorder, diagnosis, and treatment
  - the principles of a healthy diet and the importance of low alcohol intake
  - the relationship of diet, inactivity, and obesity to metabolic syndrome
  - the benefits of increased physical activity
  - prescribed medications, including administration and possible adverse reactions
  - the importance of follow-up care with the patient's health care provider to monitor weight loss, laboratory results, and blood pressure.

Methicillin-resistant *Staphylococcus aureus*

Overview

- Mutation of the very common, usually benign, bacterium *S. aureus*
- Also known by the acronym MRSA
- Resistant to the class of penicillin-like antibiotics called *beta-lactam antibiotics*
- Some strains also resistant to cephalosporins, aminoglycosides, erythromycin, tetracycline, and clindamycin
- About 90% of *S. aureus* isolates or strains penicillin resistant.
- Approximately 27% of all *S. aureus* isolates resistant to methicillin, a penicillin derivative.
- Strains resistant to penicillin first identified in 1961, to methicillin in 1968, and to vancomycin in 2002.
- Invasion, proliferation, and infection occur when natural defense systems break down (such as following invasive procedures, trauma, or chemotherapy).

- Easily spread by direct person-to-person contact
- Health care–associated MRSA (*HA-MRSA*) occurs in people who are or have recently been in the hospital with a weakened immune system
- Community-associated MRSA (*CA-MRSA*) generally occurs in healthy people who have not been in the hospital recently and among those who, have frequent close physical contact.
- CA-MRSA infections can also present as severe, invasive disease, including necrotizing pneumonia, necrotizing fasciitis, severe osteomyelitis, and sepsis.
- HA-MRSA and CA-MRSA different biologically and genetically, with CA-MRSA possibly transmitted more easily than HA-MRSA
- Endemic in nursing homes, long-term health care facilities, and community facilities
- Typically colonizes in the anterior nares; 40% of adults and most children transient nasal carriers
- Colonizes less commonly in the groin, armpits, and intestines

Causes
- Transmission from an infected patient or from a colonized patient or health care worker (symptom-free carrier of the bacteria)

Risk factors
- Burns
- Surgical or traumatic wounds
- Indwelling medical device, central venous access device, or other invasive catheter
- Abscesses, cellulitis, sepsis
- Contact dermatitis, eczema
- Impetigo
- Ulcers
- Immunosuppression
- Prolonged hospital stays

- Extended therapy with multiple or broad-spectrum antibiotics
- Proximity to others colonized or infected with MRSA
- Young age
- Participation in contact sports
- Sharing athletic equipment
- Living in crowded conditions (such as in long-term care facilities or prisons)

Assessment

History
- Possible risk factors for MRSA
- History of other household members or close contacts with skin or soft-tissue infections
- Possibly no signs or symptoms (carriers)

Physical findings
- Signs and symptoms related to the primary diagnosis (respiratory, cardiac, bone, and/or joints or other major system symptoms) in symptomatic patients
- Small, red bumps that resemble pimples, boils, or spider bites that develop into deep, painful abscesses, furuncles, or carbuncles
- Fever
- Purulent wound drainage
- Erythema
- Edema
- Pain and tenderness

Diagnostic tests
Laboratory
- Cultures from skin, urine, blood, or wounds show MRSA.
- Organism susceptibility testing identifies the best antimicrobial drug.
- D-zone disk diffusion test evaluates for inducible clindamycin resistance in CA-MRSA resistant to erythromycin.

Imaging
- Ultrasonography delineates abscesses.

Treatment
General
- Handwashing before and after patient contact
- Use gloves, as applicable.
- Transmission precautions, including contact isolation for wound, skin, and urine infections and respiratory isolation for respiratory infections
- In MRSA outbreaks, possibly surveillance and decolonization of health care personnel, consisting of a combination of topical mupirocin applied to the nares, oral antibiotics, and antimicrobial baths
- No treatment for patients with colonization only
- Removal of indwelling medical devices as soon as possible
- Moist heat for small furuncles
- Treatment of underlying conditions such as tinea pedis
- High-protein diet

Medications
- Monotherapy or combination
- Sulfamethoxazole/trimethoprim
- Clindamycin
- Doxycycline or minocycline
- Daptomycin
- Mupirocin
- Nafcillin
- Tetracycline

Surgery
- Incision and drainage of purulent lesions, including obtaining cultures and performing susceptibility testing

Nursing interventions
- Monitor vital signs.
- Administer prescribed medication(s).
- Maintain contact isolation in health care settings.
- Consider grouping infected patients together and having the same health care providers care for them.

- Employ proper hand-washing techniques (the most effective way to prevent transmission of MRSA).
- Monitor enhanced environmental cleaning.
- Obtain cultures and monitor results.
- Provide appropriate wound care.
- Evaluate the patient for adverse drug reactions.
- Provide teaching and emotional support to the patient and family members.

Patient teaching
- Be sure to cover:
  - the disorder, diagnosis, and treatment
  - the difference between MRSA infection and colonization
  - how cultures are obtained
  - how to prevent the spread of MRSA
  - the importance of proper hand-washing technique for the patient and family members
  - the purpose of contact precautions and how to comply with them
  - medication administration, dosage, and possible adverse effects
  - the importance of taking antibiotics for the full prescription period, even if the patient begins to feel better.

Multiple sclerosis

Overview
- Progressive demyelination of the white matter of the brain, spinal cord, and optic nerve because these cells are in the brain and spinal cord which are affected in this condition.
- Scar tissue develops to the damaged tissue areas producing additional damage along the nerves giving the name of "multiple sclerosis."
- Affected individuals who are 20 to 50 years of age

- Characterized by exacerbations and remissions
- In some cases, rapid progression, with death occurring within months
- Variable prognosis (Most patients with multiple sclerosis [70%] lead active lives with prolonged remissions.)

Causes

- Exact cause unknown
- Slow-acting viral infection
- Autoimmune response of the nervous system
- Allergic response
- Events that precede the onset of disease include:
  - emotional stress
  - overwork
  - fatigue
  - pregnancy
  - acute respiratory tract infections.
- Genetic factors possibly also involved
- Optic neuritis (occurs suddenly) causes vision problems that include blurred vision, graying of vision, nystagmus (may be described as a quiver) double vision, vision loss.

Risk factors

- Trauma
- Numbness or tingling of face, body or extremities
- Anoxia
- Toxins
- Nutritional deficiencies, such as vitamins D_3 and B_{12}
- Vascular lesions
- Anorexia nervosa
- Obesity in children, adolescent, and young adults

Assessment

History

- Symptoms related to the extent and site of myelin destruction, the extent of remyelination, and the adequacy of subsequent restored synaptic transmission

- Symptoms transient or lasting for hours or weeks
- Symptoms unpredictable and difficult to describe
- Visual problems and sensory impairment (the first signs)
- Blurred vision, loss of peripheral vision, diplopia, or loss of vision
- Urinary problems
- Emotional lability
- Dysphagia
- Cognitive changes that cause difficulty with focusing, problem solving, and learning new data for everyday life
- Numbness or tingling of face, body, or upper and lower extremities
- Falls
- Headache
- Pain due to spasticity of the musculoskeletal system
- Bowel disturbances (involuntary evacuation or constipation)
- Fatigue (typically the most disabling symptom)
- Intolerance to heat which can trigger symptoms

Physical findings

- Poor articulation
- Muscle weakness of the involved area
- Spasticity and hyperreflexia
- Intention tremor
- Gait ataxia
- Paralysis, ranging from monoplegia to quadriplegia
- Nystagmus and scotoma
- Optic neuritis
- Ophthalmoplegia

Diagnostic tests

- Diagnosis may require years of testing and observation.

Laboratory

- Cerebrospinal fluid analysis shows mononuclear cell pleocytosis, an elevated level of total IgG, and the presence of oligoclonal IgG.

Imaging
- MRI is the most sensitive method for detecting focal lesions associated with multiple sclerosis.

Other
- Electroencephalographic abnormalities occur in one-third of patients with multiple sclerosis.
- Evoked potential studies show slowed conduction of nerve impulses.
- Optic coherence tomography shows retinal structures, optic neuritis

Treatment

General

- Symptomatic treatment for acute exacerbations (relapses) and related signs and symptoms
- Diet high in fluid and fiber in case of constipation
- Frequent rest periods

Medications

- I.V. steroids followed by oral steroids
- Immunosuppressants
- Antimetabolites
- Alkylating drugs
- Biologic response modifiers

- Vitamins and minerals
- Complementary and alternative medicine (CAM)

Nursing interventions

- Provide emotional and psychological support.
- Assist with the physical therapy program.
- Provide adequate rest periods.
- Promote emotional stability.
- Keep the bedpan or urinal readily available because the need to void is immediate.
- Provide bowel and bladder training, if indicated.
- Give prescribed drugs.
- Monitor functional changes: speech, vision, energy, sensory impairment, and muscle dysfunction.

Patient teaching

- Be sure to cover:
  - the disease process (See *Understanding types of multiple sclerosis.*)
  - medication and adverse effects
  - the importance of avoiding stress, infections, and fatigue

---

Understanding types of multiple sclerosis

Various terms are used to describe different types of multiple sclerosis (MS).
- *Relapsing-remitting*: clear relapses (or acute attacks or exacerbations), with full recovery and lasting disability. Between attacks, the disease does not worsen.
- *Primary progressive*: steadily progressing or worsening, with minor recovery or plateaus. This form is uncommon and may involve different brain and spinal cord damage from other forms.
- *Secondary progressive*: beginning as a pattern of clear relapses and recovery but becoming steadily progressive and worsening between acute attacks
- *Progressive-relapsing*: steadily progressing from the onset but with clear, acute attacks. This form is rare. In addition, the differential diagnosis must rule out spinal cord compression, foramen magnum tumor (which may mimic the exacerbations and remissions of MS), multiple small strokes, syphilis or another infection, thyroid disease, and chronic fatigue syndrome.

– the importance of maintaining independence
– the need to avoid exposure to bacterial and viral infections
– nutritional management
– the importance of adequate fluid intake and regular urination
– the importance of adequate fiber intake and regular bowel movements
– the importance of managing relapses.

- Refer the patient to the National Multiple Sclerosis Society.
- Refer the patient to physical and occupational rehabilitation programs, as indicated.

Myocardial infarction

Overview

- Reduced blood flow through one or more coronary arteries, causing myocardial ischemia and necrosis
- Site of infarction dependent on the vessels involved
- Also called MI and heart attack
- Usually occurs in the early morning between 4:00 and 6:00 am

Causes

- Atherosclerosis
- Thrombosis
- Platelet aggregation
- Coronary artery stenosis or spasm

Risk factors

- Middle age or older (40 to 70)
- Diabetes mellitus, there could be perception impairment defecting angina warnings
- Elevated serum triglyceride, LDL, cholesterol levels, and decreased serum HDL levels
- Excessive intake of saturated fats, carbohydrates, or salt
- Hypertension
- Obesity
- Family history of CAD

- Sedentary lifestyle
- Smoking
- Stress or type A personality
- Use of drugs, such as amphetamines or cocaine

Assessment

History

- Possible CAD with increasing frequency, severity, or duration of angina
- Cardinal symptom: persistent, crushing substernal pain or pressure described as a squeezing, aching, burning, or sharp that may radiate to the left arm, jaw, neck, shoulder blades, and stomach and may persist for 12 hours or longer
- Symptom can be epigastric, a feeling of indigestion, bloating, fullness, or flatus.
- Little or no pain in an elderly patient or a patient with diabetes; pain possibly mild and confused with indigestion in other patients
- Fatigue, nausea with or without vomiting, malaise, cough, wheezing, light-headedness with or without syncope, and shortness of breath, accompanied by a feeling of impending doom
- Sudden death (may be the first and only indication of MI)
- Possible intermittent claudication
- Peripheral cyanosis, edema, pallor, diminished pulses, delayed capillary refill indicate right ventricular constriction.
- Rales or wheezes are associated with left ventricular MI.

Physical findings

- Pulse is irregular or rapid initially.
- Blood pressure is elevated.
- Extreme anxiety and restlessness
- Dyspnea
- Diaphoresis
- Tachycardia
- Hypertension

- Distension of neck veins commonly indicates failure of the right ventricle.
- Hepatojugular reflex may develop due to tricuspid decrease function.
- In inferior MI, bradycardia and hypotension
- An S_4 heart sound, an S_3 heart sound, and paradoxical splitting of the S_2 heart sound with ventricular dysfunction
- A systolic murmur of mitral insufficiency
- Pericardial friction rub with transmural MI or pericarditis

Diagnostic tests
Laboratory
- The serum creatine kinase (CK) level is elevated, especially the creatine kinase-muscle/brain (CK-MB) isoenzyme, which is the cardiac muscle fraction of CK.
- The serum lactate dehydrogenase (LD) level is elevated; the LD_1 isoenzyme level (found in cardiac tissue) is higher than the LD_2 level (in serum).
- White blood cells count elevation usually appears on the second day and lasts for 1 week.
- Platelet levels determine the need to administer medication such as heparin.
- CMP to monitor magnesium, potassium, creatinine, blood glucose, and LDH levels; also, erythrocyte sedimentation rate (ESR)
- Myoglobin (the hemoprotein found in cardiac and skeletal muscle) is detected. It is released with muscle damage, as soon as 2 hours after an MI.
- The level of troponin I is elevated only when muscle damage occurs. It is more specific than the CK-MB level. (Troponin levels increase within 4 to 6 hours of myocardial injury and may remain elevated for 5 to 11 days.)

- The BNP is elevated due to the ventricular myocardium in response to wall stress and predicts cardiac mortality.
- CRP, a nonspecific marker of inflammation, when elevated is an independent predictor of cardiac death and MI.

Imaging
- Cardiac imaging is done to determine CAD; a positive finding is used to determine when to initiate medical or surgical management.
- Nuclear medicine scans performed with I.V. technetium 99m pertechnetate can identify acutely damaged muscle by detecting accumulations of radioactive nucleotide. An area of accumulation appears as a "hot spot" on the film. Myocardial perfusion imaging with thallium 201 shows a "cold spot" (a poorly perfused area of the heart where thallium does not appear) in most patients during the first few hours after a transmural MI.
- Echocardiography shows ventricular wall dyskinesia with a transmural MI and helps evaluate the ejection fraction.

Diagnostic procedures
- Serial 12-lead ECG readings may be normal or inconclusive during the first few hours after an MI. Characteristic abnormalities include ST-segment elevation and Q waves, representing scarring and necrosis.
- Pulmonary artery catheterization may be performed to detect left- or right-sided heart failure and to monitor the response to treatment.

Treatment
General
- For arrhythmias, a pacemaker or electrical cardioversion
- Intra-aortic balloon pump for cardiogenic shock

- Low-fat, low-cholesterol diet
- Calorie restriction, if indicated
- Bed rest, with a commode available at the bedside
- Gradual increase in activity, as tolerated

Medications

- I.V. thrombolytic therapy started within 3 hours of the onset of symptoms
- Aspirin
- Antiarrhythmics and antianginals
- Calcium channel blockers
- I.V. heparin
- I.V. morphine
- Analgesics
- Antiplatelets
- Inotropic drugs
- Beta-adrenergic blockers
- Angiotensin-converting inhibitors
- Stool softeners
- Oxygen
- Human monoclonal antibody—helps to reduce levels of LDL cholesterol
- Statins

Surgery

- Surgical revascularization
- Percutaneous revascularization

Nursing interventions

- Monitor vital signs.
- Assess pain and give analgesics, as ordered. Record the severity, location, type, and duration of pain. Avoid I.M. injections.
- Check the patient's blood pressure before and after giving nitroglycerin.
- During episodes of chest pain, obtain ECG.
- Organize patient care and activities to provide periods of uninterrupted rest.
- Provide a low-cholesterol, low-sodium diet with caffeine-free beverages.
- Allow the patient to use a bedside commode.

- Assist with range-of-motion exercises.
- Provide emotional support, and help reduce stress and anxiety.
- If the patient has undergone percutaneous transluminal coronary angioplasty, sheath care is necessary. Watch for bleeding. Keep the leg with the sheath insertion site immobile. Maintain strict bed rest. Check peripheral pulses in the affected leg frequently.

Patient teaching

- Be sure to cover:
  - procedures (answering questions for the patient and family members)
  - medication dosages, adverse reactions, and signs of toxicity to watch for and report
  - not taking the NSAID, aspirin, or vitamin E when taking antiplatelet medication or anticoagulant medication.
  - dietary restrictions
  - progressive resumption of sexual activity
  - appropriate responses to new or recurrent symptoms
  - typical and atypical chest pain and the need to report pain to the health care provider
- Refer to primary care provider (PCP) for updated vaccinations, age specific.
- Refer the patient to a cardiac rehabilitation program.
- Refer the patient to a smoking-cessation program, if needed.
- Refer the patient to a weight-reduction program, if needed.

Osteoarthritis

Overview

- Chronic degeneration of joint cartilage
- Most common form of arthritis
- Range of disability, from minor limitation to near immobility

- Knees and hips most commonly affected
- The lower back, neck, finger joints, bases of thumbs, and the hallux (big toe) may be affected.
- Varying rates of progression

Causes

- Advancing age
- Possible hereditary factors
- Secondary osteoarthritis
- Traumatic injury
- Congenital abnormality
- Obesity
- Overuse
- Sedentary lifestyle
- Endocrine disorders such as diabetes mellitus
- Metabolic disorders such as chondrocalcinosis
- Repetitive use (recreational or occupational)

Risk factors

- Family members with osteoarthritis
- Obesity
- Overuse of joints
- Traumatic injury
- Joint deformity—unequal leg length
- Gender—women more likely than men
- Repetitive stress
- Occupation—sedentary

Assessment

History

- Predisposing traumatic injury
- Deep, aching joint pain
- Edema of the joint that is affected
- Pain after exercise or weight bearing or at the end of the day
- Pain that may be relieved by rest
- Stiffness in the morning and after exercise that goes away after movement
- Aching during changes in weather
- "Grating" feeling when the joint moves

- Limited movement and range of movement
- Cracking or clicking sound on movement of joints
- Difficulty walking, climbing stairs, or gripping objects in performing daily activities at home or work

Physical findings

- Contractures
- Joint swelling
- Muscle atrophy
- Deformity of the involved areas
- Gait abnormalities
- Hard nodes on the distal and proximal interphalangeal joints that may be red, swollen, and tender
- Loss of finger dexterity
- Muscle spasms, limited movement, and joint instability

Diagnostic tests

Laboratory

- Synovial fluid analysis rules out inflammatory arthritis.

Imaging

- X-rays of the affected joint may show narrowing of the joint space or margins, cyst-like bony deposits in the joint space and margins, sclerosis of the subchondral space, joint deformity or articular damage, bony growths at weight-bearing areas, and possible joint fusion.
- Radionuclide bone scan may be used to rule out inflammatory arthritis by showing normal uptake of the radionuclide.
- MRI shows the affected joint, adjacent bones, and progression of disease.

Diagnostic procedures

- Neuromuscular tests may show reduced muscle strength.

Other

- Arthroscopy shows the internal joint structures and identifies soft-tissue swelling.

Treatment
General
- Pain relief
- Improved mobility
- Minimized disability
- Activity, as tolerated
- Tai chi and yoga and/or aerobic exercise
- Physical therapy
- Occupational therapy
- Assistive mobility devices
- Alternative measures
  - Acupuncture
  - Acupressure
  - Nutritional supplements
  - Massage
- Weight reduction

Medications
- Analgesics
- NSAIDs
- Topical, oral, injection hydrotherapy
- Antispasmodics
- Selective serotonin norepinephrine reuptake inhibitor
- Hyaluronic acid joint injections
- Corticosteroids by mouth or by injection

Surgery
- Arthroplasty (partial or total)
- Arthrodesis
- Osteoplasty
- Osteotomy

Nursing interventions
- Allow adequate time for self-care.
- Adjust pain medications to allow for maximum rest.
- Identify techniques that promote rest and relaxation.
- Administer anti-inflammatory medications.
- If the hand joints are affected, use hot soaks and paraffin dips.
- If the lumbosacral spinal joints are affected, provide a firm mattress.
- If the cervical spinal joints are affected, apply a cervical collar.

- If the hip is affected, apply moist heat pads and administer antispasmodic drugs.
- If the knee is affected, help with range-of-motion exercises.
- Apply elastic supports or braces.
- Check the patient's crutches, cane, braces, or walker for proper fit.

Patient teaching
- Be sure to cover:
  - the disorder, diagnosis, and treatment
  - the need for adequate rest during the day, after exertion, and at night
  - methods to conserve energy
  - the need to take medications exactly as prescribed
  - adverse reactions to medications
  - the need to wear support shoes that fit well and the importance of repairing worn heels
  - the need to install safety devices at home
  - the importance of range-of-motion exercises and the need to perform them as gently as possible
  - the need to maintain proper body weight
  - the use of crutches or other orthopedic devices.
- Refer the patient to occupational or physical therapy, as indicated.

Osteoporosis

Overview
- Loss of calcium and phosphate from bones, causing increased vulnerability to fractures
- Primary or secondary to underlying disease
- Types of primary osteoporosis: postmenopausal osteoporosis (type I) and age-associated osteoporosis (type II)

- Secondary osteoporosis: caused by an identifiable agent or disease
- Osteoporosis is associated with constant pain.
- One in two women and one in four men over the age of 50 years develop osteoporosis.
  - 80% of those with osteoporosis are women.
- Bone breakage is most likely to occur in the hip, spine, wrist.

Causes

- Exact cause unknown
- Prolonged therapy with steroids or heparin
- Bone immobilization
- Alcoholism
- Malnutrition
- Rheumatoid arthritis
- Liver disease
- Malabsorption
- Scurvy
- Lactose intolerance
- Hyperthyroidism
- Osteogenesis imperfecta
- Sudeck's atrophy (localized in the hands and feet, with recurring attacks)
- Surgery
- Weight loss
- Lupus
- Multiple sclerosis
- Ankylosing spondylitis
- Premature menopause/menopause
- Spinal cord injury
- Diabetes mellitus
- Low levels of testosterone in men

Risk factors

- Mild, prolonged negative calcium balance
- Declining gonadal adrenal function
- Faulty protein metabolism (caused by estrogen deficiency)
- Sedentary lifestyle
- Medications that cause bone loss, for example, corticosteroids, antacids, antidepressants
- Overactive thyroid (hyperthyroidism)

- Decrease in absorption of calcium and vitamins via intestines
- Postmenopausal
- Smoking—nicotine is toxic to bones.
- Alcohol consumption
- Anorexia nervosa
- Lead exposure
- Poor calcium diet
- PPIs
- Family history of osteoporosis

Assessment

History

- Postmenopausal patient
- Condition known to cause secondary osteoporosis
- Snapping sound or sudden pain in the lower back when bending down to lift something
- Possible slow development of pain (over several years)
- With vertebral collapse, backache, and pain radiating around the trunk
- Pain aggravated by movement
- Loss of height due to curvature of the spine

Physical findings

- Humped back (hyperkyphosis)
- Markedly aged appearance
- Loss of height
- Muscle spasm
- Decreased spinal movement, with flexion more limited than extension

Laboratory

- Normal serum calcium, phosphorus, and alkaline levels
- Elevated parathyroid hormone level

Imaging

- X-ray studies show characteristic degeneration in the lower thoracolumbar vertebrae.
- CT scan assesses spinal bone loss.
- Bone scans show injured or diseased areas.

Diagnostic procedures

- Bone biopsy shows thin, porous but otherwise normal bone.
- Bone mineral density (BMD)

Other

- Dual or single photon absorptiometry (measurement of bone mass) shows loss of bone mass.
- Fracture Risk Assessment Tool (algorithm, FRAX)—a 10-year hip fracture probability

Treatment

General

- Control of bone loss
- Prevention of additional fractures
- Control of pain
- Reduction and immobilization of fractures
- Diet rich in vitamin D, calcium, and protein
- Exposure to sunlight to aid in the synthesis of vitamin D
- Physical therapy program of gentle exercise and activity
- Regular weight-bearing exercises, as indicated
- Tobacco cessation
- Alcohol—decrease amount or cessation
- Supportive devices

Medications

- Bisphosphonates
- Parathyroid hormone and analogs
- Sodium fluoride
- Calcium and vitamin D supplements
- Calcitonin
- Testosterone for men

Surgery

- Open reduction and internal fixation for femur fractures

Nursing interventions

- Encourage careful positioning, ambulation, and prescribed exercises.
- Encourage increase in fluid each day, up to 2 L/day, as tolerated.

- Promote self-care, and allow adequate time.
- Encourage mild exercise.
- Assist with walking.
- Perform passive range-of-motion exercises.
- Promote physical therapy sessions.
- Use safety precautions.
- Administer analgesia, as ordered.
- Apply heat.
- Monitor the skin for redness, warmth, and new sites of pain.
- Monitor exercise tolerance and joint mobility.
- Administer medications and vitamins and minerals, as prescribed.

Patient teaching

- Be sure to cover:
  - the disorder, diagnosis, and treatment
  - the prescribed drug regimen
  - how to recognize significant adverse reactions
  - the need to perform monthly breast self-examination while receiving estrogen therapy
  - the need to report vaginal bleeding promptly
  - the need to report new pain sites immediately
  - the importance of sleeping on a firm mattress
  - the need to avoid excessive bed rest
  - the use of a back brace, if appropriate
  - the use of proper body mechanics
  - the use of home safety devices
  - the importance of a calcium-rich diet.
- Refer the patient to physical and occupational therapy, as appropriate.

Parkinson's disease

Overview

- Brain disorder associated with decreased levels of the neurotransmitter dopamine that causes progressive deterioration, with muscle rigidity, akinesia, and involuntary tremors
- Affects age 60 years and older
- Genetic predisposition
- Men are more likely to get Parkinson's disease than women.
- Microscopic markers are Lewy bodies and are found within brain cells.
- Usual cause of death: aspiration pneumonia
- One of the most common crippling diseases in the United States
- No cure has been found.

Causes

- Usually unknown
- Exposure to toxins, such as pesticides, herbicides, as manganese dust and carbon monoxide
- Use of illegal drugs
- Type A encephalitis
- Drug-induced effect (haloperidol [Haldol], methyldopa, reserpine)

Assessment

History

- Muscle rigidity
- Bradykinesia
- Akinesia
- Insidious (unilateral pill-roll) tremor, which increases during stress either emotionally or physically or during anxiety and decreases with purposeful movement and sleep
- Dysphagia
- Loss of smell
- Pain in a specific area or all of the body
- Decrease in sexual desire or performance

- Fatigue with activities of daily living
- Muscle cramps of the legs, neck, and trunk
- Oily skin
- Increased perspiration
- Insomnia
- Mood changes
- Dysarthria
- Bladder dysfunction—unable to control urine or difficulty in urinating
- Anal sphincter dysfunction and constipation

Physical findings

- Four cardinal features
  - Tremors—typically at rest, particularly in upper extremities
  - Muscle rigidity—muscle stiffness causing resistance to passive muscle stretching
  - Bradykinesia—slow movements
  - Loss of balance—a later feature of the disorder
- High-pitched, monotonous voice
- Slurred speech
- Drooling
- Masklike facial expression
- Difficulty walking
- Lack of parallel motion in gait
- Loss of posture control with walking, sitting, standing
- Oculogyric crises (eyes fixed upward, with involuntary tonic movements)
- Muscle rigidity causing resistance to passive muscle stretching
- Difficulty pivoting
- Loss of balance
- Experiences confusion and cognitive dementia
- Changes in hand writing

Diagnostic tests

Laboratory

- CBC, CMP, urinalysis to identify other possible conditions

Imaging

- CT scan or MRI rules out other disorders such as intracranial tumors and to obtain a picture of the brain in preparation for surgery.
- Dopamine transporter scan
- PET scan
- Ultrasound of the brain

Treatment

General

- Small, frequent meals
- High-bulk foods
- Physical therapy, speech therapy, and occupational therapy
- Assistive devices to aid ambulation

Medications

- Dopamine replacement drugs
  - Dopamine precursor—Levodopa (L-dopa) is main medication.
  - Catechol-O-methyltransferase inhibitors
  - Monoamine oxidase B inhibitors
- Anticholinergics
- Antihistamines
- Antiviral agents
- Enzyme-inhibiting agents
- Tricyclic antidepressants

Surgery

- Used when drug therapy is unsuccessful
- Stereotaxic neurosurgery
- Destruction of the ventrolateral nucleus of the thalamus
- Deep brain stimulation is the most common surgery.
  - Performed after having Parkinson's disease for 4 or more years
  - Not a cure but does interrupt the abnormal signals causing motor dysfunction

Nursing interventions

- Monitor vital signs and weigh daily.
- Monitor intake and output.
- Take measures to prevent aspiration.
- Administer antiparkinsonian medication prescribed to increase dopamine in the CNS.
- Protect the patient from injury.
- Assess neurologic status.
- Stress the importance of rest periods between activities.
- Ensure adequate nutrition and monitor calorie intake.
- Monitor for constipation.
- Provide frequent warm baths and massage.
- Encourage the patient to enroll in a physical therapy program.
- Provide emotional and psychological support.
- Assess for depression.
- Assess nonverbal communication methods of communication if and when verbal communication is no longer possible.
- Encourage the patient to be independent.
- Assist with ambulation and range-of-motion exercises.
- Postoperatively, monitor for signs of hemorrhage and increased intracranial pressure.

Patient teaching

- Be sure to cover:
  - the disorder, diagnosis, and treatment
  - administration, dosages, and adverse reactions to medications
  - avoidance of vitamin B_6—due to the blocking effects of antiparkinsonian medications
  - measures to prevent pressure ulcers and contractures
  - household safety measures
  - the importance of daily bathing
  - methods to improve communication
  - balanced diet
  - exercise—aerobic

- avoidance of falls
  - Do not pivot.
  - Do not make a U-turn.
  - Avoid carrying items while walking.
  - Do not walk backward.
- the importance of a swallowing therapy regimen (aspiration precautions).
- Refer to a Parkinson's support group.
- Refer the patient to speech therapy and occupational and physical rehabilitation, as indicated.

Peptic ulcer

Overview

- Circumscribed lesion in the mucosal membrane of the lower esophagus, stomach, duodenum, or jejunum
- Occurs in two major forms: duodenal ulcer and gastric ulcer (both chronic)
- Duodenal ulcers: account for about 80% of peptic ulcers, affect the proximal part of the small intestine, and follow a chronic course characterized by remissions and exacerbations (About 5% to 10% of patients with duodenal ulcers have complications that necessitate surgery.)
- Gastric ulcers: occur in the gastric mucosa. They have a wide spectrum of clinical presentations, ranging from asymptomatic to vague epigastric pain, nausea, and iron deficiency anemia to acute life-threatening hemorrhage.

Causes

- *Helicobacter pylori*—spiral-shaped bacterium found in the stomach
- Rare occurrence—tumors— gastrinomas that form in the duodenum
  - As well as the pancreas releases large amounts of gastrin that triggers production of large amounts of acid known as Zollinger-Ellison syndrome

- Genetics—predisposition
- Use of glucocorticoids, aspirin, caffeine, medication taken to increase bone mass or NSAIDs
- Alcohol
- Smoking or chewing tobacco
- Pathologic hypersecretory states

Risk factors

- Type A blood (for gastric ulcer)
- Type O blood (for duodenal ulcer)
- Other genetic factors
- Exposure to irritants
- Cigarette smoking
- Trauma
- Psychogenic factors
- Stress
- Normal aging

Assessment

History

- Periods of symptom exacerbation and remission, with remissions lasting longer than exacerbations
- History of a predisposing factor
- Stress
- History of a dull or burning pain when stomach is empty, lasts for minutes to hours, comes and goes over days, weeks, months
- Left epigastric pain described as heartburn or indigestion and accompanied by a feeling of fullness or distention and belching often
- Severe symptoms
  - Feeling faint
  - Nausea and vomiting
  - Appetite changes
  - Dark tarry stools
  - Unexplained weight loss

Gastric ulcer

- Recent loss of weight or appetite
- Nausea or vomiting
- Pain triggered or worsened by eating

Duodenal ulcer
- Pain relieved by eating; may occur 1½ to 3 hours after food intake
- Pain that awakens the patient from sleep
- Weight gain

Physical findings
- Pallor
- Epigastric tenderness
- Hyperactive bowel sounds

Diagnostic tests
Laboratory
- CBC shows anemia.
- Testing shows occult blood in the stools.
- Venous blood sample shows *H. pylori* antibodies.
- White blood cell count is elevated.
- Urea breath test shows low levels of exhaled carbon 13.
- The fasting serum gastrin level rules out Zollinger-Ellison syndrome.

Imaging
- Barium swallow and small-bowel series may show the ulcer.
- Upper GI tract X-rays shows mucosal abnormalities.
- Upper GI series shows the shape of the upper GI tract.
- CT scan shows if the ulcer has penetrated the wall of the stomach or small intestine.

Diagnostic procedures
- Upper GI endoscopy or esophagogastroduodenoscopy confirms the ulcer and permits cytologic studies and biopsy to rule out *H. pylori* or cancer.
- Gastric secretory studies show hyperchlorhydria.

Treatment
General
- Treatment is determined by the cause of the ulcer.
- Symptomatic

- Iced saline lavage, possibly containing norepinephrine
- Laser or cautery during endoscopy
- Stress reduction
- Smoking cessation
- Avoidance of dietary irritants
- Nothing by mouth if GI bleeding is evident
- Discontinue NSAIDs or reduce the amount but must be taken after eating.

Medications
For *Helicobacter pylori*
- Amoxicillin, clarithromycin (Biaxin), and omeprazole (Prilosec), metronidazole (Flagyl)

For gastric or duodenal ulcer
- PPIs
- Antacids
- Histamine-receptor antagonists or gastric acid pump inhibitor
- Histamine-2 receptor blockers
- Protectants—coat ulcers and protect them from stomach acid such as antacids
- Coating agents—such as sucralfate, used to treat active duodenal ulcer(s)
- Antisecretory agents if the ulcer resulted from NSAID use, when NSAIDs must be continued
- Sedatives and tranquilizers (for gastric ulcer)
- Anticholinergics (for duodenal ulcers; usually contraindicated in gastric ulcers)
- Prostaglandin analogues

Surgery
- Indicated for perforation, lack of response to conservative treatment, suspected cancer, or other complications
- Type varies with the location and extent of the ulcer; major operations: bilateral vagotomy, pyloroplasty, and gastrectomy

Nursing interventions

- Assess weight daily.
- Monitor vital signs.
- Monitor lab values for protein deple-tion and anemia.
- Monitor for hematemesis and melena.
- Administer medications, as ordered.
- Provide six small meals or small hourly meals, as ordered.
- Offer emotional support.
- Monitor the patient for signs and symptoms of bleeding.
- Provide pain control.

If patient had surgery
- NG tube function and drainage
- Bowel function
- Fluid and nutritional status
- Wound site
- Signs and symptoms of metabolic alkalosis or perforation

Patient teaching

- Be sure to cover:
  - the disorder, diagnosis, and treatment
  - administration, dosage, and possi-ble reactions to medications
  - identification of medications needed to be taken before, with food, or after eating
  - warnings against using over-the-counter medications, especially aspirin, aspirin-containing products, and NSAIDs, unless the health care provider approves
  - warnings against using caffeine and alcohol during exacerbations
  - appropriate lifestyle changes such as plenty of sleep, avoid eating less than 2 hours before sleeping, do not lay down after eating a meal, including not eating any types of snacks and laying down

  - dietary modifications as indicated and may include—eat whole grains; increase intake of vitamins A and C, vegetables, and lean meat; avoid spicy foods—pepper, citrus, fried foods, high-fat foods, acidy foods such as tomatoes, carbonated beverages
  - how to decrease stress.
- Refer the patient to a smoking-cessation program, if indicated.

Pneumonia

Overview

- Acute infection of the lung paren-chyma that impairs gas exchange
- May be classified by etiology, loca-tion, or type

Causes

Bacterial and viral pneumonia
- Bacterial
  - Pneumococcal
  - *Streptococcus*
  - *Mycoplasma* are referred to as walking pneumonia.
  - *Legionella*
- Viral pneumonia
  - Influenza
  - Parainfluenza
  - Adenoviruses
  - Rhinovirus
- Chronic illness and debilitation
- Cancer
- Abdominal and thoracic surgery
- Atelectasis
- Bacterial or viral respiratory infection
- Chronic respiratory disease
- Influenza
- Smoking
- Malnutrition
- Alcoholism
- Sickle cell disease
- Tracheostomy

- Exposure to noxious gases
- Aspiration
- Immunosuppressive therapy
- Endotracheal intubation or mechanical ventilation

Aspiration pneumonia
- Caustic substance entering the airway

Risk factors
- Advanced age
- Difficulty swallowing can lead to aspiration pneumonia.
- Debilitation
- NG tube feedings
- Impaired gag reflex which can lead to aspiration pneumonia
- Poor oral hygiene

AGE ALERT
Incidence and mortality rates are highest in elderly patients.

Assessment

History

Bacterial pneumonia
- Sudden onset of:
  - pleuritic chest pain
  - cough
  - production of purulent sputum
  - chills.

Viral pneumonia
- Nonproductive cough
- Constitutional symptoms
- Fever

Aspiration pneumonia
- Fever
- Weight loss
- Malaise

Fungus pneumonia (*Pneumocystis* pneumonia)
- Fever
- Dry cough or wheezing
- Chest pain with each breath

- Shortness of breath
- Fatigue

Common signs and symptoms of pneumonia
- Cough with greenish or yellowish mucus or may have a bloody nose
- Fever—mild or high
- Chills—shacking
- Shortness of breath with activity—climbing stairs
- Headache
- Fatigue, weakness
- Loss of appetite
- Sharp or stabbing chest pain on inhalation or coughing
- Excessive perspiration
- Confusion in adults 65 years or older

Physical findings
- Fever
- Sputum production
- Dullness over the affected area
- Crackles, wheezing, or rhonchi
- Decreased breath sounds
- Decreased fremitus
- Tachypnea
- Use of accessory muscles

Diagnostic tests

Laboratory
- CBC shows leukocytosis.
- Blood culture findings are positive for the causative organism.
- Arterial blood gas values show hypoxemia.
- Fungal or acid-fast bacilli cultures identify the etiologic agent.
- Assay shows *Legionella*-soluble antigen in urine.
- Sputum culture, Gram stain, and smear show the infecting organism.

Imaging
- Chest X-rays usually show patchy or lobar infiltrates.
- CT scan to evaluate the status of the lungs

Diagnostic procedures

- Bronchoscopy or transtracheal aspiration specimens identify the etiologic agent.
- Swallowing function tests to assess the risk for aspiration pneumonia

Other

- Pulse oximetry may show decreased oxygen saturation.

Treatment

General

- Depends on the cause of the pneumonia, age, and status of immune system
- Mechanical ventilation (positive end-expiratory pressure) if there is respiratory failure
- High-calorie, high-protein diet
- Adequate fluids
- Bed rest initially and ambulate, as tolerated

Medications

- Antibiotics
- Antivirals
- Humidified oxygen
- Antitussives
- Analgesics
- Bronchodilators

Surgery

- Drainage of parapneumonic pleural effusion or lung abscess

Nursing interventions

- Monitor vital signs.
- Monitor intake and output.
- Handwashing—before and after caring for the patient
- Frequent oral hygiene to decrease dry mouth
- Monitor laboratory values.
- Administer medications, as ordered.

- Administer I.V. fluids and electrolyte replacement, as ordered.
- Maintain a patent airway and adequate oxygenation.
- Administer supplemental oxygen as ordered. Give oxygen cautiously if the patient has chronic lung disease.
- Suction the patient, as needed.
- Obtain sputum specimens, as needed.
- Provide a high-calorie, high-protein diet of soft foods.
- Administer supplemental oral feedings, NG tube feedings, or parenteral nutrition if needed.
- Take steps to prevent aspiration during NG feedings.
- Dispose of secretions properly.
- Provide a quiet, calm environment with frequent rest periods.
- Include the patient in care decisions whenever possible.

Patient teaching

- Be sure to cover:
  - the disorder, diagnosis, and treatment
  - medications and possible adverse reactions
  - the need for adequate fluid intake
  - the importance of getting adequate rest
  - deep-breathing and coughing exercises
  - chest physiotherapy
  - teaching splinting to decrease pain with coughing episodes
  - the need to avoid irritants that stimulate secretions
  - when to notify the health care provider
  - home oxygen therapy, if required
  - ways to prevent pneumonia
  - yearly influenza vaccine.
- Refer the patient to a smoking-cessation program, if indicated.

Prostate cancer

Overview

- Proliferation of cancer cells that usually takes the form of adenocarcinomas and typically originate in the posterior prostate gland
- May progress to widespread bone metastases and death
- The leading cause of cancer death in men

Causes

- Unknown

Risk factors

- Older than age 40
- Infection
- Smoking
- Family history
- Exposure to heavy metals
- Race—high incidence in African American
- High-fat diet

Assessment

History

- Symptoms rare in early stages of disease
- Later, urinary problems, such as difficulty initiating a urinary stream, dribbling, and retention of urine

Physical findings

- In early stages: a flat, firm, nodular mass with a sharp edge
- In advanced disease: edema of the scrotum or leg, with a hard lump in the prostate region

Diagnostic tests

Laboratory

- Serum prostate-specific antigen (PSA) level is elevated. (An elevated PSA level may indicate cancer with or without metastases.)

Imaging

- Transrectal prostatic ultrasonography shows the size of the prostate and the presence of abnormal growths.
- Bone scan and excretory urography determine the extent of disease.
- MRI and CT scan define the extent of the tumor.

Other

- The standard screening tests is PSA and organizations differ when to begin screening. Men should discuss screening with their PCP. Refer to screening guidelines by the USPSTF and the American Cancer Society.
- A biopsy of prostate tissue to detect cancer cells

Treatment

General

- Varies with stage of cancer
- Radiation therapy: External radiation therapy directs radiation to specific affected site or internal beam radiation. Radioactive seeds or pellets are surgically placed into or near the cancer cells to destroy them.
- High-intensity focused ultrasound—high-intensity waves directed at cancer cells to kill the cancer cells
- Cryotherapy freezes and kills cancer cells.
- Biologic therapy using the body's immune systems to fight cancer cells
- Well-balanced diet
- CAM and integrative medicine are being implemented but is not considered a standard of treatment.

Medications

- Hormonal therapy
- Chemotherapy

Surgery

- Prostatectomy
- Orchiectomy
- Radical prostatectomy
- Transurethral resection of the prostate
- Cryosurgical ablation
- Robotic-assisted laparoscopic radical prostatectomy

Nursing interventions

- Monitor vital signs.
- Monitor intake and output, noting diarrhea and/or constipation.
- Weigh daily.
- Assess consumption of a nutritious diet and for loss of appetite.
- Provide oral hygiene.
- Review laboratory results— serum transfusion, albumin, CBC, white blood cell count, platelets to detect anemia, sepsis, or myelosuppression.
- Administer medications, as ordered.
- Evaluate for pain.
- Encourage the patient to express his or her feelings.
- Assess for depression.
- Encourage rest.

Patient teaching

- Be sure to cover:
  - the disorder, diagnosis, and treatment
  - perineal exercises that decrease incontinence
  - the importance of follow-up care
  - administration, dosages, and possible adverse reaction to medication
  - tobacco cessation
  - alcohol cessation.
- Refer the patient to appropriate resources and support services, as needed.

Pulmonary embolism

Overview

- Obstruction of the pulmonary arterial bed that occurs when a mass (such as a dislodged thrombus) lodges in the main pulmonary artery or branch, partially or completely obstructing it
- Usually originates in the deep veins of the leg or pelvis
- Can be asymptomatic but sometimes causes rapid death from pulmonary infarction
- Higher incidence occurs in African Americans.

Causes

- Deep vein thrombosis
- Pelvic, renal, and hepatic vein thrombosis
- Right heart thrombus
- Upper extremity thrombosis
- Valvular heart disease
- Rarely, other types of emboli, such as bone, air, fat, amniotic fluid, tumor cells, or a foreign body

Risk factors

- Various disorders and treatments
- Ages older than 40 years
- Obesity
- Supplemental estrogen
- Pregnancy
- Hypertension
- Women—childhood-bearing years
- Smoking
- Inflammatory bowel disease
- Sedentary lifestyle
- Cancer—pancreatic, ovarian, and lung metastasis
- Surgery, venous stasis, venous injury, increased blood coagulability, and predisposing disorders, such as thromboembolism and thrombophlebitis
- Thrombophilia

Assessment
History
- Predisposing factor
- Syncope
- Increased warmth to the affected area
- Edema of the affected area
- Shortness of breath for no apparent reason
- Cough
- Sudden pleuritic pain or angina

Physical findings
- Tachycardia
- Low-grade fever
- Excessive sweating
- Weak, rapid irregular pulse
- Hypotension
- Productive cough, possibly with blood-tinged sputum
- Warmth, tenderness, and edema of the lower leg
- Dyspnea and restlessness
- Dizziness
- Transient pleural friction rub
- Rales/crackles
- S_3 and S_4 gallop, with increased intensity of the pulmonic component of S_2
- If the embolus is large, cyanosis, syncope, and distended jugular veins

Diagnostic tests
Laboratory
- Arterial blood gas values show hypoxemia.
- D-dimer level is elevated.

Imaging
- Lung ventilation-perfusion scan shows a ventilation-perfusion mismatch.
- Pulmonary angiography shows a pulmonary vessel filling defect or an abrupt vessel ending as well as the location and extent of pulmonary embolism.
- Chest X-rays may show a small infiltrate or effusion.
- Spiral chest CT scan may show central pulmonary emboli.
- CT angiography shows blood clots in the lungs and the legs.

Diagnostic procedures
- ECG may show right axis deviation, right bundle-branch block, or atrial fibrillation.
- Echocardiography may show right atrial and ventricular enlargement or thrombus.
- Duplex ultrasonography of the leg or pelvic veins may indicate the embolic source and shows the pattern of blood flow in the veins.
- MRI produces detailed images of the internal structures.

Treatment
General
- Maintenance of adequate cardiovascular and pulmonary function
- Mechanical ventilation, if indicated
- Possible fluid restriction
- Bed rest during the acute phase

Medications
- Oxygen therapy
- Thrombolytics
- Thrombin inhibitors
- Anticoagulation
- Corticosteroids (controversial)
- Diuretics
- Antiarrhythmics
- Vasopressors (for hypotension)
- Antibiotics (for septic embolus)

Surgery
- Vena caval interruption
- Vena caval filter placement
- Pulmonary embolectomy

Nursing interventions
- Administer medications, as ordered.
- Avoid I.M. injections.

- Encourage active and passive range-of-motion exercises unless contraindicated.
- Avoid massage of the lower legs.
- Apply antiembolism stockings.
- Provide adequate nutrition.
- Assist with ambulation as soon as the patient is stable.
- Encourage the use of incentive spirometry.

Patient teaching

- Be sure to cover:
  - the disease, diagnosis, and treatment
  - medications and possible adverse reactions
  - ways to prevent deep vein thrombosis and pulmonary embolism
  - signs and symptoms of abnormal bleeding
  - how to prevent abnormal bleeding
  - how to monitor anticoagulant effects
  - dietary sources of vitamin K
  - when to notify the health care provider.
- Refer the patient to a weight management program, if indicated.

Renal failure, acute (acute kidney injury)

Overview

- Sudden interruption of renal function as a result of obstruction, reduced circulation, or renal parenchymal disease
- Classified as prerenal failure, intrarenal failure (also called intrinsic or parenchymal failure), or postrenal failure
- Usually reversible with medical treatment
- If not treated, may progress to end-stage renal disease, uremia, and death
- Normally, three distinct phases: oliguric, diuretic, and recovery

Oliguric phase

- This phase may last a few days or several weeks.
- Urine output drops to less than 400 ml/day.
- Excess fluid volume, azotemia, and electrolyte imbalance occur.
- Local mediators are released, causing intrarenal vasoconstriction.
- Medullary hypoxia causes cellular swelling and adherence of neutrophils to capillaries and venules.
- Hypoperfusion occurs.
- Cellular injury and necrosis occur.
- Reperfusion causes reactive oxygen species to form, leading to further cellular injury.

Diuretic phase

- Renal function is recovered.
- Urine output gradually increases.
- The glomerular filtration rate improves, although tubular transport systems remain abnormal.

Recovery phase

- The recovery phase may last 3 to 12 months or longer.
- Renal function gradually returns to normal or near normal.

Causes

Prerenal failure

- Hypovolemia
- Diarrhea
- Hemorrhagic blood loss
- Loss of plasma volume
- Water and electrolyte losses
- Hypotension or hypoperfusion
- Renal artery or vein obstruction

Intrarenal failure

- Damage nephrons
- Acute tubular necrosis
- Glomerulopathy
- Malignant hypertension
- Coagulation defects

Postrenal failure
- Obstructive uropathy, which is usually bilateral
- Enlarged prostate
- Ureteral destruction
- Bladder neck obstruction

Risk factors
- Advanced age
- Kidney disease
- Diabetes mellitus
- Hypertension
- Liver disease/failure
- Heart failure/heart attack
- Infection
- MI
- Cholesterol blocking vessels in kidney(s)
- Blood clots in veins or arteries in or around the kidney
- Severe burns
- Severe dehydration
- Medication treatment for other conditions—chemotherapy, hypertension, antibiotics, NSAIDs

Assessment
History
- There may be no signs or symptoms and is detected through laboratory tests obtained for another medical problem.
  - Fluid retention, edema, in legs, ankles or feet
  - Shortness of breath
  - Fatigue, weakness
  - Irregular heart beat
  - Chest pain or pressure
  - Confusion
  - Seizures or coma in severe cases
  - Decreased urine output—often, the urine output will be with negative findings
- Predisposing disorder
- Recent fever, chills, or a CNS disorder
- Recent GI problem

Physical findings
- Oliguria or anuria, depending on the phase of renal failure
- Tachycardia
- Bibasilar crackles
- Irritability, drowsiness, or confusion
- Altered level of consciousness
- Bleeding abnormalities
- Dry, pruritic skin
- Dry mucous membranes
- Uremic breath odor

Diagnostic tests
Laboratory
- Blood urea nitrogen, serum creatinine, and potassium levels are elevated.
- Hematocrit, blood pH, bicarbonate, and hemoglobin levels are decreased.
- Urine casts and cellular debris are present, and the specific gravity is decreased.
- In glomerular disease, proteinuria and urine osmolality are near the serum osmolality level.
- The urine sodium level is less than 20 mEq/L if oliguria results from decreased perfusion.
- The urine sodium level is greater than 40 mEq/L if oliguria results from an intrarenal problem.
- Urine creatinine clearance is used to measure the glomerular filtration rate, 90 ml/minute, and estimate the number of remaining functioning nephrons.

Imaging
The following imaging tests may show the cause of renal failure:
- kidney ultrasonography
- kidney-ureter-bladder radiography
- excretory urography renal scan
- retrograde pyelography
- CT scan
- nephrotomography.

Diagnostic procedures
- ECG shows tall, peaked T waves; a widening QRS complex; and disappearing P waves if hyperkalemia is present.

Treatment
General

- Hemodialysis, peritoneal dialysis (if appropriate), or continuous renal replacement therapies
- High-calorie, low-protein, low-sodium, and low-potassium diet
- Fluid restriction
- Rest periods when fatigued

Medications

- Supplemental vitamins—low doses of calcium, iron, and vitamins C and D; avoid vitamins A, E, and K because, over a period of time, there could be a buildup in the body and cause nausea, dizziness, or death.
- No herbal remedies due to possible drug interactions with prescribed medications
- Diuretics, as applicable
- In hyperkalemia, hypertonic glucose and insulin infusions, sodium bicarbonate, and sodium polystyrene sulfonate to control level of potassium

Surgery

- Creation of vascular access for hemodialysis

Nursing interventions

- Administer medication, as ordered.
- Monitor for side effects of prescribed medications.
- Check for dehydration.
- Strict monitoring of intake and output, observe urine color—should not be dark.
- Monitor I.V. fluids for appropriate rate and amount.
- Monitor vital signs, focus on blood pressure.
- Check for edema.
- Monitor levels of blood urea nitrogen/creatinine for an increase and/or decrease and report findings.
- Observe for Kussmaul's breathing—a deep and labored breathing pattern associated with kidney failure.

- Give low-protein, low-potassium diet, as ordered.
- Monitor and protect from falls.
- Encourage the patient to express his or her feelings.
- Provide emotional support.
- Identify patients at risk for acute tubular necrosis, and take preventive steps.
- Monitor the patient's weight daily.
- Monitor the dialysis access site.

Patient teaching

- Be sure to cover:
  - the disorder, diagnosis, and treatment
  - administration, dosages, and possible adverse reactions to medications
  - the recommended fluid allowances
  - the importance of complying with the diet and medication regimen
  - the importance of monitoring weight daily and reporting changes of 3 lb (1.4 kg) or more immediately
  - the signs and symptoms of edema and the importance of reporting them to the health care provider.

Renal failure, chronic (chronic kidney disease)

Overview

- End result of a gradually progressive loss of renal function
- Few symptoms until more than 75% of glomerular filtration is lost, with symptoms worsening as renal function declines
- Fatal unless treated; to sustain life, maintenance dialysis or kidney transplantation may be needed.
- Anemia, bone disease, and malnutrition can develop.

- Frequently occurs in the elderly, although it can occur in all ages.
- Common in people with a family history of kidney disease

Causes

- Chronic glomerular disease
- Chronic infections such as chronic pyelonephritis
- Congenital anomalies such as polycystic kidney disease
- Vascular diseases
- Obstructive processes such as calculi
- Collagen diseases such as systemic lupus erythematosus
- Hyperkalemia
- Hypertension
- Cardiovascular diseases
- Glomerulonephritis
- Diabetes mellitus type 1 and type 2
- Decrease immune response
- Smoking
- Obesity
- Nephrotoxic agents
- Endocrine disease

Assessment

History

- Changes in frequency of urination
- Loss of appetite
- Weight loss
- Predisposing factor(s)
- Dry mouth
- Fatigue, weakness
- Nausea, vomiting
- Hiccups
- Headache
- Edema of lower extremities
- Persistent itching
- Chest pain if there is fluid retention
- Shortness of breath if there is fluid retention
- Difficulty with management of high blood pressure
- Trouble concentrating
- Chills most often of the ears, nose, hands, feet and may be due to anemia

- Muscle cramps
- Fasciculations and twitching
- Infertility and decreased libido
- Amenorrhea
- Impotence
- Pathologic fractures

Physical findings

- Decreased urine output
- Hypotension or hypertension
- Altered level of consciousness
- Peripheral edema
- Cardiac arrhythmias
- Bibasilar crackles
- Pleural friction rub
- Gum ulceration and bleeding
- Uremic fetor
- Abdominal pain on palpation
- Poor skin turgor, rash, irritation sensation
- Pale, yellow-bronze skin color
- Thin, brittle fingernails and dry, brittle hair
- Growth retardation (in children)

Diagnostic tests

Laboratory

- Blood urea nitrogen, serum creatinine, sodium, and potassium levels are elevated.
- Arterial blood gas values show decreased arterial pH and bicarbonate levels.
- Hematocrit and hemoglobin level are low; RBC survival time is decreased.
- Mild thrombocytopenia and platelet defects appear.
- Aldosterone secretion is increased.
- Hyperglycemia and hypertriglyceridemia occur.
- HDL levels are decreased.
- Arterial blood gas values show metabolic acidosis.
- Urine specific gravity is fixed at 1.010.
- Proteinuria, glycosuria, and urinary RBCs, leukocytes, casts, and crystals are detected.

Imaging

- Kidney-ureter-bladder radiography, excretory urography, nephrotomography, renal scan, and renal arteriography show reduced kidney size.

Diagnostic procedures

- Renal biopsy allows histologic identification of the underlying pathology.
- Electroencephalography shows changes that suggest metabolic encephalopathy.

Treatment

General

- Focus is on slowing progression of kidney damage and end-stage kidney failure.
- Tobacco cessation
- Hemodialysis or peritoneal dialysis
- Low-protein (with peritoneal dialysis, high-protein), high-calorie, low-sodium, low-phosphorus, and low-potassium diet
- Fluid restriction
- Rest periods when fatigued

Medications

- Loop diuretics
- Cardiac glycosides
- Antihypertensives
- Antiemetics
- Iron and folate supplements
- Erythropoietin
- Antipruritics
- Supplementary vitamins and essential amino acids

Surgery

- Creation of vascular access for dialysis
- Possible kidney transplantation

Nursing interventions

- Monitor vital signs.
- Monitor intake and output.
- Administer medication, as ordered.
- Perform meticulous skin care.
- Encourage the patient to express his or her feelings.

- Provide emotional support.
- Monitor the patient's weight and signs and symptoms of fluid overload daily.

Patient teaching

- Be sure to cover:
  - the disorder, diagnosis, and treatment
  - dietary changes
  - fluid restrictions
  - exercise/physical activity
  - care of the dialysis site, as appropriate
  - the importance of wearing or carrying medical identification.
- Refer the patient to appropriate resources and support services.

Rheumatoid arthritis

Overview

- Chronic, systemic, symmetrical inflammatory disease
- Peripheral joints and surrounding muscles, tendons, ligaments, and blood vessels primarily affected
- Skin, eyes, lungs, heart, and blood vessels can be damaged as well as the kidneys, bone marrow, salivary glands, and nerves.
- Marked by spontaneous remissions and unpredictable exacerbations
- Potentially crippling

Causes

- Unknown
- Exploration to determine if genetic components are causing an individual to be susceptible to the virus/bacteria causing the disease
- Possible effect of infection (viral or bacterial), hormonal factors, and lifestyle

Risk factors

- Gender: women more likely than men to develop rheumatoid arthritis
- Genetics: family history of disease

- Smoking cigarettes—tendency to be worse if a smoker
- Environmental factors: exposure to asbestos or silica
- Obesity

Additional factors that increase risk

- Infections
- Carpal tunnel syndrome
- Cardiovascular disease
- Pulmonary disorders
- Rheumatoid nodules
- Sjögren's syndrome

Assessment

History

- Insidious onset of nonspecific symptoms including fatigue, malaise, persistent low-grade fever, anorexia, weight loss, and vague articular symptoms
- Later, more specific localized articular symptoms, commonly in the fingers
- Bilateral, symmetrical symptoms that may extend to the wrists, elbows, knees, hips, shoulders, and ankles
- Stiff joints, worse in the mornings for 30 minutes or longer and with no activity
- Stiff, weak, or painful muscles
- Numbness or tingling in toes, feet, or weakness or loss of sensation in fingers
- Flares occur that can last for days or months.
- Pain on inspiration
- Shortness of breath

Physical findings

- Joint deformities and contractures
- Red, painful, swollen arms
- Foreshortened hands
- Boggy wrists
- Rheumatoid nodules
- Leg ulcers
- Eye redness
- Joints that are warm to the touch

- Pericardial friction rub
- Positive Babinski's sign

Diagnostic tests

Laboratory

- Rheumatoid factor (RF) test result is positive in 75% to 80% of patients, as indicated by a titer of 1:160 or higher.
- Synovial fluid analysis shows increased volume and turbidity but decreased viscosity and complement (C3 and C4) levels; white blood cell count may exceed 10,000/µl.
- Serum globulin levels are elevated.
- ESR is elevated.
- CBC shows moderate anemia and slight leukocytosis. (See *Classifying rheumatoid arthritis*.)
- CRP is elevated.

Imaging

- In early stages of the disease, X-rays show bone demineralization and soft-tissue swelling. Later, they help determine the extent of cartilage and bone destruction, erosion, subluxations, and deformities, and show the characteristic pattern of these abnormalities.
- MRI and CT scans may provide information about the extent of damage and severity.

Other

- Synovial tissue biopsy shows inflammation.

Treatment

General

- Adequate sleep (8 to 10 hours every night)
- Splinting
- Range-of-motion exercises and carefully individualized muscle-strengthening exercises
- Application of moist heat
- Frequent rest periods between activities
- Assistive devices

Classifying rheumatoid arthritis

A patient who meets four of the seven American College of Rheumatology criteria is classified as having rheumatoid arthritis. The patient must experience the first four criteria for at least 6 weeks, and a health care provider must observe the second through fifth criteria.

Criteria
1. Morning stiffness in and around the joints that lasts for 1 hour before full improvement
2. Arthritis in three or more joint areas, with at least three joint areas (as observed by a health care provider) exhibiting soft-tissue swelling or joint effusions, not just bony overgrowth (The 14 possible areas involved include the right and left proximal interphalangeal, metacarpophalangeal, wrist, elbow, knee, ankle, and metatarsophalangeal joints.)
3. Arthritis of the hand joints, including the wrist, metacarpophalangeal joint, or proximal interphalangeal joint
4. Arthritis that involves the same joint areas on both sides of the body
5. Subcutaneous rheumatoid nodules over bony prominences
6. The finding of abnormal amounts of serum rheumatoid factor by any method that produces a positive result in fewer than 5% of patients without rheumatoid arthritis
7. Radiographic changes, usually on posteroanterior radiographs of the hand and wrist, that show erosions or unequivocal bony decalcification localized in or most noticeable adjacent to the involved joints

Medications
- Disease-modifying antirheumatic drugs (DMARDs)
- Biologic response modifiers
- Janus kinase (JAK) inhibitor
- Salicylates
- NSAIDs
- Antimalarials (hydroxychloroquine)
- Gold salts
- Penicillamine
- Corticosteroids
- Antineoplastic agents

Other methods
- Complementary and alternative treatments have been shown to be helpful, as prescribed.
  - Fish oil—reduces inflammation and reduces stiffness
  - Plant oils—borage or black currant
  - Tai chi—reduces pain

Surgery
- Metatarsal head and distal ulnar re-sectional arthroplasty and insertion of a silicone prosthesis between the metacarpophalangeal and proximal interphalangeal joints
- Arthrodesis (joint fusion)
- Synovectomy
- Osteotomy
- Repair of ruptured tendon
- In advanced disease, joint reconstruction or total joint arthroplasty

Nursing interventions
- Administer analgesics as ordered, and watch for adverse reactions.
- Perform meticulous skin care.
- Supply adaptive devices, such as a zipper-pull, easy-to-open beverage cartons, lightweight cups, and unpackaged silverware.
- Assess for depression.

After total knee or hip arthroplasty

- Monitor vital signs.
- Administer blood replacement products, antibiotics, and pain medication, as ordered.
- Have the patient perform active dorsiflexion; immediately report inability to do so.
- Supervise isometric exercises every 2 hours.
- After total hip arthroplasty, check traction for pressure areas and keep the head of the bed raised 30 to 45 degrees.
- Change or reinforce dressings, as needed, using aseptic technique.
- Have the patient turn, cough, and breathe deeply every 2 hours.
- After total knee arthroplasty, keep the leg extended and slightly elevated.
- After total hip arthroplasty, keep the hip in abduction. Watch for and immediately report inability to rotate the hip or bear weight on hip, increased pain, or a leg that appears shorter than the other leg.
- Assist the patient in activities, keeping his or her weight on the unaffected side.

Patient teaching

- Be sure to cover:
  - the disorder, diagnosis, and treatment
  - the chronic nature of rheumatoid arthritis and the possible need for major lifestyle changes
  - importance to avoid falls
  - the importance of a balanced diet and weight control
  - the importance of adequate sleep
  - sexual concerns.
- If the patient requires total knee or hip arthroplasty, be sure to cover:
  - preoperative and surgical procedures
  - postoperative exercises, with supervision of the patient's practice to ensure that he or she is performing the exercises correctly
  - deep-breathing and coughing exercises to perform after surgery
  - the need to perform frequent range-of-motion leg exercises after surgery
  - the use of a constant passive-motion device after total knee arthroplasty or placement of an abduction pillow between the legs after total hip arthroplasty
  - how to use a trapeze to move about in bed
  - fall prevention
  - dosages and possible adverse reactions to medications.
- Refer the patient to the Arthritis Foundation.
- Refer the patient to a support group.
- Refer the patient to physical and occupational therapy.

Seizure disorder

Overview

- Neurologic condition characterized by recurrent seizures
- Seizure is a single surge of electrical activity of the brain due to excess electrical activity and often occurs as a one-time event.
- Intelligence not affected
- Good seizure control achieved in about 80% of patients with strict adherence to prescribed treatment
- Classified as two main types: partial and generalized

Causes

- Idiopathic in half of cases—one seizure

Nonidiopathic epilepsy in half the cases

- Nonidiopathic—more than one seizure is known as epilepsy.
- Birth trauma
- Anoxia
- Perinatal infection or injury

- Genetic abnormalities (tuberous sclerosis and phenylketonuria)
- Metabolic abnormalities (hypoglycemia, pyridoxine deficiency, hypoparathyroidism)
- Brain tumors or other space-occupying lesions
- Meningitis, encephalitis, or brain abscess
- Traumatic injury
- Ingestion of toxins, such as mercury, lead, or carbon monoxide
- Stroke
- Apparent familial incidence in some seizure disorders

Seizure disorder
- Partial (focal)
  - Starts on one side of the brain
- Simple partial seizure
  - Spreads to all parts of the brain
- Complex partial seizures
  - Affects the consciousness
- Generalized seizure
  - Affects both sides of the brain

Assessment

History

- Seizure occurrence unpredictable and unrelated to activities
- Precipitating factors or events possibly reported
- Headache
- Mood changes
- Lethargy
- Myoclonic jerking
- Description of an aura
- Description of a pungent smell
- GI distress
- Rising or sinking feeling in the stomach
- Dreamy feeling
- Unusual taste in the mouth
- Visual disturbance
- Partial (focal)
  - Involuntary muscle twitching
  - Vision changes
  - Dizziness
  - Sensory changes

- Simple partial seizure
  - Involuntary muscle twitching
  - Vision changes
  - Dizziness
- Complex partial seizures
  - Muscle spasms
  - Limb twitching
  - Loss of consciousness
- Generalized seizures
  - Aura—the experience of abnormal sensations as a precursor to a seizure—a smell or sounds, dizziness, anxiety moment
  - Absence—brief, are motionless, starring off
  - Myoclonic—twitching of both sides of the body—arms and legs
  - Tonic-clonic also known as grand mal seizure—lasts up to 20 minutes, uncontrolled movements, may lose bladder control, may lose consciousness
  - Tonic—may have a moan or a cry, may be saliva or form from the mouth, may bite their tongue or cheek, chest stiffness interferes with breathing and the person may turn blue and make gasping or gurgling sounds
  - Clonic—jerky movements of arms and legs that are rapid that may last up to 3 minutes and the movements relax; there may be loose stools noticed and will return to normal breathing
- Febrile
  - Occurs in presence of fever, most often in children 6 months to 5 years

Physical findings

- Findings possibly normal while the patient is not having a seizure and when the cause is idiopathic
- Findings related to the underlying cause of the seizure

Diagnostic tests

Laboratory

- Serum glucose and calcium test results rule out other diagnoses.

Imaging

- CT scan and MRI may indicate abnormalities in internal structures.
- Skull radiography may show skull fractures or certain neoplasms within the brain.
- Brain scan may show malignant lesions when the X-ray findings are normal or questionable.
- Cerebral angiography may show cerebrovascular abnormalities, such as aneurysm or tumor.

Other

- Electroencephalogram shows paroxysmal abnormalities. (A negative finding does not rule out epilepsy because paroxysmal abnormalities occur intermittently.)

Treatment

General

- Protection of the airway during seizures
- Stimulation of the vagal nerve by a pacemaker
- Detailed presurgical evaluation to characterize the seizure type, frequency, and site of onset and the patient's psychological functioning and degree of disability to select candidates for surgery when medical treatment is unsuccessful
- No dietary restrictions
- Safety measures
- Activity, as tolerated

Medications

- Anticonvulsants

Surgery

- Removal of a demonstrated focal lesion
- Implanted neurostimulation device that for epilepsy detects abnormal electrical activity of the brain and the implant delivers electrical stimulation to prevent seizures.
- Correction of the underlying problem

Nursing interventions

- Institute seizure precautions.
- Actions
  - Protect patient from injury.
  - Gently guide to the floor.
  - Do not hold the patient still.
  - Do not put anything in the mouth.
  - Time the seizure.
  - Calm support.
- Prepare the patient for surgery if indicated.
- Give prescribed anticonvulsants.
- Monitor seizure activity.

Patient teaching

- Be sure to cover:
  - the disorder, diagnosis, and treatment
  - the importance of maintaining a normal lifestyle
  - the importance of complying with the prescribed drug schedule
  - adverse drug effects
  - care during a seizure
  - the importance of regular meals and checking with the health care provider before dieting
  - the importance of carrying a medical identification card or wearing medical identification jewelry.
- Refer the patient to the Epilepsy Foundation.
- Refer the patient to his or her state's motor vehicle department for information about obtaining a driver's license.

Stroke (cerebrovascular accident)

Overview

- Sudden impairment of circulation in the blood vessels to the brain
- Third most common cause of death in the United States
- 700,000 people affected each year; half of cases result in death.
- Most common cause of neurologic disability
- About 50% of stroke survivors permanently disabled
- Recurrence possible within weeks, months, or years
- Also known as cerebrovascular accident or brain attack

Causes

Cerebral thrombosis (thrombotic stroke)

- Most common cause of stroke
- Obstruction of a blood vessel in the extracerebral vessels by formation of a blood clot
- Site possibly intracerebral

Cerebral embolism (ischemic stroke)

- Second most common cause of stroke
- Formation of an embolus, a blood clot, blocks or closes a blood vessel or an artery of the brain or that gets trapped in the arteries outside of the brain
- History of rheumatic heart disease
- Endocarditis
- Posttraumatic valvular disease
- Cardiac arrhythmias
- Atrial fibrillation is considered a common cause.
- After open heart surgery

Cerebral hemorrhage

- Third most common cause of stroke
- A blood vessel breaks and bleeds into the brain.

- Extravasated blood present most often near an embolus
- Chronic hypertension
- Cerebral aneurysms
- Arteriovenous malformation
- Trauma

Intracerebral stroke

- A damaged or disease blood vessel(s) bursts within the brain.

Subarachnoid stroke

- A severe headache with popping or snapping feeling due to anticoagulants or head injury

Transient ischemic attacks (mini strokes)

- The blood supply to the brain is briefly interrupted and symptoms resolve.

Risk factors

- History of transient ischemic attack
- Heart disease
- Stress
- Lack of physical activity
- Use of illegal drugs
- Hypertension
- Smoking
- Familial history of cerebrovascular disease
- Gender—young men more likely than women; for older ages, women more likely than men
- Obesity
- Excessive alcohol use
- High RBC count
- Cardiac arrhythmias
- Diabetes mellitus
- Sickle cell disease
- Vasculitis
- Poor diet
- Sleep apnea
- Gout
- High serum triglyceride levels
- Use of hormonal contraceptives in conjunction with smoking and hypertension
- Elevated cholesterol and triglyceride levels

Assessment

History

- Varying clinical features, depending on:
  - the artery affected
  - the severity of damage
  - the extent of collateral circulation
  - FAST (via American Stroke Association)
    - F—face dropping, numbness, and weakness on one side
    - A—arm weakness or numbness on one side of the body
    - S—speech difficulty, slurred speech or difficulty speaking or not being understood when speaking, confusion
    - T—time—what is the time for any of the symptoms
- Severe headache with unknown cause
- One or more risk factors
- Trouble walking, balance/coordination, unexplained falls
- Sudden onset of hemiparesis or hemiplegia
- Gradual onset of dizziness, mental disturbances, or seizures
- Loss of consciousness, sudden aphasia, or loss of vision in one eye or both eyes

Physical findings

- With stroke in the left hemisphere, signs and symptoms on the right side
- With stroke in the right hemisphere, signs and symptoms on the left side
- With stroke that causes cranial nerve damage, signs and symptoms on the same side
- Change in the level of consciousness
- With a conscious patient, anxiety along with communication and mobility difficulties
- Urinary incontinence
- Loss of voluntary muscle control
- Hemiparesis or hemiplegia on one side of the body
- Decreased deep tendon reflexes
- Hemianopia on the affected side of the body
- With left-sided hemiplegia, problems with visuospatial relations
- Sensory losses

Diagnostic tests

Laboratory

- Laboratory tests—including levels of anticardiolipin antibodies, antiphospholipid, factor V (Leiden) mutation, antithrombin III, protein S, and protein C—may show increased risk of thrombosis
- PT and partial thromboplastin time (PTT) levels to measure length of time for blood to clot

Imaging

- MRI and magnetic resonance angiography allow the size and location of the lesion to be evaluated.
- Cerebral angiography details the disruption of cerebral circulation and is the test of choice for examining the entire cerebral blood flow.
- CT scan detects structural abnormalities.
- PET provides data on cerebral metabolism and changes in cerebral blood flow.
- Carotid ultrasound displays a picture of carotid arteries internal flow of blood and buildup of cholesterol plaques.

Other

- Transcranial Doppler studies are used to evaluate the velocity of blood flow.
- Carotid Doppler is used to measure flow through the carotid and vertebral arteries.

- Two-dimensional echocardiogram is used to evaluate the heart for dysfunction.
- Cerebral blood flow studies are used to measure blood flow to the brain.
- Echocardiography displays size and shape of the heart, function of chambers and valves, detects blood clots inside the heart, and the functioning of the aorta.
- ECG shows reduced electrical activity in an area of cortical infarction.

Treatment

General

- Careful management of blood pressure
- Varies, depending on the cause and clinical manifestations
- Pureed dysphagia diet or tube feedings, if indicated
- Physical, speech, and occupational rehabilitation
- Care measures to help the patient adapt to specific deficits

Medications

- Alert: tissue plasminogen activator (tPA) when the cause is not hemorrhagic (emergency care within 3 hours of onset of the symptoms)
- Anticonvulsants
- Stool softeners
- Anticoagulants
- Antiplatelets
- Analgesics
- Antidepressants
- Antiplatelets
- Lipid-lowering agents
- Antihypertensives
  Note: Antiplatelets stop

platelets from clumping together; anticoagulants keep blood clots from getting large if tPA cannot be given within the first 3 hours of stroke symptoms.

Surgery

- Craniotomy
- Carotid endarterectomy
- Extracranial-intracranial bypass
- Ventricular shunts
- Carotid artery angioplasty
- Intra-arterial thrombolysis
- Mechanical embolus removal in cerebral ischemia (MERCI)—removes clots from an artery

Nursing interventions

- Monitor vital signs.
- Monitor for edema.
- Monitor intake and output.
- Maintain a patent airway and oxygenation.
- Offer the urinal or bedpan every 2 hours.
- Insert an indwelling urinary catheter if necessary.
- Ensure adequate nutrition.
- Provide careful mouth care.
- Provide meticulous eye care.
- Follow the physical therapy program, and assist the patient with exercise.
- Establish and maintain communication with the patient.
- Provide psychological support.
- Set realistic short-term goals.
- Protect the patient from injury.
- Provide careful positioning to prevent aspiration and contractures.
- Take steps to prevent complications.
- Administer medications, as ordered.
- Monitor the patient for the development of deep vein thrombosis and pulmonary embolus.

Patient teaching

- Be sure to cover:
  - the disorder, diagnosis, and treatment
  - occupational and speech therapy programs
  - dietary regimen

– medication regimen
– adverse drug reactions
– stroke prevention.
- Refer the patient to home care services.
- Refer the patient to outpatient services, speech, and occupational rehabilitation programs, as indicated.

Thrombophlebitis

Overview

- Development of a thrombus that may cause vessel occlusion or embolization
- Acute condition characterized by inflammation and thrombus formation
- May occur in deep or superficial veins or iliofemoral
- Typically occurs at the valve cusps because venous stasis encourages accumulation and adherence of platelet and fibrin

Causes

- Smoking
- May be idiopathic
- Prolonged bed rest
- Trauma
- Surgery
- Pregnancy and childbirth
- Hormonal contraceptives such as estrogens
- Neoplasms
- Fracture of the spine, pelvis, femur, or tibia
- Venous insufficiency
- Pacemaker could irritate blood vessel wall
- Venulitis
- Thrombophilias

Risk factors

- Age older than 60 years
- Obesity
- Stroke
- Inactivity
- Family history of blood clots
- Polycythemia vera
- Smoking
- Traveling in a car or airplane for long distances

Assessment

History

- Asymptomatic in up to 50% of patients with deep vein thrombophlebitis
  - Superficial: vein near the surface of the skin, warm, tenderness, pain in the affected area
  - Deep: pain deep within a muscle, edema of affected area
- Possible tenderness, edema in affected area, skin erythema occurs sometimes, aching, or severe pain in the affected leg or arm; fever, chills, and malaise

Physical findings

- Redness, swelling, and tenderness of the affected leg or arm
- Possible positive Homans' sign
- Positive cuff sign
- Possible sensation of warmth in the affected leg or arm
- Lymphadenitis in patients with extensive vein involvement
- Nonpitting edema with deep vein thrombosis

Diagnostic tests

Laboratory

- CBC, CMP, antithrombin level, blood coagulation studies, homocysteine level

Diagnostic procedures

- Duplex ultrasonography shows reduced blood flow to a specific area and obstruction to venous flow, particularly in iliofemoral deep vein thrombophlebitis.
- Use venography to visualize veins in the legs and identify, and locate blood clots in veins of the legs and check adequacy of blood flow.
- Phlebography shows filling defects and diverted blood flow but is rarely used.

Treatment

General

- Apply no pressure over affected area
- Application of warm, moist compresses to the affected area
- Antiembolism stockings
- Bed rest, with elevation of the affected extremity

Medications

- Anticoagulants
- Thrombolytics
- NSAIDs for superficial thrombophlebitis if not taking an antiplatelet or anticoagulant
- Analgesics

Surgery

- Simple ligation to vein plication or clipping
- Embolectomy
- Caval interruption with transvenous placement of a vena cava filter

Nursing interventions

- Enforce bed rest as ordered and elevate the patient's affected arm or leg but avoid compressing the popliteal space.
- Apply warm compresses or a covered aquathermia pad.
- Give analgesics, as ordered.
- Mark, measure, and record the circumference of the affected arm or leg daily, and compare this measurement with that of the other arm or leg.
- Administer anticoagulants, as ordered.
- Perform or encourage range-of-motion exercises.
- Use pneumatic compression devices.
- Apply antiembolism stockings.
- Monitor the results of laboratory tests.
- Monitor for signs and symptoms of pulmonary embolism.
- Monitor for worsening signs and symptoms of a stroke.

Patient teaching

- Be sure to cover:
  - the disorder, diagnosis, and treatment
  - the importance of follow-up blood studies to monitor anticoagulant therapy
  - how to give injections (if the patient requires subcutaneous anticoagulation therapy after discharge)
  - the need to avoid prolonged sitting or standing to help prevent a recurrence
  - the proper application and use of antiembolism stockings
  - the importance of adequate hydration
  - the need to use an electric razor and to avoid products that contain aspirin.

Tuberculosis

Overview

- Acute or chronic lung infection characterized by pulmonary infiltrates and the formation of granulomas with caseation, fibrosis, and cavitation
- Tuberculosis (TB):
  - is a systemic disease
  - is a latent infection
  - has an incubation period after infection of 2 to 4 weeks.
- TB of the lungs spreads by air via coughing, talking, singing, sneezing, and not by touch.
- May affect the kidney, spine, brain, or other body parts
  - There is a no spread to others if the TB is in these body parts.
- Excellent prognosis with proper treatment and compliance
- Increase in cases related to emergence of multidrug-resistant strains of TB

Causes

- Exposure to *Mycobacterium tuberculosis*—latent TB
- In some cases, exposure to other strains of mycobacteria

Risk factors

- Close contact with a patient newly diagnosed with TB
- History of previous exposure to TB
- Weakened immune system due to illness(es)
- Multiple sexual partners
- Recent immigration from Africa, Asia, Mexico, or South America
- Gastrectomy
- History of silicosis, diabetes, malnutrition, severe kidney disease, organ transplant, HIV, cancer, Hodgkin's disease, or leukemia
- Drug and alcohol abuse
- Residence in a nursing home, mental health facility, or prison
- Immunosuppression and use of corticosteroids
- Homelessness
- Working in health care

Assessment

History

In primary infection

- Usually asymptomatic after a 4- to 8-week incubation period
- Weakness and fatigue
- Anorexia and weight loss
- Low-grade fever or chills
- Night sweats
- With latent TB
  - No symptomatology
  - No feelings of being ill
  - Cannot be spread to others
  - There is a positive skin test or blood test.
- There is:
  - a negative chest X-ray
  - a negative sputum smear and/or culture
  - no need for a treatment plan.

- TB disease
  - Feelings of being sick exact
  - Becomes active when the immune system is weak and is not able to be resistant
  - There is a moderate to severe cough with expectorant of sputum or blood that lasts 3 weeks or longer.
- There is:
  - loss of appetite
  - weight loss
  - chills, fever, night sweats
  - a positive sputum smear and/or culture
  - a positive skin test and blood test
  - an abnormal chest X-ray
  - contagious.
- A treatment plan is activated.

In reactivated infection

- Chest pain
- Productive cough (blood or mucopurulent or blood-tinged sputum)
- Low-grade fever

Physical findings

- Dullness over the affected area
- Crepitant crackles
- Bronchial breath sounds
- Enlarged lymph nodes
- Wheezes
- Whispered pectoriloquy

Diagnostic tests

Laboratory

- Tuberculin skin test result is positive in both active and inactive TB.
- TB blood test is preferred for individuals who have been vaccinated with bacillus Calmette-Guérin (BCG) because a TB skin tests will yield a false positive.
- Genotyping to identify TB strains
- Stains and cultures of sputum, cerebrospinal fluid, urine, abscess drainage, or pleural fluid show heat-sensitive, nonmotile, aerobic, acid-fast bacilli

Imaging

- Chest X-rays show nodular lesions, patchy infiltrates, cavity formation, scar tissue, and calcium deposits.
- CT or MRI shows the presence and extent of lung damage.

Diagnostic procedures

- Bronchoscopy specimens show heat-sensitive, nonmotile, aerobic, acid-fast bacilli.

Treatment

General

- After 2 to 4 weeks, when the disease is no longer infectious, resumption of normal activities while continuing to take medication
- Well-balanced, high-calorie diet
- Rest initially, with resumption of activity, as tolerated

Medications

- Antitubercular therapy for at least 6 months with daily oral doses of:
  - isoniazid (INH)
  - rifampin (RIF)
  - pyrazinamide (PZA)
  - ethambutol (EMB) added in some cases.
- Second-line drugs include:
  - capreomycin
  - streptomycin
  - aminosalicylic acid (para-aminosalicylic acid)
  - pyrazinamide (PZA)
  - cycloserine.
- Latent *M. tuberculosis*
  - Isoniazid (INH)
  - Rifapentine (RPT)
  - Rifampin (RIF)
  - Rifadin
- HIV with positive TB
  - Ethambutol (EMB)
  - Isoniazid (INH)
  - Pyrazinamide (PZA)
  - Rifampin (RIF)

Surgery

- For complications that require invasive or surgical intervention

Nursing interventions

- Monitor vital signs.
- Administer drug therapy.
- Isolate the patient in a quiet, properly ventilated room, and maintain TB precautions.
- Provide diversional activities.
- Dispose secretions properly.
- Provide adequate rest periods.
- Provide a well-balanced, high-calorie diet.
- Provide small, frequent meals.
- Consult with a dietitian if oral supplements are needed.
- Perform chest physiotherapy.
- Provide supportive care.
- Include the patient in care decisions.
- Monitor for drug resistance and drug-drug interaction signs and symptoms.
- Monitor visual acuity if the patient is taking ethambutol.

Patient teaching

- Be sure to cover:
  - the disorder, diagnosis, and treatment
  - medications and potential adverse reactions
  - when to notify the health care provider
  - the need for isolation
  - the importance of postural drainage and chest percussion
  - the importance of coughing and deep-breathing exercises, including a demonstration, if needed
  - the importance of regular follow-up examinations
  - the signs and symptoms of recurring TB
  - the possibility that rifampin may decrease the effectiveness of hormonal contraceptives

Preventing tuberculosis

Explain respiratory and standard precautions to a hospitalized patient with tuberculosis. Before discharge, tell him or her that he or she must take precautions to prevent spreading the disease, such as wearing a mask around others, until his or her health care provider tells him or her that he or she is no longer contagious. He or she should tell all health care providers he or she sees, including his or her dentist and optometrist, that he or she has tuberculosis so that they can institute infection-control precautions.

Teach the patient other specific precautions to avoid spreading the infection. Tell him or her to cough and sneeze into tissues and to dispose of the tissues properly. Stress the importance of washing his or her hands thoroughly in hot, soapy water after handling his or her own secretions. Also instruct him or her to wash his or her eating utensils separately in hot, soapy water.

- – the need for a balanced, high-calorie, high-protein diet
- – measures to prevent TB.
  (See *Preventing tuberculosis*.)
- Refer anyone exposed to an infected patient for testing and follow-up.
- Refer the patient to a support group, such as the American Lung Association.
- Refer the patient to a smoking-cessation program, if indicated.

Vancomycin-resistant enterococci

Overview

- Other names—superbug-VRE; gastroenteritis-VRE; hospital-acquired infection–VRE; colitis-VRE
- Mutation of a common bacterium normally found in the GI tract
- Vancomycin-resistant enterococci (VRE) first identified in the United States in 1989
- Easily spread by direct person-to-person contact
- Also called glycopeptide-resistant enterococci
- Resistance mediated by enzymes that substitute a different molecule for the terminal amino acid so that vancomycin cannot bind

- Rare strains with intrinsic resistance have inherited, low-level resistance to vancomycin
- More commonly found strains have acquired resistance to vancomycin and have the ability to acquire and share genetic information with other bacteria.
- Can survive on dry surfaces from 7 days to 4 months
- Most likely to cause urinary tract infection, bacteremia, endocarditis, or meningitis
- Has been reported in facilities in more than 40 states
- Incidence as high as 14% in oncology units

Causes

- Direct contact with an infected patient or colonized patient or health care worker
- Contact with a contaminated surface, such as an overbed table

Risk factors

- Immunocompromised condition
- Severe underlying illness
- Older age
- Indwelling medical device, central venous access device, or other types of invasive catheter
- Major surgery

- Open wounds
- History of taking vancomycin or a third-generation cephalosporin, antibiotics targeted at anaerobic bacteria, or multiple courses of antibiotics
- History of enterococcal bacteremia, often linked to endocarditis
- Organ transplantation
- Long-term facilities
  - Chronic infection
  - Weak immune system
- Prolonged or repeated hospital admissions
- Cancer
- Cardiothoracic or intra-abdominal surgery
- Wounds draining into the pelvic or intra-abdominal area
- Pressure ulcers
- Chronic renal failure
- Exposure to contaminated equipment or a VRE-positive patient

Assessment
History
- Possible breach in the immune system, surgery, or condition predisposing the patient to infection
- Multiple antibiotic use
- Possible risk factors for VRE

Physical findings
- Carrier commonly asymptomatic

Diagnostic tests
Laboratory
- Culture and susceptibility testing performed on stool samples or rectal swabs confirms VRE.

Treatment
General
- Possibly no treatment with an asymptomatic infection
- Contact isolation for a colonized patient until patient is culture negative or is discharged
- No known method to decolonize VRE carrier

Medications
- Antimicrobials (VRE isolates not susceptible to vancomycin are generally susceptible to other antimicrobial drugs.)
- Linezolid
- Quinupristin/dalfopristin

Nursing interventions
- Consider grouping infected patients together and having the same health care providers care for them.
- Institute contact precautions.
- Use infection-control practices, such as wearing gloves and employing proper hand-washing techniques, to reduce the spread of VRE.
- Consider chlorhexidine baths, which have shown reduction in skin contamination of patients with VRE.
- Ensure judicious and careful use of antibiotics. Encourage health care providers to limit the use of antibiotics.
- Monitor the patient's response to treatment and watch for complications.

Patient teaching
- Be sure to cover:
  - the disorder, diagnosis, and treatment (See *Taking precautions at home*, page 278.)
  - the importance of family and visitors using personal protective equipment when visiting the patient
  - the importance of proper hand-washing technique for the patient and family members
  - how to dispose of protective equipment
  - medication administration, dosage, and possible adverse effects
  - the importance of taking antibiotics for the full prescription period, even if the patient begins to feel better.

Taking precautions at home

Tell the patient's caregivers to:
* wash their hands with soap and water after physical contact with the patient and before leaving the home
* use towels only once when drying hands after contact
* wear disposable gloves if they expect to come in contact with the patient's body fluids and to wash hands after removing the gloves
* change linens routinely and whenever they become soiled
* clean the patient's environment routinely and when it becomes soiled with body fluids
* tell health care provider and other health care personnel caring for the patient that the patient is infected with an organism resistant to multiple drugs.

Selected references

American Academy of Allergy Asthma & Immunology. (2015). *Biologics in asthma: The next step towards personalized treatment.* Retrieved from https://www.aaaai.org/global/latest-research-summaries/New-Research-from-JACI-In-Practice/biologics-asthma

American Cancer Society. (2018). *About colorectal cancer.* Retrieved from https://www.cancer.org/cancer/colon-rectal-cancer/about.html

American Cancer Society. (2018). *American Cancer Society guideline for colorectal cancer screening.* Retrieved from https://www.cancer.org/cancer/colon-rectal-cancer/detection-diagnosis-staging/acs-recommendations.html

Centers for Disease Control and Prevention. (2018). *What is viral hepatitis?* Retrieved from https://www.cdc.gov/hepatitis/abc/index.html

Dauby, P. (2017). *Eosinophilic gastroenteritis and eosinophilic esophagitis.* Retrieved from http://www.allergyexpert.us/food/eosinophilicgastroenteritis.html

MedicineNet. (2017). *Diabetes symptoms (type 1 and type 2).* Retrieved from https://www.medicinenet.com/diabetes_mellitus/article.htm#what_is_the_prognosis_for_a_person_with_diabetes

MedlinePlus. (2017). *Gastroesophageal reflux disease.* Retrieved from https://medlineplus.gov/ency/article/000265.htm

National Cancer Institute. (2018). *Male breast cancer treatment (PDQ®)—health professional version.* Retrieved from https://www.cancer.gov/types/breast/hp/male-breast-treatment-pdq

National Heart, Lung, and Blood Institute. (2017). *Heart failure: Also known as congestive heart failure.* Retrieved from https://www.nhlbi.nih.gov/health-topics/heart-failure#HeartHealthyLifestyle

National Institutes of Health. (2017). *What causes Alzheimer's disease?* Retrieved from https://www.nia.nih.gov/health/what-causes-alzheimers-disease

National Institutes of Health. (2018). *Alzheimer's disease fact sheet.* Retrieved from https://www.nia.nih.gov/health/alzheimers-disease-fact-sheet

National Institutes of Health. (2019). *Ischemic heart disease: Also known as coronary artery disease, coronary heart disease, coronary microvascular disease.* Retrieved from https://www.nhlbi.nih.gov/health-topics/ischemic-heart-disease

Papadakis, M. A., McPhee, S. J., & Rabow, M. W. (2019). *Current medical diagnosis & treatment.* New York, NY: McGraw Hill Education.

Ratini, M. (2018). *Coronary artery disease.* Retrieved from https://www.webmd.com/heart-disease/guide/heart-disease-coronary-artery-disease#1

Schiffman, G., & Davis, C. P. (2017). *Emphysema.* Retrieved from https://www.emedicinehealth.com/emphysema/article_em.htm#what_is_emphysema

WebMD. (2018). *What is eosinophilic asthma?* Retrieved from https://www.webmd.com/asthma/eosinophilic-asthma-causes#1

6 Common Procedures

Performing them safely and accurately

Arterial pressure monitoring

Direct monitoring of arterial pressure permits continuous measurement of systolic, diastolic, and mean pressures and allows sampling of arterial blood. Direct measurement, which reflects systemic vascular resistance and blood flow, is generally more accurate than indirect methods, which are based on blood flow.

Direct monitoring is indicated when highly accurate or frequent blood pressure measurements are required—for example, in patients with low cardiac output (CO) and high systemic vascular resistance. It may be used for hospitalized patients if obesity or edema makes indirect measurement difficult. It may also be used for patients who are receiving titrated doses of vasoactive drugs or who need frequent blood sampling.

Indirect monitoring, which carries few associated risks, is commonly performed by applying pressure to an artery (such as by inflating a blood pressure cuff around the arm or using an automated noninvasive system) to decrease blood flow. As pressure is released, flow resumes and can be palpated or auscultated. Korotkoff's sounds presumably result from a combination of blood flow and vibrations of the arterial wall; with reduced flow, these vibrations may be less pronounced.

Equipment and preparation

Sheet protector • gloves, gown, mask, protective eyewear

For arterial catheter insertion

Sterile gloves • 20G catheter (type and length depend on the insertion site, the patient's size, and other anticipated uses of the line) • preassembled preparation kit (if available) • sterile drapes • sterile towels • prepared pressure transducer system • ordered local anesthetic • sutures • syringe and 21G to 25G 1″ needle • tubing and medication labels • site-care kit (containing sterile dressing, antimicrobial ointment, and hypoallergenic tape) • arm board and soft wrist restraint (for a femoral site, an ankle restraint) • sterile marker and label • optional: electric clippers (for femoral artery insertion)

For blood sample collection from an open system

Sterile 4″ × 4″ gauze pads • Vacutainer • needleless Vacutainer Luer Lok adapter needle • appropriate blood specimen collection tubes • laboratory requests, labels and transport bag

For blood sample collection from a closed system

Syringes with attached cannulae of appropriate size and number for ordered laboratory tests • laboratory requests, labels, and transport bag • alcohol swabs • blood transfer unit • Vacutainers

For arterial line tubing changes

Sheet protector • preassembled arterial pressure tubing with flush device and disposable pressure transducer • sterile gloves • 500-ml bag of I.V. flush solution (usually normal saline solution) • 500 or 1,000 units of heparin • syringe and 21G to 25G 1″ needle • I.V. pole • alcohol swabs • medication and tubing labels • pressure bag • site-care kit (containing a sterile dressing)

For arterial catheter removal

Sterile 4″ × 4″ gauze pad • sheet protector • sterile suture removal set • dressing • alcohol swabs • hypoallergenic tape

For femoral line removal

Additional four sterile 4″ × 4″ gauze pads • small sandbag (which you may wrap in a towel or place in a pillowcase) • adhesive bandage

For a catheter-tip culture

Sterile 4″ × 4″ gauze pad • sterile scissors • sterile container • specimen label

Before setting up and priming the monitoring system, wash your hands thoroughly. Maintain asepsis by wearing personal protective equipment throughout preparation. Label all medications, medication containers, and other solutions on and off the sterile field.

After you have prepared the equipment, set the alarms on the bedside monitor according to facility policy.

Implementation

- Confirm the patient's identity using at least two patient identifiers.
- Explain the procedure to the patient and his or her family, including the purpose of arterial pressure monitoring and the anticipated duration of catheter placement. Verify that a consent form has been signed.
- Check the patient's history for an allergy or a hypersensitivity to iodine, the ordered local anesthetic, or latex.
- Maintain asepsis by wearing personal protective equipment throughout all of the procedures described here.
- Position the patient for easy access to the catheter insertion site. Place a sheet protector under the site.
- If the catheter will be inserted into the radial artery, perform Allen's test to assess collateral circulation in the hand.

Inserting an arterial catheter

- Using a preassembled preparation kit, the health care provider prepares and anesthetizes the insertion site. He or she covers the surrounding area with either sterile drapes or sterile towels. The health care provider inserts the catheter into the artery using sterile gloves and other protective equipment. Then the fluid-filled pressure tubing is attached.
- While the health care provider holds the catheter in place, activate the fast-flush release to flush blood from the catheter. After each fast-flush operation, observe the drip chamber to verify that the continuous flush rate is as desired. A waveform should appear on the bedside monitor.
- The health care provider may suture the catheter in place, or you may secure it with hypoallergenic tape. Apply antimicrobial ointment and cover the insertion site with a sterile dressing, as specified by facility policy.

- Immobilize the insertion site. With a radial or brachial site, use an arm board and a soft wrist restraint (if required by the patient's condition). Adhere to facility policy. With a femoral site, assess the need for an ankle restraint. Keep the patient on bed rest, with the head of the bed raised no more than 15 to 30 degrees, to prevent the catheter from kinking. Level the zeroing stopcock of the pressure transducer with the phlebostatic axis. Then zero the system to atmospheric pressure.
- Activate the monitor alarms as appropriate.

Obtaining a blood sample from an open system

- Assemble the equipment, taking care not to contaminate the nonvented cap, stopcock, and syringes. Attach the needleless Luer Lok adapter to the Vacutainer. Turn off or temporarily silence the monitor alarms, depending on facility policy. (Some facilities require that alarms be left on.)
- Locate the blood sampling port of the stopcock nearest the patient. Open a sterile 4″ × 4″ gauze pad. Remove the nonvented cap from the stopcock and place it on the gauze pad.
- Connect the needleless adapter of the Vacutainer into the sampling port of the stopcock and turn the stopcock off to the flush solution. Attach a blood specimen collection tube for the discard sample into the stopcock. (This sample is discarded because it is diluted with flush solution.) Follow facility policy on how much discard blood to collect. In most cases, you will withdraw 5 to 10 ml.
- Remove the discard-specimen blood collection tube from the Vacutainer.
- Next, attach each blood specimen collection tube to the Vacutainer, keeping the stopcock turned off to the flush solution. Because the

Vacutainer is a nonvented system, there will not be any backflow of blood from the patient.
- If the health care provider has ordered coagulation tests, obtain blood for this sample from the final syringe to prevent dilution from the flush device.
- After you have obtained blood for the final sample, turn the stopcock off to the sampling port and activate the fast-flush release to clear the tubing. Turn off the stopcock to the patient and attach an empty blood specimen collection tube or place a sterile 4″ × 4″ gauze pad beneath the sampling port of the stopcock and activate the fast-flush release to clear the stopcock port of any remaining blood.
- Turn the stopcock off to the stopcock port and remove the Vacutainer. Put a new sterile nonvented cap on the blood sampling port. Reactivate the monitor alarms. Label all blood specimen collection tubes with correct labels and send all samples to the laboratory in a laboratory transport bag with the laboratory request.
- Check the monitor for return of the arterial waveform and the pressure reading. (See *Understanding the arterial waveform.*)

Obtaining a blood sample from a closed system

- Assemble the equipment, maintaining aseptic technique. Locate the closed-system reservoir and the blood-sampling site. Turn off or temporarily silence the monitor alarms, depending on facility policy. (Some facilities require that alarms be left on.)
- Holding the reservoir upright, grasp the flexures and slowly fill the reservoir with blood over 3 to 5 seconds. (This blood is the discard blood.) If you feel resistance, reposition the affected extremity and check the

Understanding the arterial waveform

Normal arterial blood pressure produces a characteristic waveform that represents ventricular systole and diastole. The waveform has five distinct components: the anacrotic limb, systolic peak, dicrotic limb, dicrotic notch, and end diastole.

The anacrotic limb marks the initial upstroke of the waveform, which results as blood is rapidly ejected from the ventricle through the open aortic valve into the aorta. The rapid ejection causes a sharp rise in arterial pressure, which appears as the highest point of the waveform (called the systolic peak).

As blood continues to flow into the peripheral vessels, arterial pressure falls and the waveform begins a downward trend. This part is called the dicrotic limb. Arterial pressure usually continues to fall until pressure in the ventricle is less than pressure in the aortic root. When this occurs, the aortic valve closes. This event appears as a small notch (dicrotic notch) on the downside of the waveform. When the aortic valve closes, diastole begins and it progresses until the aortic root pressure gradually descends to its lowest point. On the waveform, this point is known as end diastole.

Normal arterial waveform

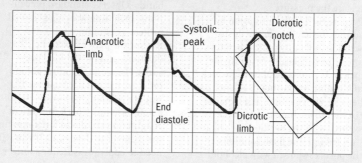

catheter site for obvious problems (such as kinking). Then withdraw the blood.

- Turn off the one-way valve to the reservoir by turning the handle perpendicular to the tubing. Clean the sampling site with an alcohol swab. Using a syringe with an attached cannula, insert the cannula into the sampling site. (Make sure that the plunger is depressed to the bottom of the syringe barrel.) Slowly fill the syringe. Then grasp the cannula near the sampling site and remove the syringe and cannula as one unit. Repeat the procedure as needed to fill the required number of syringes. If the health care provider has ordered coagulation tests, obtain blood for those tests from the final syringe to prevent dilution from the flush solution.

- After you fill the syringes, turn the one-way valve to its original position, parallel to the tubing. Smoothly and evenly, push down on the plunger until the flexures lock in place in the fully closed position and all fluid has been reinfused. The fluid should be reinfused over a 3- to 5-second period. Then activate the fast-flush release to clear blood from the tubing and the reservoir.

- Clean the sampling site with an alcohol swab. Reactivate the monitor alarms. Using the blood-transfer unit, transfer blood samples to the appropriate Vacutainers, labeling them according to facility policy. Send all of the samples to the laboratory with the appropriate documentation.

Changing arterial line tubing

- Wash your hands and follow standard precautions.
- Consult facility policy to determine the appropriate length of tubing to change.
- Inflate the pressure bag to 300 mm Hg and check it for air leaks. Then release the pressure.
- Prepare the I.V. flush solution by adding the heparin to the flush solution as facility policy dictates and following health care providers' orders. If your patient has a history of bleeding or clotting problems, use heparin with caution. The heparin should be drawn up into the syringe with the needle attached and injected into the flush solutions after the port is swabbed with alcohol. Prime the pressure tubing and transducer system. Add medication and tubing labels. Apply 300 mm Hg of pressure to the system. Then hang the I.V. bag on a pole.
- Place the sheet protector under the affected extremity. Remove the dressing from the catheter insertion site, taking care not to dislodge the catheter or cause vessel trauma. Turn off or temporarily silence the monitor alarms, depending on facility policy. (Some facilities require that alarms be left on.)
- Turn off the flow clamp of the tubing segment that you will change. Disconnect the tubing from the catheter hub, taking care not to dislodge the catheter. Immediately insert the primed pressure tubing with the transducer system into the catheter hub. Secure the tubing and activate the fast-flush release to clear it.
- Reactivate the monitor alarms. Apply an appropriate sterile dressing according to facility protocol.
- Level the zeroing stopcock of the transducer with the phlebostatic axis and zero the system to atmospheric pressure.

Removing an arterial line

- Consult facility policy to determine whether you are permitted to perform this procedure.
- Explain the procedure to the patient.
- Assemble all equipment. Wash your hands. Observe standard precautions, including wearing personal protective equipment.
- Record the patient's systolic, diastolic, and mean blood pressures. If a manual, indirect blood pressure has not been assessed recently, obtain one now to establish a new baseline. Check the patient's coagulation studies before removing the catheter to determine if you will need to apply pressure for a longer time to achieve hemostasis.
- Turn off the monitor alarms and the flow clamp to the flush solution.
- Carefully remove the dressing over the insertion site. Remove any sutures, using the sterile suture removal set, and carefully check that all sutures have been removed.
- Withdraw the catheter with a gentle, steady motion. Keep the catheter parallel to the artery during withdrawal to reduce the risk of traumatic injury.
- Immediately after you withdraw the catheter, apply pressure to the site with a sterile 4″ × 4″ gauze pad. Maintain constant pressure for at least 15 minutes (longer if bleeding or oozing persists). Apply additional

pressure if a femoral site was used or if the patient has coagulopathy or is receiving an anticoagulant. In some facilities, a compression device may be used to apply pressure to the femoral site.

- Cover the site with an appropriate dressing and secure it with hypoallergenic tape. If stipulated by facility policy, make a pressure dressing by folding in half four sterile 4″ × 4″ gauze pads and apply the dressing. Cover the dressing tightly with an adhesive bandage. For a patient with a femoral site, refer to your facility's policy for maintaining bed rest after the procedure.
- Avoid raising the head of the bed higher than 30 to 45 degrees and avoid flexing the affected hip during this time.
- If the health care provider has ordered a culture of the catheter tip to diagnose a suspected infection, culture the tip by swiping it across a solid growth medium such as an agar plate. (Do not cut the catheter tip and send it to the laboratory in a sterile container because that method of organism isolation may be unreliable.)
- Observe the site for bleeding. Assess circulation in the extremity distal to the site by evaluating color, pulses, and sensation. Repeat this assessment every 15 minutes for the first 4 hours, every 30 minutes for the next 2 hours, and then hourly for the next 6 hours, and per facility policy.

Special considerations

- Observing the pressure waveform on the monitor can enhance the assessment of arterial pressure. An abnormal waveform may reflect an arrhythmia (such as atrial fibrillation) or other cardiovascular problems, such as aortic stenosis, aortic insufficiency, alternating pulse, or

paradoxical pulse. (See *Recognizing abnormal arterial waveforms*, page 286.)

- Following facility policy regarding frequency, change the pressure tubing (usually every 2 to 3 days) and change the dressing at the catheter site. Regularly assess the site for signs of infection, such as redness and swelling, and notify the health care provider immediately if you find any.
- Erroneous pressure readings may be caused by a catheter that is clotted or by positional or loose connections; added stopcocks or extension tubing; inadvertent entry of air into the system; or improper calibration, leveling, or zeroing of the monitoring system. If the catheter lumen clots, the flush system may be improperly pressurized. Regularly assess the amount of flush solution in the I.V. bag and maintain 300 mm Hg of pressure in the pressure bag.
- Monitor the patient for complications, such as arterial bleeding, infection, air embolism, arterial spasm, and thrombosis.

Documentation

Document the date of system setup. Document the systolic, diastolic, and mean pressure readings as well. Record circulation in the extremity distal to the site by assessing color, pulses, and sensation. Carefully document the amount of flush solution infused to ensure accurate assessment of the patient's fluid status. Document the date and time the catheter was removed, how long pressure was held, the condition of the site, and any complications that occurred.

Document the patient's position when obtaining blood pressure readings to help determine trends.

Recognizing abnormal arterial waveforms

Understanding a normal arterial waveform is relatively straightforward. An abnormal waveform, however, is more difficult to decipher. Abnormal patterns and markings may provide important diagnostic clues to the patient's cardiovascular status, or they may simply signal trouble in the monitor. Use this chart to help you recognize and resolve waveform abnormalities.

Abnormality	Possible causes	Nursing interventions
Alternating high and low waves in a regular pattern	Ventricular bigeminy	• Check the electrocardiogram to confirm ventricular bigeminy. The tracing should reflect premature ventricular contractions every second beat.
	Cardiac tamponade	• Assess the patient for signs of tamponade.
Flattened waveform	Overdamped waveform or a patient with hypotension	• Check the blood pressure with a sphygmomanometer. If the reading is high, suspect overdamping. Correct the problem by trying to aspirate the arterial line. If you succeed, flush the line. If the reading is very low or absent, suspect hypotension.
Slightly rounded waveform with consistent variations in systolic height	Patient on ventilator with positive end-expiratory pressure	• Check the systolic blood pressure regularly. The difference between the highest systolic pressure and the lowest systolic pressure should be less than 10 mm Hg. If the difference exceeds that amount, suspect paradoxical pulse, possibly from cardiac tamponade.
Slow upstroke	Aortic stenosis	• Check the heart sounds for signs of aortic stenosis. Also, notify the health care provider, who will document suspected aortic stenosis.
Diminished amplitude on inspiration	Paradoxical pulse, possibly from cardiac tamponade, constrictive pericarditis, or lung disease	• Note the systolic pressure during inspiration and expiration. If the inspiratory pressure is at least 10 mm Hg less than the expiratory pressure, call the health care provider. • If you are also monitoring pulmonary artery pressure, watch for a diastolic plateau. This occurs when the mean central venous pressure (right atrial pressure), mean pulmonary artery pressure, and mean pulmonary artery wedge pressure (pulmonary artery obstructive pressure) are within 5 mm Hg of one another.

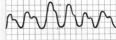

Automated external defibrillation

Automated external defibrillators (AEDs) are commonly used to meet the need for early defibrillation, which is considered the most effective treatment for ventricular fibrillation. Some facilities require an AED in every noncritical care unit. Their use is also common in such public places as shopping malls, sports stadiums, and airplanes. Instruction in using an AED is required as part of basic life support (BLS) and advanced cardiac life support (ACLS) training.

The 2016 American Heart Association (AHA) guidelines for cardiopulmonary resuscitation (CPR) and emergency cardiovascular care recommend the integration of high-quality CPR with the use of an AED.

AGE ALERT

AEDs can be used in children ages 1 to 8. For this age-group, an AED with a pediatric dose attenuator system should be used, if available.

AEDs are used increasingly to provide early defibrillation, even when no health care provider is present. The AED interprets the victim's cardiac rhythm and gives the operator step-by-step directions on how to proceed if defibrillation is indicated. Most AEDs have a "quick look" feature that allows you to see the rhythm with the paddles before the electrodes are connected.

The AED is equipped with a microcomputer that senses and analyzes a patient's heart rhythm at the push of a button. Then it audibly or visually prompts you to deliver a shock.

All models have the same basic function, but they operate differently. For example, all AEDs communicate directions through messages shown on a display screen, by voice commands, or both. Some AEDs display a patient's heart rhythm simultaneously.

All devices record your interactions with the patient during defibrillation, either on a cassette tape or in a solid-state memory module. Some AEDs have an integral printer that allows immediate documentation of the event. Facility policy determines who is responsible for reviewing all AED interactions; the patient's health care provider always has that option. Local and state regulations govern who is responsible for collecting AED case data for reporting purposes.

Equipment

AED • two prepackaged electrodes • electrode connector cables

Implementation

- After you discover that your patient is unresponsive to your questions, pulseless, and apneic, follow BLS and ACLS protocols. Ask a colleague to bring the AED into the patient's room and set it up before the code team arrives.
- Firmly press the ON button and wait while the machine performs a brief self-test. Most AEDs indicate their readiness by sounding a computerized voice that says "Stand clear" or by emitting a series of loud beeps. (If the AED is not functioning properly, it conveys the message "Don't use the AED. Remove and continue cardiopulmonary resuscitation [CPR].") Remember to report any AED malfunctions according to facility procedure.
- Open the foil packets that contain the two electrode pads. Attach the electrode cable to the AED.

- Expose the patient's chest. Remove the plastic backing film from the electrode pads and place one electrode pad on the right upper portion of the patient's chest, just beneath his or her clavicle.
- Place the second pad to the left of the apex of the heart. (Placement for the electrode pads is the same for both manual defibrillation and cardioversion.)
- Now, the machine is ready to analyze the patient's heart rhythm. Ask everyone to stand clear and press the ANALYZE button when you are prompted by the machine. Be careful not to touch or move the patient while the AED is in analysis mode. (If you get the message "Check electrodes," make sure that the electrodes are correctly placed and that the patient cable is securely attached and then press the ANALYZE button again.)
- In 15 to 30 seconds, the AED will analyze the patient's rhythm. When the patient needs a shock, the AED will display a "Stand clear" message and emit a beep that changes into a steady tone as it is charging.
- When an AED is fully charged and ready to deliver a shock, it prompts you to press the SHOCK button after informing everyone to "clear" the victim. (Some fully automatic AED models automatically deliver a shock within 15 seconds after analyzing the patient's rhythm and informing you to "clear" the victim. If a shock is not needed, the AED displays a "No shock indicated" message and prompts you to "Check patient.")
- Make sure that no one is touching the patient or his or her bed and call out "Stand clear." Then press the SHOCK button on the AED. Most AEDs are ready to deliver a shock within 15 seconds.
- After the first shock, continue CPR, beginning with five cycles of chest compression for about 2 minutes.

Do not delay compressions to recheck rhythm or pulse. After five cycles of CPR, the AED should analyze the rhythm and deliver another shock, if indicated.

- If a nonshockable rhythm is detected, the AED should instruct you to resume CPR. Then continue the algorithm sequence until the code team leader arrives.

Special considerations

- AEDs vary from one manufacturer to another, so familiarize yourself with the equipment at your facility.
- The operation of the AED should be checked according to your facility's policy.
- Defibrillation can cause accidental electric shock to those providing care.

Documentation

After the code, remove and transcribe the computer memory module or tape, or prompt the AED to print a rhythm strip with the code data. Follow facility policy for analyzing and storing the code data. Document the code on the appropriate form, including such information as the patient's name, age, medical history, and reason for seeking care; the time that you found the patient in arrest; the time that CPR began; the time that the AED was applied; the number of shocks that the patient received; the time that the pulse was regained; the postarrest care that was given; and the findings of physical assessment.

Bladder irrigation, continuous

Continuous bladder irrigation can help to prevent obstruction of the urinary tract by flushing out small blood clots that form after prostate or bladder surgery. It may also be used to treat an irritated, inflamed, or infected bladder lining.

This procedure requires placement of a triple-lumen catheter. One lumen controls balloon inflation, one allows irrigant inflow, and one allows irrigant outflow. The continuous flow of irrigating solution through the bladder also creates a mild tamponade that may help to prevent venous hemorrhage. Although a catheter is typically inserted while the patient is in the operating room after prostate or bladder surgery, a catheter may be inserted at the bedside in nonsurgical patients.

Equipment and preparation

One 4,000-ml container or two 2,000-ml containers of sterile irrigating solution (usually normal saline solution) or the prescribed amount of medicated solution • Y-type tubing made specifically for bladder irrigation • alcohol or antiseptic pad • I.V. pole or bedside pole attachment • drainage bag and tubing

Normal saline solution is usually prescribed for bladder irrigation after prostate or bladder surgery. Large volumes of irrigating solution are usually required during the first 24 to 48 hours after surgery. Y-type tubing is used because it allows immediate irrigation with reserve solution.

Before you start continuous bladder irrigation, double-check the irrigating solution against the health care provider's order. If the solution contains an antibiotic, check the patient's chart to make sure that he or she is not allergic to the drug. Unless specified otherwise, the patient should remain on bed rest while receiving continuous bladder irrigation.

Implementation

- Confirm the patient's identity using at least two patient identifiers.
- Wash your hands. Assemble all equipment at the patient's bedside. Explain the procedure and provide privacy.
- Insert the spike of the Y-type tubing into the container of irrigating solution. (If you have a two-container system, insert one spike into each container.) (See *Setup for continuous bladder irrigation*, page 290.)
- Squeeze the drip chamber on the spike of the tubing.
- Open the flow clamp and flush the tubing to remove air, which could cause bladder distention. Then close the clamp.
- To begin, hang the irrigating solution on the I.V. pole.
- Clean the opening to the inflow lumen of the catheter with the alcohol or antiseptic pad.
- Insert the distal end of the Y-type tubing securely into the inflow lumen (third port) of the catheter.
- Make sure that the outflow lumen is securely attached to the tubing of the drainage bag.
- Open the flow clamp under the container of irrigating solution and set the drip rate as ordered.
- To prevent air from entering the system, replace the primary container before it empties completely.
- If you have a two-container system, simultaneously close the flow clamp under the nearly empty container and open the flow clamp under the reserve container. This prevents reflux of irrigating solution from the reserve container into the nearly empty one. Hang a new reserve container on the I.V. pole and insert the tubing, maintaining asepsis.
- Empty the drainage bag about every 4 hours or as often as needed. Use sterile technique to avoid the risk of contamination.
- Monitor the patient's vital signs at least every 4 hours during irrigation, increasing the frequency if the patient's condition becomes unstable.
- Monitor urine output at least hourly for the first 4 hours and according to facility policy. Check for bladder distention or abdominal pain.

Setup for continuous bladder irrigation

During continuous bladder irrigation, a triple-lumen catheter allows irrigating solution to flow into the bladder through one lumen and to flow out through another, as shown in the inset. The third lumen is used to inflate the balloon that holds the catheter in place.

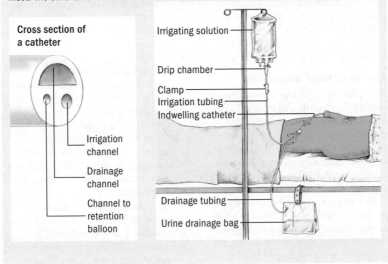

Cross section of a catheter

Irrigation channel

Drainage channel

Channel to retention balloon

Irrigating solution

Drip chamber

Clamp

Irrigation tubing

Indwelling catheter

Drainage tubing

Urine drainage bag

Special considerations

- Check the inflow and outflow lines periodically for kinks to make sure that the solution is running freely. If the solution flows rapidly, check the lines frequently.
- Measure the outflow volume accurately. It should, allowing for urine production, exceed inflow volume. If the inflow volume exceeds the outflow volume postoperatively, suspect bladder rupture at the suture lines or renal damage and notify the health care provider immediately.
- Assess outflow for changes in appearance and for blood clots, especially if irrigation is being performed postoperatively to control bleeding. If the drainage is bright red, irrigating solution is usually infused rapidly, with the clamp wide open, until the drainage clears.

Notify the health care provider at once if you suspect hemorrhage. If the drainage is clear, the solution is usually given at a rate of 40 to 60 drops per minute. The health care provider typically specifies the rate for antibiotic solutions.

- Encourage oral fluid intake of 2 to 3 qt/day (2 to 3 L/day), unless contraindicated.
- Watch for interruptions in the continuous irrigation system; these can predispose the patient to infection.
- Check frequently for obstruction in the outflow lumen of the catheter. Obstruction can lead to bladder distention.

Documentation

Each time you finish a container of solution, record the date, the time, and the amount of fluid given on the intake and output record. Also, record the time and the amount of fluid each time you empty the drainage bag. Note the appearance of the drainage as well as any complaints that the patient reports.

Cardiac monitoring

Because it allows continuous observation of the electrical activity of the heart, cardiac monitoring is used for patients who have conduction disturbances and for those who are at risk for life-threatening arrhythmias. Like other forms of electrocardiogram (ECG), cardiac monitoring uses electrodes that are placed on the patient's chest to transmit electrical signals that are converted into a tracing of cardiac rhythm on an oscilloscope.

Two types of monitoring may be performed: hardwire or telemetry. With hardwire monitoring, the patient is connected to a monitor at his or her bedside, where the rhythm display appears; it may also be transmitted to a console at a remote location. With telemetry monitoring, the patient is connected to a small transmitter that sends electrical signals to a monitor in another location. Battery-powered and portable, telemetry frees the patient from cumbersome wires and cables. In addition to being able to walk around, the patient is safely isolated from the electrical leakage and accidental shock occasionally associated with hardwire monitoring. Telemetry is especially useful for monitoring arrhythmias that occur during sleep, rest, exercise, or stressful situations. However, unlike hardwire monitoring, telemetry can monitor only cardiac rate and rhythm.

Regardless of the type of monitor used, cardiac monitors can display the patient's heart rate and rhythm, produce a printed record of the cardiac rhythm, and sound an alarm if the heart rate exceeds or falls below specified limits. Monitors also recognize and count abnormal heartbeats as well as changes. For example, a relatively new technique, ST-segment monitoring, helps to detect myocardial ischemia, electrolyte imbalance, coronary artery spasm, and hypoxic events. The ST segment represents early ventricular repolarization, and changes in this waveform component reflect alterations in myocardial oxygenation. Any monitoring lead that views an ischemic heart region will show ST-segment changes. The software establishes a template of the patient's normal QRST pattern from the selected leads. Then the monitor displays ST-segment changes. Some monitors display these changes continuously, and others show them only on command.

Equipment and preparation

For hardwire monitoring

Cardiac monitor • leadwires • patient cable • disposable pregelled electrodes (3 to 5 electrodes, depending on the patient's needs) • alcohol pad • 4″ × 4″ gauze pads • optional: clippers and washcloth

For telemetry monitoring

Transmitter • pouch for transmitter • telemetry battery pack, leadwires, and disposable pregelled electrodes

For hardwire monitoring, plug the cardiac monitor into an electrical outlet and turn it on to warm up the unit while you prepare the equipment and the patient. Insert the cable into the appropriate socket in the monitor. Connect the leadwires to the cable. In most systems, the leadwires are permanently secured to the cable. Each leadwire should indicate the location for attachment to the patient: right arm (RA), left arm (LA), right leg (RL), left leg (LL), and ground (C or V). This designation should appear on the leadwire—if it is permanently connected—or at the connection of the leadwires and cable to the patient. Connect an electrode to each leadwire, checking carefully that each leadwire is in its correct outlet.

For telemetry monitoring, insert a new battery into the transmitter. Make sure that the poles on the battery match the polar markings on the transmitter case. Some units have a battery test feature. If this feature is available, test the unit to check that the battery is operational. If the leadwires are not permanently affixed to the telemetry unit, attach them securely. If they must be attached individually, make sure that you connect each one to the correct outlet.

Implementation

Hardwire monitoring

- Confirm the patient's identity using at least two patient identifiers.
- Explain the procedure to the patient, provide privacy, and ask him or her to expose his or her chest. Wash your hands.
- Determine the positions of the electrodes on the patient's chest, based on which system and lead you are using. (See *Positioning monitoring leads.*)
- If the leadwires and patient cable are not permanently attached, verify that the electrode placement corresponds to the label on the patient cable.
- If necessary, clip an area about 4″ (10 cm) in diameter around each electrode site. Clean the area with an alcohol pad and dry it completely to remove skin secretions that may interfere with electrode function. Gently abrade the dried area by rubbing it briskly until it reddens to remove dead skin cells and to promote better electrical contact with living cells. (Some electrodes have a small, rough patch for abrading the skin; otherwise, use a dry washcloth or a dry gauze pad.)

- Remove the backing from the disposable pregelled electrode. Check the gel for moistness. If the gel is dry, discard it and replace it with a fresh electrode.
- Apply the electrode to the site and press firmly to ensure a tight seal. Repeat with the remaining electrodes.
- When all of the electrodes are in place, check for a tracing on the cardiac monitor. Assess the quality of the ECG.
- To verify that the monitor is detecting each beat, compare the digital heart rate display with your count of the patient's heart rate.
- If necessary, use the gain control to adjust the size of the rhythm tracing. Use the position control to adjust the position of the waveform on the recording paper.
- Set the upper and lower limits of the heart rate alarm, based on facility policy. Turn the alarm on.

Telemetry monitoring

- Confirm the patient's identity using at least two patient identifiers.
- Wash your hands. Explain the procedure to the patient and provide privacy.
- Expose the patient's chest and select the lead arrangement. Remove the backing from one of the disposable pregelled electrodes. Check the gel for moistness. If it is dry, discard the electrode and obtain a new one.
- Apply the electrode to the appropriate site by pressing one side of the electrode against the patient's skin, pulling gently, and then pressing the other side against the skin. Press your fingers in a circular motion around the electrode to fix the gel and stabilize the electrode. Repeat this procedure for each electrode.

(Text continues on page 295.)

Positioning monitoring leads

These illustrations show the correct electrode positions for the monitoring leads you will use most often. For each lead, you will see electrode placement for a five-leadwire system, a three-leadwire system, and a telemetry system.

In the two-hardwire systems, the electrode positions for one lead may be identical to those for another lead. In this case, you simply change the lead selector switch to the setting that corresponds to the lead you want. In some cases, you will need to reposition the electrodes.

In the telemetry system, you can create the same lead with two electrodes that you do with three, simply by eliminating the ground electrode.

The illustrations below use these abbreviations: RA, right arm; LA, left arm; RL, right leg; LL, left leg; C, chest; and G, ground.

Five-leadwire system	**Three-leadwire system**	**Telemetry system**

Lead I

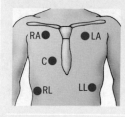 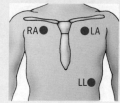 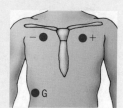

Lead II

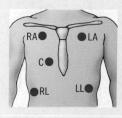 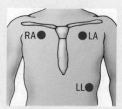 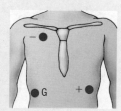

Lead III

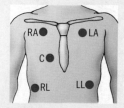 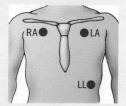 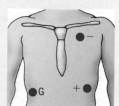

(continued)

Positioning monitoring leads *(continued)*

Five-leadwire system	Three-leadwire system	Telemetry system

Lead MCL₁

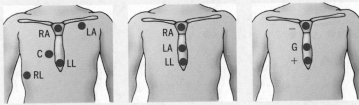

Lead MCL₆

Sternal lead

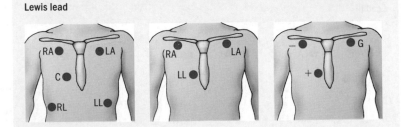

Lewis lead

- Attach an electrode to the end of each leadwire.
- Place the transmitter in the pouch. Tie the pouch strings around the patient's neck and waist, making sure that the pouch fits snugly but comfortably. If no pouch is available, place the transmitter in the patient's bathrobe pocket.
- Check the patient's waveform for clarity, position, and size. Adjust the gain and baseline as needed. (If necessary, ask the patient to remain resting or sitting in his or her room while you locate his or her telemetry monitor at the central station.)
- To obtain a rhythm strip, press the RECORD key at the central station. Label the strip with the patient's name and room number, the date, and the time. Also, identify the rhythm. Place the rhythm strip in the appropriate location in the patient's chart.

Special considerations

- Make sure that all electrical equipment and outlets are grounded to avoid electric shock and interference (artifacts). Ensure that the patient is clean and dry to prevent electric shock.
- Avoid opening the electrode packages until just before using them, to prevent the gel from drying out.
- Avoid placing the electrodes on bony prominences, hairy locations, areas where defibrillator pads will be placed, or areas where the chest will be compressed.
- If the patient's skin is very oily, scaly, or diaphoretic, rub the electrode site with a dry 4″ × 4″ gauze pad before applying the electrode to help reduce interference in the tracing. Instruct the patient to breathe normally during the procedure. If respirations distort the recording, ask the patient to hold his or her breath briefly to reduce baseline wander in the tracing.

- Assess the integrity of the patient's skin and reposition the electrodes every 24 hours or as needed.

 Patient Teaching Tip

If the patient is being monitored by telemetry, show him or her how the transmitter works. If applicable, show the patient the button that can produce a recording of his or her ECG at the central station. Teach the patient how to push the button whenever there are symptoms. Explain that pushing the button causes the central console to print a rhythm strip. Tell the patient to remove the transmitter to take a shower or bath, but explain that you should be informed before he or she removes the unit.

Documentation

Record in your nurses' notes the date and time that monitoring begins and the monitoring lead used. Document a rhythm strip at least every 8 hours and if any changes occur in the patient's condition (or as stated by facility policy). Label the rhythm strip with the patient's name and room number, the date, and the time.

Cardiac output measurement

CO—the amount of blood ejected by the heart in 1 minute—helps to evaluate cardiac function. The most widely used method of calculating this measurement is the bolus thermodilution technique. Performed at the patient's bedside, the thermodilution technique is the most practical method of evaluating the cardiac status of critically ill patients and those suspected of having cardiac disease. Other methods include the Fick's method and the dye dilution test.

To measure CO, a quantity of solution that is colder than the patient's blood is injected into the right atrium via a port on a pulmonary artery (PA) catheter. This indicator solution mixes with the blood as it travels through the right ventricle into the PA. A thermistor on the catheter registers the change in the temperature of the flowing blood. A computer plots the temperature change over time as a curve and calculates the flow based on the area under the curve.

Iced or room-temperature injectant may be used. The choice is based on facility policy as well as the patient's status. The accuracy of the bolus thermodilution technique depends on the ability of the computer to differentiate the temperature change that the injectant causes in the PA as well as the temperature changes in the artery. Because it is colder than room-temperature injectant, iced injectant provides a stronger signal and thus is more easily detected.

Typically, however, room-temperature injectant is more convenient to use and provides equally accurate measurements. Iced injectant may be more accurate for patients with high or low CO, hypothermic patients, or patients with volume restrictions.

Equipment and preparation
For the thermodilution method

Thermodilution PA catheter in position • CO computer, temperature injectate probe, and cable (or a module for the bedside cardiac monitor) • closed or open injectant delivery system • 10-ml syringe • 500-ml bag of I.V. solution (dextrose 5% in water [D_5W] or normal saline solution) • crushed ice and water and Styrofoam container (if iced injectant is used)

Newer bedside cardiac monitors measure CO continuously, either invasively or noninvasively. If your bedside monitor does not have this capability, you will need a freestanding CO computer.

Wash your hands thoroughly and assemble the equipment at the patient's bedside. Insert the closed injectant system tubing into the 500-ml bag of I.V. solution. Connect the 10-ml syringe to the system tubing and prime the tubing with I.V. solution until all of the air is out. Then clamp the tubing. The steps that follow differ, depending on the temperature of the injectant.

For room-temperature injectant in a closed-delivery system

After you clamp the tubing, connect the primed system to the stopcock of the proximal injectant lumen of the thermodilution PA catheter. Next, connect the temperature probe from the CO computer to the flow-through housing device. Connect the CO computer cable to the thermistor connector on the PA catheter and verify the blood temperature reading. Finally, turn on the CO computer and enter the correct computation constant, as provided by the catheter manufacturer. The constant is determined by the volume and temperature of the injectant as well as the size and type of catheter.

AGE ALERT

For children, you will need to adjust the computation constant to reflect a smaller volume and a smaller catheter size.

For iced injectant in a closed-delivery system

After you clamp the tubing, place the coiled segment into the Styrofoam container and add crushed ice and water to cover the entire coil. Let the solution cool for 15 to 20 minutes. The rest of the steps are the same as those for room-temperature injectant in a closed-delivery system.

Implementation

- Confirm the patient's identity using at least two patient identifiers.
- Place the patient in a supine position, with the head of the bed elevated not more than 20 degrees. Tell him or her not to move during the procedure.
- Explain to the patient that the procedure will cause no discomfort.

For room-temperature injectant in a closed-delivery system

- Verify the presence of a PA waveform on the cardiac monitor.
- Unclamp the I.V. tubing and withdraw exactly 10 ml of solution. Reclamp the tubing.
- Turn the stopcock at the catheter injectant hub to open a fluid path between the injectant lumen of the thermodilution PA catheter and the syringe.
- Press the START button on the CO computer or wait for an INJECT message to flash.
- Inject the solution smoothly within 4 seconds, making sure that it does not leak at the connectors.
- If available, analyze the contour of the thermodilution washout curve on a strip chart recorder. It should show a rapid upstroke and a gradual, smooth return to the baseline.
- Repeat these steps until three values are within 10% to 15% of the median value. Compute the average and record the patient's CO.
- Return the stopcock to its original position and make sure that the injectant delivery system tubing is clamped.
- Verify the presence of a PA waveform on the cardiac monitor.

- Discontinue CO measurements when the patient's condition is hemodynamically stable and the patient has been weaned from vasoactive and inotropic medications. You can leave the PA catheter in place for pressure measurements.
- Disconnect and discard the injectant delivery system and the I.V. bag. Cover exposed stopcocks with air-occlusive caps.
- Monitor the patient for signs and symptoms of inadequate perfusion, including restlessness; fatigue; changes in the level of consciousness (LOC); decreased capillary refill time; diminished peripheral pulses; oliguria; and pale, cool skin.

For iced injectant in a closed-delivery system

- Unclamp the I.V. tubing and withdraw 5 ml of solution into the syringe.

AGE ALERT

With children, withdraw 3 ml or less.

- Inject the solution to flow past the temperature sensor while you observe the injectant temperature that registers on the computer. Verify that the injectant temperature is between 43° and 54° F (6.1° and 12.2° C).
- Verify the presence of a PA waveform on the cardiac monitor.
- Withdraw exactly 10 ml of cooled solution before you reclamp the tubing.
- Turn the stopcock at the catheter injectant hub to open a fluid path between the injectant lumen of the PA catheter and the syringe.

- Press the START button on the CO computer or wait for the INJECT message to flash.
- Inject the solution smoothly within 4 seconds, making sure that it does not leak at the connectors.
- If available, analyze the contour of the thermodilution washout curve. It should show a rapid upstroke and a gradual, smooth return to the baseline.
- Wait 1 minute between injections and repeat the procedure until three values are within 10% to 15% of the median value. Compute the average and record the patient's CO.
- Return the stopcock to its original position and make sure that the injectant delivery system tubing is clamped.
- Verify the presence of a PA waveform on the cardiac monitor.

Special considerations

- The normal range for CO is 4 to 8 L/minute. The adequacy of a patient's CO is better assessed by calculating his or her cardiac index (CI), adjusted for his or her body size.
- To calculate the patient's CI, divide his or her CO by his or her body surface area (BSA), which is a function of height and weight. For example, a CO of 4 L/minute might be adequate for a 5'5", 120-lb (1.65-m, 54.4-kg) patient (normally, a BSA of 1.59 and a CI of 2.5) but would be inadequate for a 6'2", 230-lb (1.88-m, 104.3-kg) patient (normally, a BSA of 2.26 and a CI of 1.8). The normal CI for adults ranges from 2.5 to 4.2 L/minute/m²; for pregnant women, it is 3.5 to 6.5 L/minute/m².

AGE ALERT

The normal CI for infants and children is 3.5 to 4 L/minute/m²; for elderly adults, it is 2 to 2.5 L/minute/m².

- Add the fluid volume injected for CO determinations to the patient's total intake. Injectant delivery of 30 ml/hour will contribute 720 ml to the patient's 24-hour intake.
- After CO is measured, make sure that the clamp on the injectant bag is secured to prevent inadvertent delivery of the injectant to the patient.

Documentation

Document your patient's CO, CI, and other hemodynamic values and vital signs at the time of measurement. Note the patient's position during measurement as well as any other unusual occurrences, such as bradycardia or neurologic changes.

Cardiopulmonary resuscitation, adult

Cardiopulmonary resuscitation (CPR) aims to restore and maintain the patient's respirations and circulation after his or her heartbeat and breathing have stopped. A BLS procedure performed on patients in cardiac arrest, CPR should be performed according to the 2016 AHA guidelines.

Most adults in sudden cardiac arrest develop ventricular fibrillation and require defibrillation, and CPR alone does not improve survival rates. However, early activation of emergency medical services (EMS), high-quality CPR, and defibrillation as well as early ACLS all contribute to an improved survival rate.

Basic CPR consists of assessing the patient, calling for help, and then following the ABC protocol: open the *airway*, restore *breathing*, and restore *circulation*. After the patient's airway has been opened and his or her breathing and circulation restored, defibrillation, drug therapy, and diagnosis by ECG may follow. If possible, find out if the patient has a *Do Not Resuscitate* order before beginning CPR.

Equipment

A hard surface on which to place the patient • optional: protective equipment such as a disposable airway device

Implementation

- Follow these step-by-step CPR guidelines as currently recommended by the AHA.

One-person rescue

- Assess the patient to determine if he or she is unconscious. To ensure you do not start CPR on a person who is conscious, shake his or her shoulders and shout, "Are you okay?" If there is no response, check whether the patient has an injury, particularly to the head or neck.

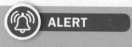

ALERT

If you suspect a head or neck injury, move the patient as little as possible to reduce the risk of paralysis.

- Call out for help, send someone to activate EMS, or call a code as appropriate. Get the AED. If no one is available, activate EMS or call a code yourself, get the AED, and return to the patient.
- Put the patient in the supine position on a hard, flat surface. When moving the patient, roll his or her head and torso as a unit. Avoid twisting or pulling his or her neck, shoulders, or hips.
- Kneel near the patient's shoulders to gain easy access to his or her head and chest.

Open the airway: Head-tilt, chin-lift maneuver

- If the patient does not appear to have a neck injury, use the head-tilt, chin-lift maneuver to open his or her

airway. To do this, place one hand on patient's forehead and apply pressure to tilt his or her head back. Be aware that, frequently, the muscles controlling the patient's tongue will be relaxed, causing the tongue to obstruct the airway; this maneuver opens the airway.

- Place the fingertips of your other hand under the bony part of the patient's lower jaw near his or her chin. Lift the patient's chin while keeping his or her mouth partially open. Do not place your fingertips on the soft tissue under his or her chin because this maneuver may obstruct the airway.

Open the airway: Jaw-thrust maneuver

- If you suspect a neck injury, use the jaw-thrust maneuver instead of the head-tilt, chin-lift maneuver.
- Kneel at the patient's head with your elbows on the ground.
- Rest your thumbs on the patient's lower jaw near the corners of the mouth, pointing your thumbs toward his or her feet. Place your fingertips around the lower jaw.
- To open the airway, lift the lower jaw with your fingertips.

Check for breathing

- While maintaining the open airway, place your ear over the patient's mouth and nose. Listen for air moving and note whether his or her chest rises and falls. You may also feel for airflow on your cheek.
- If the patient starts to breathe, keep the airway open and continue checking breathing until help arrives.
- If the patient does not start breathing within 10 seconds after you open his or her airway, begin rescue breathing. Pinch the patient's nostrils shut using the hand you had on his or her forehead.

- Take a regular (not deep) breath and place your mouth over his or hers, creating a tight seal.
- Give two full breaths that have enough volume to produce a visible chest rise. Each ventilation should last over 1 second.
- If your first attempt at ventilation is not successful, reposition the patient's head and try again. If you still are not successful, the patient may have a foreign-body obstruction. Check for dentures or another foreign-body airway obstruction. If you see dentures or any other object blocking the airway, remove the object.

Assess circulation

- Keep your hand on the patient's forehead so that his or her airway remains open.
- Palpate the carotid artery closest to you. To do this, place your index and middle fingers in the groove between the trachea and the sternocleidomastoid muscle.
- Palpate for 10 seconds to detect a pulse and observe for signs of circulation.

If you detect a pulse, do not start chest compressions. Instead, do rescue breathing, giving 10 to 12 breaths (one for every 5 to 6 seconds). After 2 minutes, recheck the pulse. You should give each breath over 1 second, and the breath should cause the chest to rise visibly. After 2 minutes, recheck the patient's pulse, but spend no more than 10 seconds doing so.

- If the patient has no pulse, start giving chest compressions. Make sure that the patient is lying on a

hard surface and that your knees are far enough apart to provide you with a wide base of support.
- Put the heel of one hand on the center of the patient's chest at the nipple line. Place the other hand directly on top of the first hand, making sure your fingers are not on his or her chest. This position will keep the compression force on the sternum and reduce the risk of rib fracture, lung puncture, or liver laceration.
- With elbows locked, arms straight, and shoulders directly over your hands, you are ready to give chest compressions. Compress the sternum 1½″ to 2″ (3.8 to 5 cm), using your upper body weight and delivering pressure through the heels of your hands.
- After each compression, release pressure completely and allow the patient's chest to return to a normal position so that the heart can fill with blood.

Do not change hand position during compressions; you might injure the patient.

- Give 30 chest compressions at a rate of about 100 per minute. Push hard and fast.
- Open the airway and give two ventilations. Find the proper hand position again and give 30 more compressions.
- Continue chest compressions until EMS arrives or another rescuer arrives with the AED.
- Interrupt chest compressions as infrequently as possible and make sure interruptions last no longer

than 10 seconds, except for special interventions such as use of an AED or insertion of an airway.

Two-person rescue

- If another rescuer arrives and the EMS team has not arrived, tell the second rescuer to repeat the call for help.
- If the second rescuer is not a health care professional, ask him or her to stand by. Then, after about 2 minutes or five cycles of compressions and ventilations, you can switch. The switch should occur within 5 seconds.
- If the rescuer is another health care professional, you can perform two-person CPR. He or she should start assisting after you have finished five cycles of 30 compressions, 2 ventilations, and a pulse check.
- The second rescuer should get into place opposite you. While you are checking for a pulse, he or she should find the proper hand placement for delivering chest compressions.
- If you do not detect a pulse, say, "No pulse, continue CPR," and give two ventilations.
- The second rescuer should begin giving compressions at a rate of 100 per minute. Compressions and ventilations should be given at a ratio of 30 compressions to 2 ventilations. The "compressor" (at this point, the second rescuer) should count out loud so that the "ventilator" can anticipate when to give ventilations.
- To ensure ventilations are effective, make sure they cause a visible chest rise.
- As the "ventilator," you must check for breathing and a pulse.
- The compressor role should switch after five cycles of compressions and ventilations. The switch should take no more than 5 seconds.

- Both rescuers should continue giving CPR until an AED or defibrillator arrives, the ACLS providers take over, or the patient starts to move.

Special considerations

- Some health care professionals may hesitate to give mouth-to-mouth breaths. For this reason, the AHA recommends that all health care professionals learn how to use disposable airway equipment.
- If you are a single rescuer activating EMS, getting an AED, and returning to the patient to perform CPR, tailor your response to take into account the cause of the arrest. For instance, if you are rescuing an unresponsive patient with a likely hypoxic arrest, perform five cycles of CPR before activating EMS and getting an AED.
- Lay rescuers should use the head-tilt, chin-lift maneuver for all patients, whether or not they appear injured, because the jaw thrust is difficult to perform. Lay rescuers are also taught to give two rescue breaths and immediately begin 30 chest compressions without stopping to check for a pulse. This is because research has shown they cannot reliably check for a pulse within 10 seconds or accurately assess for other signs of circulation.

 ALERT

CPR can cause complications, especially if the compressor's hands are placed improperly on the sternum. Such complications include fractured ribs, liver laceration, and punctured lungs. Gastric distention may result from giving too much air during ventilation.

Documentation

Note why you initiated CPR; report whether the patient suffered cardiac or respiratory arrest. Record when you found the patient and started CPR and how long the patient received CPR. Note the patient's response and any complications. Also include any interventions taken to correct complications.

If the patient also received ACLS, document which interventions were performed, who performed them, when they were performed, and what equipment was used. Document if the patient was moved to an intensive care unit.

Central venous access device insertion and removal

A central venous access device (CVAD), also known as a central venous (CV) catheter, is a sterile catheter made of polyurethane or silicone rubber (Silastic). It is inserted through a large vein, such as the subclavian vein, the jugular vein, or peripheral veins. The tip of the catheter must be placed in the superior vena cava for the catheter to be considered a CVAD.

By providing access to the central veins, CV therapy offers several benefits. It allows monitoring of CV pressure (CVP), which indicates blood volume or pump efficiency, and permits aspiration of blood samples for diagnostic tests. It also allows administration of I.V. fluids (in large amounts, if needed) when an emergency arises, when decreased peripheral circulation makes peripheral vein access difficult, when prolonged I.V. therapy reduces the number of accessible peripheral veins, when solutions must be diluted (for large fluid volumes or for irritating or hypertonic fluids such as total parenteral nutrition solutions), and when a patient requires long-term venous access. Because multiple blood samples can be drawn without repeated venipuncture, the CVAD decreases the patient's anxiety and preserves the peripheral veins.

A peripherally inserted central catheter (PICC) usually enters at the basilic vein and terminates in the superior vena cava. PICCs may be inserted by a specially trained nurse, radiologist, or surgeon. New catheters have longer needles and smaller lumens, facilitating this procedure. PICCs are typically used for long-term I.V. antibiotic therapy and can be safely used in the home care and long-term care settings. They may also be used in a patient who has a chest injury; neck, chest, or shoulder burns; compromised respiratory function; or a surgical site that is close to a CV line placement site.

CV therapy increases the risk of certain life-threatening complications, such as pneumothorax, sepsis, thrombus formation, and perforation of blood vessels and adjacent organs. Also, a CVAD may decrease patient mobility, is difficult to insert, and is more expensive than a peripheral I.V. catheter.

At the end of therapy or at the onset of complications, a health care provider or nurse removes the CVAD. CVAD removal is a sterile procedure. A PICC-trained nurse may remove a peripherally inserted central line. If the patient has an infection, the removal procedure includes swabbing the catheter tip over an agar plate for culture.

Equipment and preparation

For inserting a CVAD

Cap, sterile gloves, and gowns • blanket • linen-saver pad • sterile towel • large sterile drape, marker, and labels • masks • alcohol pad • chlorhexidine swab • normal saline solution • 3-ml syringe with 25G 1″ needle • 1% or 2% injectable lidocaine • D_5W • syringes for blood sample collection • suture material • two 14G or 16G CVADs • I.V. solution with administration set prepared for use • infusion pump or controller as needed • transparent semipermeable dressing • 1″ adhesive tape • sterile scissors • heparin or normal saline flushes as needed • portable X-ray machine • optional: clippers

For flushing a catheter

Normal saline solution or heparin flush solution • alcohol pad

For changing an injection cap

Alcohol pad • injection cap • padded clamp

For removing a CVAD

Clean gloves • mask • sterile suture removal set • alcohol pad • sterile 2″ × 2″ gauze pads • forceps • tape • sterile, plastic adhesive-backed dressing or transparent semipermeable dressing • agar plate, if needed for culture • antimicrobial swab

The type of catheter (tunneled, implanted, or percutaneously inserted) selected depends on the type of therapy to be used. The Centers for Disease Control and Prevention recommends using antimicrobial-impregnated catheters in adults who expect to keep the catheter in place longer than 5 days to decrease the risk of catheter-related bloodstream infections. Some facilities have prepared trays containing most of the equipment needed for catheter insertion. Before insertion of a CVAD, confirm the catheter type and size with the health care provider; usually, a 14G or 16G catheter is selected. Set up the I.V. solution and prime the administration set using strict aseptic technique. Recheck all connections to make sure that they are tight. As ordered, notify the radiology department that a chest X-ray is required.

Implementation

- Confirm the patient's identity using at least two patient identifiers.
- Wash your hands thoroughly to prevent the spread of microorganisms.

Inserting a CVAD

- Reinforce the health care provider's explanation of the procedure and answer the patient's questions. Make sure that the patient has signed a consent form and check his or her history for hypersensitivity to iodine, latex, or the local anesthetic.
- Place the patient in Trendelenburg's position to dilate the veins and reduce the risk of an air embolism.
- For subclavian access, place a rolled blanket lengthwise between the patient's shoulders to increase venous distention. For jugular access, place a rolled blanket under the opposite shoulder to extend the neck, making anatomic landmarks more visible. Place a linen-saver pad under the patient to prevent soiling of the bed.
- Turn the patient's head away from the site to prevent possible contamination from airborne pathogens and to make the site more accessible. Or if dictated by facility policy, place a mask on the patient unless this increases his or her anxiety or is contraindicated due to his or her respiratory status.
- Prepare the insertion site. Make sure that the skin is free from hair because hair can harbor microorganisms. Clip the hair close to the skin rather than shaving and according to facility policy. You may also need to wash the skin with soap and water.
- Establish a sterile field on a table, using a sterile towel or the wrapping from the instrument tray. Label all medications, medication containers, and other solutions on and off the sterile field.
- Put on a mask and sterile gloves and gown (maximum barrier precautions). Clean the area around the insertion site with a chlorhexidine swab using a vigorous side-to-side motion.
- After the health care provider puts on a cap, mask, sterile gown, and sterile gloves and drapes the area with a large sterile drape to create

a sterile field, open the packaging of the 3-ml syringe and the 25G 1″ needle. Give the syringe to the health care provider using sterile technique.

- Wipe the top of the lidocaine vial with an alcohol pad and invert it. The health care provider then fills the 3-ml syringe and injects the anesthetic into the site.

- Open the catheter package and give the catheter to the health care provider using aseptic technique. The health care provider then inserts the catheter.

- During this time, prepare the I.V. administration set for immediate attachment to the catheter hub. Ask the patient to perform Valsalva's maneuver while the health care provider attaches the I.V. line to the catheter hub. This maneuver increases intrathoracic pressure, reducing the possibility of an air embolus.

- After the health care provider attaches the I.V. line to the catheter hub, set the flow rate at a keep-vein-open rate to maintain venous access. (Alternatively, the catheter may be capped and flushed with heparin.) The health care provider then sutures the catheter in place.

- After an X-ray confirms correct catheter placement in the superior vena cava, set the flow rate as ordered.

- Use antimicrobial solution to remove dried blood that could harbor microorganisms. Secure the catheter with a catheter securement device, sterile tape, or sterile surgical strips and use a transparent semipermeable dressing.

- Expect some serosanguineous drainage during the first 24 hours. Label the dressing with the date and time of catheter insertion and the length and gauge of the catheter.

- Place the patient in a comfortable position and reassess his or her status.

Flushing a catheter

- To maintain patency, flush the catheter routinely, according to facility policy. If the system is being maintained as a heparin lock and the infusions are intermittent, the flushing procedure will vary according to facility policy, the medication administration schedule, and the type of catheter.

- All lumens of a multilumen catheter must be flushed regularly. Verify that tip placement is in the superior vena cava. Flush vigorously, using only low-pressure 10-ml syringes. It is important to be able to obtain 3 to 5 ml of free-flowing blood before each flush. If you cannot obtain 3 to 5 ml of blood, follow facility policy regarding catheter occlusion or malfunction. Most facilities use a heparin flush solution, available in premixed 10-ml multidose vials. Recommended concentrations vary from 10 to 100 units of heparin per milliliter. Use normal saline solution instead of heparin to maintain patency in two-way valve devices, such as the Groshong type. Research suggests that heparin is not always needed to keep the line open.

- The recommended frequency for flushing CVADs varies from once every 8 hours to once weekly.

- The recommended amount of flushing solution also varies. If the volume of the cannula and the add-on devices is known, Infusion Nurses Society standards require using twice that amount. All catheters have the same internal volume of less than 1 ml. Most facilities recommend using 3 to 5 ml of solution to flush the catheter, although some facility policies call for as much as 10 ml of solution.

- Before flushing, clean the cap with an alcohol pad. Allow the cap to dry. If you are using a needleless system when flushing, follow manufacturer guidelines.

- Access the cap and aspirate 3 to 5 ml of blood to confirm the proper function and patency of the CVAD.

- Inject the recommended type and amount of flush solution.
- After you flush the catheter, maintain positive pressure by keeping your thumb on the plunger of the syringe while you withdraw the syringe. This prevents blood backflow and clotting in the line. If you are flushing a valved catheter, close the clamp just before the last of the flush solution leaves the syringe.

Changing an injection cap

- CVADs that are used for intermittent infusions have needle-free injection caps (short Luer Lok devices similar to the heparin lock adapters that are used for peripheral I.V. therapy). These caps must be Luer Lok types to prevent inadvertent disconnection and an air embolism. These caps contain a minimal amount of empty space, so do not preflush the cap before you connect it.
- The frequency of cap changes varies according to facility policy and frequency of use. Changing the cap once weekly is recommended. Use strict aseptic technique when changing the cap.
- Clean the connection site with an alcohol pad.
- Instruct the patient to perform Valsalva's maneuver while you quickly disconnect the old cap and connect the new injection cap using aseptic technique. If he or she cannot perform this maneuver, use a padded clamp or pinch off the catheter to prevent air from entering the catheter.

Removing a CVAD

- Before starting, check the patient's record for the most recent placement (confirmed by X-ray) to trace the catheter's path as it exits the body.
- Make sure that assistance is available if a complication (such as uncontrolled bleeding) occurs during

catheter removal. Some vessels, such as the subclavian vein, can be difficult to compress. Before you remove the catheter, explain the procedure to the patient.
- Place the patient in a supine position to prevent an air embolism.
- Wash your hands and put on clean gloves and a mask.
- Turn off all infusions and prepare a sterile field using a sterile drape.
- Remove and discard the old dressing and change to sterile gloves.
- Inspect the site for signs of drainage and inflammation.
- Clip the sutures and use forceps to remove the catheter in a slow, even motion. Have the patient perform Valsalva's maneuver as the catheter is withdrawn to prevent an air embolism.
- Apply pressure with a dry sterile gauze pad immediately after you remove the catheter.
- Apply antiseptic ointment to the catheter exit site to seal the site and prevent an air embolism. Cover the site with a sterile 2″ × 2″ gauze pad and place a transparent semipermeable dressing over the gauze. Write the date and time of removal and your initials on the dressing with indelible ink. Keep the site covered until epithelialization has occurred. Follow up with the patient's family health care provider if the patient is discharged.
- Measure the length of the removed PICC catheter to ensure that the catheter has been completely removed. If you suspect that the catheter has not been completely removed, notify the health care provider immediately and monitor the patient closely for signs of distress. If you suspect an infection, swab the catheter on a fresh agar plate and send the specimen to the laboratory for culture.
- Dispose the I.V. tubing and equipment properly.

Special considerations

- Chest X-ray confirmation of proper catheter placement should be obtained before administering fluid and medication
- Watch for signs of air embolism, including sudden onset of pallor, cyanosis, dyspnea, coughing, and tachycardia that progresses to syncope and shock. If any of these signs occur, place the patient on his or her left side in Trendelenburg's position and notify the health care provider. Make sure that the exit site is covered with an occlusive dressing.
- After the catheter is inserted, monitor the patient for signs and symptoms of pneumothorax, such as shortness of breath, uneven chest movement, tachycardia, and chest pain. Notify the health care provider immediately if these signs appear.
- If a gauze dressing is used, change it at least every 48 hours or according to facility policy. If a transparent semipermeable dressing is used, change it every 7 days, according to facility policy, or whenever it becomes moist or soiled. Change the tubing every 72 hours and the solution every 24 hours, according to facility policy. Dressing, tubing, and solution changes for a CVAD should be performed using aseptic technique. (See *Key steps in changing a central venous dressing*.) Assess the site daily for signs and symptoms of complications, such as discharge, inflammation, and tenderness, and document your observations.

Key steps in changing a central venous dressing

Appropriate dressing changes and site care are needed to remove *Staphylococcus epidermidis*, the major organism causing infection in central venous catheters. Expect to change your patient's central venous dressing weekly. Many facilities specify dressing changes whenever the dressing becomes soiled, moist, or loose. The following illustrations show the key steps you will perform.

First, put on clean gloves and remove the old dressing by pulling it toward the exit site of a long-term catheter or toward the insertion site of a short-term catheter. This technique helps you to avoid pulling out the line. Remove and discard your gloves.

Next, put on sterile gloves and clean the skin around the site using an antimicrobial solution. Start at the center and move outward using a circular motion.

Allow the skin to dry. Use chlorhexidine swabs as recommended by the Centers for Disease Control and Prevention to clean the site using a vigorous side-to-side motion. Do not use circular motion.

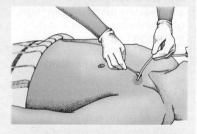

After the solution has dried, cover the site with a dressing such as the transparent semipermeable dressing shown below. Write the time and date on the dressing.

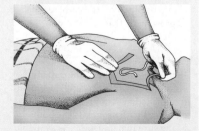

- To prevent an air embolism, close the catheter clamp or have the patient perform Valsalva's maneuver each time that the catheter hub is open to air. A Groshong catheter does not require clamping because it has a closed, valved-tip catheter.
- Long-term use of a CVAD, such as a Hickman catheter, a Broviac catheter, a port, or a PICC, allows patients to receive all types of infusion therapies at home. These catheters have a much longer life than short-term devices because they are less thrombogenic and less prone to infection.

Patient Teaching Tip

A candidate for home therapy may have a family member or friend who can safely and competently administer the I.V. fluids—a backup helper; a suitable home environment; transportation; and the ability to prepare, handle, store, and dispose of the equipment. The care procedures used in the home are the same as those used in the facility.

The overall goal of home therapy is patient safety, so patient teaching must begin well before discharge. Most patients who receive home therapy learn to care for the catheter themselves and infuse their own medications and solution.

- Complications can occur at any time during infusion therapy. Traumatic complications such as pneumothorax typically occur at the time of catheter insertion but may not be noticed until after the procedure is completed. Systemic complications such as sepsis typically occur later, during infusion therapy.

Other complications include thrombus formation and air embolism.

Documentation

Record the date and time of insertion, the length and location of the catheter, the solution infused, the health care provider's name, and the patient's response to the procedure. Also document the time of the X-ray, its results, and your notification of the health care provider.

Finally, record the date and time of catheter removal and the type of antimicrobial ointment and dressing applied. Note the condition of the catheter insertion site.

Central venous pressure monitoring

In central venous pressure (CVP) monitoring, the health care provider inserts a catheter through a vein and advances it until its tip lies in or near the right atrium. Because no major valves lie at the junction of the vena cava and the right atrium, pressure at end diastole reflects back to the catheter. When connected to a manometer, the catheter measures CVP, an index of right ventricular function.

CVP monitoring helps you to assess cardiac function, evaluate venous return to the heart, and indirectly gauge how well the heart is pumping. The CV line also provides access to a large vessel for rapid, high-volume fluid administration and allows frequent blood withdrawal for laboratory samples.

CVP monitoring can be done intermittently or continuously. The catheter is inserted percutaneously or using a cutdown method. Typically, a single-lumen CVP line is used for intermittent pressure readings. To measure the patient's volume status, a disposable plastic water manometer is attached between the I.V. line and the central catheter with a three- or four-way stopcock. CVP is recorded in centimeters of water (cm H_2O) or millimeters of mercury (mm Hg) and read from manometer markings.

CVP is highly individualized but usually ranges from 5 to 10 cm H_2O. Any condition that alters venous return, circulating blood volume, or cardiac performance can affect CVP. If the circulating volume increases (such as with enhanced venous return to the heart), CVP rises. If the circulating volume decreases (such as with reduced venous return), CVP drops.

Equipment

For intermittent CVP monitoring

Disposable CVP manometer set • leveling device (such as a rod from a reusable CVP pole holder or a carpenter's level or rule) • stopcock (to attach the CVP manometer to the catheter) • I.V. pole • I.V. solution, drip chamber, and tubing

For continuous CVP monitoring

Pressure monitoring kit with disposable pressure transducer • leveling device • bedside pressure module • continuous I.V. flush solution • 1 unit/1 to 2 ml of heparin flush solution • pressure bag

For removing a CV catheter

Gloves • suture removal set • sterile gauze pads • antimicrobial ointment • dressing • tape

Implementation

- Confirm the patient's identity using at least two patient identifiers.
- Gather the necessary equipment. Explain the procedure to the patient to reduce his or her anxiety.
- Assist the health care provider as he or she inserts the CV catheter. The procedure is similar to that used for PA pressure monitoring, except that the catheter is advanced only as far as the superior vena cava.

Monitoring CVP intermittently with a water manometer

- With the CV line in place, position the patient flat. Use a leveling device to align the base of the disposable CVP manometer with the previously determined zero reference point. Because CVP reflects right atrial pressure, you must align the right atrium (zero reference point) with the zero mark on the manometer. To find the right atrium, locate the fourth intercostal space at the midaxillary line; this is the phlebostatic axis. Mark the appropriate place on the patient's chest so that all subsequent recordings are made using the same location.
- If the patient cannot tolerate a flat position, place him or her in semi-Fowler's position. When the head of the bed is elevated, the phlebostatic axis remains constant, but the midaxillary line changes. Use the same degree of elevation for all subsequent measurements.
- Attach the manometer to an I.V. pole or place it next to the patient's chest. Make sure that the zero reference point is level with the right atrium. (See *Measuring CVP with a water manometer*.)
- Verify that the manometer is connected to the I.V. tubing. Typically, the markings on the manometer range from −2 to 38 cm H_2O. However, manufacturer's markings may differ, so read the directions before setting up the manometer and obtaining readings.
- Turn the stopcock off to the patient. Slowly fill the manometer with I.V. solution until the fluid level is 10 to 20 cm H_2O higher than the expected CVP value. Do not overfill the tube because fluid that spills over the top can become a source of contamination.
- Turn the stopcock off to the I.V. solution and open to the patient.

Measuring CVP with a water manometer

To ensure accurate central venous pressure (CVP) readings, make sure that the base of the manometer is aligned with the patient's right atrium (the zero reference point). The manometer set usually contains a leveling rod to allow you to determine this alignment quickly.

After you adjust the position of the manometer, examine the typical three-way stopcock. By turning it to any position shown below, you can control the direction of fluid flow. Four-way stopcocks are also available.

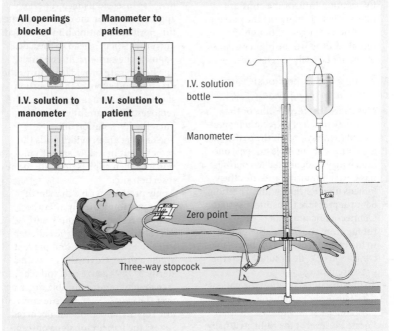

The fluid level in the manometer will drop. When the fluid level comes to rest, it will fluctuate slightly with respirations. Expect it to drop during inspiration and to rise during expiration.

- Record CVP at the end of expiration, when intrathoracic pressure has a negligible effect. Depending on the type of water manometer used, note the value either at the bottom of the meniscus or at the midline of the small floating ball.

- After obtaining the CVP value, turn the stopcock to resume the I.V. infusion. Adjust the drip rate as needed.
- Place the patient in a comfortable position.

Monitoring CVP continuously with a water manometer

Follow the procedure as outlined for monitoring CVP intermittently with a water manometer, except that the CVP system will be continuously hooked up for use.

- Make sure that the stopcock is turned so that the I.V. solution port, the CVP column port, and the patient port are open. With this stopcock position, infusion of the I.V. solution increases CVP. Therefore, expect higher readings than those taken with the stopcock turned off to the I.V. solution. If the I.V. solution infuses at a constant rate, CVP will change as the patient's condition changes, although the initial reading will be higher. Assess the patient closely for changes.

Monitoring CVP continuously with a pressure monitoring system

- Make sure that the CV line or the proximal lumen of a PA catheter is attached to the system. If the patient has a CV line with multiple lumens, one lumen may be dedicated to continuous CVP monitoring and the other lumens used for fluid administration.
- Set up a pressure transducer system. Connect noncompliant pressure tubing from the CVP catheter hub to the transducer. Then connect the continuous I.V. flush solution to the pressure tubing.
- To obtain values, position the patient flat. If he or she cannot tolerate this position, use semi-Fowler's position. Locate the level of the right atrium by identifying the phlebostatic axis. Zero the transducer, leveling the transducer air–fluid interface stopcock with the right atrium. Read the CVP value from the digital display on the monitor and note the waveform. Make sure that the patient is still when the reading is taken to prevent artifact. (See *Identifying hemodynamic pressure monitoring problems.*) Use this position for all subsequent readings.

Removing a CV access device

- You may assist the health care provider in removing a CV access device. (In some states, a nurse is permitted to remove the catheter when acting under a health care provider's order or under advanced collaborative standards of practice.)
- If the head of the bed is elevated, minimize the risk of air embolism during catheter removal—for instance, by placing the patient in Trendelenburg's position if the line was inserted using a superior approach. If he or she cannot tolerate this position, position him or her flat.
- Turn the patient's head to the side opposite the catheter insertion site. The health care provider removes the dressing and exposes the insertion site. If sutures are in place, he or she removes them carefully.
- Turn the I.V. solution off.
- The health care provider pulls the catheter out in a slow, smooth motion and then applies pressure to the insertion site.
- Apply pressure with a dry sterile gauze pad immediately after the catheter is removed. Apply antimicrobial ointment to the catheter exit site to seal the site and prevent air embolism. Cover the site with a sterile 2″ × 2″ gauze pad and place a transparent semipermeable dressing over the gauze. Keep the site covered until epithelialization has occurred.
- Assess the patient for signs of respiratory distress, which may indicate an air embolism.

Special considerations

- As ordered, arrange for daily chest X-rays to check the placement of the catheter.
- Care for the insertion site according to facility policy. Typically, you will change the dressing weekly.
- Wash your hands before performing dressing changes and use aseptic technique and sterile gloves when redressing the site. When removing the old dressing, observe the patient for signs of infection, such as

Identifying hemodynamic pressure monitoring problems

Problem	Possible causes	Interventions
No waveform	• Power supply turned off • Monitor screen pressure range set too low	• Check the power supply. • Raise the monitor screen pressure range, if necessary. • Rebalance and recalibrate the equipment.
	• Loose connection in the line • Transducer not connected to the amplifier • Stopcock off to the patient • Catheter occluded or out of the blood vessel	• Tighten loose connections. • Check and tighten the connection. • Position the stopcock correctly. • Use the fast-flush valve to flush the line or try to aspirate blood from the catheter. If the line remains blocked, notify the health care provider and prepare to replace the line.
Drifting waveforms	• Improper warm-up • Electrical cable kinked or compressed • Temperature change in room air or I.V. flush solution	• Allow the monitor and transducer to warm up for 10 to 15 minutes. • Place the monitor's cable where it cannot be stepped on or compressed. • Routinely zero and calibrate the equipment 30 minutes after setting it up. This allows I.V. fluid to warm to room temperature.
Line that does not flush	• Stopcocks positioned incorrectly • Inadequate pressure from a pressure bag • Kink in the pressure tubing • Blood clot in the catheter	• Make sure that the stopcocks are positioned correctly. • Make sure that the pressure bag gauge reads 300 mm Hg. • Check the pressure tubing for kinks. • Try to aspirate the clot with a syringe. If the line still will not flush, notify the health care provider and prepare to replace the line, if necessary. *Important:* Never use a syringe to flush a hemodynamic line.

(continued)

Identifying hemodynamic pressure monitoring problems *(continued)*

Problem	Possible causes	Interventions
Artifact (waveform interference)	• Patient movement	• Wait until the patient is quiet before taking a reading.
	• Electrical interference	• Make sure that the electrical equipment is connected and grounded correctly.
	• Catheter fling (tip of the pulmonary artery [PA] catheter moving rapidly in a large blood vessel or heart chamber)	• Notify the health care provider, who may try to reposition the catheter.
	• Transducer balancing port positioned below the patient's right atrium	• Position the balancing port level with the patient's right atrium.
	• Flush solution flow rate too fast	• Check the flush solution flow rate. Maintain it at 3 to 4 ml/hour.
	• Air in the system	• Remove air from the lines and the transducer.
False-high readings	• Transducer balancing port positioned above the right atrium	• Position the balancing port level with the patient's right atrium.
	• Transducer imbalance	• Make sure that the flow system of the transducer is not kinked or occluded and rebalance and recalibrate the equipment.
	• Loose connection	• Tighten loose connections.
		• Secure all connections.
False-low readings	• Air bubbles	• Remove air from the lines and the transducer.
	• Blood clot in the catheter	• Check for and replace cracked equipment.
	• Blood flashback in the line	• Refer to "Line that does not flush" on page 311.
	• Incorrect transducer position	• Make sure that the stopcock positions are correct, tighten loose connections, replace cracked equipment, flush the line with the fast-flush valve, and replace the transducer dome if blood backs up into it.
		• Make sure that the transducer is kept at the level of the right atrium at all times. Improper levels give false-high or false-low pressure readings.

Identifying hemodynamic pressure monitoring problems *(continued)*

Problem	Possible causes	Interventions
Damped waveform	• Arterial catheter out of the blood vessel or pressed against the vessel wall	• Reposition the catheter if it is against the vessel wall. • Try to aspirate blood to confirm proper placement in the vessel. If you cannot aspirate blood, notify the health care provider and prepare to replace the line. *Note:* Bloody drainage at the insertion site may indicate catheter displacement. Notify health care provider.
	• Ruptured balloon	• Notify health care provider immediately for catheter replacement.
PA wedge pressure tracing unobtainable	• Incorrect amount of air in the balloon	• If you feel no resistance when injecting air or if you see blood leaking from the balloon inflation lumen, stop injecting air and notify the health care provider. If the catheter is left in, label the inflation lumen with a warning not to inflate.
	• Catheter malpositioned	• Deflate the balloon. Check the label on the catheter for the correct volume. Reinflate slowly with the correct amount. To avoid rupturing the balloon, never use more than the stated volume. • Notify the health care provider. Obtain a chest X-ray.

redness, and note patient complaints of tenderness. Cover the site with a clear, transparent semipermeable dressing.

• After the initial CVP reading, reevaluate readings frequently to establish a baseline for the patient. Authorities recommend obtaining readings at 15-, 30-, and 60-minute intervals to establish a baseline. If the patient's CVP fluctuates by more than 2 cm H_2O, suspect a change in his or her clinical status and report this finding to the health care provider.

• Change the I.V. solution every 24 hours and the I.V. tubing every 96 hours, according to facility policy.

Label the I.V. solution, tubing, and dressing with the date, the time, and your initials.

• Assess the patient for complications of CVP monitoring, including pneumothorax (which typically occurs on catheter insertion), sepsis, thrombus, puncture of a vessel or an adjacent organ, and air embolism.

Documentation

Document all dressing, tubing, and solution changes. Also document the patient's tolerance of the procedure, the date and time of catheter removal, and the type of dressing applied. Note the condition of the catheter insertion site and whether a culture specimen was collected. Note any complications as well as actions taken.

Chest physiotherapy

Chest physiotherapy (PT) includes postural drainage, coughing and deep-breathing exercises, and chest percussion and vibration. Together, these techniques mobilize and eliminate secretions, reexpand lung tissue, and promote efficient use of the respiratory muscles. Of critical importance to the bedridden patient, chest PT helps to prevent or treat atelectasis and may also help to prevent pneumonia, two respiratory complications that can seriously impede recovery.

Postural drainage performed with percussion and vibration encourages peripheral pulmonary secretions to empty by gravity into the major bronchi or trachea and is accomplished by sequential repositioning of the patient. Usually, secretions drain best with the patient positioned so that the bronchi are perpendicular to the floor. Lower and middle lobe bronchi usually empty best with the patient in the head-down position; upper lobe bronchi, in the head-up position. Percussing the chest with cupped hands mechanically dislodges thick, tenacious secretions from the bronchial walls. Vibration can be used with percussion or as an alternative to it in a patient who is frail, is in pain, or is recovering from thoracic surgery or trauma.

Candidates for chest PT include patients who expectorate large amounts of sputum, such as those with bronchiectasis or cystic fibrosis. The procedure has not been proven effective in treating patients with status asthmaticus, lobar pneumonia, or acute exacerbations of chronic bronchitis when the patient has scant secretions and is being mechanically ventilated. Chest PT has little value in the treatment of patients with stable, chronic bronchitis.

Contraindications include active pulmonary bleeding with hemoptysis and the immediate posthemorrhage stage, fractured ribs or an unstable chest wall, lung contusions, pulmonary tuberculosis, untreated pneumothorax, acute asthma or bronchospasm, lung abscess or tumor, bony metastasis, head injury, and recent myocardial infarction.

Equipment and preparation

Stethoscope • emesis basin • facial tissues • pillows or folded towels for positioning • gloves, face shield, and gown • suction equipment as needed • equipment for oral care • trash bag

Gather the equipment at the bedside. Set up suction equipment, if needed, and test its function.

Implementation

- Confirm the patient's identity using at least two patient identifiers.
- Check the order.
- Explain the procedure to the patient, provide privacy, and wash your hands.
- Put on gloves, face shield, and gown and follow standard precautions.
- Auscultate the patient's lungs with a stethoscope to determine the patient's baseline respiratory status.
- Position the patient as necessary using pillows. For patients with generalized disease, drainage usually begins with the lower lobes, continues with the middle lobes, and ends with the upper lobes. For patients with localized disease, drainage begins with the affected lobes and proceeds to the other lobes to avoid spreading the disease to uninvolved areas.
- Instruct the patient to remain in each position for 10 to 15 minutes. During this time, perform percussion and vibration as ordered. (See *Performing percussion and vibration.*)

Performing percussion and vibration

To perform percussion, instruct the patient to breathe slowly and deeply, using the diaphragm, to promote relaxation. Hold your hands in a cupped shape, with your fingers flexed and your thumbs pressed tightly against your index fingers. Percuss each segment for 1 to 2 minutes by alternating your hands against the patient in a rhythmic manner. Listen for a hollow sound on percussion to verify that you are performing the technique correctly.

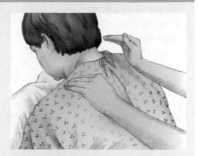

To perform vibration, ask the patient to inhale deeply and then to exhale slowly through pursed lips. While the patient exhales, firmly press your fingers and the palms of your hands against the chest wall. Tense the muscles of your arms and shoulders in an isometric contraction to send fine vibrations through the chest wall. Vibrate during five exhalations over each chest segment.

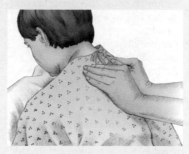

- After you perform postural drainage, percussion, or vibration, instruct the patient to cough to remove loosened secretions. First, tell the patient to inhale deeply through his or her nose and then to exhale in three short huffs. Then instruct him or her to inhale deeply again and then to cough through a slightly open mouth. Three consecutive coughs are highly effective. An effective cough sounds deep, low, and hollow; an ineffective one, high-pitched. Have the patient exercise for about 1 minute and then have him or her rest for 2 minutes. Gradually progress to 10-minute exercise periods done four times daily.
- If coughing is ineffective, suction the patient.

- Provide oral hygiene because secretions may have a foul taste or a stale odor. Dispose secretions with suction equipment or tissues and a trash bag. Provide an emesis basin if needed.
- Monitor the patient's response to treatment and auscultate his or her lungs to evaluate the effectiveness of therapy.

Special considerations

- For optimal effectiveness and safety, modify chest PT according to the patient's condition. For example, initiate or increase the flow of supplemental oxygen, if indicated. Also, suction the patient who has an ineffective cough reflex. If the patient tires quickly during therapy, shorten the sessions. Fatigue leads to shallow respirations and increased hypoxia. Chest PT should be limited to 30 minutes or less, as tolerated. Drainage of different lobes may need to be done during separate PT sessions.

- If the patient is receiving chest PT to prevent dehydration of mucus and promote easier mobilization, make sure that he or she takes in plenty of fluids. Avoid performing postural drainage immediately before or within 1½ hours after meals to avoid nausea and aspiration of food or vomitus.

- Because chest percussion can induce bronchospasm, adjunct treatment (for example, intermittent positive-pressure breathing, aerosol, or nebulizer therapy) should precede chest PT.

- Do not perform percussion over the spine, liver, kidneys, or spleen to avoid injury to the spine or internal organs. Also, avoid performing percussion on bare skin or on a female patient's breasts. Percuss over soft clothing (but not over buttons, snaps, or zippers) or place a thin towel over the chest wall. Remove jewelry that might scratch or bruise the patient.

Patient Teaching Tip

Teach the patient splinting while coughing, and deep-breathing preoperatively. This allows the patient to concentrate and practice when he or she is pain free. Postoperatively, instruct the patient to cough and deep breath, while splinting, to minimize pain.

- Observe the patient for complications. During postural drainage in head-down positions, pressure on the diaphragm by abdominal contents can impair respiratory excursion and lead to hypoxia or postural hypotension. The head-down position may also lead to increased intracranial pressure (ICP), which precludes the use of chest PT in a patient with acute neurologic impairment. Vigorous percussion or vibration can cause rib fracture, especially if the patient has osteoporosis. In a patient with emphysema and blebs, coughing can lead to pneumothorax.

Documentation

Record the date and time of chest PT. Note the positions used to drain secretions and the length of time that each position is maintained. Also record the chest segments that are percussed or vibrated; the color, amount, odor, and viscosity of secretions produced and the presence of blood; complications that occur and nursing actions that are taken; and the patient's tolerance of treatment.

Colostomy and ileostomy care

A patient with an ascending or transverse colostomy or an ileostomy must wear an external pouch to collect emerging fecal matter, which is typically watery or pasty. In addition to collecting waste matter, the pouch helps to control odor and protect the stoma and peristomal skin. Most disposable pouching systems can be used for 2 to 7 days; some models last even longer.

All pouching systems must be changed immediately if a leak develops, and every pouch must be emptied when it is one-third to one-half full. The patient with an ileostomy may need to empty his or her pouch four or five times daily.

Naturally, the best time to change the pouching system is when the bowel is least active, usually 2 to 4 hours after meals. After a few months, most patients can predict the best changing time.

The selection of a pouching system should take into consideration which system provides the best adhesive seal and skin protection for the individual patient. The type of pouch selected also depends on the location and structure of the stoma, the availability of supplies, the wear time, the consistency of effluent, personal preference, and cost.

Equipment

Pouching system • stoma measuring guide • stoma paste (if drainage is watery to pasty or stoma secretes excess mucus) • scissors • water or pouch-cleaning solution • washcloth and towel • closure clamp • toilet or bedpan • gloves • facial tissue • optional: ostomy belt, paper tape, mild nonmoisturizing soap, electric clippers • prepared skin barrier • gauze pad

Pouching systems may be drainable or closed-bottomed, disposable or reusable, adhesive-backed, and one- or two-piece. (See *Comparing ostomy pouching systems*, page 318.)

Implementation

- Provide privacy and emotional support.

Fitting the pouch and skin barrier

- For a pouch with an attached skin barrier, measure the stoma with the stoma-measuring guide. Select the opening size that matches the stoma.
- For an adhesive-backed pouch with a separate skin barrier, measure the stoma with the measuring guide and select the opening that matches

the stoma. Trace the selected size opening onto the paper back of the skin barrier. Cut out the opening. (If the pouch has precut openings, which can be handy for a round stoma, select an opening that is ⅛″ [3 mm] larger than the stoma. If the pouch comes without an opening, cut the hole ⅛″ wider than the measured tracing.) The cut-to-fit system works best for an irregularly shaped stoma.

- For a two-piece pouching system with flanges, see *Applying a skin barrier and pouch*, page 319.
- Avoid fitting the pouch too tightly because the stoma has no pain receptors. A constrictive opening could injure the stoma or the skin without the patient feeling the warning of discomfort. Avoid cutting the opening too big because a large opening may expose the skin to fecal matter and moisture.
- A patient with a descending or sigmoid colostomy who has formed stools and whose ostomy does not secrete much mucus may choose to wear only a pouch. In this case, make sure that the pouch opening closely matches the stoma size.
- Between 6 weeks and 1 year after surgery, the stoma will shrink to its permanent size. At that point, pattern-making preparations will not be needed unless the patient gains weight, has additional surgery, or injures the stoma.

Applying or changing the pouch

- Collect all equipment.
- Wash your hands and provide privacy.
- Explain the procedure to the patient. As you perform each step, explain what you are doing and why because the patient will eventually perform the procedure himself or herself.
- Put on gloves.

Comparing ostomy pouching systems

Manufactured in many shapes and sizes, ostomy pouches are fashioned for comfort, safety, and easy application. For example, a disposable, closed-end pouch may meet the needs of a patient who irrigates, who wants added security, or who wants to discard the pouch after each bowel movement. Another patient may prefer a reusable, drainable pouch. Some commonly available pouches are described below.

Disposable pouches

The patient who must empty his or her pouch often (because of diarrhea or a new colostomy or ileostomy) may prefer a one-piece, drainable, disposable pouch with a closure clamp attached to a skin barrier (below left).

These transparent or opaque, odor-proof, plastic pouches come with attached adhesive or Karaya seals. Some pouches have microporous adhesive or belt tabs. The bottom opening allows for easy draining. This pouch may be used permanently or temporarily, until the stoma size stabilizes.

Also disposable and made of transparent or opaque, odor-proof plastic, a one-piece, disposable, closed-end pouch (below right) may come in a kit with an adhesive seal, belt tabs, a skin barrier, or a carbon filter for gas release. A patient with a regular bowel elimination pattern may choose this style for added security and confidence.

A two-piece, disposable, drainable pouch with a separate skin barrier (shown below) permits frequent changes and minimizes skin breakdown. Also made of transparent or opaque, odor-proof plastic, this style comes with belt tabs and usually snaps to the skin barrier with a flange mechanism.

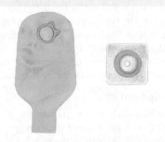

Reusable pouches

Typically manufactured from sturdy, opaque, hypoallergenic plastic, the reusable pouch comes with a separate, custom-made faceplate and O-ring (as shown below). Some pouches have a pressure valve for releasing gas. The device has a 1- to 2-month life span, depending on how frequently the patient empties the pouch.

Reusable equipment may benefit a patient who needs a firm faceplate or who wishes to minimize cost. However, many reusable ostomy pouches are not odor proof.

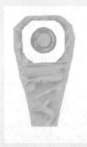
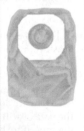
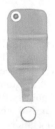
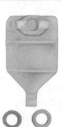

Applying a skin barrier and pouch

Fitting a skin barrier and an ostomy pouch properly can be done in a few steps. The commonly used, two-piece pouching system with flanges is shown below.

Measure the stoma using a measuring guide.

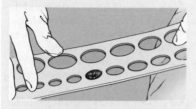

Trace the appropriate circle carefully on the back of the skin barrier.

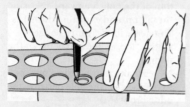

Cut the circular opening in the skin barrier. Bevel the edges to prevent them from irritating the patient.

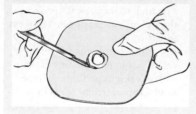

Remove the backing from the skin barrier and moisten it or apply barrier paste as needed along the edge of the circular opening.

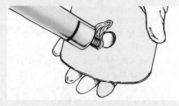

Center the skin barrier over the stoma, with the adhesive side down, and gently press it to the skin.

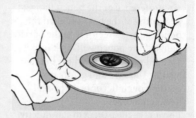

Gently press the pouch opening onto the ring until it snaps into place.

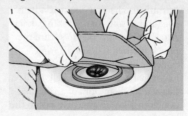

- Remove and discard the old pouch. Wipe the stoma and the peristomal skin gently with a facial tissue.
- Carefully wash the stoma with mild nonmoisturizing soap and water and dry the peristomal skin by patting it gently. Allow the skin to dry

thoroughly. Inspect the peristomal skin and stoma. If necessary, clip the surrounding hair (in a direction away from the stoma) to promote a better seal and avoid skin irritation from hair pulling against the adhesive.

- If you are applying a separate skin barrier, peel off the paper backing of the prepared skin barrier, center the barrier over the stoma, and press gently to ensure adhesion.
- You may want to outline the stoma on the back of the skin barrier (depending on the product) with a thin ring of stoma paste to provide extra skin protection. Skip this step if the patient has a sigmoid or descending colostomy, formed stools, and little mucus.
- Remove the paper backing from the adhesive side of the pouching system and center the pouch opening over the stoma. Press gently to secure.
- For a pouching system with flanges, align the lip of the pouch flange with the bottom edge of the skin barrier flange. Gently press around the circumference of the pouch flange, beginning at the bottom, until the pouch adheres securely to the barrier flange. (The pouch will click into its secured position.) Hold the barrier against the skin and gently pull on the pouch to confirm the seal between flanges.
- Encourage the patient to stay quietly in position for about 5 minutes to improve adherence. The patient's body warmth also helps to improve adherence and to soften a rigid skin barrier.
- Attach an ostomy belt to secure the pouch further, if desired. (Some pouches have belt loops and others have plastic adapters for belts.)
- Leave a small amount of air in the pouch to allow drainage to fall to the bottom.
- Apply the closure clamp, if needed.
- If desired, apply paper tape in a picture-frame fashion to the pouch edges for additional security.

Emptying the pouch
- Put on gloves.
- Tilt the bottom of the pouch upward and remove the closure clamp.

- Turn up a cuff on the lower end of the pouch and allow the pouch to drain into the toilet or bedpan.
- Wipe the bottom of the pouch with a gauze pad and reapply the closure clamp.
- The bottom portion of the pouch can be rinsed with cool tap water. Do not aim water up near the top of the pouch because the water may loosen the seal on the skin.
- A two-piece flanged system can also be emptied by unsnapping the pouch. Let the drainage flow into the toilet.
- Release flatus through the gas release valve, if the pouch has one. Otherwise, release flatus by tilting the bottom of the pouch upward, releasing the clamp, and expelling the flatus. To release flatus from a flanged system, loosen the seal between the flanges.
- Never make a pinhole in a pouch to release gas. The hole destroys the odor-proof seal.
- Remove and discard gloves.

Special considerations

- After you perform the procedure and explain it to the patient, encourage the patient's increasing involvement in self-care.
- Use adhesive solvents and removers only after patch testing of the patient's skin is performed. Some products may irritate the skin or produce hypersensitivity reactions. Consider using a liquid skin sealant, if available, to give the skin added protection from drainage and adhesive irritants.
- Remove the pouching system if the patient reports burning or itching beneath it or purulent drainage around the stoma. Notify the health care provider or therapist of skin irritation, breakdown, rash, or unusual appearance of the stoma or peristomal area.

- Use commercial pouch deodorants, if desired. However, most pouches are odor-free, and odor should be evident only when you empty the pouch or if it leaks. Before the patient is discharged, suggest that he or she avoid odor-causing foods, such as fish, eggs, onions, and garlic.
- If the patient wears a reusable pouching system, suggest that he or she obtains two or more systems so that he or she can wear one while the other dries after it is cleaned with soap and water or a commercially prepared cleaning solution.
- Failure to fit the pouch properly over the stoma or improper use of a belt can injure the stoma. Be alert for a possible allergic reaction to adhesives or other ostomy products.

Documentation

Record the date and time of the pouching system change and note the character of drainage, including color, amount, type, and consistency. Describe the appearance of the stoma and the peristomal skin. Document patient teaching and describe the teaching content. Record the patient's response to self-care and evaluate his or her learning progress.

Colostomy irrigation

Irrigation of a colostomy can serve two purposes: It allows a patient with a descending or sigmoid colostomy to regulate bowel function and it cleans the large bowel before and after tests, surgery, or other procedures.

Colostomy irrigation may begin as soon as bowel function resumes after surgery. However, most clinicians recommend waiting until the patient's bowel movements are more predictable. Initially, the nurse or the patient irrigates the colostomy at the same time every day, recording the amount of output and any spillage that occurs between irrigations. Between 4 and 6 weeks may pass before colostomy irrigation establishes a predictable pattern of elimination.

Equipment and preparation

Colostomy irrigation set (contains an irrigation drain or sleeve, an ostomy belt [if needed] to secure the drain or sleeve; water-soluble lubricant; drainage pouch clamp; and irrigation bag with clamp, tubing, and cone tip) • 1 L of tap water irrigant warmed to about 105° F (40.6° C) • warmed normal saline solution (for cleansing enemas) • I.V. pole or wall hook • washcloth and towel • water • ostomy pouching system • linen-saver pad • gloves • optional: bedpan or chair; mild nonmoisturizing soap; rubber band or clip; and small dressing, bandage, or commercial stoma cap

Depending on the patient's condition, irrigation of the colostomy may be performed in bed using a bedpan or in the bathroom using the toilet or a chair. Set up the irrigation bag with tubing and a cone tip. For irrigation with the patient in bed, place the bedpan beside the bed and elevate the head of the bed to between 45 and 90 degrees, if allowed. For irrigation in the bathroom, have the patient sit on the toilet or on a chair facing the toilet, whichever he or she finds more comfortable.

Fill the irrigation bag with warmed tap water (or normal saline solution, if the irrigation is to clean the bowel). Hang the bag on the I.V. pole or a wall hook. The bottom of the bag should be at the patient's shoulder level to prevent fluid from entering the bowel too quickly. Most irrigation sets also have a clamp that regulates the flow rate.

Prime the tubing with irrigant to prevent air from entering the colon and possibly causing cramps and gas pains.

Implementation

- Confirm the patient's identity using at least two patient identifiers.
- Explain each step of the procedure to the patient because he or she will probably be irrigating the colostomy himself or herself.
- Provide privacy and wash your hands.
- If the patient is in bed, place a linen-saver pad under him or her to protect the sheets from getting soiled.
- Put on gloves.
- If the patient uses an ostomy pouch, remove it.
- Place the irrigation sleeve over the stoma. If the sleeve does not have an adhesive backing, secure the sleeve with an ostomy belt. If the patient has a two-piece pouching system with flanges, snap off the pouch and save it. Snap on the irrigation sleeve.
- Place the open-ended bottom of the irrigation sleeve in the bedpan or toilet to promote drainage by gravity. If necessary, cut the sleeve so that it meets the water level inside the bedpan or toilet. Effluent may splash from a short sleeve or may not drain from a long sleeve.
- Lubricate your gloved small finger with water-soluble lubricant and insert the gloved finger into the stoma. If you are teaching the patient, have him or her do this to determine the bowel angle at which to insert the cone safely. Expect the stoma to tighten when the finger enters the bowel and then to relax in a few seconds.
- Lubricate the cone with water-soluble lubricant to prevent it from irritating the mucosa.
- Insert the cone into the top opening of the irrigation sleeve and then into the stoma. Angle the cone to match the bowel angle. Insert the cone gently but snugly; never force it into place.

- Unclamp the irrigation tubing and allow the water to flow slowly. If you do not have a clamp to control the flow rate of the irrigant, pinch the tubing to control the flow. The water should enter the colon over a period of 5 to 10 minutes. (If the patient reports cramping, slow or stop the flow, keep the cone in place, and have the patient take a few deep breaths until the cramping stops.) Cramping during irrigation may result from a bowel that is ready to empty, water that is too cold, a rapid flow rate, or air in the tubing.
- Have the patient remain stationary for 15 to 20 minutes to allow the initial effluent to drain.
- If the patient is ambulatory, he or she can stay in the bathroom until all effluent empties, or he or she can clamp the bottom of the drainage sleeve with a rubber band or clip and return to bed. Explain that ambulation and activity stimulate elimination. Suggest that the nonambulatory patient lean forward or massage his or her abdomen to stimulate elimination.
- Wait about 45 minutes for the bowel to finish eliminating the irrigant and effluent. Then remove the irrigation sleeve.
- If the irrigation was intended to clean the bowel, repeat the procedure with warmed normal saline solution until the return solution appears clear.
- Using a washcloth, mild nonmoisturizing soap, and water, gently clean the area around the stoma. Rinse and dry the area thoroughly with a clean towel.
- Inspect the skin and stoma for changes in appearance. Although it is usually dark pink to red, the color of the stoma may change with the patient's status. Notify the health care provider of marked changes in stoma color. A pale hue may result from anemia. Substantial darkening

suggests a change in blood flow to the stoma.

- Apply a clean pouch. If the patient has a regular pattern of bowel elimination, he or she may prefer a small dressing, bandage, or commercial stoma cap.
- If the irrigation sleeve is disposable, discard it. If the irrigation sleeve is reusable, rinse it and hang it to dry along with the irrigation bag, tubing, and cone.

Special considerations

- Irrigating a colostomy to establish a regular bowel elimination pattern is not successful in all patients. If the bowel continues to move between irrigations, try decreasing the volume of irrigant. Increasing the volume of irrigant will not help because it only stimulates peristalsis. Keep a record of results. Also consider irrigating every other day.
- Irrigation may help regulate bowel function in patients with a descending or sigmoid colostomy because this is the bowel's stool storage area. However, a patient with an ascending or transverse colostomy will not benefit from irrigation. A patient with a descending or sigmoid colostomy who is missing part of the ascending or transverse colon may not be able to irrigate successfully because his or her ostomy may function as an ascending or transverse colostomy.
- If diarrhea develops, discontinue irrigations until stools form again. Irrigation alone will not achieve regularity for the patient. He or she must also observe a complementary diet and exercise regimen.
- If the patient has a strictured stoma that prohibits cone insertion, remove the cone from the irrigation tubing and replace it with a soft silicone catheter. Angle the catheter gently

2″ to 4″ (5 to 10 cm) into the bowel to instill the irrigant. Do not force the catheter into the stoma and do not insert it farther than the recommended length because you may perforate the bowel.

- Observe the patient for complications. Bowel perforation may occur if a catheter is incorrectly inserted into the stoma. Fluid and electrolyte imbalances may result from using too much irrigant.

Documentation

Record the date and time of irrigation and the type and amount of irrigant used. Note the color of the stoma and the character of drainage, including its color, consistency, and amount. Record patient teaching. Describe the teaching content and the patient's response to self-care instruction. Evaluate the patient's learning progress.

Defibrillation

The 2016 AHA guidelines identify defibrillation as the standard treatment for ventricular fibrillation after CPR. CPR prolongs the time that defibrillation can occur, but CPR alone is not likely to correct ventricular fibrillation, so early defibrillation is critical.

Defibrillation involves using electrode paddles to direct an electric current through the patient's heart. The current causes the myocardium to depolarize, which in turn encourages the sinoatrial node to resume control of the electrical activity of the heart. The electrode paddles that deliver the current may be placed on the patient's chest or, during cardiac surgery, directly on the myocardium.

Because ventricular fibrillation leads to immediate death if it is not corrected, the success of defibrillation depends on early recognition and quick treatment of this arrhythmia.

In addition to treating ventricular fibrillation, defibrillation may be used to treat ventricular tachycardia that does not produce a pulse.

Patients with a history of ventricular fibrillation may be candidates for an implantable cardioverter-defibrillator, a sophisticated device that automatically discharges an electric current when it senses a ventricular tachyarrhythmia. (See *Understanding the ICD*.)

Equipment

Defibrillator with ECG monitor and recorder • external paddles • conductive medium pads • oxygen therapy equipment • handheld resuscitation bag • emergency cardiac medications

Understanding the ICD

The implantable cardioverter-defibrillator (ICD) has a programmable pulse generator and lead system that monitors the activity of the heart, detects ventricular bradyarrhythmias and tachyarrhythmias, and responds with appropriate therapies. The range of therapies includes antitachycardia and bradycardia pacing, cardioversion, and defibrillation. Newer defibrillators can also provide dual-chamber or biventricular pacing.

Implantation of an ICD is similar to that of a permanent pacemaker. The cardiologist positions the lead (or leads) transvenously in the endocardium of the right ventricle (and the right atrium, if both chambers require pacing). The lead connects to a generator box, which is implanted on the left or right side of the upper chest, near the clavicle.

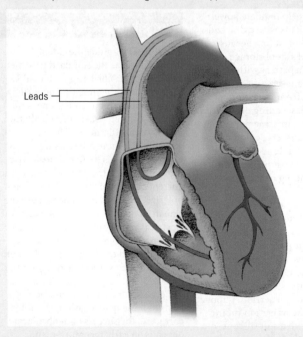

Leads

Implementation

- Assess the patient to determine if he or she lacks a pulse. Call for help and perform CPR until the defibrillator and other emergency equipment arrive.
- If the defibrillator has "quick look" capability, place the external paddles on the patient's chest to view his or her cardiac rhythm quickly. Otherwise, connect the monitoring leads of the ECG monitor with recorder to the patient and assess his or her cardiac rhythm. If ventricular fibrillation or pulseless ventricular tachycardia occurs, prepare to defibrillate the patient.
- Expose the patient's chest and apply conductive medium pads at the paddle placement positions. For anterolateral placement, place one paddle to the right of the upper sternum, just below the right clavicle, and the other over the fifth or sixth intercostal space at the left anterior axillary line. For anteroposterior placement, place the anterior paddle directly over the heart at the precordium, to the left of the lower sternal border. Place the flat posterior paddle under the patient's body, beneath the heart and immediately below the scapulae, but not under the vertebral column.

ALERT

Never place defibrillator paddles over an implanted pacemaker.

- Turn on the defibrillator. For external defibrillation in an adult patient, set the energy level to 360 joules, unless using a biphasic defibrillator, which uses lower energy settings. (See *Biphasic defibrillators.*)
- Charge the paddles by pressing the CHARGE buttons, which are located either on the machine or on the paddles.

Biphasic defibrillators

Most facility defibrillators are monophasic; they deliver a single current of electricity that travels in one direction between the two pads or paddles on the patient's chest. To be effective, they require a high amount of electric current.

Recently, new biphasic defibrillators have been introduced into facilities. Placement of the pads or paddles is the same as with monophasic defibrillators. The difference is that the electric current discharged from the pads or paddles travels in a positive direction for a specified duration and then reverses and flows in a negative direction for the remaining time of the electrical discharge. This type of defibrillator delivers two currents of electricity and lowers the defibrillation threshold of the heart muscle, making it possible to defibrillate ventricular fibrillation successfully with smaller amounts of energy. Instead of 360 joules, an initial shock of 120 to 200 joules is usually effective. The biphasic defibrillator adjusts for differences in impedance (the resistance of the current through the chest). This helps reduce the number of shocks needed to terminate ventricular fibrillation. Biphasic technology uses lower energy levels and fewer shocks. Thus, it reduces the damage to the myocardial muscle. Biphasic defibrillators, when used at the clinically appropriate energy level, may be used for defibrillation and—when placed in the synchronized mode—for synchronized cardioversion.

- Place the paddles over the conductive pads and press firmly against the patient's chest using 25 lb (11.4 kg) of pressure.
- Reassess the patient's cardiac rhythm.
- If the patient remains in ventricular fibrillation or pulseless ventricular tachycardia, instruct all personnel to stand clear of the patient and the bed.
- Discharge the current by pressing both paddle CHARGE buttons simultaneously.
- Resume CPR immediately. Perform five cycles of CPR and then reassess the patient's rhythm.
- If necessary, prepare to defibrillate a second time. Instruct a colleague to set the energy level on the defibrillator to 360 joules. Announce that you are preparing to defibrillate and follow the procedure described earlier.
- Resume CPR immediately. Perform five cycles of CPR and reassess the patient. If defibrillation is needed again, instruct a colleague to set the energy level to 360 joules. Then follow the same procedure as before.
- If the patient still has no pulse after three initial defibrillations, resume CPR, give supplemental oxygen, and begin administration of appropriate emergency cardiac medications such as antiarrhythmics. Also, consider possible causes for failure of the patient's rhythm to convert, such as acidosis or hypoxia.
- If defibrillation restores a normal rhythm, check the patient's central and peripheral pulses and measure the patient's blood pressure, heart rate, and respiratory rate. Assess the patient's LOC, cardiac rhythm, breath sounds, skin color, and urine output. Obtain baseline arterial blood gas (ABG) values and a 12-lead ECG. Provide supplemental oxygen, ventilation, and medications as needed. Check the patient's chest for electrical burns and treat them

as ordered with corticosteroid or lanolin-based creams. Also, prepare the defibrillator for immediate reuse.

Special considerations

- Defibrillators vary from one manufacturer to the next, so familiarize yourself with the equipment. Defibrillator operation should be checked at least every 8 hours and after each use.
- Defibrillation can be affected by several factors, including the size and placement of the paddles, the condition of the patient's myocardium, the duration of the arrhythmia, chest resistance, and the number of countershocks.
- Remove any transdermal medications from the chest (and back if using anteroposterior placement) because the medium may interfere with current conduction or produce a burn.
- Defibrillation can cause accidental electric shock to those providing care. The use of an insufficient amount of conductive medium can lead to skin burns.

Documentation

Document the procedure, including the patient's ECG rhythms before and after defibrillation; the number of times that defibrillation was performed; the voltage used during each attempt; whether a pulse returned; the dosage, route, and time of drug administration; whether CPR was used; the way that the airway was maintained; and the patient's outcome.

Doppler use

More sensitive than palpation for determining pulse rate, the Doppler ultrasound blood flow detector is especially useful when a pulse is weak. Unlike palpation, which detects expansion and retraction of the arterial walls, this instrument detects the motion of red blood cells (RBCs).

Equipment

Doppler ultrasound blood flow detector • coupling or transmission gel • soft cloth • antiseptic solution

Implementation

- Apply a small amount of coupling or transmission gel (not water-soluble lubricant) to the ultrasound probe.
- Position the probe on the skin directly over the selected artery.
- When using a Doppler ultrasound blood flow detector model with a speaker, turn the instrument on. Moving counterclockwise, set the volume control to the lowest setting. If your model does not have a speaker, plug in the earphones and slowly raise the volume. The Doppler ultrasound stethoscope is basically a stethoscope fitted with an audio unit, a volume control, and a transducer, which amplifies the movement of RBCs.
- To obtain the best signals with either device, tilt the probe 45 to 60 degrees from the artery and apply gel between the skin and the probe. Slowly move the probe in a circular motion to locate the center of the artery and the Doppler signal—a hissing noise at the heartbeat.
- Avoid moving the probe rapidly because it distorts the signal.
- Count the signals for 60 seconds to determine the pulse rate.
- After you have measured the pulse rate, clean the probe with an approved antiseptic solution. Do not immerse the probe or bump it against a hard surface.

Documentation

Record the location and quality of the pulse, the pulse rate, and the time of measurement.

Feeding tube insertion and removal

Inserting a feeding tube nasally or orally into the stomach or duodenum provides nourishment to a patient who cannot or will not eat. The feeding tube also permits administration of supplemental feedings to a patient who has very high nutritional requirements, such as an unconscious patient or one with extensive burns. Typically, a nurse inserts the feeding tube as ordered. The preferred route for a feeding tube is nasal, but the oral route may be used for patients with such conditions as a deviated septum or an injury of the head or nose.

The health care provider may order duodenal feeding when the patient cannot tolerate gastric feeding or when he or she expects gastric feeding to produce aspiration. The absence of bowel sounds or possible intestinal obstruction contraindicates the use of a feeding tube.

Feeding tubes differ somewhat from standard nasogastric (NG) tubes. Made of silicone, rubber, or polyurethane, feeding tubes have small diameters and great flexibility. These qualities reduce oropharyngeal irritation, necrosis resulting from pressure on the tracheoesophageal wall, irritation of the distal esophagus, and discomfort from swallowing. To facilitate passage, some feeding tubes are weighted with tungsten. Some tubes need a guide wire to keep them from curling in the back of the throat.

These small-bore tubes usually have radiopaque markings and a water-activated coating that provides a lubricated surface.

Equipment and preparation

For insertion

Feeding tube (#6 to #18 French, with or without a guide wire) • linen-saver pad • gloves • hypoallergenic tape

• water-soluble lubricant • skin preparation (such as tincture of benzoin) • facial tissues • penlight • small cup of water with straw or ice chips • emesis basin • 60-ml syringe • pH test strip

For removal

Linen-saver pad • tube clamp • bulb syringe

Have a tube of the proper size available. Usually, the health care provider orders the smallest bore tube that will allow free passage of the liquid feeding formula. Read the instructions on the tubing package carefully because the characteristics of feeding tubes vary according to the manufacturer. (For example, some tubes have marks at the appropriate lengths for gastric, duodenal, and jejunal insertion.)

Examine the tube to make sure that it is free from defects, such as cracks or rough or sharp edges. Next, run water through the tube to check for patency, activate the coating, and facilitate removal of the guide wire.

Implementation

• Confirm the patient's identity using at least two patient identifiers.
• Explain the procedure to the patient and show him or her the feeding tube so that he or she knows what to expect and can cooperate more fully.
• Provide privacy. Wash your hands and put on gloves.
• Assist the patient into semi-Fowler's or high Fowler's position.
• Place a linen-saver pad across the patient's chest in case of spills.
• To determine the tube length needed to reach the stomach, extend the distal end of the tube from the tip of the patient's nose to his or her earlobe. Coil this portion of the tube around your fingers so that the end will remain curved until you insert it. Extend the uncoiled portion from the earlobe to the xiphoid process.

Use a small piece of hypoallergenic tape to mark the total length of the two portions.

Inserting the tube nasally

• Using the penlight, assess nasal patency. Inspect the nasal passages for a deviated septum, polyps, or other obstructions. Occlude one nostril, and then the other, to determine which has the better airflow. Assess the patient's history of nasal injury or surgery.
• Lubricate the curved tip of the tube (and the guide wire, if appropriate) with a small amount of water-soluble lubricant to ease insertion and prevent tissue injury.
• Ask the patient to hold the emesis basin and facial tissues in case he or she needs them.
• To advance the tube, insert the curved, lubricated tip into the more patent nostril and direct it along the nasal passage toward the ear on the same side. When it passes the nasopharyngeal junction, turn the tube 180 degrees to aim it downward into the esophagus. Tell the patient to lower his or her chin to his or her chest to close the trachea. Then give him or her a small cup of water with a straw or ice chips. Direct him or her to sip the water or suck on the ice and swallow frequently to ease passage of the tube. Advance the tube as he or she swallows.

Inserting the tube orally

• Have the patient lower his or her chin to close his or her trachea and then to open his or her mouth.
• Place the tip of the tube at the back of the patient's tongue, give him or her water, and instruct him or her to swallow. Remind the patient to avoid clamping his or her teeth down on the tube. Advance the tube as the patient swallows.

Positioning the tube

- Continue to pass the tube until the tape marking of the appropriate length reaches the patient's nostril or lips. Tube placement should be confirmed by X-ray.
- Once each shift or before administering liquids or medications, you can check tube placement by measuring the exposed portion of the tube and documenting its length. Any increase from the original measurement may signal that the tube has dislodged.
- You may also check tube placement by examining the aspirate and placing a small amount on the pH test strip. Probability of gastric placement is increased if the aspirate has a typical gastric fluid appearance (grassy green, clear and colorless with mucous shreds, or brown) and the pH is ≤5.
- After you confirm the initial proper tube placement, remove the tape marking of the tube length.
- Tape the tube to the patient's nose and remove the guide wire.
- To advance the tube to the duodenum, especially a tungsten-weighted tube, position the patient on his or her right side. This allows gravity to assist in passage of the tube through the pylorus. Move the tube forward 2″ to 3″ (5 to 7.5 cm) hourly until X-ray studies confirm duodenal placement. (An X-ray must confirm placement before feeding begins because duodenal feeding can cause nausea and vomiting if it is accidentally delivered to the stomach.)
- Apply a skin preparation to the patient's cheek before securing the tube with tape. This helps the tube to adhere to the skin and prevents irritation.
- Tape the tube securely to the patient's cheek to avoid excessive pressure on his or her nostrils.

Removing the tube

- Protect the patient's chest with a linen-saver pad.
- Flush the tube with air with the bulb syringe, clamp or pinch it to prevent aspiration of fluid during withdrawal, and withdraw the tube gently but quickly.
- Promptly cover and discard the used tube.

Special considerations

- Check gastric residual contents before each feeding. Withhold the feeding if residual volumes are greater than 200 ml on two successive assessments.
- Flush the feeding tube every 4 hours with 20 to 30 ml of normal saline solution or water to maintain patency, if there are no contraindications and according to facility policy. Retape the tube at least daily and as needed. Alternate taping of the tube toward the inner and the outer side of the nose to avoid constant pressure on the same nasal area. Inspect the skin for redness and breakdown.
- Provide nasal hygiene daily using cotton-tipped applicators and water-soluble lubricant to remove crusted secretions. Help the patient to brush his or her teeth, gums, and tongue with mouthwash or a mild salt water solution at least twice daily.
- If the patient cannot swallow the feeding tube, use a guide to aid insertion.
- Precise placement of the feeding tube is especially important because small-bore feeding tubes may slide into the trachea without causing immediate signs or symptoms of respiratory distress, such as coughing, choking, gasping, or cyanosis. However, the patient will usually cough if the tube enters the larynx. To make sure that the tube clears the larynx, ask the patient to speak. If he or she cannot,

the tube is in the larynx. Withdraw the tube at once and reinsert it.

- When aspirating gastric contents to check tube placement, pull gently on the syringe plunger to prevent trauma to the stomach lining or bowel. If you meet resistance during aspiration, stop the procedure because resistance may result simply from the tube lying against the stomach wall. If the tube coils above the stomach, you will not be able to aspirate the stomach contents. To rectify this situation, change the patient's position or withdraw the tube a few inches, readvance it, and try to aspirate again. If the tube was inserted with a guide wire, do not use the guide wire to reposition the tube. However, the health care provider may do so, using fluoroscopic guidance.

 Patient Teaching Tip

If the patient will use a feeding tube at home, make appropriate nursing referrals for home care and teach the patient and his or her caregivers how to use and care for a feeding tube. Teach them how to obtain equipment, insert and remove the tube, prepare and store feeding formula, and solve problems regarding tube position and patency.

Teach the patient to watch for complications related to prolonged intubation, such as skin erosion at the nostril, sinusitis, esophagitis, esophagotracheal fistula, gastric ulceration, and pulmonary and oral infection.

Documentation

For tube insertion, record the date and time, tube type and size, insertion site, exposed length of tube, area of placement, and confirmation of proper placement. Also record the name of the person performing the procedure. Record flushes on the patient's record of intake and output. For tube removal, record the date, time, and the patient's tolerance of the procedure.

Gastric lavage

After poisoning or drug overdose, especially in patients who have central nervous system depression or an inadequate gag reflex, gastric lavage flushes the stomach and removes ingested substances through a gastric lavage tube. The procedure is also used to empty the stomach in preparation for endoscopic examination. For patients with gastric or esophageal bleeding, lavage with tepid or iced water or normal saline solution may be used to stop bleeding. However, some controversy exists over the effectiveness of iced lavage for this purpose.

Gastric lavage can be continuous or intermittent. Typically, this procedure is done in the emergency department or intensive care unit by a health care provider, gastroenterologist, or nurse. A wide-bore lavage tube is usually inserted by a gastroenterologist.

Gastric lavage is contraindicated after ingestion of a corrosive substance (such as lye, a petroleum distillate, ammonia, an alkali, or a mineral acid) because the lavage tube may perforate the already compromised esophagus.

Correct placement of the lavage tube is essential for patient safety. Accidental misplacement of the tube (in the lungs, for example) followed by lavage can be fatal. Other complications of gastric lavage include bradyarrhythmias and aspiration of gastric fluids.

Equipment and preparation

Lavage setup • two graduated containers for drainage • clamp or smooth hemostat • 2 to 3 L of normal saline solution, tap water, or appropriate

Preparing for gastric lavage

Prepare the lavage setup as follows:
- Connect one of the three pieces of large-lumen tubing to the irrigant container.
- Insert the stem of the Y-connector in the other end of the tubing.
- Connect the remaining two pieces of tubing to the free ends of the Y-connector.
- Place the unattached end of one of the tubes into one of the drainage containers. (Later, you will connect the other piece of tubing to the patient's gastric tube.)
- Clamp the tube that leads to the irrigant.
- Suspend the entire setup from the I.V. pole, hanging the irrigant container at the highest level.

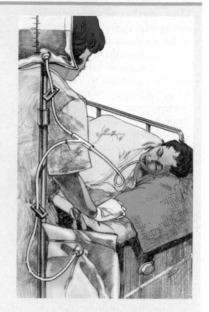

antidote as ordered • basin of ice, if ordered • Ewald's tube or any large-lumen gastric or lavage tube, typically #36 to #40 French • water-soluble lubricant or anesthetic ointment • stethoscope • ½″ hypoallergenic tape • 50-ml bulb or catheter-tip syringe • gloves • face shield • linen-saver pad or towel • tonsillar suction device • labeled specimen container • laboratory requests • norepinephrine • optional: patient restraints and charcoal

A prepackaged, syringe-type irrigation kit may be used for intermittent lavage. For poisoning or a drug overdose, however, the continuous lavage setup may be more appropriate because it is a faster and more effective means of diluting and removing the harmful substance.

Set up the lavage equipment. (See *Preparing for gastric lavage.*) If iced lavage is ordered, chill the desired irrigant (water or normal saline solution) in a basin of ice. Lubricate the end of the lavage tube with the water-soluble lubricant or anesthetic ointment.

Implementation

- Confirm the patient's identity using at least two patient identifiers.
- Explain the procedure to the patient, provide privacy, and wash your hands.
- Put on gloves and a face shield.
- Drape the towel or linen-saver pad over the patient's chest to protect him or her from spills.
- The health care provider inserts the lavage tube nasally and advances it slowly and gently. Forceful insertion

may injure tissues and cause epistaxis. He or she checks the placement of the tube by injecting about 30 cc of air into the tube with the bulb syringe and then auscultating the abdomen with a stethoscope. If the tube is in place, he or she will hear air entering the stomach.

- Because the patient may vomit when the lavage tube reaches the posterior pharynx during insertion, be prepared to suction the airway immediately with a tonsillar suction device.
- When the lavage tube passes the posterior pharynx, help the patient into Trendelenburg's position and turn him or her toward his or her left side in a three-quarter prone posture. This position minimizes passage of gastric contents into the duodenum and may prevent the patient from aspirating vomitus.
- After securing the lavage tube nasally or orally with hypoallergenic tape and making sure that the irrigant inflow tube on the lavage setup is clamped, connect the unattached end of this tube to the lavage tube. Allow the stomach contents to empty into a graduated drainage container before you instill irrigant. This confirms proper tube placement and decreases the risk of overfilling the stomach with irrigant and inducing vomiting. If you are using a syringe irrigation kit, aspirate the stomach contents with a 50-ml bulb or catheter-tip syringe before instilling the irrigant.
- When you confirm proper tube placement, begin gastric lavage by instilling about 250 ml of irrigant to assess the patient's tolerance and prevent vomiting. Use water or normal saline solution, preferably warmed to 68° F (20.2° C) to avoid the risk of hypothermia.
- Clamp the inflow tube with a smooth hemostat and unclamp the outflow tube to allow the irrigant to flow out. If you are using the syringe irrigation kit, aspirate the irrigant with the syringe and empty it into a graduated container. Measure the amount of outflow to make sure that it equals at least the amount of irrigant that you instilled. This prevents accidental stomach distention and vomiting. If the drainage amount is significantly less than the instilled amount, reposition the tube until sufficient solution flows out. Gently massage the abdomen over the stomach to promote outflow.
- Repeat the inflow–outflow cycle until the returned fluids appear clear. This signals that the stomach no longer holds harmful substances or that bleeding has stopped.
- Assess the patient's vital signs, urine output, and LOC every 15 minutes. Notify the health care provider of any changes.
- If ordered, remove the lavage tube.

Special considerations

- To control gastrointestinal (GI) bleeding, the health care provider may order continuous irrigation of the stomach with an irrigant and a vasoconstrictor such as norepinephrine. After the stomach absorbs norepinephrine, the portal system delivers the drug directly to the liver, where it is metabolized. This prevents the drug from circulating systemically and initiating a hypertensive response. Alternatively, the health care provider may direct you to clamp the outflow tube for a prescribed period after you instill the irrigant and the vasoconstrictor and before you withdraw it. This allows the mucosa time to absorb the drug.
- Never leave a patient alone during gastric lavage. Observe him or her continuously for changes in LOC and monitor vital signs frequently. The natural vagal response to

intubation can depress the patient's heart rate.

- If you must restrain the patient, secure the restraints on the same side of the bed or stretcher so that you can free them quickly without moving to the other side of the bed.
- Remember to keep tracheal suctioning equipment nearby and to watch closely for airway obstruction caused by vomiting or excess oral secretions. Throughout gastric lavage, you may need to suction the oral cavity frequently to ensure an open airway and prevent aspiration. For the same reasons, and if he or she does not exhibit an adequate gag reflex, the patient may require an endotracheal (ET) tube before the procedure.
- When you aspirate the stomach for ingested poisons or drugs, save the contents in a labeled specimen container to send to the laboratory for analysis with the appropriate laboratory request. If ordered, after lavage to remove poisons or drugs, administer charcoal, as directed, through the NG tube. The charcoal will absorb remaining toxic substances. The tube may be clamped temporarily, allowed to drain via gravity, attached to intermittent suction, or removed.
- When you perform gastric lavage to stop bleeding, keep precise records of intake and output to determine the amount of bleeding. When large volumes of fluid are instilled and withdrawn, serum electrolyte and ABG levels may be measured during or at the end of lavage.
- Assess the patient for complications during gastric lavage. Vomiting and subsequent aspiration, the most common complications of gastric lavage, occur more commonly in a groggy patient. Bradyarrhythmias may also occur. Especially after iced lavage, the patient's body

temperature may drop, thereby triggering cardiac arrhythmias.

Documentation

Record the date and time of lavage, the size and type of NG tube used, the volume and type of irrigant, and the amount of gastric contents drained. Document this information on the record of intake and output and include your observations, including the color and consistency of drainage. Keep precise records of the patient's vital signs and LOC, drugs instilled through the tube, the time that the tube was removed, and the patient's response to the procedure.

Gastrostomy feeding button care

A gastrostomy feeding button is an alternative feeding device for an ambulatory patient who is receiving long-term enteral feedings. Approved by the U.S. Food and Drug Administration for 6-month implantation, feeding buttons can be used to replace gastrostomy tubes, if necessary.

The feeding button has a mushroom dome at one end and two wing tabs and a flexible safety plug at the other. When inserted into an established stoma, the button lies almost flush with the skin, with only the top of the safety plug visible.

The button can usually be inserted into a stoma in less than 15 minutes. In addition to its cosmetic appeal, the device is easily maintained, reduces skin irritation and breakdown, and is less likely to become dislodged or to migrate than an ordinary feeding tube. A one-way antireflux valve mounted just inside the mushroom dome prevents accidental leakage of gastric contents. The device usually is replaced after 3 to 4 months because the antireflux valve wears out.

Equipment

Gastrostomy feeding button of the correct size (all three sizes, if correct one is not known) • gloves • feeding accessories, including adapter, feeding catheter, food syringe or bag, and formula • catheter clamp • cleaning equipment, including water, cotton-tipped applicator, pipe cleaner, and mild soap or antiseptic solution • optional: pump to provide continuous infusion over several hours

Implementation

- Confirm the patient's identity using two patient identifiers.
- Explain the insertion, reinsertion, and feeding procedure to the patient. Tell him or her that the health care provider will perform the initial insertion.
- Wash your hands and put on gloves.
- Check for residual with the syringe. If you find more than 50 ml of residual, inform the health care provider and withhold the feeding until reassessment.
- Attach the adapter and feeding catheter to the food syringe or bag. Clamp the catheter and fill the syringe or bag and catheter with formula. Refill the syringe before it is empty. These steps prevent air from entering the stomach and distending the abdomen.
- Open the safety plug and attach the adapter and feeding catheter to the gastrostomy feeding button. Elevate the food syringe or bag above the patient's stomach level and gravity-feed the formula for 15 to 30 minutes, varying the height as needed to alter the flow rate. Use a pump for continuous infusion or for feedings that last several hours.
- After the feeding, flush the button with 10 ml of water. Clean the inside of the feeding catheter with a cotton-tipped applicator and water to preserve its patency and to dislodge formula or food particles.

Lower the food syringe or bag below the patient's stomach level to allow belching. Remove the adapter and feeding catheter. The antireflux valve should prevent gastric reflux. Snap the safety plug into place to keep the lumen clean and prevent leakage if the antireflux valve fails. If the patient feels nauseated or vomits after the feeding, vent the button with the adapter and feeding catheter to help control the vomiting.

- Wash the catheter and food syringe or bag in mild soap and rinse thoroughly. Clean the catheter and adapter with a pipe cleaner. Rinse the equipment well before using it for the next feeding. Soak the equipment once per week according to the manufacturer's recommendations.

Special considerations

- If the button pops out during feeding, reinsert it, estimate the amount of formula already delivered, and resume feeding. (See *How to reinsert a gastrostomy feeding button.*)
- Once daily, clean the peristomal skin with mild soap and water or povidone-iodine solution and let the skin air-dry for 20 minutes to minimize skin irritation. Also clean the site whenever spillage from the feeding bag occurs.

 Patient Teaching Tip

Before discharge, make sure that the patient can insert and care for the gastrostomy feeding button. If necessary, teach him or her or a family member or caregiver how to reinsert the button by first practicing on a model. Offer written instructions and answer the patient's questions about obtaining replacement supplies.

How to reinsert a gastrostomy feeding button

If your patient's gastrostomy feeding button pops out (with coughing, for instance), you or the patient will need to reinsert the device. Here are some steps to follow.

Prepare the equipment

Collect the feeding button, an obturator, and water-soluble lubricant. If the button will be reinserted, wash it with soap and water and rinse it thoroughly.

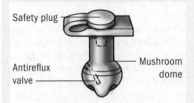

Insert the button

- Check the depth of the patient's stoma to make sure that you have a feeding button of the correct size. Then clean around the stoma.
- Lubricate the obturator with a water-soluble lubricant and distend the button several times to ensure the patency of the antireflux valve within the button.
- Lubricate the mushroom dome and the stoma. Gently push the button through the stoma into the stomach.

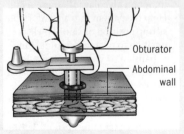

- Remove the obturator by gently rotating it as you withdraw it, to keep the antireflux valve from adhering to it. If the valve sticks, gently push the obturator back into the button until the valve closes.
- After you remove the obturator, make sure that the valve is closed. Then close the flexible safety plug, which should be relatively flush with the skin surface.

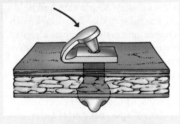

- If you need to administer a feeding right away, open the safety plug and attach the feeding adapter and feeding tube. Deliver the feeding as ordered.

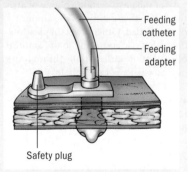

Documentation

Record the feeding time and duration, the amount and type of feeding formula used, and patient tolerance. Maintain records of intake and output as needed. Note the appearance of the stoma and surrounding skin.

Incentive spirometry

Incentive spirometry involves the use of a breathing device to help the patient achieve maximal ventilation. The device measures respiratory flow or respiratory volume and induces the patient to take a deep breath and hold it for several seconds. This deep breath increases lung volume, boosts alveolar inflation, and promotes venous return. This exercise also establishes alveolar hyperinflation for a longer time than is possible with a normal deep breath, thus preventing and reversing the alveolar collapse that causes atelectasis and pneumonitis.

Devices used for incentive spirometry provide a visual incentive to breathe deeply. Some are activated when the patient inhales a certain volume of air; the device then estimates the amount of air inhaled. Others contain plastic floats that rise according to the amount of air that the patient pulls through the device when he or she inhales.

Patients who are at low risk for atelectasis may use a flow incentive spirometer. Patients who are at high risk may need a volume incentive spirometer, which measures lung inflation more precisely.

Incentive spirometry benefits the patient who requires prolonged bed rest, especially the postoperative patient, who may regain his or her normal respiratory pattern slowly because of such predisposing factors such as abdominal or thoracic surgery, advanced age, inactivity, obesity, smoking, and decreased ability to cough effectively and expel lung secretions.

Equipment and preparation

Flow or volume incentive spirometer, as indicated, with sterile disposable tube and mouthpiece (The tube and mouthpiece are sterile on first use and clean on subsequent uses.) • stethoscope • warm water

Assemble the ordered equipment at the patient's bedside. Read the manufacturer's instructions for spirometer setup and operation. Remove the sterile disposable tube and mouthpiece from the package and attach them to the device. Set the flow rate or volume goal, as determined by the health care provider or respiratory therapist and based on the patient's preoperative performance. Turn on the machine, if necessary.

Implementation

- Confirm the patient's identity using at least two patient identifiers.
- Wash your hands and follow standard precautions.
- Assess the patient's condition.
- Explain the procedure to the patient, making sure that he or she understands the importance of performing incentive spirometry regularly to maintain alveolar inflation.
- Help the patient into a comfortable sitting position or semi-Fowler's position to promote optimal lung expansion. If you are using a flow incentive spirometer and the patient cannot assume or maintain this position, he or she can perform the procedure in any position as long as the device remains upright. Tilting a flow incentive spirometer decreases the required patient effort and reduces the effectiveness of the exercise.
- Auscultate the patient's lungs with a stethoscope to provide a baseline for comparison with posttreatment auscultation.

- Instruct the patient to insert the sterile mouthpiece and to close his or her lips tightly around it. A weak seal may alter flow or volume readings.
- Instruct the patient to exhale normally and then to inhale as slowly and deeply as possible. If the patient has difficulty with this step, tell him or her to suck as he or she would through a straw but more slowly. Ask the patient to retain the entire volume of air that he or she inhaled for 3 seconds or, if you are using a device with a light indicator, until the light turns off. This deep breath creates sustained transpulmonary pressure near the end of inspiration and is sometimes called a sustained maximal inspiration.
- Tell the patient to remove the mouthpiece and exhale normally. Allow him or her to relax and take several normal breaths before attempting another breath with the spirometer. Repeat this sequence 5 to 10 times during every waking hour. Note tidal volumes (V_T).
- Evaluate the patient's ability to cough effectively. Encourage him or her to cough after each effort because deep lung inflation may loosen secretions and facilitate their removal. Examine the expectorated secretions.
- Auscultate the patient's lungs and compare the findings with those of the first auscultation.
- Instruct the patient to remove the mouthpiece. Wash the mouthpiece in warm water and shake it dry. Avoid immersing the spirometer itself because this enhances bacterial growth and impairs the effectiveness of the internal filter in preventing inhalation of extraneous material.
- Place the mouthpiece in a plastic storage bag between exercises. Label it and the spirometer, if applicable, with the patient's name so that

another patient does not inadvertently use the equipment.

Special considerations

- If the patient is scheduled for surgery, assess beforehand his or her respiratory pattern and ability to meet appropriate postoperative goals. Teach the patient how to use the spirometer before surgery so that he or she can concentrate on your instructions and practice the exercise. A preoperative evaluation will also help in establishing postoperative therapeutic goals.
- Avoid exercising at mealtime to prevent nausea. If the patient has difficulty breathing only through his or her mouth, provide a noseclip to measure each breath fully. Provide paper and a pencil so that the patient can note exercise times. Exercise frequency varies with the patient's condition and ability.
- Immediately after surgery, monitor the patient's exercise frequently to ensure compliance and assess achievement.

Documentation

Record preoperative teaching. Document preoperative flow or volume levels, the date and time of the procedure, the type of spirometer used, the flow or volume levels achieved, and the number of breaths taken. Note the patient's condition before and after the procedure, his or her tolerance of the procedure, and the results of both auscultations.

If you used a flow incentive spirometer, compute the volume by multiplying the setting by the duration that the patient kept the ball (or balls) suspended, as follows. If the patient suspended the ball for 3 seconds at a setting of 500 cc during each of 10 breaths, multiply 500 cc by 3 seconds and then record this total (1,500 cc) and the number of breaths, as follows: 1,500 cc × 10 breaths. If you used a volume incentive spirometer, take the volume reading directly from the spirometer. For example, record 1,000 cc × 5 breaths.

Latex allergy protocol

Latex, a natural product of the rubber tree, is commonly used in barrier protection products and medical equipment—and more and more nurses and patients are becoming hypersensitive to it. Those who are at increased risk for latex allergy include people who have had or will undergo multiple surgical procedures (especially those with a history of spina bifida), health care workers (especially those in the emergency department and operating room), workers who manufacture latex and latex-containing products, and people with a genetic predisposition to latex allergy.

People who are allergic to certain cross-reactive foods—including apricots, cherries, grapes, kiwis, passion fruit, bananas, avocados, chestnuts, tomatoes, and peaches—may also be allergic to latex. Exposure to latex elicits an allergic response similar to the response elicited by these foods.

For people with latex allergy, latex becomes a hazard when the protein in latex comes in direct contact with the mucous membranes or is inhaled, as occurs when powdered latex surgical gloves are used. People with asthma are at greater risk for worsening symptoms from airborne latex.

The diagnosis of latex allergy is based on the patient's history and findings on physical examination. Laboratory testing should be performed to confirm or exclude the diagnosis. Skin testing can be done. The radioallergosorbent test measures the serum level of latex-specific immunoglobulin E in the blood. Other blood tests include the AlaSTAT test, Hycor assay, and Pharmacia CAP test.

Latex allergy can produce various signs and symptoms, including generalized itching (on the hands and arms, for example); itchy, watery, or burning eyes; sneezing and coughing (hay fever–type signs and symptoms); rash; hives; bronchial asthma, scratchy throat, or difficulty breathing; edema of the face, hands, or neck; and anaphylaxis.

To help identify people who are at risk, ask specific questions about latex allergy during the health history. (See *Latex allergy screening.*) If the patient's history shows a latex sensitivity, the health care provider assigns him or her to one of three categories based on the extent of his or her sensitization. Group 1 patients have a history of anaphylaxis or a systemic reaction when exposed to a natural latex product. Group 2 patients have a clear history of a nonsystemic allergic reaction. Group 3 patients do not have a history of latex hypersensitivity but are considered high risk because of an associated medical condition, occupation, or crossover allergy.

If you determine that the patient is sensitive to latex, make sure that he or she does not come in contact with it because such contact could result in a life-threatening hypersensitivity reaction. Creating a latex-free environment is the only way to safeguard the patient. Many facilities now designate latex-free equipment that is usually kept on a cart that can be moved into the patient's room.

Equipment and preparation

Latex allergy patient identification wristband • latex-free equipment, including room contents

After you have determined that the patient has a latex allergy or is sensitive to latex, arrange for him or her to be placed in a private room. If that is not possible, make the room latex-free, even if his or her roommate has not

Latex allergy screening

To determine if your patient has a latex sensitivity or allergy, ask the following screening questions:
- What is your occupation?
- Have you experienced an allergic reaction, local sensitivity, or itching after exposure to any latex products, such as balloons or condoms?
- Do you have shortness of breath or wheezing after blowing up balloons or after a dental visit? Do you have itching in or around your mouth after eating a banana?

If your patient answers "yes" to any of these questions, proceed with the following questions:
- Do you have a history of allergies, dermatitis, or asthma? If so, what type of reaction do you have?

- Do you have any congenital abnormalities? If yes, explain.
- Do you have any food allergies? If so, what specific allergies do you have? Describe your reaction.
- If you experience shortness of breath or wheezing when blowing up latex balloons, describe your reaction.
- Have you had any previous surgical procedures? Did you experience associated complications? If so, describe them.
- Have you had previous dental procedures? Did you have any complications? If so, describe them.
- Are you exposed to latex in your occupation? Do you experience a reaction to latex products at work? If so, describe your reaction.

been designated as hypersensitive to latex, to prevent the spread of airborne particles from latex products used on the other patient.

Implementation
For all patients in groups 1 and 2
- Assess all patients who are being admitted to the delivery room or short procedure unit or having a surgical procedure for latex allergy.
- If the patient has a confirmed latex allergy, bring a cart with latex-free equipment into the room.
- Document in the patient's chart (according to facility policy) that the patient has a latex allergy. If policy requires that the patient wear a latex allergy patient identification wristband, place it on the patient.
- Post a LATEX ALLERGY sign in the patient's room.
- If the patient will be receiving anesthesia, make sure that LATEX

ALLERGY is clearly visible on the front of the chart. (See *Anesthesia induction and latex allergy*, page 340.) Notify the circulating nurse in the surgical unit, the nurses in the postanesthesia care unit, and all other team members that the patient has a latex allergy.
- If the patient must be transported to another area of the facility, make sure that the latex-free cart accompanies him or her and that all health care workers who come in contact with the patient are wearing nonlatex gloves. The patient should wear a mask with cloth ties when leaving his or her room to protect him or her from inhaling airborne latex particles.
- Notify central supply, dietary services, and the pharmacy about the patient's allergy.
- If the patient will have an I.V. line, make sure that only latex-free products are used to establish I.V. access.

Anesthesia induction and latex allergy

Causes of intraoperative reaction	Signs and symptoms in a conscious patient	Signs and symptoms in an anesthetized patient
• Latex contact with mucous membranes • Latex contact with the intraperitoneal serosal lining • Inhalation of airborne latex particles during anesthesia • Injection of antibiotics and anesthetic agents through latex ports	• Abnormal cramping • Anxiety • Bronchoconstriction • Diarrhea • Faintness • Generalized pruritus • Itchy eyes • Nausea • Shortness of breath • Swelling of soft tissue (hands, face, and tongue) • Vomiting • Wheezing	• Bronchospasm • Cardiopulmonary arrest • Facial edema • Flushing • Hypotension • Laryngeal edema • Tachycardia • Urticaria • Wheezing

- Be sure that you use only latex-free I.V. products and supplies.
- Use a nonlatex tourniquet. If none are available, use a latex tourniquet over clothing.
- Use latex-free equipment for oxygen administration. Remove the elastic and tie the equipment on with gauze.
- Wrap your stethoscope, blood pressure cuff and tubing, and ECG wires with a nonlatex product to protect the patient from latex contact.
- Wrap a transparent semipermeable dressing over the patient's finger before using pulse oximetry.
- Use latex-free syringes when administering medication.
- If the patient has an allergic reaction to latex, act immediately. (See *Managing a latex allergy reaction.*)

Special considerations

- The signs and symptoms of latex allergy usually occur within 30 minutes after anesthesia is induced. However, the time of onset can range from 10 minutes to several hours.
- As a health care worker, you are in a position to develop latex hypersensitivity. If you suspect that you are sensitive to latex, contact the employee health services department about facility protocol for latex-sensitive employees. Use latex-free products whenever possible to help reduce your exposure to latex.
- Patients who do not have a history of latex hypersensitivity but have an associated medical condition, occupation, or crossover allergy should be aware of the potential for latex hypersensitivity.

 ALERT

Do not assume that if something does not look like rubber, it is not latex. Latex is found in various types of equipment, including electrocardiograph leads, oral and nasal airway tubing, tourniquets, nerve stimulation pads, temperature strips, and blood pressure cuffs.

Managing a latex allergy reaction

If you determine that your patient is having an allergic reaction to a latex product, act immediately. Make sure that you perform emergency interventions using latex-free equipment. If the latex product that caused the reaction is known, remove it and perform the following measures:

- If the allergic reaction develops during medication administration or during a procedure, stop the medication or procedure immediately.
- Assess the patient's airway, breathing, and circulation.
- Administer 100% oxygen with continuous pulse oximetry.
- Start I.V. volume expanders with lactated Ringer's solution or normal saline solution.

- Administer epinephrine according to the patient's symptoms.
- Administer famotidine, as ordered.
- If bronchospasm is evident, treat it with nebulized albuterol, as ordered.
- Secondary treatment for latex allergy reaction is aimed at treating the swelling and tissue reaction to the latex as well as breaking the chain of events associated with the allergic reaction. It includes:
  - diphenhydramine
  - methylprednisolone
  - famotidine.
- Document the event and the exact cause (if known). If latex particles have entered the I.V. line, insert a new I.V. line with a new catheter, new tubing, and new infusion attachments as soon as possible.

Lumbar puncture

Lumbar puncture involves inserting a sterile needle into the subarachnoid space of the spinal canal, usually between the third and fourth lumbar vertebrae. This procedure is used to detect the presence of blood in the cerebrospinal fluid (CSF), to obtain CSF specimens for laboratory analysis, and to inject dyes or gases for contrast in radiologic studies. It is also used to administer drugs or anesthetics and to relieve ICP by removing CSF.

Performed by a health care provider or an advanced practice nurse, lumbar puncture requires sterile technique and careful patient positioning. This procedure is contraindicated in patients with a lumbar deformity or an infection at the puncture site. Lumbar puncture is not recommended if the patient has an intracranial mass lesion because the rapid reduction in pressure

that follows lumbar puncture can lead to tonsillar herniation and medullary compression.

Equipment and preparation

Overbed table • two pairs of sterile gloves • antiseptic solution • sterile gauze pads • alcohol pad • sterile fenestrated drape • 3-ml syringe for local anesthetic • 25G ¾" sterile needle for injecting anesthetic • local anesthetic (usually 1% lidocaine) •18G or 20G 3½" spinal needle with stylet (22G needle for children) • three-way stopcock • manometer • small adhesive bandage • three sterile collection tubes with stoppers • laboratory requests • labels • light source such as a gooseneck lamp • sterile marker and labels • optional: patient-care reminder

Disposable lumbar puncture trays contain most of the needed sterile equipment.

Implementation

- Confirm the patient's identity using at least two patient identifiers.
- Explain the procedure to the patient to ease anxiety and ensure cooperation. Make sure that the patient has signed a consent form.
- Inform the patient that he or she may experience a headache after lumbar puncture, but reassure him or her that cooperating during the procedure minimizes this effect.
- Check the patient's history for hypersensitivity to local anesthetic.
- Immediately before the procedure, provide privacy and instruct the patient to void.
- Wash your hands thoroughly.
- Open the disposable lumbar puncture tray on an overbed table, being careful not to contaminate the sterile field when you open the wrapper. Label all medications, medication containers, and other solutions on and off the sterile field.
- Provide an adequate light source at the puncture site and adjust the height of the patient's bed to allow the procedure to be performed comfortably.
- Position the patient and reemphasize the importance of remaining as still as possible to minimize discomfort and trauma. (See *Positioning for lumbar puncture*.)
- The health care provider cleans the puncture site with sterile gauze pads soaked in antiseptic solution, wiping in a circular motion away from the puncture site. He or she uses three different pads to prevent contamination of spinal tissues by normal skin flora. Next, he or she drapes the area with the sterile fenestrated drape to provide a sterile field. (If the health care provider uses povidone-iodine pads instead of sterile gauze pads, he or she may remove his or her sterile gloves and put on another pair to avoid introducing antiseptic solution

Positioning for lumbar puncture

To position a patient for a lumbar puncture, have him or her lie on his or her side at the edge of the bed, with the chin tucked to the chest and knees drawn up to the abdomen. Make sure that the patient's spine is curved and his or her back is at the edge of the bed (as shown below). This position widens the spaces between the vertebrae, easing insertion of the needle.

To help the patient maintain this position, place one of your hands behind his or her neck and the other hand behind the knees, and pull gently. Hold the patient firmly in this position throughout the procedure to prevent accidental displacement of the needle.

Patient positioning

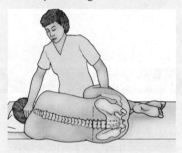

Typically, the health care provider inserts the needle between the third and fourth lumbar vertebrae (as shown below).

Needle positioning

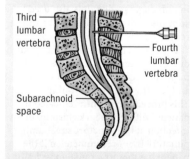

Third lumbar vertebra

Fourth lumbar vertebra

Subarachnoid space

into the subarachnoid space with the lumbar puncture needle.)

- If no ampule of anesthetic is included on the equipment tray, clean the injection port of a multidose vial of anesthetic with an alcohol pad. Invert the vial 45 degrees so that the health care provider can insert a 25G needle and syringe and withdraw the anesthetic for injection.

- Before the health care provider injects the anesthetic, tell the patient that he or she will experience a transient burning sensation and local pain. Ask the patient to report other persistent pain or sensations because they may indicate irritation or puncture of a nerve root, requiring repositioning of the needle.

- When the health care provider inserts the spinal needle with stylet into the subarachnoid space, instruct the patient to remain still and to breathe normally. If necessary, hold the patient firmly in position to prevent sudden movement that may displace the needle.

- If the lumbar puncture is being performed to administer contrast media for radiologic studies or spinal anesthetic, the health care provider injects the dye or anesthetic at this time.

- When the needle is in place, the health care provider attaches a manometer with a three-way stopcock to the needle hub to read the CSF pressure. If ordered, help the patient extend his or her legs to provide a more accurate pressure reading.

- The health care provider detaches the manometer and allows CSF to drain from the needle hub into the collection tubes. When he or she has collected 2 to 3 ml in each tube, mark the tubes in sequence, insert stoppers to secure them, and label them.

- If the health care provider suspects an obstruction in the spinal subarachnoid space, he or she may check for Queckenstedt's sign. After he or she

takes an initial CSF pressure reading, compress the patient's jugular vein for 10 seconds, as ordered. This increases ICP and—if no subarachnoid block is present—causes the CSF pressure to rise. The health care provider takes pressure readings every 10 seconds until the pressure stabilizes.

- After the health care provider collects the specimens and removes the spinal needle, clean the puncture site with antiseptic solution and apply a small adhesive bandage.

- Send the CSF specimens to the laboratory immediately, with the completed laboratory request.

Special considerations

- During lumbar puncture, watch the patient closely for signs of an adverse reaction: elevated pulse rate, pallor, and clammy skin. Alert the health care provider immediately if any significant changes occur.

- The patient may be ordered to lie flat for 8 to 12 hours after the procedure. If necessary, place a patient-care reminder on his or her bed.

- Collected CSF specimens must be sent to the laboratory immediately; they cannot be refrigerated for later transport.

- If ordered, encourage the patient to drink fluids after the procedure to reduce the risk of spinal headache.

- Check the puncture site for redness, swelling, and drainage every hour for the first 4 hours and then every 4 hours for the next 24 hours.

- Assess the patient for complications after lumbar puncture. Headache is the most common adverse effect. Others include a reaction to the anesthetic, meningitis, epidural and subdural abscess, bleeding into the spinal canal, leakage of CSF through the dural defect that remains after the needle is withdrawn, local pain caused by irritation of the nerve root, edema and hematoma at the puncture site, transient difficulty voiding, and fever. The most serious complications (tonsillar herniation and medullary compression) are rare.

Documentation

Record the initiation and completion times of the procedure; the patient's response; the drugs administered; the number of specimen tubes collected; the time at which specimens were transported to the laboratory; and the color, consistency, and any other characteristics of the collected specimens.

Manual ventilation

Manual ventilation involves using a handheld resuscitation bag, which is an inflatable device that can be attached to a face mask or directly to an ET or a tracheostomy tube to allow manual delivery of oxygen or room air to the lungs of a patient who cannot breathe by himself or herself. Usually used in an emergency, manual ventilation can also be performed while the patient is disconnected temporarily from a mechanical ventilator, such as during a tubing change, during transport, or before suctioning. In these cases, use of the handheld resuscitation bag maintains ventilation. Administration of oxygen with a resuscitation bag can help improve a compromised cardiorespiratory system.

Equipment and preparation

Handheld resuscitation bag • mask • oxygen source (wall unit or tank) • oxygen tubing • nipple adapter attached to oxygen flowmeter • gloves • goggles or face shield (if needed) • optional: oxygen accumulator and positive end-expiratory pressure (PEEP) valve • optional: oropharyngeal airway or nasopharyngeal airway

Unless the patient is intubated or has a tracheostomy, select a mask that fits snugly over the patient's mouth and nose. Attach the mask to the resuscitation bag. If oxygen is readily available, connect the handheld resuscitation bag to the oxygen source. Attach one end of the oxygen tubing to the bottom of the bag and the other end to the nipple adapter on the flowmeter of the oxygen source.

Turn on the oxygen and adjust the flow rate according to the patient's condition. For example, if the patient has a low partial pressure of arterial oxygen, he or she will need a higher fraction of inspired oxygen (FIO_2). To increase the concentration of inspired oxygen, you can add an oxygen accumulator (also called an oxygen reservoir). This device, which attaches to an adapter on the bottom of the bag, permits an FIO_2 of up to 100%. If time allows, set up suction equipment.

Implementation

- Put on gloves and other personal protective equipment and follow standard precautions.
- Turn the oxygen flow rate to 15 L/minute.
- Before you use the handheld resuscitation bag, remove any objects from the patient's upper airway. Also, suction the patient to remove secretions that may obstruct the airway. If necessary, insert an oropharyngeal or nasopharyngeal airway to maintain airway patency. If the patient has a tracheostomy or an ET tube in place, suction the tube.
- If appropriate, remove the headboard and stand at the head of the bed to help keep the patient's neck extended and to free space at the side of the bed for other activities such as CPR.
- Tilt the patient's head backward, if not contraindicated, and pull his or her jaw forward to move the tongue away from the base of the pharynx and prevent obstruction of the airway. (See *How to apply a handheld resuscitation bag and mask*.)

How to apply a handheld resuscitation bag and mask

Circle the edges of the mask with the index and first finger of one hand while lifting the jaw with the other fingers. Make sure there is a tight seal.

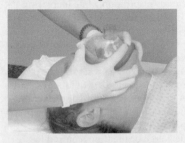

Make sure that the patient's mouth remains open underneath the mask. Attach the bag to the mask and to the tubing that leads to the oxygen source.

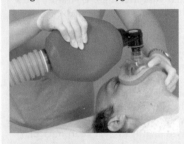

If the patient has a tracheostomy tube or an endotracheal tube in place, remove the mask from the bag and attach the handheld resuscitation bag directly to the tube.

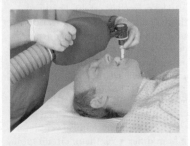

- Keeping your nondominant hand on the patient's mask, exert downward pressure to seal the mask against his or her face. For an adult patient, use your dominant hand to compress the bag to deliver 500 to 600 cc of air over 1 second.

AGE ALERT

For infants and children, use a pediatric handheld resuscitation bag. For a child, deliver 15 breaths/minute, or one compression of the bag every 4 seconds; for an infant, 20 breaths/minute, or one compression every 3 seconds. Infants and children should receive 250 to 500 cc of air with each compression.

- Deliver breaths with the patient's own inspiratory effort, if any is present. Do not attempt to deliver a breath as the patient exhales.
- Observe the patient's chest to ensure that it rises and falls with each compression. If ventilation does not occur, check the fit of the mask and the patency of the patient's airway. If necessary, reposition the patient's head and ensure patency with an oral airway.

Special considerations

- Add PEEP to manual ventilation by attaching a PEEP valve to the resuscitation bag. This may improve oxygenation if the patient has not responded to an increased FIO_2 levels. Always use a PEEP valve to manually ventilate a patient who has been receiving PEEP on the ventilator.
- If the patient has a possible cervical injury, avoid neck hyperextension; instead, use the jaw-thrust technique

to open the airway. If you need both hands to keep the patient's mask in place and maintain hyperextension, use the lower part of your arm to compress the bag against your side.

- Observe the patient for vomiting through the clear part of the mask. If vomiting occurs, stop the procedure immediately, lift the mask, wipe and suction the vomitus, and resume resuscitation.
- Underventilation commonly occurs because it is difficult to keep the handheld resuscitation bag positioned tightly on the patient's face while ensuring an open airway. In addition, the volume of air delivered to the patient varies with the type of bag used and the hand size of the person who is compressing the bag. For these reasons, have someone assist with the procedure, if possible.
- Aspiration of vomitus can result in pneumonia, and gastric distention may occur if air is forced into the patient's stomach.

Documentation

In an emergency, record the date and time of the procedure, the manual ventilation efforts, complications that occurred and the nursing action taken, and the patient's response to treatment, according to facility protocol for respiratory arrest.

In a nonemergency situation, record the date and time of the procedure, the reason and the length of time that the patient was disconnected from mechanical ventilation and received manual ventilation, complications that occurred and nursing actions taken, and the patient's tolerance of the procedure.

Mechanical ventilation

Mechanical ventilation involves using a mechanical ventilator that moves air into and out of the patient's lungs. Although the equipment serves to ventilate the patient, it does not ensure adequate gas exchange. Mechanical ventilators may use either positive or negative pressure to ventilate patients.

Positive-pressure ventilators exert a positive pressure on the airway, which causes inspiration while increasing V_T. The inspiratory cycles of these ventilators may vary in volume, pressure, or time. For example, a volume-cycle ventilator—the type most commonly used—delivers a preset volume of air each time, regardless of lung resistance. A pressure-cycle ventilator generates flow until the machine reaches a preset pressure, regardless of the volume delivered or the time required to achieve the pressure. A time-cycle ventilator generates flow for a preset amount of time. A high-frequency ventilator uses high respiratory rates and low V_T to maintain alveolar ventilation.

Negative-pressure ventilators act by creating negative pressure, which pulls the thorax outward and allows air to flow into the lungs. Examples of such ventilators are the iron lung, the cuirass (chest shell), and the body wrap. Negative-pressure ventilators are used mainly to treat neuromuscular disorders, such as Guillain-Barré's syndrome, myasthenia gravis, and poliomyelitis.

Other indications for ventilator use include central nervous system disorders, such as cerebral hemorrhage and spinal cord transsection, adult respiratory distress syndrome, pulmonary edema, chronic obstructive pulmonary disease, flail chest, and acute hypoventilation.

Equipment and preparation

Oxygen source • air source that can supply 50 psi • mechanical ventilator • humidifier • ventilator circuit tubing, connectors, and adapters • condensation collection trap • spirometer, respirometer, or electronic device to measure flow and volume • in-line thermometer • probe for gas sampling and measuring airway pressure • gloves • handheld resuscitation bag with reservoir • suction equipment • sterile distilled water • equipment for ABG analysis • soft restraints, if indicated • optional: oximeter

In most facilities, respiratory therapists assume responsibility for setting up the ventilator. If necessary, check the manufacturer's instructions for setting it up. In most cases, you will need to add sterile distilled water to the humidifier and connect the ventilator to the appropriate gas source.

Implementation

- Verify the health care provider's order for ventilator support. If the patient is not already intubated, prepare him or her for intubation.
- When possible, explain the procedure to the patient and family to help reduce anxiety and fear. Assure the patient and family that staff members are nearby to provide care.
- Perform a complete physical assessment and draw blood for ABG analysis to establish a baseline.
- Suction the patient, if necessary.
- Plug the mechanical ventilator into an uninterruptable, emergency power, electrical outlet; connect it to the oxygen source; and turn it on. Adjust the settings on the ventilator as ordered. (See *Ventilator modes and settings*, page 348.) Make sure that the alarms are set as ordered and that the humidifier is filled with sterile distilled water. Attach a capnographic device that measures carbon dioxide levels to confirm ET tube placement, detect disconnection from the ventilator, and allow early detection of complications.

- Put on gloves if you have not done so already. Connect the ET tube to the ventilator. Observe the patient for chest expansion and auscultate for bilateral breath sounds to verify that the patient is being ventilated.
- Monitor the patient's ABG values after the initial ventilator setup (usually 20 to 30 minutes), after changes in the ventilator settings, and as the patient's clinical condition indicates to determine if the patient is being ventilated adequately and to prevent oxygen toxicity. Be prepared to adjust the ventilator settings based on the ABG analysis.
- Check the ventilator circuit tubing frequently for condensation, which can cause airflow resistance and infection if the patient aspirates it. As needed, drain the condensate into a collection trap or briefly disconnect the patient from the ventilator (ventilating him or her with a handheld resuscitation bag, if necessary) and empty the water into a receptacle. Do not drain the condensate into the humidifier because the condensate may be contaminated with the patient's secretions.
- Check the in-line thermometer to make sure that the temperature of the air delivered to the patient is close to body temperature. Monitor flow volume and airway pressure according to facility policy.
- When monitoring the patient's vital signs, count spontaneous breaths as well as ventilator-delivered breaths.
- Change, clean, or dispose the ventilator tubing and equipment according to facility policy to reduce the risk of bacterial contamination. Typically, the ventilator tubing is changed every 48 to 72 hours and sometimes more often.
- When ordered, begin to wean the patient from the ventilator.

Ventilator modes and settings

Although a respiratory therapist usually initiates mechanical ventilation and adjusts the ventilator modes or settings based on the health care provider's orders, you should understand all of the following terms.

Mode or setting	Function
Assist-control (A/C) ventilation	• Delivers a breath at a preset tidal volume (V_T) if patient fails to initiate a breath within a preset time period • Ventilator triggered to deliver a breath at a preset V_T if patient initiates a breath
Continuous positive airway pressure (CPAP)	• Can only be used with patients who are breathing spontaneously and effectively • Maintains a preset positive pressure in the airways to decrease resistance
Control ventilation (CV)	• Delivers a preset V_T at a fixed rate, regardless of whether patient initiates any breaths • Used for apneic patients
High-frequency ventilation (HFV)	• Delivers a small amount of gas at a rapid rate, ranging from 60 to 100 breaths/minute • Requires sedation and drug-induced paralysis • Used for hemodynamically unstable patients during short-term procedures or for patients at risk for pneumothorax
Independent lung ventilation (ILV)	• Uses two ventilators to ventilate each lung separately • Uses a double-lumen endotracheal tube and requires sedation and drug-induced paralysis • Useful for patients with different disease processes in each lung
Inverse ratio ventilation (IRV)	• Reverses normal inspiratory-expiratory (I:E) ratio of 1:2, delivering an I:E ratio of 2:1 or greater to allow longer inspiration • Requires sedation and drug-induced paralysis • Helps improve oxygenation in patient who is hypoxic even while on positive end-expiratory pressure
Positive end-expiratory pressure	• Setting triggers ventilator to apply positive pressure at the end of each expiration to keep alveoli open and increase area for oxygen exchange.
Pressure support ventilation (PSV)	• Allows ventilator to apply a preset amount of positive pressure when patient inspires spontaneously • Increases V_T while decreasing patient's breathing workload
Synchronous intermittent mandatory ventilation (SIMV)	• Delivers a preset number of breaths at a specific V_T • Allows patient to supplement mechanical ventilations with his or her own breaths; V_T and rate determined by patient's own inspiratory ability

Special considerations

- Provide the patient with emotional support during all phases of mechanical ventilation to reduce anxiety and promote successful treatment. Even if the patient is unresponsive, continue to explain all procedures and treatments to him or her.
- Make sure that the ventilator alarms are on at all times. These alarms alert nursing staff to potentially hazardous conditions and changes in patient status. If an alarm sounds and the problem cannot be identified easily, disconnect the patient from the ventilator and use a handheld resuscitation bag to ventilate him or her.
- Unless contraindicated, turn the patient from side to side every 1 to 2 hours to facilitate lung expansion and removal of secretions. Perform active or passive range-of-motion (ROM) exercises for all extremities to reduce the hazards of immobility. If the patient's condition permits, position him or her upright at regular intervals to increase lung expansion. When moving the patient or the ventilator tubing, make sure that condensation in the tubing does not flow into the lungs. Aspiration of this contaminated moisture can cause infection. Provide care for the artificial airway as needed.
- Assess the patient's peripheral circulation and monitor urine output for signs of decreased CO. Watch for signs and symptoms of excess fluid volume or dehydration.
- Place the call light within the patient's reach and establish a method of communication, such as a communication board, because intubation and mechanical ventilation impair the patient's ability to speak. An artificial airway may help the patient to speak by allowing air to pass through his or her vocal cords.

- Administer a sedative or a neuromuscular blocker as ordered to relax the patient or to eliminate spontaneous breathing efforts that can interfere with the action of the ventilator. A patient who is receiving a neuromuscular blocker requires close observation because of inability to breathe or communicate.
- If the patient is receiving a neuromuscular blocker, make sure that a sedative is also administered. Neuromuscular blockers cause paralysis without altering the patient's LOC. Reassure the patient and his or her family that the paralysis is temporary. Make sure that emergency equipment is readily available in case the ventilator malfunctions or the patient is accidentally extubated. Continue to explain all procedures to the patient and take additional steps to ensure safety, such as raising the side rails of the bed while turning him or her and covering and lubricating his or her eyes.
- Make sure that the patient gets adequate rest and sleep because fatigue can delay weaning from the ventilator. Provide subdued lighting, safely muffle equipment noises, and restrict staff access to the area to promote quiet during rest periods.
- When weaning the patient, watch for signs of hypoxia. Schedule weaning to fit comfortably and realistically within the patient's daily regimen. Avoid scheduling sessions after meals, baths, or lengthy therapeutic or diagnostic procedures. Have the patient help you set up the schedule to give him or her some sense of control over the procedure. As the patient's tolerance for weaning increases, help him or her sit up while out of bed to improve breathing and sense of well-being. Suggest diversionary activities to take his or her mind off his or her breathing.

Patient Teaching Tip

If the patient will be discharged while using a ventilator, evaluate the family's or the caregiver's ability and motivation to provide such care. Well before discharge, develop a teaching plan to address the patient's needs. For example, teaching should include information about ventilator care and settings, artificial airway care, suctioning, respiratory therapy, communication, nutrition, therapeutic exercise, the signs and symptoms of infection, and ways to troubleshoot minor equipment malfunctions.

- Evaluate the patient's need for adaptive equipment, such as a hospital bed, a wheelchair or walker with a ventilator tray, a patient lift, and a bedside commode. Determine whether the patient needs to travel; if so, select appropriate portable and backup equipment.
- Before discharge, have the patient's caregiver demonstrate his or her ability to use the equipment. At discharge, contact a durable medical equipment vendor and a home health nurse to follow up with the patient. Refer the patient to community resources, if available.
- Assess the patient for complications. Mechanical ventilation can cause tension pneumothorax; decreased CO; oxygen toxicity; excess fluid volume caused by humidification; infection; and GI complications, such as distention or bleeding from stress ulcers.

Documentation

Document the date and time that mechanical ventilation is initiated. Note the type of ventilator used as well as its settings. Describe the patient's subjective and objective responses to mechanical ventilation, including vital signs, breath sounds, use of accessory muscles, intake and output, and weight. List complications that occurred and nursing actions taken. Record all pertinent laboratory data, including the results of ABG analysis and oxygen saturation levels.

During weaning, record the date and time of each session; the weaning method used; and the baseline and subsequent vital signs, oxygen saturation levels, and ABG values. Describe the patient's subjective and objective responses, including LOC, respiratory effort, arrhythmias, skin color, and need for suctioning.

List all complications and nursing actions taken. If the patient was receiving pressure support ventilation or using a T-piece or tracheostomy collar, note the duration of spontaneous breathing and the patient's ability to maintain the weaning schedule. If intermittent mandatory ventilation was used, with or without pressure support ventilation, record the control breath rate, the time of each breath reduction, and the rate of spontaneous respirations.

Nasogastric tube insertion and removal

Usually inserted to decompress the stomach, an NG tube can prevent vomiting after major surgery. An NG tube is typically in place for 48 to 72 hours after surgery by which time peristalsis usually resumes. However, the tube may remain in place for shorter or longer periods, depending on its use.

The NG tube has other diagnostic and therapeutic applications, especially in assessing and treating upper GI bleeding, collecting gastric contents for analysis, performing gastric lavage, aspirating gastric secretions, and administering medications and nutrients.

Inserting an NG tube requires close observation of the patient and verification of proper placement. An NG tube must be inserted with extra care in pregnant patients and in those with an increased risk of complications. For example, a health care provider will order an NG tube for a patient with aortic aneurysm, myocardial infarction, gastric hemorrhage, or esophageal varices only if he or she believes that the benefits outweigh the risks. The tube must be removed carefully to prevent injury or aspiration.

Most NG tubes have a radiopaque marker or strip at the distal end to allow the position of the tube to be verified by X-ray. If an X-ray does not confirm placement, the health care provider may order fluoroscopy.

The most common types of NG tubes are the Levin tube, which has one lumen, and the Salem Sump tube, which has two lumens, one for suction and drainage and a smaller one for ventilation. Air flows through the vent lumen continuously. This protects the delicate gastric mucosa by preventing a vacuum from forming should the tube adhere to the stomach lining. The Moss tube, which has a triple lumen, is usually inserted during surgery. (See *Types of NG tubes.*)

Types of NG tubes

The health care provider will choose the type and diameter of the nasogastric (NG) tube that best suits the patient's needs, including lavage, aspiration, enteral therapy, or stomach decompression. Choices may include the Levin tube and the Salem Sump tube.

Levin tube

The Levin tube is a rubber or plastic tube that has a single lumen, a length of 42″ to 50″ (106.7 to 127 cm), and holes at the tip and along the side.

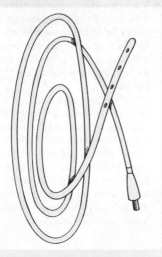

Salem Sump tube

The Salem Sump tube is a double-lumen tube that is made of clear plastic and has a blue sump port (pigtail) that allows atmospheric air to enter the patient's stomach. Thus, the tube floats freely and does not adhere to or damage the gastric mucosa. The larger port of this 48″ (122-cm) tube serves as the main suction conduit. The tube has openings at 45, 55, 65, and 75 cm as well as a radiopaque line to verify placement.

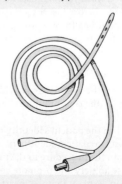

Equipment and preparation

For inserting an NG tube

NG tube (usually #12, #14, #16, or #18 French for a normal adult) • towel or linen-saver pad • facial tissues • emesis basin • penlight • 1″ or 2″ hypoallergenic tape • gloves • water-soluble lubricant • cup of water with straw (if appropriate) • pH test strip • tongue blade • catheter-tip or bulb syringe or irrigation set • safety pin • ordered suction equipment • optional: ice, alcohol pad, warm water, and rubber band

For removing an NG tube

Gloves • catheter-tip syringe • normal saline solution • towel or linen-saver pad • adhesive remover • optional: clamp

Inspect the NG tube for defects, such as rough edges or partially closed lumens. Check the patency of the tube by flushing it with water. To ease insertion, increase the flexibility of a stiff tube by coiling it around your gloved fingers for a few seconds or by dipping it into warm water. Stiffen a limp rubber tube by briefly chilling it in ice.

Implementation

- Whether you are inserting or removing an NG tube, provide privacy, wash your hands, and put on gloves before inserting the tube. Check the health care provider's order to determine the type of tube that should be inserted.

Inserting an NG tube

- Confirm the health care provider's order for the type of tube to be inserted.
- Confirm the patient's identity using at least two patient identifiers.
- Explain the procedure to the patient to ease anxiety and promote cooperation. Explain that the insertion may cause some nasal discomfort, gagging, and watery eyes. Tell the patient that swallowing will ease advancement of the tube.
- Agree on a signal that the patient can use if he or she wants you to stop briefly during the procedure.
- Gather and prepare all necessary equipment.
- Help the patient into high Fowler's position, unless contraindicated.
- Put on gloves and drape the towel or linen-saver pad over the patient's chest to protect his or her gown and bed linens from spills.
- Have the patient blow his or her nose gently to clear his or her nostrils.
- Place the facial tissues and emesis basin within the patient's reach.
- Help the patient to face forward with the neck in a neutral position.
- To determine how long the NG tube must be to reach the patient's stomach, hold the end of the tube at the tip of his or her nose, then extend the tube to his or her earlobe and then down to the xiphoid process.
- Mark this distance on the tubing with the tape. (Average measurements for an adult range from 22″ to 26″ [56 to 66 cm].) You may need to add 2″ (5 cm) to this measurement for tall patients to ensure entry into the stomach.
- To determine which nostril will allow easier access, use a penlight and inspect for a deviated septum or other abnormalities. Ask the patient if he or she has had nasal surgery or a nasal injury. Assess airflow in both nostrils by occluding one nostril at a time while the patient breathes through his or her nose. Choose the nostril with better airflow.

- Lubricate the first 3″ (7.6 cm) of the tube with a water-soluble lubricant to minimize injury to the nasal passages. Using a water-soluble lubricant prevents lipoid pneumonia, which may result from aspiration of an oil-based lubricant or from accidental slippage of the tube into the trachea.
- Instruct the patient to hold his or her head straight and upright.
- Grasp the tube with the end pointing downward; curve it, if necessary; and carefully insert it into the more patent nostril (as shown below).

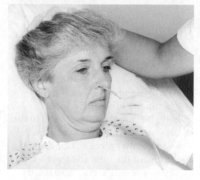

- Aim the tube downward and toward the ear closer to the chosen nostril. Advance it slowly to avoid pressure on the turbinates and resultant pain and bleeding.
- When the tube reaches the nasopharynx, you will feel resistance. Instruct the patient to lower his or her head slightly to close the trachea and open the esophagus. Rotate the tube 180 degrees toward the opposite nostril to redirect it so that it will not enter the patient's mouth.
- Unless contraindicated, offer the patient a cup of water with a straw. Direct the patient to sip and swallow as you slowly advance the tube (as shown at the top of the next column). This helps the tube to pass to the esophagus. If you are not using water, ask the patient to swallow.

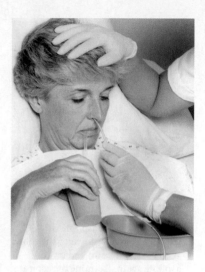

Ensuring proper tube placement

- Use a tongue blade and penlight to examine the patient's mouth and throat for signs of a coiled section of tubing (especially in an unconscious patient). Coiling indicates an obstruction.
- Keep an emesis basin and facial tissues readily available for the patient.
- As you carefully advance the tube and the patient swallows, watch for signs of respiratory distress, which may indicate that the tube is in the bronchus and must be removed immediately.
- Stop advancing the tube when the tape mark reaches the patient's nostril.
- Attach a catheter-tip or bulb syringe to the tube and try to aspirate the stomach contents. If you do not obtain stomach contents, position the patient on the left side to move the tube into the greater curvature of the stomach and aspirate again.

ALERT

When confirming tube placement, never place the end of the tube in a container of water. If the tube is mispositioned in the trachea, the patient may aspirate water. Furthermore, water without bubbles does not confirm proper placement. Instead, the tube may be coiled in the trachea or the esophagus.

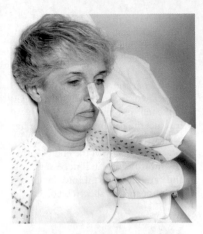

- If you still cannot aspirate the stomach contents, advance the tube 1″ to 2″ (2.5 to 5 cm) and try to aspirate again. Examine the aspirate and place a small amount on the pH test strip. If the aspirate has a gastric fluid appearance (grassy green, clear and colorless with mucous shreds, or brown) and the pH is ≤5, probability of gastric placement is increased.
- If possible, have tube placement confirmed by X-ray.
- Secure the NG tube to the patient's nose with hypoallergenic tape (or another designated tube holder). If the patient's skin is oily, wipe the bridge of her nose with an alcohol pad and allow it to dry. You will need about 4″ (10.2 cm) of 1″ tape. Split one end of the tape up the center about 1½″ (3.8 cm). Make tabs on the split ends by folding the sticky sides together. Stick the uncut end of the tape on the patient's nose so that the split in the tape starts about ½″ (1.3 cm) to 1½″ (3.8 cm) from the tip of his or her nose. Crisscross the tabbed ends around the tube (as shown at the top of the next column). Apply another piece of tape over the bridge of the nose to secure the tube.

- Alternatively, stabilize the tube with a prepackaged product that secures and cushions it at the nose.
- To reduce discomfort from the weight of the tube, tie a slipknot around the tube with a rubber band. Secure the rubber band to the patient's gown with a safety pin or wrap another piece of tape around the end of the tube and leave a tab. Fasten the tape tab to the patient's gown.
- Attach the tube to suction equipment, if ordered, and set the designated suction pressure.
- Provide frequent nose and mouth care while the tube is in place.

Removing an NG tube

- Explain the procedure to the patient, informing him or her that it may cause some nasal discomfort and sneezing or gagging.
- Assess the patient's bowel function by auscultating for peristalsis or flatus.
- Help the patient into semi-Fowler's position. Drape a towel or linen-saver pad across the patient's chest to protect his or her gown and bed linens from spills.
- Wash your hands and put on gloves.

- Using a catheter-tip syringe, flush the tube with 10 ml of normal saline solution to make sure that the tube does not contain stomach contents that could irritate tissues during tube removal.
- Untape the tube from the patient's nose and unpin it from his or her gown.
- Clamp the tube by folding it in your hand.
- Ask the patient to hold his or her breath to close the epiglottis. Withdraw the tube gently and steadily. When the distal end of the tube reaches the nasopharynx, you can pull it quickly.
- As soon as possible, cover and remove the tube. Its sight and odor may nauseate the patient.
- Assist the patient with thorough mouth care and clean the tape residue from his or her nose with adhesive remover.
- For the next 48 hours, monitor the patient for signs and symptoms of GI dysfunction, including nausea, vomiting, abdominal distention, and food intolerance. GI dysfunction may necessitate reinsertion of the tube.

Special considerations

- If the patient has a deviated septum or other nasal condition that prevents nasal insertion, pass the tube orally after removing dentures if necessary. Slide the tube over the tongue; proceed as you would for nasal insertion.
- When using the oral route, coil the end of the tube around your hand. This helps to curve and direct the tube downward at the pharynx.
- If the patient is unconscious, tilt his or her chin toward his or her chest to close the trachea. Advance the tube between respirations to make sure that it does not enter the trachea.

- While advancing the tube in an unconscious patient or in a patient who cannot swallow, stroke the patient's neck to encourage the swallowing reflex and facilitate passage down the esophagus.
- While advancing the tube, watch for signs that it has entered the trachea, such as choking or breathing difficulties in a conscious patient and cyanosis in an unconscious patient or a patient without a cough reflex. If these signs occur, remove the tube immediately. Allow the patient time to rest and then try to reinsert the tube.
- Vomiting after tube placement suggests tubal obstruction or incorrect position. Assess the patient immediately to determine the cause.
- An NG tube may be inserted or removed at home. Indications for insertion include gastric decompression and short-term feeding. A home care nurse or the patient may insert the tube, deliver the feeding, and remove the tube.
- Assess the patient for potential complications of prolonged intubation, such as skin erosion at the nostril, sinusitis, esophagitis, esophagotracheal fistula, gastric ulceration, and pulmonary and oral infection. Additional complications that may result from suction include electrolyte imbalances and dehydration.

Documentation

Record the type and size of the NG tube and the date, time, and route of insertion. Note the type and amount of suction, if used, and describe the drainage, including the amount, color, character, consistency, and odor. Note the patient's tolerance of the procedure.

When you remove the tube, record the date and time. Describe the color, consistency, and amount of gastric drainage. Note the patient's tolerance of the procedure.

Obstructed airway, adult

Sudden obstructed airway can occur when a foreign body lodges in the throat or bronchus; when the patient aspirates blood, mucus, or vomitus; when the tongue blocks the pharynx; or when the patient experiences traumatic injury, bronchoconstriction, or bronchospasm. The patient will display such symptoms as grabbing his or her throat with his or her hand, being unable to speak, coughing weakly and ineffectively, or making high-pitched sounds while inhaling.

A completely obstructed airway causes anoxia, which leads to brain damage and death in 4 to 6 minutes. An upper abdominal thrust creates diaphragmatic pressure in the static lung below the foreign body sufficient to expel the obstruction.

Use abdominal thrusts on a conscious adult patient who cannot speak, cough, or breathe; if the patient is unconscious, instead start CPR immediately. For a pregnant or markedly obese patient or for a patient who has recently undergone abdominal surgery, use a chest thrust instead of an abdominal thrust. The chest thrust forces air out of the lungs to create an artificial cough.

These maneuvers are contraindicated in a patient with incomplete or partial airway obstruction or when the patient can maintain adequate ventilation to dislodge the foreign body by effective coughing. However, a patient who cannot speak, cough, or breathe requires immediate action to dislodge the obstruction.

Equipment

• No specific equipment needed

Implementation

Conscious adult

• Determine the patient's LOC by tapping his or her shoulder and asking, "Are you choking? Can you speak?" If the patient has complete airway obstruction, he or she will not be able to answer. If the patient makes crowing sounds, the airway is partially blocked and you should encourage him or her to cough. This will either clear the airway or make the obstruction complete. Intervene for a complete obstruction.
• Tell the patient that you will try to dislodge the foreign body.
• Stand behind the patient and wrap your arms around his or her waist. Make a fist with one hand and place the thumb side of your fist against his or her abdomen, at the midline, slightly above the umbilicus, and well below the xiphoid process. Grasp your fist with the other hand.
• Press your fist into the patient's abdomen with quick inward and upward thrusts five times. Each thrust should be a separate and distinct movement; each should be forceful enough to create an artificial cough that will dislodge the object.
• Repeat thrusts until the object is expelled from the airway or the patient becomes unresponsive. Make sure you have a firm grasp on the patient because he or she may lose consciousness and need to be lowered to the floor.
• If the patient loses consciousness, lower him or her to the floor, support the head and neck to prevent injury, and place him or her in the supine position. Call for help, activate EMS, begin CPR, and follow the interventions for relieving an obstructed airway in an unconscious person.

Obese or pregnant conscious adult

• If the patient is conscious, stand behind the patient and place your arms under the armpits and around the chest.

- Place the thumb side of your clenched fist against the middle of the sternum, avoiding the margins of the ribs and the xiphoid process. Grasp your fist with your other hand and perform a chest thrust with enough force to expel the foreign body. Continue until the patient expels the obstruction or loses consciousness.
- If the patient loses consciousness, carefully lower the patient to the floor and place in a supine position. Establish unresponsiveness, call for help, activate EMS, and begin CPR.

Unconscious adult

- If you come upon an unconscious patient, establish unresponsiveness. Call for help or activate EMS.
- If you are rescuing a conscious patient with an obstructed airway and the patient loses consciousness, lower the patient to the ground and immediately activate EMS. Place the patient in a supine position and begin CPR.
- Each time the airway is opened using the head-tilt, chin-lift maneuver, look for an object in the patient's mouth. Remove the object if present.
- Attempt to ventilate the patient and follow with 30 chest compressions.

 ALERT

The blind finger-sweep is no longer taught by the AHA. A finger-sweep should only be used when a foreign body can be seen in the mouth. Studies have shown that blind finger-sweeps may result in injury to the patient's mouth and throat or to the rescuer's fingers, and there is no evidence of its effectiveness. In addition, the tongue-jaw lift is no longer used. The patient's mouth should be opened using a head-tilt, chin-lift maneuver.

Special considerations

- If the patient vomits during chest or abdominal thrusts, wipe out the mouth to prevent additional obstruction and resume the maneuver as necessary.
- Even if efforts to clear the airway do not seem to be effective, keep trying. As oxygen deprivation increases, smooth and skeletal muscles relax, making your maneuvers more likely to succeed.
- Explain what you are doing as needed to gain the patient's cooperation.
- Complications such as nausea, regurgitation, and achiness may develop after the patient regains consciousness and can breathe independently. Assess the patient for injuries such as ruptured or lacerated abdominal or thoracic viscera, which may result from improper placement of the rescuer's hands or because of osteoporosis or metastatic lesions.

Documentation

Record the date and time of the procedure. Note the patient's actions before the obstruction, document the approximate length of time it took to clear the airway, and record the type and size of object removed.

Note the patient's vital signs after the procedure and his or her tolerance of the procedure. Document any complications that occurred and nursing actions taken.

Peripheral I.V. catheter insertion

Peripheral I.V. catheter insertion involves selection of a venipuncture device and an insertion site, application of a tourniquet, preparation of the site, and venipuncture. Selection of a venipuncture device and site depends on the type of solution to be used; the frequency and duration of infusion; the patency and location of accessible veins; the patient's age, size, and condition; and, when possible, the patient's preference.

If possible, choose a vein in the nondominant arm or hand. The preferred venipuncture sites are the cephalic and basilic veins in the lower arm and the veins in the dorsum of the hand. The least favorable sites are the veins in the leg and the foot because of the increased risk of thrombophlebitis. Antecubital veins can be used if no other venous access is available.

A peripheral catheter allows administration of fluids, medication, blood, and blood components and maintains I.V. access to the patient. Insertion is contraindicated in a sclerotic vein, an edematous or impaired arm or hand, or a postmastectomy arm with axillary node dissection and in patients with a mastectomy, burns, or an arteriovenous fistula. Subsequent venipunctures should be performed proximal to a previously used or injured vein.

Equipment and preparation

Alcohol pads or other approved antimicrobial solution such as chlorhexidine swabs • gloves • disposable tourniquet (latex-free tubing) • I.V. access devices • I.V. solution with attached and primed administration set • I.V. pole • sharps container • transparent semipermeable dressing • commercial catheter-securement device, sterile 1″ hypoallergenic gauze tape, or sterile surgical strips • 1″ hypoallergenic tape • optional: arm board, roller gauze, and warm packs • adhesive bandage

Commercial venipuncture kits come with or without an I.V. access device. In many facilities, venipuncture equipment is kept on a tray or cart, allowing a choice of the correct access devices and easy replacement of contaminated items.

Check the information on the label of the I.V. solution container, including the patient's name and room number, the type of solution, the date and time of its preparation, the preparer's name,

and the ordered infusion rate. Compare the health care provider's orders with the solution label to verify that the solution is correct. Select the smallest gauge device that is appropriate for the infusion (unless subsequent therapy will require a larger one). Smaller gauges cause less trauma to the veins, allow greater blood flow around their tips, and reduce the risk of phlebitis.

If you are using a winged infusion set, connect the adapter to the administration set and unclamp the line until fluid flows from the open end of the needle cover. Then close the clamp and place the needle on a sterile surface, such as the inside of its packaging.

Take the catheter device and open its package to allow easy access.

Implementation

- Confirm the patient's identity using at least two patient identifiers.
- Place the I.V. pole in the proper slot in the patient's bed frame. If you are using a portable I.V. pole, position it close to the patient.
- Hang the I.V. solution with the attached primed administration set on the I.V. pole.
- Verify the patient's identity by comparing the information on the solution container with the two patient identifiers on the patient's wristband.
- Wash your hands thoroughly. Explain the procedure to the patient to ensure his or her cooperation and reduce anxiety. Anxiety can cause a vasomotor response that results in venous constriction.

Selecting the site

- Select the puncture site. If long-term therapy is anticipated, start distal on the selected vein so that you can move proximally, as needed, for subsequent I.V. insertion sites. For infusion of an irritating medication, choose a large vein. Make sure that the intended vein can accommodate the I.V. access device.

- Place the patient in a comfortable, reclining position, leaving the arm in a dependent position to increase venous fill of the lower arms and hands. If the patient's skin is cold, warm it by rubbing and stroking the arm, covering the entire arm with warm packs, or submerging it in warm water for 5 to 10 minutes.

Applying the tourniquet

- Apply a tourniquet above the antecubital fossa to dilate the vein. Check for a radial pulse. If it is not present, release the tourniquet and reapply it with less tension to prevent arterial occlusion.
- To locate veins, lower the arm below heart level. Have the patient pump his or her fist. Tap gently over the vein.
- Lightly palpate the vein with the index and middle fingers of your nondominant hand. Once the vein is identified and secure, stretch the skin to anchor the vein. If the vein feels hard or ropelike, select another vein.
- Leave the tourniquet in place for no longer than 3 minutes. If you cannot find a suitable vein and prepare the site in that time, release the tourniquet for a few minutes. Then reapply it and continue the procedure.

Preparing the site

- Put on gloves. Clip the hair around the insertion site, if needed, and according to facility policy. Clean the site with a chlorhexidine swab using a vigorous side-to-side motion to remove flora that would otherwise be introduced into the vascular system with the venipuncture. Allow the antimicrobial solution to dry.
- If ordered, administer a local anesthetic. Make sure that the patient is not sensitive to lidocaine.
- Lightly press the vein with the thumb of your nondominant hand about 1½″ (3.8 cm) from the intended insertion site. The vein should feel round, firm, fully engorged, and resilient.
- Grasp the access cannula. If you are using a winged infusion set, hold the short edges of the wings (with the bevel of the needle facing upward) between the thumb and forefinger of your dominant hand. Squeeze the wings together. If you are using an over-the-needle cannula, grasp the plastic hub with your dominant hand, remove the cover, and examine the cannula tip. If the edge is not smooth, discard and replace the device.
- Use the thumb of your nondominant hand to stretch the skin taut below the puncture site to stabilize the vein (as shown below).

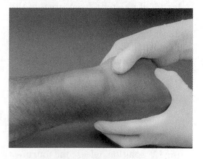

- Tell the patient that you are about to insert the device.
- Hold the needle with the bevel up and enter the skin directly over the vein at a 0- to 15-degree angle (as shown below).

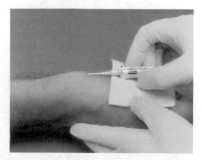

- Aggressively push the needle directly through the skin about ⅓″ (1 cm) and into the vein in one motion. Check the flashback chamber behind the hub for blood return, signifying that the vein has been properly accessed. You may not see blood return in a small vein.
- Level the insertion device slightly by lifting its tip to prevent puncturing the back wall of the vein with the access device.
- If you are using a winged infusion set, advance the needle fully, if possible, and hold it in place. Release the tourniquet, open the administration set clamp slightly, and check for free flow or infiltration.
- If you are using an over-the-needle cannula, advance the device to at least half its length to ensure that the cannula itself—not just the introducer needle—has entered the vein. Remove the tourniquet.
- Grasp the cannula hub to hold it in the vein and withdraw the needle. As you withdraw it, press lightly on the catheter tip to prevent bleeding.
- Advance the cannula up to the hub or until you meet resistance.
- To advance the cannula while infusing I.V. solution, release the tourniquet and remove the inner needle. Using aseptic technique, attach the I.V. tubing and begin the infusion. Stabilize the vein with one hand and use the other to advance the catheter into the vein. When the catheter is advanced, decrease the I.V. flow rate. This method reduces the risk of puncturing the opposite wall of the vein because the catheter is advanced without the steel needle and because the rapid flow dilates the vein.
- To advance the cannula before starting the infusion, release the tourniquet. Stabilize the vein with one hand and use the other hand to advance the catheter up to the hub (as shown in the next column).

Remove the inner needle and, using aseptic technique, quickly attach the I.V. tubing. This method typically results in less blood being spilled.

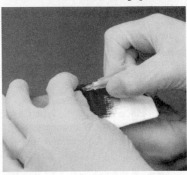

Dressing the site

- After the venous access device has been inserted, clean the skin completely. If necessary, dispose the stylet in a sharps container. Regulate the flow rate.
- If possible, use a commercial catheter-securement device to secure the catheter. Or use sterile 1″ hypoallergenic tape or sterile surgical strips to secure the device.
- Apply a transparent semipermeable dressing to the site.
- Loop the I.V. tubing on the patient's limb and secure the tubing with hypoallergenic tape. The loop allows some slack to prevent dislodgment of the cannula because of tension on the line. (See *Methods of taping a venous access site*.)
- Label the last piece of tape with the type and gauge of the needle and the length of the cannula, the date and time of insertion, and your initials. Adjust the flow rate as ordered.
- If needed, place an arm board under the joint and secure it with roller gauze or tape to provide stability. Make sure that the insertion site is visible and that the tape is not constricting the patient's circulation.

Methods of taping a venous access site

When using tape to secure the venous access device to the insertion site, use one of the basic methods described below. Only sterile tape should be used under a transparent semipermeable dressing.

Chevron method

- Cut a long strip of ½" tape. With the sticky side up, place it under the cannula.
- Cross the ends of the tape over the cannula so that the tape sticks to the patient's skin (as shown below).
- Apply a piece of 1" tape across the two wings of the chevron.
- Loop the tubing and secure it with another piece of 1" tape. When the dressing is secured, apply a label. On the label, write the date and time of insertion, the type and gauge of the needle, and your initials.

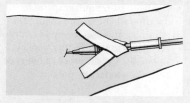

H method

- Cut three strips of 1" tape.
- Place one strip of tape over each wing, keeping the tape parallel to the cannula (as shown below).
- Place the other strip of tape perpendicular to the first two strips. Put it either directly on top of the wings or just below the wings, directly on top of the tubing.
- Make sure that the cannula is secure. Then apply a dressing and a label. On the label, write the date and time of insertion, the type and gauge of the needle or cannula, and your initials.

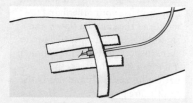

U method

- Cut a 2" (5-cm) strip of ½" tape. With the sticky side up, place the tape under the hub of the cannula.
- Bring each side of the tape up, folding it over the wings of the cannula in a U shape (as shown below). Press it down parallel to the hub.
- Apply tape to stabilize the catheter.
- When a dressing is secured, apply a label. On the label, write the date and time of insertion, the type and gauge of the needle or cannula, and your initials.

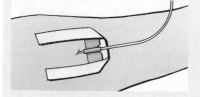

Check frequently for impaired circulation distal to the infusion site.

Removing a peripheral I.V. catheter

- A peripheral I.V. catheter is removed at the completion of therapy, for cannula site changes, and for suspected infection or infiltration. The procedure usually requires gloves, a sterile gauze pad, and an adhesive bandage.
- To remove the I.V. catheter, clamp the I.V. tubing to stop the flow of solution. Gently remove the transparent dressing and all tape from the skin.
- Using aseptic technique, open the gauze pad and adhesive bandage and place them within reach. Put on gloves. Hold the sterile gauze pad over the puncture site with one hand and use your other hand to withdraw the cannula slowly and smoothly, keeping it parallel to the skin. Inspect the tip of the cannula; if it is not smooth, assess the patient immediately and notify the health care provider.
- Using the gauze pad, apply firm pressure over the puncture site for 1 to 2 minutes after removal or until bleeding has stopped.
- Clean the site and apply the adhesive bandage or, if blood oozes, apply a pressure bandage.
- If drainage appears at the puncture site, swab the tip across an agar plate and send it to the laboratory to be cultured, according to facility policy. Clean the area, apply a sterile dressing, and notify the health care provider.
- Instruct the patient to restrict activity for about 10 minutes and to leave the dressing in place for at least 1 hour. If the patient has lingering tenderness at the site, apply warm packs and notify the health care provider.

Special considerations

AGE ALERT

Apply the tourniquet carefully to avoid pinching the skin. If necessary, apply it over the patient's gown. Make sure that skin preparation materials are at room temperature to avoid vasoconstriction because of lower temperatures.

- If the patient is allergic to chlorhexidine, clean the skin with alcohol.
- If you do not see blood flashback, remove the cannula and try again or proceed according to facility policy.
- Change a gauze or transparent dressing whenever you change the administration set (every 48 hours or according to your facility's policy).
- Rotate the I.V. site every 72 hours or according to facility policy.

Patient Teaching Tip

Many patients who receive I.V. therapy at home have a CV line. If you are caring for a patient who is going home with a peripheral line, teach him or her how to care for the I.V. site and how to identify certain complications. If the patient has movement restrictions, make sure that he or she understands them.

- Teach the patient how to examine the site. Instruct him or her to notify the health care provider or home care nurse if he or she has redness, swelling, or discomfort or if the dressing becomes moist.

- Tell the patient to report all problems with the I.V. line (for instance, if the solution stops infusing or if an alarm goes off on an infusion pump). Explain that a home care nurse will change the I.V. site at established intervals.
- If the patient is using an intermittent infusion device, teach him or her how and when to flush it.
- Teach the patient about possible complications related to peripheral lines. Complications can result from the needle or the catheter (infection and phlebitis) or from the solution (circulatory overload, infiltration, sepsis, and allergic reaction). (See *Risks of peripheral I.V. therapy*, pages 364 to 371.)

Documentation

In your notes or on the appropriate I.V. sheets, record the date and time of the venipuncture; the type, gauge, and length of the cannula; the anatomic location of the insertion site; and the reason the site was changed.

Document the number of attempts at venipuncture, the type and flow rate of I.V. solution, the name and amount of medication in the solution (if any), all adverse reactions and the actions taken to correct them, patient teaching and evidence of patient understanding, and your initials.

Peripheral I.V. line maintenance

Routine maintenance of I.V. sites and systems includes regular assessment and rotation of the site and periodic changes of the dressing, tubing, and solution. These measures help to prevent complications, such as thrombophlebitis and infection. They should be performed according to facility policy.

Typically, gauze I.V. dressings are changed every 48 hours or when the dressing becomes wet, soiled, or nonocclusive. Transparent semipermeable dressings are changed whenever I.V. tubing is changed. I.V. tubing is changed every 72 hours or according to facility policy, and I.V. solution is changed every 24 hours or as needed. The site should be assessed every 2 hours if a transparent semipermeable dressing is used. Otherwise, the site is assessed with every dressing change and should be rotated every 72 hours.

Equipment and preparation

For dressing changes

Gloves • chlorhexidine swab • adhesive bandage, sterile 2″ × 2″ gauze pad, or transparent semipermeable dressing • 1″ adhesive tape

For solution changes

Solution container as ordered (bag or bottle) • alcohol pad

For tubing changes

I.V. administration set • gloves • sterile 2″ × 2″ gauze pad • adhesive tape for labeling • hypoallergenic tape

For I.V. site changes

Commercial kits containing the equipment for dressing changes are available.

If the facility keeps I.V. equipment and dressings in a tray or cart, have it nearby, if possible, because you may need to select a new venipuncture site, depending on the condition of the current site. If you are changing the solution and tubing, attach and prime the I.V. administration set before you enter the patient's room.

Implementation

- Confirm the patient's identity using at least two patient identifiers.

(*Text continues on page 372.*)

Risks of peripheral I.V. therapy

Complications	Signs and symptoms
Local complications	
Cannula dislodgment	• Cannula partially backed out of vein • Solution infiltrating
Hematoma	• Tenderness at the venipuncture site • Bruised area around the site • Inability to advance or flush the I.V. line
Infiltration	• Swelling at and above the I.V. site (may extend along the entire limb) • Discomfort, burning, or pain at the site (may be painless) • Tight feeling at the site • Skin cool to the touch around the I.V. site • Blanching at the site • Continuing fluid infusion, even when the vein is occluded, although the rate may decrease
Nerve, tendon, or ligament damage	• Extreme pain (similar to electrical shock when the nerve is punctured) • Numbness and muscle contraction • Delayed effects, including paralysis, numbness, and deformity

Possible causes	Nursing interventions
• Loosened tape or tubing snagged in the bed linens, resulting in partial retraction of the cannula; cannula pulled out by a confused patient	• If no infiltration occurs, retape without pushing the cannula back into the vein. If it has pulled out, apply pressure to the I.V. site with a sterile dressing. *Prevention* • Tape the venipuncture device securely on insertion.
• Puncture of the vein through the opposite wall at the time of insertion • Leakage of blood as a result of needle displacement • Application of inadequate pressure when the cannula is discontinued	• Remove the venous access device. • Apply pressure and warm soaks to the affected area. • Recheck for bleeding. • Document the patient's condition and your interventions. *Prevention* • Choose a vein that can accommodate the size of the venous access device. • Release the tourniquet as soon as insertion is successful.
• Venous access device dislodged from the vein or perforation of the vein	• Stop the infusion and infiltrate the site with antidote, if ordered. • Check the patient's pulse and capillary refill periodically to assess circulation. • Apply ice (early) or warm soaks (later) to aid absorption and elevate the patient's limb. • Restart the infusion above the infiltration site or in another limb. • Document the patient's condition and your interventions. *Prevention* • Check the I.V. site frequently. • Do not obscure the area above the site with tape. • Teach the patient to observe the I.V. site and to report pain or swelling.
• Improper venipuncture technique that causes injury to the surrounding nerves, tendons, or ligaments • Tight taping or improper splinting with an arm board	• Stop the procedure. *Prevention* • Do not penetrate the tissues repeatedly with the venous access device. • Do not apply excessive pressure when taping; do not encircle the limb with tape. • Pad the arm boards and secure them with tape, if possible.

(continued)

Risks of peripheral I.V. therapy *(continued)*

Complications	Signs and symptoms
Local complications (continued)	
Occlusion	• Infusion that does not flow • Pump alarms indicating occlusion • Discomfort at infusion site
Phlebitis	• Tenderness proximal to the venous access device • Redness at the tip of the cannula and along the vein • Vein that is hard on palpation • Pain during infusion • Possible blanching if vasospasm occurs • Elevated temperature • Puffy area over vein
Severed cannula	• Leakage from the shaft of the cannula
Thrombophlebitis	• Severe discomfort • Reddened, swollen, and hardened vein

Possible causes	Nursing interventions
• Interruption of the I.V. flow • Failure to flush the saline lock • Backflow of blood in the line when the patient walks • Line clamped for too long	• Use a mild flush injection. Do not force it. If it is unsuccessful, remove the I.V. line and insert a new one. *Prevention* • Maintain the I.V. flow rate. • Flush promptly after intermittent piggyback administration. • Have the patient walk with his or her arm bent at the elbow to reduce the risk of blood backflow.
• Poor blood flow around the venous access device • Friction from movement of the cannula along the vein wall • Venous access device left in the vein for too long • Drug or solution with high or low pH or high osmolarity, such as phenytoin and some antibiotics (erythromycin, nafcillin, and vancomycin)	• Remove the venous access device. • Apply warm soaks. • Notify the health care provider if the patient has a fever. • Document the patient's condition and your interventions. *Prevention* • Restart the infusion using a larger vein for an irritating solution or restart it with a smaller gauge device to ensure adequate blood flow. • Tape the device securely to prevent motion.
• Inadvertent cutting of the cannula by scissors • Reinsertion of the needle into the cannula	• If the broken part is visible, attempt to retrieve it. If you are unsuccessful, notify the health care provider. • If a portion of the cannula enters the bloodstream, place a tourniquet above the I.V. site to prevent progression of the broken part. • Notify the health care provider and the radiology department. • Document the patient's condition and your interventions. *Prevention* • Do not use scissors near the I.V. site. • Never reinsert the needle into the cannula. • Remove the unsuccessfully inserted cannula and the needle together.
• Thrombosis and inflammation	• Remove the device; restart the infusion in the opposite limb if possible. • Apply warm soaks. • Notify the health care provider. • Watch for I.V. therapy–related infection (thrombi provide an excellent environment for bacterial growth). *Prevention* • Check the site frequently. Remove the venous access device at the first sign of redness and tenderness.

(continued)

Risks of peripheral I.V. therapy *(continued)*

Complications	Signs and symptoms
Local complications (continued)	
Thrombosis	• Painful, reddened, and swollen vein • Sluggish or stopped I.V. flow
Vasovagal reaction	• Sudden pallor, sweating, faintness, dizziness, and nausea • Decreased blood pressure
Venous spasm	• Pain along the vein • Sluggish flow rate when the clamp is completely open • Blanched skin over the vein
Systemic complications	
Air embolism	• Respiratory distress • Unequal breath sounds • Weak pulse • Increased central venous pressure • Decreased blood pressure • Confusion, disorientation, loss of consciousness

Possible causes	Nursing interventions
• Injury to the endothelial cells of the vein wall, allowing platelets to adhere and thrombi to form	• Remove the venous access device; restart infusion in the opposite limb, if possible. • Apply warm soaks. • Watch for I.V. therapy–related infection (thrombi provide an excellent environment for bacterial growth). *Prevention* • Use proper venipuncture techniques to reduce injury to the vein.
• Vasospasm as a result of anxiety or pain	• Lower the head of the bed. • Instruct the patient to take deep breaths. • Check the patient's vital signs. *Prevention* • Prepare the patient for therapy to relieve his or her anxiety. • Use a local anesthetic to prevent pain.
• Severe irritation of the vein from irritating drugs or fluids • Administration of cold fluids or blood • Very rapid flow rate (with fluids at room temperature)	• Apply warm soaks over the vein and the surrounding area. • Decrease the flow rate. *Prevention* • Use a blood warmer for blood or packed red blood cells.
• Solution container that is empty • Solution container that is emptying and an added container that is pushing air down the line (if the line is not purged first) • Tubing that is disconnected	• Discontinue the infusion. • Place the patient on his or her left side in Trendelenburg's position to allow air to enter the right atrium and disperse by way of the pulmonary artery. • Administer oxygen. • Notify the health care provider. • Document the patient's condition and your interventions. *Prevention* • Purge the tubing of air completely before starting the infusion. • Use an air-detection device on the pump or an air-eliminating filter proximal to the I.V. site. • Secure the connections.

(continued)

Risks of peripheral I.V. therapy *(continued)*

Complications	Signs and symptoms
Systemic complications (continued)	
Allergic reaction	• Itching • Watery eyes and nose • Bronchospasm • Wheezing • Urticarial rash • Edema at I.V. site • Anaphylactic reaction (flushing, chills, anxiety, itching, palpitations, paresthesia, wheezing, seizures, cardiac arrest) within minutes or up to 1 hour after exposure
Circulatory overload	• Discomfort • Engorgement of the jugular veins • Respiratory distress • Increased blood pressure • Crackles • Increased difference between fluid intake and output
Systemic infection (septicemia or bacteremia)	• Fever, chills, and malaise for no apparent reason • Contaminated I.V. site, usually with no visible signs of infection at the site

Possible causes	Nursing interventions
• Allergens such as medications	• If a reaction occurs, stop the infusion immediately. • Maintain a patent airway. • Notify the health care provider. • Administer an antihistaminic steroid, an anti-inflammatory, and an antipyretic as prescribed. • Give 0.2 to 0.5 ml of 1:1,000 aqueous epinephrine subcutaneously as prescribed. Repeat at 3-minute intervals and as needed and prescribed. *Prevention* • Obtain the patient's allergy history. Be aware of cross-allergies. • Assist with test dosing and document any new allergies. • Monitor the patient carefully during the first 15 minutes of administration of a new drug.
• Loosening of the roller clamp to allow run-on infusion • Flow rate that is too rapid • Miscalculation of fluid requirements	• Raise the head of the bed. • Administer oxygen as needed. • Notify the health care provider. • Administer medications (probably furosemide) as prescribed. *Prevention* • Use a pump, volume-control set, controller, or rate minder for elderly or compromised patients. • Recheck calculations of the fluid requirements. • Monitor the infusion frequently.
• Failure to maintain aseptic technique during insertion of the device or site care • Severe phlebitis, which can set up ideal conditions for the growth of organisms • Poor taping that permits the venous access device to move, which can introduce organisms into the bloodstream • Prolonged indwelling time of the device • Weak immune system	• Notify the health care provider. • Administer medications as prescribed. • Culture the site and the device. • Monitor the patient's vital signs. *Prevention* • Use aseptic technique when handling solutions and tubing, inserting the venous access device, and discontinuing infusion. • Secure all connections. • Change the I.V. solutions, tubing, and venous access device at the recommended times. • Use I.V. filters.

(continued)

- Wash your hands thoroughly to prevent the spread of microorganisms. Wear gloves whenever you are working near the venipuncture site.
- Explain the procedure to the patient to allay fears and ensure cooperation.

Changing the dressing

- Remove the old dressing, open all supply packages, and put on gloves.
- Hold the cannula in place with your nondominant hand to prevent accidental movement or dislodgment, which could puncture the vein and cause infiltration.
- Assess the venipuncture site for signs and symptoms of infection (redness and pain), infiltration (coolness, blanching, and edema), and phlebitis (redness, firmness, pain along the path of the vein, and edema). If such signs and symptoms are present, cover the area with a sterile 2″ × 2″ gauze pad and remove the catheter or needle. Apply pressure to the area until the bleeding stops and apply an adhesive bandage. Using fresh equipment, start the I.V. line in another appropriate site, preferably on the opposite extremity.
- If the venipuncture site is without complications, stabilize the cannula and carefully clean around the puncture site with a chlorhexidine swab, using a circular motion outward from the site to avoid introducing bacteria into the clean area. Allow the area to dry completely.
- Cover the site with a transparent semipermeable dressing. This type of dressing allows visibility of the insertion site and maintains sterility. It is placed over the insertion site to halfway up the cannula. Label the dressing with the date and time of the procedure.

Changing the solution

- Wash your hands.
- Inspect the new solution container for cracks, leaks, and other damage. Check the solution for discoloration, turbidity, and particulates. Note the date and time that the solution was mixed as well as its expiration date.
- When inverting the tubing, clamp it to prevent air from entering it. Keep the drip chamber half full.
- If you are replacing a bag, remove the seal or tab from the new bag and remove the old bag from the pole. Remove the spike, insert it into the new bag, and adjust the flow rate.
- If you are replacing a bottle, remove the cap and seal from the new bottle and wipe the rubber port with an alcohol pad. Clamp the line, remove the spike from the old bottle, and insert the spike into the new bottle. Then hang the new bottle and adjust the flow rate.

Changing the tubing

- Reduce the I.V. flow rate, remove the old spike from the container, and hang it on the I.V. pole. Place the cover of the new spike loosely over the old one.
- Keeping the old spike in an upright position above the patient's heart level, insert the new spike into the I.V. container.
- Prime the system. Hang the new I.V. container and the primed set on the pole and grasp the new adapter in one hand. Stop the flow rate in the old tubing.
- Put on sterile gloves.
- Place a sterile gauze pad under the needle or cannula hub to create a sterile field. Press one finger over the cannula to prevent bleeding.
- Gently disconnect the old tubing (as shown in the next page), taking care to avoid dislodging or moving

the I.V. device. If you have trouble disconnecting the old tubing, use a hemostat to hold the hub securely while you twist the tubing to remove it. Alternatively, use one hemostat on the venipuncture device and another on the hard plastic end of the tubing. Pull the hemostats in opposite directions. Do not clamp the hemostats shut; this could crack the tubing adapter or the venipuncture device.

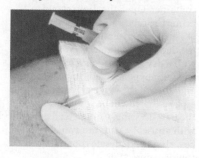

- Remove the protective cap from the new tubing and connect the new adapter to the cannula. Hold the hub securely to prevent dislodging the needle or the cannula tip.
- Observe for blood backflow into the new tubing to verify that the needle or cannula is still in place. (You may not be able to do this with small-gauge cannulas.)
- Adjust the clamp to maintain the appropriate flow rate.
- Retape the cannula hub and I.V. tubing and recheck the I.V. flow rate because taping may alter it.
- Label the new tubing and container with the date and time. Label the solution container with a time strip.

Special considerations

Check the prescribed I.V. flow rate before each solution change to prevent errors. If you crack the adapter or hub or if you accidentally dislodge the cannula from the vein, remove the cannula. Apply pressure and an adhesive bandage to stop bleeding. Perform a venipuncture at another site and restart the I.V. line.

Documentation

Record the time, date, and the rate and type of solution (and any additives) in the I.V. flowchart. Also record dressing or tubing changes and the appearance of the site in your notes.

Peritoneal dialysis, continuous ambulatory

Continuous ambulatory peritoneal dialysis (CAPD) requires insertion of a permanent peritoneal catheter (such as a Tenckhoff catheter) to constantly circulate dialysate in the peritoneal cavity. Inserted under local anesthetic, the catheter is sutured in place and its distal portion is tunneled subcutaneously to the skin surface. There it serves as a port for the dialysate, which flows into and out of the peritoneal cavity by gravity.

CAPD is usually used for patients with end-stage renal disease. CAPD can be a welcome alternative to hemodialysis because it gives the patient more independence and requires less travel for treatments. It also provides more stable fluid and electrolyte levels than conventional hemodialysis.

Patients or family members can usually learn to perform CAPD after only 2 weeks of training. Because the patient can resume normal daily activities between solution changes, CAPD helps to promote independence and a return to a near-normal lifestyle. It also costs less than hemodialysis.

Conditions that may prohibit CAPD include recent abdominal surgery, abdominal adhesions, an infected abdominal wall, diaphragmatic tears, ileus, and respiratory insufficiency.

Equipment

To infuse dialysate

Prescribed amount of dialysate (usually in 2-L bags) • basin of hot water or commercial warmer • three surgical masks • 42″ (106.7-cm) connective tubing with drain clamp • six to eight packages of sterile 4″ × 4″ gauze pads • medication, if ordered • antiseptic pads • hypoallergenic tape • plastic snap-top container • antiseptic solution • sterile basin • container of alcohol • sterile gloves • belt or small fabric pouch • two sterile waterproof paper drapes (one fenestrated) • optional: syringes and labeled specimen container

To temporarily discontinue dialysis

Three sterile waterproof paper drapes (two fenestrated) • 4″ × 4″ gauze pads (for cleaning and dressing the catheter) • two surgical masks • sterile basin • hypoallergenic tape • antiseptic solution • sterile gloves • sterile rubber catheter cap

All equipment for infusing the dialysate and discontinuing the procedure must be sterile. Commercially prepared sterile CAPD kits are available. Check the concentration of the dialysate against the health care provider's order. Also check the expiration date and the appearance of the solution. It should be clear, not cloudy. Warm the solution to body temperature with a heating pad or a commercial warmer, if one is available. Do not warm the solution in a microwave oven because the temperature is unpredictable.

To minimize the risk of contaminating the port, leave the wrapper of the dialysate container in place. This also keeps the bag dry, which makes it easier to examine for leakage after the wrapper is removed.

Wash your hands and put on a surgical mask. Remove the dialysate container from the warming setup and remove its protective wrapper. Squeeze the bag firmly to check for leaks.

If ordered, use a syringe to add any prescribed medication to the dialysate, using sterile technique to avoid contamination. (The ideal approach is to add medication under a laminar flow hood.) Disinfect multidose vials in a 5-minute povidone-iodine soak. Insert the connective tubing into the dialysate container. Open the drain clamp to prime the tube and close the clamp.

Place an antiseptic pad on the port of the dialysate container. Cover the port with a dry gauze pad and secure the pad with hypoallergenic tape. Remove and discard the surgical mask. Tear the tape so that it will be ready to secure the new dressing. Commercial devices with antiseptic pads are available for covering the dialysate container and tubing connection.

Implementation

- Weigh the patient to establish a baseline level. Weigh him or her at the same time each day to help monitor fluid balance.

Infusing dialysate

- Assemble all equipment at the patient's bedside and explain the procedure. Prepare the sterile field by placing a sterile waterproof paper drape on a dry surface near the patient. Take care to maintain the sterility of the drape.
- Fill the plastic snap-top container with antiseptic solution and place it on the sterile field. Place the basin of hot water on the sterile field. Place four pairs of sterile gauze pads in the sterile basin and saturate them with the antiseptic solution. Drop the remaining gauze pads on the sterile field. Loosen the cap on the alcohol container and place it next to the sterile field.

- Put on a surgical mask and provide one for the patient.
- Carefully remove the dressing covering the peritoneal catheter and discard it. Avoid touching the catheter or the skin. Check the integrity of the skin at the catheter site and look for signs of infection such as purulent drainage. If drainage is present, obtain a specimen, put it in a labeled specimen container, and notify the health care provider.
- Put on the sterile gloves and palpate the insertion site and the subcutaneous tunnel route for tenderness or pain. If these symptoms occur, notify the health care provider.

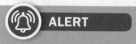

ALERT

If the patient has drainage, tenderness, or pain, do not proceed with the infusion without specific orders.

- Wrap one gauze pad saturated with antiseptic solution around the distal end of the catheter and leave it in place for 5 minutes. Clean the catheter and the insertion site with the rest of the gauze pads, moving in concentric circles away from the insertion site. Use straight strokes to clean the catheter, beginning at the insertion site and moving outward. Use a clean area of the pad for each stroke. Loosen the catheter cap one notch and clean the exposed area. Place each used pad at the base of the catheter to help support it. After you use the third pair of pads, place the sterile waterproof, fenestrated paper drape around the base of the catheter. Continue to clean the catheter for another minute with one of the remaining pads soaked with antiseptic solution.

- Remove the antiseptic solution pad on the catheter cap, remove the cap, and use the remaining antiseptic pad to clean the end of the catheter hub. Attach the connective tubing from the dialysate container to the catheter. Make sure to secure the Luer Lok connector tightly.
- Open the drain clamp on the dialysate container to allow the solution to enter the peritoneal cavity by gravity over a period of 5 to 10 minutes. Leave a small amount of fluid in the bag to make the bag easier to fold. Close the drain clamp.
- Fold the bag and secure it with a belt or tuck it into the patient's clothing or a small fabric pouch.
- After the prescribed dwell time (usually 4 to 6 hours), unfold the bag, open the clamp, and allow peritoneal fluid to drain back into the bag by gravity.
- When drainage is complete, attach a new bag of dialysate. Repeat the infusion.
- Discard the used supplies appropriately.

Discontinuing dialysis temporarily

- Wash your hands, put on a surgical mask, and provide a mask for the patient. Explain the procedure to the patient.
- Using sterile gloves, remove and discard the dressing over the peritoneal catheter.
- Set up a sterile field next to the patient by covering a clean, dry surface with a sterile waterproof paper drape. Take care to maintain the sterility of the drape. Place all equipment on the sterile field and place the 4″ × 4″ gauze pads in the sterile basin. Saturate them with the antiseptic solution. Open the 4″ × 4″ gauze pads to be used as the dressing and drop them onto the sterile field.

Tear pieces of hypoallergenic tape as needed.

- Tape the dialysate tubing to the side rail of the bed to keep the catheter and tubing off the patient's abdomen.

- Change to another pair of sterile gloves. Place one of the fenestrated drapes around the base of the catheter.

- Use a pair of antiseptic pads to clean about 6″ (15 cm) of the dialysis tubing. Clean the tubing for 1 minute, moving in one direction only, away from the catheter. Then clean the catheter, moving from the insertion site to the junction of the catheter and the dialysis tubing. Place used pads at the base of the catheter to prop it up. Use two more pairs of pads to clean the junction for a total of 3 minutes.

- Place the second fenestrated drape over the first at the base of the catheter. With the fourth pair of pads, clean the junction of the catheter and 6″ (15.2 cm) of the dialysate tubing for another minute.

- Disconnect the dialysate tubing from the catheter. Pick up the sterile rubber catheter cap and fasten it to the catheter, making sure that it fits securely over both notches of the hard plastic tip of the catheter.

- Clean the insertion site and a 2″ (5 cm) radius around it with antiseptic pads, working from the insertion site outward. Let the skin air-dry before applying the dressing.

- Properly dispose the used supplies.

Special considerations

- If inflow and outflow are slow or absent, check the tubing for kinks. You can also try raising the solution or repositioning the patient to increase the inflow rate. Repositioning the patient or applying manual pressure to the lateral aspects of the patient's abdomen may also help to increase drainage.

- Make sure that the patient keeps an accurate record of fluid intake and output. Excessive fluid loss may result from a concentrated (4.25%) dialysate solution, improper or inaccurate monitoring of inflow and outflow, or inadequate oral fluid intake. Excessive fluid retention may result from improper or inaccurate monitoring of inflow and outflow or excessive salt or oral fluid intake.

 Patient Teaching Tip

Teach the patient and family how to use sterile technique throughout the procedure, especially for cleaning the insertion site and changing the dressing, to prevent complications such as peritonitis. Also teach them the signs and symptoms of peritonitis—cloudy fluid, fever, abdominal pain, and tenderness—and emphasize the importance of notifying the health care provider immediately if such signs and symptoms arise. Encourage them to call the health care provider immediately if redness and drainage occur; these are also signs of infection. Peritonitis is the most common complication of CAPD. Although it is treatable, it can permanently scar the peritoneal membrane, decreasing its permeability and reducing the efficiency of dialysis. Untreated peritonitis can cause septicemia and death. Inform the patient about the advantages of an automated continuous cycler system for home use. (See *Continuous-cycle peritoneal dialysis.*) Instruct the patient to record his or her weight and blood pressure daily and to check regularly for swelling of the extremities.

Continuous-cycle peritoneal dialysis

Continuous-cycle peritoneal dialysis (CCPD) is an easy method for the patient who uses an automated continuous cycler system. When set up, this system runs the dialysis treatment automatically until all of the dialysate is infused. The system remains closed throughout the treatment, which reduces the risk of contamination. CCPD can be performed while the patient is awake or asleep. The system's alarms warn about general system, dialysate, and patient problems.

The cycler can be set to an intermittent or continuous dialysate schedule at home or in a health care facility. The patient typically initiates CCPD at bedtime and undergoes three to seven exchanges, depending on individual prescriptions. On awakening, the patient infuses the prescribed dialysis volume, disconnects himself or herself from the unit, and carries the dialysate in his or her peritoneal cavity during the day.

The continuous cycler requires the same aseptic care and maintenance procedures as the manual method.

Documentation

Record the type and amount of fluid instilled and returned for each exchange, the time and duration of the exchange, and any medications added to the dialysate. Note the color and clarity of the returned exchange fluid and check it for mucus, pus, and blood. Also note any discrepancy in the balance of fluid intake and output as well as any signs of fluid imbalance, such as weight changes, decreased breath sounds, peripheral edema, ascites, and changes in skin turgor. Record the patient's weight, blood pressure, and pulse rate after his or her last fluid exchange for the day.

Pulse oximetry

Performed intermittently or continuously, oximetry is a relatively simple procedure that is used to monitor arterial oxygen saturation noninvasively. Pulse oximeters usually denote arterial oxygen saturation values with the symbol Spo_2. Invasively measured arterial oxygen saturation values are denoted by the symbol Sao_2.

Two diodes send red and infrared light through a pulsating arterial vascular bed such as the one in the fingertip. A photodetector that is slipped over the finger measures the transmitted light as it passes through the vascular bed, detects the relative amount of color absorbed by the arterial blood, and calculates the exact mixed venous oxygen saturation without interference from surrounding venous blood, skin, connective tissue, or bone. Ear oximetry works by monitoring the transmission of light waves through the vascular bed of a patient's earlobe. The results will be inaccurate if the patient's earlobe is poorly perfused, as from low CO.

Equipment

Oximeter • transducer (photodetector) for finger or ear probe • alcohol pads • nail polish remover, if needed

Implementation

• Explain the procedure to the patient.

Finger pulse oximetry

• Select a finger for the test. Although the index finger is commonly used, a smaller finger may be selected if the patient's fingers are too large for the equipment. Make sure that the patient is not wearing false fingernails and remove any nail polish from the test finger with nail polish remover. Place the transducer (photodetector) finger probe over the patient's finger so that light beams and sensors oppose each other and attach to the oximeter. If the patient has long fingernails, position the probe perpendicular to the finger, if possible, or clip the fingernail. Always position the patient's hand at heart level to eliminate venous pulsations and to promote accurate readings.

AGE ALERT

If you are testing a neonate or a small infant, wrap the probe around the foot so that light beams and detectors oppose each other. For a large infant, use a probe that fits on the great toe and secure it to the foot.

- Turn on the power switch. If the device is working properly, a beep will sound, a display will light momentarily, and the pulse searchlight will flash. The SpO_2 and pulse rate displays will show stationary zeros. After four to six heartbeats, the SpO_2 and pulse rate displays will supply information with each beat, and the pulse amplitude indicator will begin to track the pulse.

Ear pulse oximetry

- Using an alcohol pad, massage the patient's earlobe for 10 to 20 seconds. Mild erythema indicates adequate vascularization. Following the manufacturer's instructions, attach the ear probe to the patient's earlobe or pinna. Use the ear probe stabilizer for prolonged or exercise testing. Be sure to establish good contact on the ear; an unstable probe may set off the low-perfusion alarm. After the probe has been attached for a few seconds, a saturation reading and pulse waveform will appear on the screen.

- Leave the ear probe in place for 3 minutes or more, until readings stabilize at the highest point, or take three separate readings and average them, revascularizing the patient's earlobe each time.

- After the procedure, remove the probe, turn off and unplug the unit, and clean the probe by gently rubbing it with an alcohol pad.

Special considerations

- If oximetry has been performed properly, the readings are typically accurate. However, certain factors may interfere with accuracy. For example, elevated carboxyhemoglobin or methemoglobin levels, such as occurring in heavy smokers and urban dwellers, can cause a falsely elevated SpO_2 reading. (See *Diagnosing pulse oximeter problems*.)

- Certain intravascular substances, such as lipid emulsions and dyes, can also prevent accurate readings. Other factors that may interfere with accurate results include excessive light (for example, from phototherapy, surgical lamps, direct sunlight, and excessive ambient lighting), excessive patient movement, excessive ear pigment, hypothermia, hypotension, and vasoconstriction.

- If the patient has compromised circulation in the extremities, you can place a photodetector across the bridge of his or her nose.

- If SpO_2 is used to guide weaning of the patient from forced inspiratory oxygen, obtain ABG analysis occasionally to correlate SpO_2 readings with SaO_2 levels.

Diagnosing pulse oximeter problems

To maintain a continuous display of arterial oxygen saturation levels, you will need to keep the monitoring site clean and dry. Make sure that the skin does not become irritated from adhesives used to keep disposable probes in place. You may need to change the site if this happens. Disposable probes that irritate the skin can be replaced by nondisposable models that do not need tape.

Another common problem with pulse oximeters is the failure of the devices to obtain a signal. If this happens, your first reaction should be to check the patient's vital signs. If they are sufficient to produce a signal, check for the following problems.

Venous pulsations

Erroneous readings may result if the pulse oximeter detects venous pulsations. These may occur in patients with tricuspid regurgitation or pulmonary hypertension or if a finger probe is taped on too tightly.

Poor connection

See if the sensors are properly aligned. Make sure that the wires are intact and securely fastened and that the pulse oximeter is plugged into a power source.

Inadequate or intermittent blood flow to the site

Check the patient's pulse rate and capillary refill time and take corrective action if blood flow to the site is decreased. This may mean loosening restraints, removing tight-fitting clothes, taking off a blood pressure cuff, or checking arterial and I.V. lines. If none of these interventions works, you may need to find an alternate site. Finding a site with proper circulation may prove challenging when a patient is receiving a vasoconstrictor.

Equipment malfunction

Remove the pulse oximeter from the patient, set the alarm limits according to your facility's policy, and try the instrument on yourself or another healthy person. This will tell you if the equipment is working correctly.

- If an automatic blood pressure cuff is used on the same extremity that is used to measure SpO_2, the cuff will interfere with SpO_2 readings during inflation.
- If light is a problem, cover the probes; if patient movement is a problem, move the probe or select a different probe; and if ear pigment is a problem, reposition the probe, revascularize the site, or use a finger probe.
- Normal SpO_2 levels for ear and pulse oximetry are 90% to 100% for adults and 93.8% to 100% by 1 hour after birth for healthy, full-term neonates. Lower levels may indicate hypoxemia that warrants intervention. For such patients, follow facility policy or the health care provider's orders, which may include increasing oxygen

therapy. If SaO_2 levels decrease suddenly, you may need to resuscitate the patient immediately. Notify the health care provider of any significant change in the patient's condition.

Documentation

Document the procedure, including the date, time, and type of procedure; the oximetric measurement; and the actions taken. Record the reading in appropriate flowcharts, if indicated.

Seizure management

Seizures are paroxysmal events that are associated with abnormal electrical discharges of neurons in the brain. Partial seizures are usually unilateral, involving a localized or focal, area of the brain. Generalized seizures involve the entire brain. When a patient has a generalized seizure, the goal of nursing care is to protect him or her from injury and prevent serious complications. Appropriate care also includes observation of the characteristics of the seizure to help determine the area of the brain involved.

Patients who are considered at risk for seizures are those with a history of seizures and those with conditions that predispose them to seizures. These conditions include metabolic abnormalities, such as hypocalcemia, hypoglycemia, and pyridoxine deficiency; brain tumors or other space-occupying lesions; infections, such as meningitis, encephalitis, and brain abscess; traumatic injury, especially if the dura mater was penetrated; ingestion of toxins, such as mercury, lead, or carbon monoxide; genetic abnormalities, such as tuberous sclerosis and phenylketonuria; perinatal injuries; and stroke. Patients at risk for seizures need precautionary measures to help prevent injury if a seizure occurs. (See *Precautions for generalized seizures*.)

Precautions for generalized seizures

By taking appropriate precautions, you can help to protect a patient from injury, aspiration, and airway obstruction in case he or she has a seizure. Plan your precautions using information obtained from the patient's history. What kind of seizure has the patient previously had? Is he or she aware of exacerbating factors? Sleep deprivation, missed doses of an anticonvulsant, and even upper respiratory tract infections can increase seizure frequency in some people who have had seizures. Was his or her previous seizure an acute episode or did it result from a chronic condition?

Gather the equipment

Based on answers provided in the patient's history, you can tailor your precautions to his or her needs. Start by gathering the appropriate equipment, including a hospital bed with full-length side rails, commercial side rail pads or six bath blankets (four for a crib), adhesive tape, an oral airway, and oral or nasal suction equipment.

Bedside preparations

Carry out the precautions that you think are appropriate for the patient. Remember that a patient with preexisting seizures who is being admitted for a change in medication, treatment of an infection, or detoxification may have an increased risk of seizures.

- Explain the reasons for the precautions to the patient.
- To protect the patient's limbs, head, and feet from injury if he or she has a seizure while in bed, cover the side rails, headboard, and footboard with side rail pads or bath blankets. If you use blankets, keep them in place with adhesive tape. Be sure to keep the side rails raised while the patient is in bed to prevent falls. Keep the bed in a low position to minimize injuries that may occur if the patient climbs over the side rails.
- Place an airway at the patient's bedside or tape it to the wall above the bed according to facility policy. Keep suction equipment nearby in case you need to establish a patent airway. Explain to the patient how the airway will be used.
- If the patient has frequent or prolonged seizures, prepare an I.V. heparin lock to facilitate the administration of emergency medications.

Equipment

Oral airway • suction equipment • side rail pads • seizure activity record • optional: I.V. line and normal saline solution, oxygen as ordered, ET intubation, dextrose 50% in water, thiamine

Implementation

- If you are with a patient when he or she experiences an aura, help him or her get into bed, raise the side rails, and adjust the bed flat. Use side rail pads and blankets to pad the rails securely. If the patient is away from his or her room, lower him or her to the floor and place a pillow, blanket, or other soft material under his or her head to keep it from hitting the floor.
- Stay with the patient during the seizure and be ready to intervene if complications such as airway obstruction develop. If necessary, have another staff member obtain the appropriate equipment and notify the health care provider of the obstruction.
- Provide privacy, if possible.

ALERT

During a seizure do not try to hold the patient's mouth open or place your hands inside his or her mouth because the patient may bite you. After the patient's jaw becomes rigid, do not force an airway into place because you could break his or her teeth or cause another injury. If needed, insert an oral airway after the seizure subsides.

- Move hard or sharp objects out of the patient's way and loosen his or her clothing.
- Do not forcibly restrain the patient or restrict movements during the seizure. The force of movements against restraints could cause muscle strain or even joint dislocation.
- Time the seizure activity from beginning to end and continually assess the patient during the seizure. Observe the earliest sign, such as head or eye deviation, as well as how the seizure progresses, what form it takes, and how long it lasts. Document the seizure on the hospital seizure activity record. Your description may help determine the type and cause of the seizure.
- If this is the patient's first seizure, notify the health care provider immediately. If the patient has had seizures before, notify the health care provider only if the seizure activity is prolonged or if the patient does not regain consciousness. (See *Understanding status epilepticus*, page 382.)
- If ordered, establish an I.V. line and infuse normal saline solution at a keep-vein-open rate.
- If the seizure is prolonged and the patient becomes hypoxemic, administer oxygen, as ordered. Some patients may require ET intubation.
- If the patient has diabetes and hypoglycemia, administer dextrose 50% in water by I.V. push, if ordered. If the patient has alcoholism, a bolus of thiamine may be ordered to stop the seizure.
- After the seizure, turn the patient on his or her side and apply suction, if needed, to facilitate drainage of secretions and maintain a patent airway. Insert an oral airway, if needed.
- Check the patient for injuries.
- Reorient and reassure the patient, as needed.
- When the patient is comfortable and safe, document what happened during the seizure.
- After the seizure, monitor the patient's vital signs and mental status every 15 to 20 minutes for 2 hours.

Understanding status epilepticus

Status epilepticus is a continuous seizure state, unless it is interrupted by emergency interventions. It can occur with all types of seizures. The most life-threatening example is generalized tonic-clonic status epilepticus, which is a continuous generalized tonic-clonic seizure without intervening return of consciousness.

Status epilepticus, which is always an emergency, is accompanied by respiratory distress. It can result from abrupt withdrawal of an anticonvulsant, hypoxic or metabolic encephalopathy, acute head trauma, or septicemia as a result of encephalitis or meningitis.

Emergency treatment of status epilepticus usually consists of phenobarbital, diazepam, lorazepam, or phenytoin; I.V. dextrose 50% (when seizures are caused by hypoglycemia); and I.V. thiamine (in patients with chronic alcoholism or withdrawal).

● Ask the patient about aura and activities preceding the seizure. The type of aura (auditory, visual, olfactory, gustatory, or somatic) helps to pinpoint the site in the brain where the seizure originated.

Special considerations

● Because a seizure commonly indicates an underlying disorder, such as meningitis or a metabolic or electrolyte imbalance, a complete diagnostic workup will be ordered if the cause of the seizure is not evident.
● The patient who has a seizure may experience an injury, respiratory difficulty, and decreased mental capability. Common injuries include scrapes and bruises that occur when the patient hits objects during the seizure and traumatic injury to the tongue caused by biting. If you suspect a serious injury, such as a fracture or deep laceration, notify the health care provider and arrange for appropriate evaluation and treatment.
● Changes in respiratory function include aspiration, airway obstruction, and hypoxemia. After the seizure, complete a respiratory assessment and notify the health care provider if

you suspect a problem. Expect most patients to experience a postictal period of decreased mental status lasting 30 minutes to 24 hours. Reassure the patient that this does not indicate incipient brain damage.

Documentation

Document that the patient requires seizure precautions and record all precautions taken. Record the date and the time that the seizure began as well as its duration and any precipitating factors. Identify any sensation that may be considered an aura. If the seizure was preceded by an aura, have the patient describe what he or she experienced.

Record any involuntary behavior that occurred at the onset of the seizure, such as lip smacking, chewing movements, or hand and eye movements. Describe where the movement began and the parts of the body involved. Note if the activity showed any progression or pattern. Document whether the patient's eyes deviated to one side and whether the pupils changed in size, shape, equality, or reaction to light. Note if the patient's teeth were clenched or open. Record incontinence, vomiting, or salivation that occurred during the seizure.

Note the patient's response to the seizure. Was the patient aware of what happened? Did he or she fall into a deep sleep after the seizure? Was he or she upset or ashamed? Document all medications given, all complications experienced during the seizure, and all interventions performed. Record the patient's mental status after the seizure.

Sequential compression therapy

Safe, effective, and noninvasive, sequential compression therapy helps prevent deep vein thrombosis (DVT) in surgical patients. This therapy massages the legs in a wavelike, milking motion that promotes blood flow and deters thrombosis.

Typically, sequential compression therapy complements other preventive measures, such as antiembolism stockings and anticoagulant therapy. Although patients who are at low risk for DVT may require only antiembolism stockings, those who are at moderate to high risk may require both antiembolism stockings and sequential compression therapy. These preventive measures are continued for as long as the patient remains at risk.

Both antiembolism stockings and sequential compression sleeves are commonly used preoperatively and postoperatively because blood clots tend to form during surgery. About 20% of blood clots form in the femoral vein. Sequential compression therapy counteracts blood stasis and coagulation changes, two of the three major factors that promote DVT. It reduces stasis by increasing peak blood flow velocity, helping to empty the femoral vein's valve cusps of pooled or static blood. The compressions cause an anticlotting effect by increasing fibrinolytic activity, which stimulates the release of a plasminogen activator.

Equipment

Measuring tape and sizing chart for brand of sleeves being used • pair of compression sleeves in correct size • connecting tubing • compression controller

Implementation

- Explain the procedure to the patient to increase his or her cooperation.
- Wash your hands.

Determining proper sleeve size

- Before applying the compression sleeve, determine the proper size of sleeve that you need. Wash your hands.
- Measure the circumference of the patient's upper thigh while he or she rests in bed. Do this by placing the measuring tape under the thigh at the gluteal furrow (as shown below).

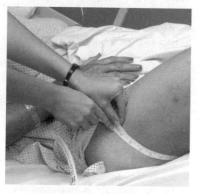

- Hold the tape snugly, but not tightly, around the patient's leg. Note the exact circumference.
- Find the patient's thigh measurement on the sizing chart and locate the corresponding size of the compression sleeve.

- Remove the compression sleeves from the package and unfold them.
- Lay the unfolded sleeves on a flat surface with the cotton lining facing up (as shown below).

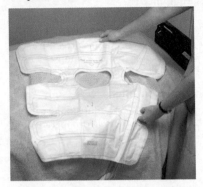

- Notice the markings on the lining denoting the ankle and the area behind the knee at the popliteal pulse point. Use these markings to position the sleeves at the appropriate landmarks.

Applying the sleeves

- Place the patient's leg on the lining of one of the sleeves. Position the back of the knee over the popliteal opening.
- Make sure that the back of the ankle is over the ankle marking.
- Starting at the side opposite the clear plastic tubing, wrap the sleeve snugly around the patient's leg.
- Fasten the sleeve securely with the Velcro fasteners. For the best fit, secure the ankle and calf sections, followed by the thigh section.
- The sleeve should fit snugly, but not tightly. Check the fit by inserting two fingers between the sleeve and the patient's leg at the knee opening. Loosen or tighten the sleeve by readjusting the Velcro fastener.
- Using the same procedure, apply the second sleeve (as shown at the top of the next column).

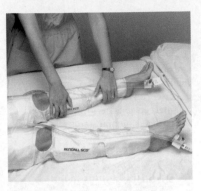

Operating the system

- Connect each sleeve to the tubing leading to the controller. Both sleeves must be connected to the compression controller for the system to operate. Line up the blue arrows on the sleeve connector with the arrows on the tubing connectors and firmly push the ends together. Listen for a click, which signals a firm connection. Make sure that the tubing is not kinked.
- Plug the compression controller into the proper wall outlet. Turn on the power.
- The controller automatically sets the compression sleeve pressure at 45 mm Hg, which is the midpoint of the normal range (35 to 55 mm Hg).
- Observe the patient to see how well he or she tolerates the therapy and the controller as the system completes its first cycle.
- Check the AUDIBLE ALARM key. The green light should be lit, indicating that the alarm is working.
- The compression sleeves should function continuously (24 hours/day) until the patient is fully ambulatory. Check the sleeves at least once each shift to ensure proper fit and inflation.

Removing the sleeves

- You may remove the sleeves when the patient is walking, bathing, or leaving the room for tests or other procedures, as long as you reapply the sleeves immediately after the tests and procedures are over. To disconnect the sleeves from the tubing, press the latches on each side of the connectors and pull the connectors apart.
- Store the tubing and the compression controller according to facility policy. This equipment is not disposable.

Special considerations

- Remove the sleeves and assess and document skin integrity every 8 hours to avoid skin breakdown.
- The compression controller also has a mechanism to help cool the patient.
- If you are applying only one sleeve— for example, if the patient has a cast—leave the unused sleeve folded in the plastic bag. Cut a small hole in the sealed bottom edge of the bag and pull the sleeve connector (the part that holds the connecting tubing) through the hole. Then you can join both sleeves to the compression controller.
- If a malfunction triggers the instrument alarm, you will hear beeping. The system shuts off whenever the alarm is activated.
- To respond to the alarm, remove the operator's card from the slot on the top of the compression controller. Follow the instructions printed on the card next to the matching code.
- Do not use this therapy in patients with any of the following conditions:
  - Acute DVT or DVT diagnosed within the last 6 months
  - Severe peripheral arterial occlusive disease
  - Lower extremity bypass

  - Massive edema of the legs because of pulmonary edema or heart failure
  - Any local condition that would likely be aggravated by the compression sleeves, such as dermatitis, vein ligation, gangrene, and recent skin grafting. A patient with a pronounced leg deformity would also be unlikely to benefit from the compression sleeves.

Documentation

Document the procedure, the patient's understanding of the procedure, the patient's response, and the status of the alarm and cooling settings.

Surgical site verification

Wrong-site surgery is a general term that refers to a surgical procedure that is performed on the wrong body part or side of the body, or even the wrong patient. This error may occur in the operating room or in other settings, such as during ambulatory care or interventional radiology.

Several factors may contribute to an increased risk of wrong-site surgery, including inadequate assessment of the patient, inadequate review of the medical records, inaccurate communication among members of the health team, the involvement of multiple surgeons in the procedure, failure to include the patient in the site-identification process, and the practice of relying solely on the health care provider for site identification.

Because serious consequences may result from wrong-site surgery, the nurse must confirm that the correct site has been identified before surgery begins.

Equipment

Surgical consent • medical record • procedure schedule • hypoallergenic, nonlatex permanent marker

Implementation

- Confirm the patient's identity using at least two patient identifiers.
- Before the procedure, check the patient's chart for documentation. Compare the information on the chart with the history and physical examination form, the nursing assessment, the preprocedure verification checklist, the signed informed consent form with the exact procedure site identified, the procedure schedule, and the patient's verbal confirmation of the correct site.
- After you verbally confirm the site with the patient, the person performing the surgery or a member of the surgical team who is fully informed about the patient and the procedure marks the site with a permanent marker. The mark needs to be visible after the patient has been prepped and draped.
- Make sure that the surgical team (surgeon, operating room or procedure staff, and anesthesia personnel) identifies the patient and verifies the correct procedure and the correct site before they begin the surgery.

Special considerations

If the patient's condition prevents him or her from verifying the correct site, the surgeon will identify and mark the site using history and physical examination forms, signed informed consent form, preprocedure verification checklist, procedure schedule, X-rays, and other imaging studies.

Documentation

Complete the preprocedure verification checklist used by the facility. Record that the correct site was verified and note who marked the correct site with a permanent marker.

Synchronized cardioversion

Used to treat tachyarrhythmias, cardioversion delivers an electric charge to the myocardium at the peak of the R wave. This charge causes immediate depolarization, interrupting reentry circuits and allowing the sinoatrial node to resume control. Synchronizing the electric charge with the R wave ensures that the current will not be delivered on the vulnerable T wave and thus will not disrupt repolarization.

Synchronized cardioversion is the treatment of choice for arrhythmias that do not respond to vagal massage or drug therapy, such as atrial tachycardia, atrial flutter, atrial fibrillation, and symptomatic ventricular tachycardia.

Cardioversion should be performed according to the 2016 AHA guidelines and should be preceded by an assessment of the patient's cardiac and metabolic status if possible. This assessment should include electrolyte values and renal function tests.

Cardioversion may be an elective or an urgent procedure, depending on how well the patient tolerates the arrhythmia. For example, if the patient is hemodynamically unstable, he or she requires urgent cardioversion. When preparing for cardioversion, the patient's condition can deteriorate quickly, necessitating immediate defibrillation.

Indications for cardioversion include stable paroxysmal atrial tachycardia, unstable paroxysmal supraventricular tachycardia, atrial fibrillation, atrial flutter, and ventricular tachycardia with a pulse.

Equipment

Cardioverter-defibrillator • conductive medium pads • anterior, posterior, or transverse paddles • ECG monitor with recorder • sedative • oxygen therapy equipment • airway

• handheld resuscitation bag • emergency cardiac medication • automatic blood pressure cuff (if available) • pulse oximeter (if available)

Implementation

• Confirm the patient's identity using at least two patient identifiers.
• Explain the procedure to the patient and make sure that he or she has signed a consent form.
• Check the patient's recent serum potassium and magnesium levels and ABG values. Also check recent digoxin levels. Although patients receiving digoxin may undergo cardioversion, they tend to require lower energy levels to convert. If ordered, withhold the dose on the day of the procedure.
• Withhold all food and fluids for 6 to 12 hours before the procedure. If the cardioversion is urgent, withhold the previous meal.
• Obtain a 12-lead ECG to serve as a baseline.
• Check to see if the health care provider has ordered the administration of any cardiac drugs before the procedure. Verify that the patient has a patent I.V. site in case drug administration becomes necessary.
• Connect the patient to a pulse oximeter and an automatic blood pressure cuff, if available.
• Consider administering oxygen for 5 to 10 minutes before the cardioversion to promote myocardial oxygenation. If the patient wears dentures, evaluate whether they support his or her airway or might cause an airway obstruction. If they might cause an obstruction, remove them.
• Place the patient in the supine position and assess his or her vital signs, LOC, cardiac rhythm, and peripheral pulses.
• Remove any oxygen delivery device just before cardioversion to avoid possible combustion.

• Have emergency cardiac medication at the patient's bedside.
• Administer a sedative as ordered. The patient should be heavily sedated but should still able to breathe adequately.
• Carefully monitor the patient's blood pressure and respiratory rate until recovery.
• Apply the ECG monitor with recorder and press the POWER button to turn on the cardioverter-defibrillator. Push the SYNC button to synchronize the machine with the patient's QRS complexes. Make sure that the SYNC button flashes with each of the patient's QRS complexes. You should also see a bright green flag flash on the ECG monitor.
• Turn the ENERGY SELECT dial to the ordered amount of energy. ACLS protocols call for 50 to 100 joules for a patient with unstable supraventricular tachycardia, 100 to 200 joules for a patient with atrial fibrillation, 50 to 100 joules for a patient with atrial flutter, and 100 joules for a patient who has monomorphic ventricular tachycardia with a pulse.
• Remove the paddles from the machine and prepare them as you would if you were defibrillating the patient. Place the conductive medium pads or the appropriate paddles in the same positions as you would to defibrillate.
• Make sure that everyone stands away from the bed and then push the discharge buttons. Hold the paddles in place and wait for the energy to be discharged—the machine must synchronize the discharge with the QRS complex.
• Check the waveform on the monitor. If the arrhythmia does not convert, repeat the procedure two or three more times at 3-minute intervals. Gradually increase the energy level with each additional countershock.

- After the cardioversion, frequently assess the patient's LOC and respiratory status, including airway patency, respiratory rate and depth, and the need for supplemental oxygen. Because the patient will be heavily sedated, he or she may require airway support with a hand-held resuscitation bag.
- Record a postcardioversion 12-lead ECG and monitor the patient's ECG rhythm for 2 hours. Check the patient's chest for electrical burns.

Special considerations

- If the patient is attached to a bedside or telemetry monitor, disconnect the unit before cardioversion. The electric current that it generates could damage the equipment.
- Improper synchronization may result if the patient's ECG tracing contains artifact-like spikes, such as peaked T waves or bundle-branch blocks when the R″ wave may be taller than the R wave.
- Although the electric shock of cardioversion will not usually damage an implanted pacemaker, avoid placing the paddles directly over the pacemaker.
- Remove any patches with metallic backings such as nitroglycerin patches. This backing may cause a ring during cardioversion.
- Reset the synchronization mode after each cardioversion because many defibrillators automatically default back to the unsynchronized mode.
- Common complications after cardioversion include transient, harmless arrhythmias, such as atrial, ventricular, and junctional premature beats. Serious ventricular arrhythmias, such as ventricular fibrillation, may also occur. However, this type of arrhythmia is more likely to result from digoxin toxicity, high amounts

of electrical energy, severe heart disease, electrolyte imbalance, or improper synchronization with the R wave.

Documentation

Document the procedure, including the voltage delivered with each attempt, the rhythm strips obtained before and after the procedure, and the patient's tolerance of the procedure.

Temporary pacemaker insertion and care

Usually inserted in an emergency, a temporary pacemaker consists of an external, battery-powered pulse generator and a lead or electrode system. The four types of temporary pacemakers include transcutaneous, transvenous, transthoracic, and epicardial.

In a life-threatening situation, when time is critical, a transcutaneous pacemaker is the best choice. This device sends an electrical impulse from the pulse generator to the patient's heart by way of two electrodes, which are placed on the front and back of the patient's chest. Transcutaneous pacing is quick and effective, but it is used only until the health care provider can institute transvenous pacing.

Transcutaneous pacing is recommended by the 2016 AHA guidelines for CPR and emergency cardiovascular care for symptomatic bradycardia when a pulse is present. If transcutaneous pacing does not correct the problem, transvenous pacing is indicated. Transvenous pacing involves threading an electrode catheter through a vein into the patient's right atrium or right ventricle. The electrode attaches to an external pulse generator. As a result, the pulse generator can provide an electrical stimulus directly to the endocardium. This is the most common type of pacemaker.

However, the health care provider may choose to insert a transthoracic pacemaker as an elective surgical procedure or as an emergency measure during CPR. To insert this type of pacemaker, the health care provider performs a procedure similar to pericardiocentesis in which he or she uses a cardiac needle to pass an electrode through the chest wall and into the right ventricle. This procedure carries a significant risk of coronary artery laceration and cardiac tamponade.

During cardiac surgery, the surgeon may insert electrodes through the epicardium of the right ventricle and, if he or she wants to institute atrioventricular sequential pacing, the right atrium. From there, the electrodes pass through the chest wall, where they remain available if temporary pacing becomes necessary. This is called epicardial pacing.

In addition to helping to correct conduction disturbances, a temporary pacemaker may help to diagnose conduction abnormalities. For example, during a cardiac catheterization or electrophysiology study, a health care provider may use a temporary pacemaker to localize conduction defects. In the process, he or she may also learn whether the patient is at risk for an arrhythmia.

Contraindications to pacemaker therapy include electromechanical dissociation and ventricular fibrillation.

Equipment

For transcutaneous pacing

Transcutaneous pacing generator • transcutaneous pacing electrodes • cardiac monitor • clippers

For all other types of temporary pacing

Temporary pacemaker generator with new battery • guide wire or introducer • electrode catheter • sterile gloves • sterile dressings • adhesive tape • antiseptic solution • sterile marker

and labels • nonconducting tape or rubber surgical glove • pouch for external pulse generator • emergency cardiac drugs • intubation equipment • defibrillator • cardiac monitor with strip chart recorder • equipment to start a peripheral I.V. line, if appropriate • I.V. fluids • sedative • optional: elastic bandage or gauze strips, restraints

For transvenous pacing

All equipment listed for temporary pacing • bridging cable • percutaneous introducer tray or venous cutdown tray • sterile gowns • linen-saver pad • antimicrobial soap • alcohol pads • vial of 1% lidocaine • 5-ml syringe • fluoroscopy equipment, if needed • fenestrated drape • prepackaged cutdown tray (for antecubital vein placement only) • sutures • receptacle for infectious wastes

For transthoracic pacing

All equipment listed for temporary pacing • transthoracic or cardiac needle

For epicardial pacing

All equipment listed for temporary pacing • atrial epicardial wires • ventricular epicardial wires • sterile rubber finger cot • sterile dressing materials (if the wires will not be connected to a pulse generator)

Implementation

- Confirm the patient's identity using at least two patient identifiers.
- If applicable, explain the procedure to the patient.

For transcutaneous pacing

- If necessary, clip the patient's hair over the areas of electrode placement. Do not shave the areas. If you nick the skin, the current from the pulse generator could cause discomfort and the nicks could become irritated or infected after the electrodes are applied.

- Attach monitoring electrodes to the patient in the lead I, II, or III position. Do this even if the patient is already on a bedside or telemetry monitor because you will need to connect the electrodes to the pacemaker. If you select the lead II position, adjust the LL electrode placement to accommodate the anterior pacing electrode and the patient's anatomy.
- Plug the patient cable into the ECG input connection on the front of the pacing generator. Set the selector switch to the MONITOR ON position.
- You should see the ECG waveform on the monitor. Adjust the R-wave beeper volume to a suitable level and activate the alarm by pressing the ALARM ON button. Set the alarm for 10 to 20 beats lower and 20 to 30 beats higher than the intrinsic rate.
- Press the START/STOP button to obtain a printout of the waveform.
- Now you are ready to apply the two pacing electrodes. First, make sure that the patient's skin is clean and dry to ensure good skin contact.
- Pull off the protective strip from the posterior electrode (marked BACK) and apply the electrode on the left side of the back, just below the scapula and to the left of the spine.
- The anterior pacing electrode (marked FRONT) has two protective strips—one covering the jellied area and one covering the outer rim. Expose the jellied area and apply it to the skin in the anterior position—to the left side of the precordium in the usual V_2 to V_5 position. Move this electrode around to obtain the best waveform. Then expose the outer rim of the electrode and firmly press it to the skin.
- Now you are ready to pace the heart. After making sure that the energy output in milliamperes (mA) is 0, connect the electrode cable to the monitor output cable.

- Check the waveform, looking for a tall QRS complex in lead II.
- Turn the selector switch to PACER ON. Tell the patient that he or she may feel a thumping or twitching sensation. Reassure the patient that you will give medication if he or she cannot tolerate the discomfort.
- Set the rate dial to 10 to 20 beats higher than the patient's intrinsic rhythm. Look for pacer artifact or spikes, which will appear as you increase the rate. If the patient does not have an intrinsic rhythm, set the rate at 60.
- Slowly increase the amount of energy delivered to the heart by adjusting the OUTPUT mA dial. Do this until capture is achieved—you will see a pacer spike followed by a widened QRS complex that resembles a premature ventricular contraction. This is the pacing threshold. To ensure consistent capture, increase the output by 10%. Do not go any higher because you could cause the patient needless discomfort.
- With full capture, the patient's heart rate should be approximately the same as the pacemaker rate set on the machine. The usual pacing threshold is between 40 and 80 mA.

For transvenous pacing

- Check the patient's history for hypersensitivity to local anesthetics. Attach the cardiac monitor to the patient and obtain a baseline assessment, including the patient's vital signs, skin color, LOC, heart rate and rhythm, and emotional state. Insert a peripheral I.V. line if the patient does not already have one. Begin an I.V. infusion of D_5W at a keep-vein-open rate.
- Insert a new battery into the external pacemaker generator and test it to make sure that it has a strong charge. Connect the bridging cable to the

generator and align the positive and negative poles. This cable allows slack between the electrode catheter and the generator, reducing the risk of accidental displacement of the catheter.

- Place the patient in the supine position. If necessary, clip the hair around the insertion site. Open the supply tray while maintaining a sterile field. Label all medications, medication containers, and other solutions on and off the sterile field. Using sterile technique, clean the insertion site with antimicrobial soap and then wipe the area with antiseptic solution. Cover the insertion site with a fenestrated drape. Because fluoroscopy may be used during the placement of leadwires, put on a protective apron.
- Provide the health care provider with the local anesthetic.
- After anesthetizing the insertion site, the health care provider will puncture the brachial, femoral, subclavian, or jugular vein. Then he or she will insert a guide wire or an introducer and advance the electrode catheter.
- As the catheter advances, watch the cardiac monitor. When the electrode catheter reaches the right atrium, you will notice large P waves and small QRS complexes. Then, as the catheter reaches the right ventricle, the P waves become smaller whereas the QRS complexes enlarge. When the catheter touches the right ventricular endocardium, expect to see elevated ST segments, premature ventricular contractions, or both.
- When the electrode catheter is in the right ventricle, it will send an impulse to the myocardium, causing depolarization. If the patient needs atrial pacing, alone or with ventricular pacing, the health care provider may place an electrode in the right atrium.
- Meanwhile, continuously monitor the patient's cardiac status and treat

any arrhythmias, as appropriate. Assess the patient for jaw pain and earache; these symptoms indicate that the electrode catheter has missed the superior vena cava and has moved into the neck instead.

- When the electrode catheter is in place, attach the catheter leads to the bridging cable, lining up the positive and negative poles.
- Set the pacemaker as ordered.
- The health care provider will then suture the catheter to the insertion site. Afterward, put on sterile gloves and apply a sterile dressing to the site. Label the dressing with the date and time of application.

For transthoracic pacing

- Clean the skin to the left of the xiphoid process with povidone-iodine solution. Work quickly because CPR must be interrupted for the procedure.
- After interrupting CPR, the health care provider will insert a transthoracic needle through the patient's chest wall to the left of the xiphoid process and into the right ventricle. He or she will follow this needle with the electrode catheter.
- Connect the electrode catheter to the generator, lining up the positive and negative poles. Watch the cardiac monitor for signs of ventricular pacing and capture.
- After the health care provider sutures the electrode catheter into place, use sterile technique to apply a sterile $4'' \times 4''$ gauze dressing to the site. Tape the dressing securely and label it with the date and time of application.
- Check the patient's peripheral pulses and vital signs to assess CO. If you cannot palpate a pulse, continue to perform CPR.
- If the patient has a palpable pulse, assess his or her vital signs, ECG reading, and LOC.

For epicardial pacing

- During preoperative teaching, inform the patient that epicardial pacemaker wires may be placed during cardiac surgery.
- Just before the end of cardiac surgery, the health care provider will hook epicardial wires into the epicardium. Depending on the patient's condition, the health care provider may insert atrial wires, ventricular wires, or both.
- If indicated, connect the electrode catheter to the generator, lining up the positive and negative poles. Set the pacemaker as ordered.
- If the wires will not be connected to an external pulse generator, place them in a sterile rubber finger cot. Cover both the wires and the insertion site with a sterile, occlusive dressing to help protect the patient from microshock and infection.

Special considerations

- Take care to prevent microshock. Warn the patient not to use any electrical equipment that is not grounded, such as telephones, electric shavers, televisions, or lamps.
- Other safety measures include placing a plastic cover (supplied by the manufacturer) over the pacemaker controls to avoid an accidental setting change. Insulate the pacemaker by covering all exposed metal parts, such as the electrode connections and pacemaker terminals, with nonconducting tape, or place the pacing unit in a dry rubber surgical glove. If the patient is disoriented or uncooperative, use restraints to prevent accidental removal of the pacemaker wires. If the patient needs emergency defibrillation, make sure that the pacemaker can withstand the procedure. If you are unsure, disconnect the pulse generator to avoid damage.
- When using a transcutaneous pacemaker, do not place the electrodes over a bony area because bone conducts current poorly. With female patients, place the anterior electrode under the patient's breast but not over the diaphragm. If the health care provider inserts the electrode through the brachial or femoral vein, immobilize the patient's arm or leg to avoid putting stress on the pacing wires.
- After insertion of any temporary pacemaker, assess the patient's vital signs, skin color, LOC, and peripheral pulses to determine the effectiveness of the paced rhythm. Perform a 12-lead ECG to serve as a baseline and perform additional ECGs daily or with clinical changes. If possible, obtain a rhythm strip before, during, and after pacemaker placement; whenever the pacemaker settings are changed; and whenever the patient receives treatment because of a complication related to the pacemaker.
- Continuously monitor the ECG reading, noting the capture, sensing, rate, intrinsic beats, and competition of paced and intrinsic rhythms. If the pacemaker is sensing correctly, the sense indicator on the pulse generator should flash with each beat.
- Record the date and time of pacemaker insertion, the type of pacemaker, the reason for insertion, and the patient's response. Note the pacemaker settings. Document all complications and the interventions taken.
- If the patient has epicardial pacing wires in place, clean the insertion site with antiseptic solution and change the dressing daily. At the same time, monitor the site for signs of infection. Keep the pulse generator nearby in case pacing becomes necessary.

Complications

Complications associated with pacemaker therapy include microshock, equipment failure, and competitive or fatal arrhythmias. Transcutaneous pacemakers may also cause skin breakdown and muscle pain and twitching when the pacemaker fires. Transvenous pacemakers may cause such complications as pneumothorax or hemothorax, cardiac perforation and tamponade, diaphragmatic stimulation, pulmonary embolism, thrombophlebitis, and infection. Also, if the health care provider threads the electrode through the antecubital or femoral vein, venous spasm, thrombophlebitis, or lead displacement may result.

Complications associated with transthoracic pacemakers include pneumothorax, cardiac tamponade, emboli, sepsis, lacerations of the myocardium or coronary artery, and perforation of a cardiac chamber. Epicardial pacemakers carry a risk of infection, cardiac arrest, and diaphragmatic stimulation.

Documentation

Record the reason for pacing, the time it started, and the locations of the electrodes. For a transvenous or transthoracic pacemaker, note the date, the time, and the reason for the temporary pacemaker.

For any temporary pacemaker, record the pacemaker settings. Note the patient's response to the procedure along with all complications and the interventions taken. If possible, obtain rhythm strips before, during, and after pacemaker placement; whenever pacemaker settings are changed; and when the patient is treated for a complication caused by the pacemaker. As you monitor the patient, record his or her response to temporary pacing and note changes in his condition.

Thoracic drainage

Thoracic drainage uses gravity and possibly suction to restore negative pressure and remove material that collects in the pleural cavity. An underwater seal in the drainage system allows air and fluid to escape from the pleural cavity but does not allow air to reenter.

The system combines drainage collection, a water seal, and suction control into a single unit. (See *Disposable drainage systems*, page 394.)

Specifically, thoracic drainage may be ordered to remove accumulated air, fluids (blood, pus, chyle, serous fluids), or solids (blood clots) from the pleural cavity; to restore negative pressure in the pleural cavity; or to reexpand a partially or totally collapsed lung.

Equipment and preparation

Thoracic drainage system (Pleur-evac, Argyle, Atrium, or Thora-Klex systems, which may function as gravity draining systems or may be connected to suction to enhance chest drainage) • sterile distilled water (usually 1 L) • adhesive tape • sterile clear plastic tubing • two rubber-tipped Kelly clamps • sterile 50-ml catheter-tip syringe • suction source, if ordered • optional: alcohol pad, lotion

Check the health care provider's order to determine the type of drainage system to be used and the specific procedural details. If appropriate, request the drainage and suction systems from the central supply department. Collect the appropriate equipment and take it to the patient's bedside.

Implementation

- Explain the procedure to the patient and wash your hands.
- Maintain sterile technique throughout the procedure and whenever you make changes in the system or alter any of the connections to avoid introducing pathogens into the pleural space.

Setting up a commercially prepared disposable system

- Open the thoracic drainage system. Place it on the floor in the rack that the manufacturer supplied to avoid accidentally knocking it over or dislodging the components. After the system is prepared, it may be hung from the side of the patient's bed.

Disposable drainage systems

Commercially prepared disposable drainage systems combine drainage collection, water seal, and suction control in one unit (as shown below). These systems ensure patient safety with positive- and negative-pressure relief valves and have a prominent air-leak indicator. Some systems produce no bubbling sound.

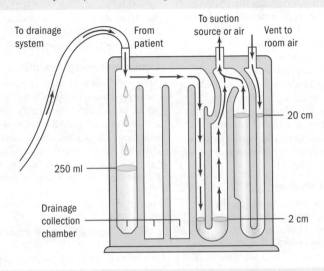

- Remove the plastic connector from the short tube that is attached to the water-seal chamber. Using a sterile 50-ml catheter-tip syringe, instill sterile distilled water into the water-seal chamber until it reaches the 2-cm mark or the mark specified by the manufacturer. The Ohio and Thora-Klex systems are ready to use, but with the Pleur-evac and Thora-Klex systems, 15 ml of sterile water may be added to help detect air leaks. Replace the plastic connector.
- If suction is ordered, remove the cap (also called the muffler, or the atmosphere vent cover) on the suction-control chamber to open the vent. Instill sterile distilled water until it reaches the 20-cm mark or the ordered level and recap the suction-control chamber.
- Using the long tube, connect the patient's chest tube to the closed drainage collection chamber. Secure the connection with adhesive tape.
- Using the sterile clear plastic tubing, connect the short tube on the drainage system to the suction source and turn on the suction. Gentle bubbling should begin in the suction chamber, indicating that the correct level of suction has been reached.

Managing closed-chest underwater seal drainage

- Monitor the patient every 2 hours.
- Monitor the character, consistency, and amount of drainage in the drainage collection chamber.
- Mark the drainage level in the drainage collection chamber by noting the date and time at the drainage level on the chamber every 8 hours (or more often if there is a large amount of drainage).
- Check the water level in the water-seal chamber every 8 hours. If necessary, carefully add sterile distilled water until the level reaches the 2-cm mark indicated on the water-seal chamber of the commercial system.
- Check for fluctuation in the water-seal chamber as the patient breathes. Normal fluctuations of 2″ to 4″ (5 to 10 cm) reflect changes in pressure in the pleural space during respiration. To check for fluctuation when a suction system is being used, momentarily disconnect the suction system so that the air vent is opened and observe for fluctuation.
- Check for intermittent bubbling in the water-seal chamber. This occurs normally when the system is removing air from the pleural cavity. If bubbling is not readily apparent during quiet breathing, have the patient cough or take a deep breath. Absence of bubbling indicates that the pleural space has sealed.
- Check the water level in the suction-control chamber. Detach the chamber or bottle from the suction source; when bubbling ceases, observe the water level. If necessary, add sterile distilled water to bring the level to the 20-cm line, or as ordered.
- Check for gentle bubbling in the suction-control chamber because it indicates that the proper level of suction has been reached. Vigorous bubbling in this chamber increases the rate of water evaporation.
- Periodically check that the air vent in the system is working properly. Occlusion of the air vent results in a buildup of pressure in the system that could cause the patient to have tension pneumothorax.
- Coil the tubing and secure it to the edge of the bed with a rubber band or tape. Avoid creating dependent loops or kinks or placing pressure on the tubing. Avoid lifting the drainage system above the patient's chest because fluid may flow back into the pleural space.
- Keep two rubber-tipped Kelly clamps at the patient's bedside to clamp the chest tube in case the commercially prepared system cracks or to locate an air leak.
- Encourage the patient to cough frequently and to breathe deeply to help drain the pleural space and expand the lungs.
- Tell him or her to sit upright to allow optimal lung expansion and to splint the insertion site while coughing to minimize pain.
- Check the rate and quality of the patient's respirations and auscultate his or her lungs periodically to assess air exchange in the affected lung. Diminished or absent breath sounds may indicate that the lung has not reexpanded.
- Tell the patient to report breathing difficulty immediately. Notify the health care provider immediately if the patient has cyanosis, rapid or shallow breathing, subcutaneous emphysema, chest pain, or excessive bleeding.
- When clots are visible, you may be able to strip (or milk) the tubing, depending on facility policy. This procedure is controversial because it creates high negative pressure that could suck viable lung tissue into the drainage ports of the tube, with

subsequent ruptured alveoli and pleural air leak. Strip the tubing only when clots are visible. Use an alcohol pad or lotion as a lubricant on the tube and pinch the tube between your thumb and index finger about 2″ (5 cm) from the insertion site. Using your other thumb and index finger, compress the tubing as you slide your fingers down the tube or use a mechanical stripper. After the tube has been stripped, release your thumb and index finger and pinch the tube near the insertion site.

- Check the chest tube dressing at least every 8 hours. Palpate the area surrounding the dressing for crepitus or subcutaneous emphysema, which indicates that air is leaking into the subcutaneous tissue surrounding the insertion site. Change the dressing, if necessary, or according to facility policy.

- Encourage active or passive ROM exercises for the patient's arm on the affected side if he or she has been splinting the arm. Usually, a patient who has undergone thoracotomy will splint his or her arm to decrease his or her discomfort.

- Give ordered pain medication as needed to provide comfort and to help with deep breathing, coughing, and ROM exercises.

- Remind the ambulatory patient to keep the drainage system below chest level and to be careful not to disconnect the tubing to maintain the water seal. With a suction system, the patient must stay within range of the length of tubing attached to a wall outlet or portable pump.

Special considerations

- Instruct staff and visitors to avoid touching the equipment to prevent complications from separated connections.

- If excessive continuous bubbling is present in the water-seal chamber, especially if suction is being used, make sure that there is not a leak in the drainage system. Try to locate a leak by clamping the tube momentarily at various points along its length. Begin clamping at the proximal end of the tube and work down toward the drainage system, paying special attention to the seal around the connections. If any connection is loose, push it back together and tape it securely. The bubbling will stop when a clamp is placed between the air leak and the water seal. If you clamp along the entire length of the tube and the bubbling does not stop, the drainage unit may be cracked and need replacement.

- If a commercially prepared drainage collection chamber fills, replace it. Double-clamp the tube close to the insertion site (use two clamps facing in opposite directions), exchange the system, remove the clamps, and retape the connection.

 ALERT

Never leave the tubes clamped for longer than 1 minute to prevent tension pneumothorax, which may occur when clamping stops air and fluid from escaping.

- If a commercially prepared system cracks, clamp the chest tube momentarily with the two rubber-tipped clamps at the bedside (placed there at the time of tube insertion). Place the clamps close to each other near the insertion site; they should face in opposite directions to provide a more complete seal. Observe the patient for altered respirations while the tube is clamped. Replace the damaged equipment. (Prepare the new unit before you clamp the tube.)

- Instead of clamping the tube, you can submerge the distal end of the tube in a container of normal saline solution to create a temporary water seal while you replace the drainage system. Check facility policy for the proper procedure.
- Tension pneumothorax may result from excessive accumulation of air, drainage, or both. Eventually, it may exert pressure on the heart and aorta, causing a precipitous fall in CO.

Documentation

Record the date and time that thoracic drainage began, the type of system used, the amount of suction applied to the pleural cavity, the presence or absence of bubbling or fluctuation in the water-seal chamber, the initial amount and type of drainage, and the patient's respiratory status.

At the end of each shift, record how frequently the system is inspected and the chest tubes are milked or stripped as well as the amount, color, and consistency of drainage; the presence or absence of bubbling or fluctuation in the water-seal chamber; the patient's respiratory status; the condition of the chest dressings; any pain medication given; and all complications and the nursing action taken.

Tracheal suction

Tracheal suction involves the removal of secretions from the trachea or bronchi by means of a catheter inserted through the mouth or nose, a tracheal stoma, a tracheostomy tube, or an ET tube. In addition to removing secretions, tracheal suctioning stimulates the cough reflex. This procedure helps maintain a patent airway to promote optimal exchange of oxygen and carbon dioxide and to prevent pneumonia that results from pooling of secretions. Performed as frequently as the patient's condition warrants, tracheal suction calls for strict aseptic technique.

Equipment and preparation

Supplemental oxygen source (wall or portable unit, such as nasal cannula or aerosol source, and handheld resuscitation bag with mask, 15-mm adapter, or PEEP valve, if indicated) • wall or portable suction apparatus • collection container • connecting tube • suction catheter kit (or sterile suction catheter, one sterile glove, one clean glove, and disposable sterile solution container) • 1-L bottle of sterile water or normal saline solution • sterile water-soluble lubricant (for nasal insertion) • syringe for deflating cuff of ET or tracheostomy tube • waterproof trash bag • goggles and face mask or face shield • optional: sterile towel

Choose a suction catheter of the appropriate size. The diameter should be no larger than half of the inside diameter of the tracheostomy or ET tube to minimize hypoxia during suctioning. (A #12 or #14 French catheter may be used for an 8-mm or larger tube.) Place the suction apparatus on the patient's overbed table or bedside stand. Position the table or stand on your preferred side of the bed to facilitate suctioning.

Attach the collection container to the suction unit and the connecting tube to the collection container. Label and date the normal saline solution or sterile water. Open the waterproof trash bag.

Implementation

- Before suctioning, determine whether the facility requires a health care provider's order and obtain one, if necessary.
- Assess the patient's vital signs, breath sounds, and general appearance to establish a baseline for

comparison after suctioning. Review the patient's ABG values and oxygen saturation levels if they are available. Evaluate the patient's ability to cough and deep-breathe because they will help to move secretions up the tracheobronchial tree. If you will be performing nasotracheal suctioning, check the patient's history for a deviated septum, nasal polyps, nasal obstruction, nasal trauma, epistaxis, or mucosal swelling.

- Wash your hands. Put on personal protective equipment. Explain the procedure to the patient, even if he or she is unresponsive. Tell him or her that suctioning usually causes transient coughing or gagging but that coughing helps to remove the secretions. If the patient has been suctioned previously, summarize the reasons for suctioning. Continue to reassure the patient throughout the procedure to minimize anxiety, promote relaxation, and decrease oxygen demand.

- Assemble all equipment, making sure that the suction apparatus is connected to a collection container and connecting tube.

- Unless contraindicated, place the patient in semi-Fowler's or high Fowler's position to promote lung expansion and productive coughing.

- Remove the top from the normal saline solution or sterile water bottle.

- Open the package containing the disposable sterile solution container.

- Using strictly aseptic technique, open the suction catheter kit and put on the gloves. If you are using individual supplies, open the suction catheter and the gloves, placing the clean glove on your nondominant hand and then the sterile glove on your dominant hand.

- Using your nondominant (nonsterile) hand, pour the normal saline solution or sterile water into the solution container.

- Place a small amount of sterile water-soluble lubricant on the sterile area. Lubricant may be used to facilitate passage of the catheter during nasotracheal suctioning.

- Place a sterile towel over the patient's chest, if desired, to provide an additional sterile area.

- Using your dominant (sterile) hand, remove the catheter from its wrapper. Keep it coiled so that it will not touch a nonsterile object. Using your other hand to manipulate the connecting tubing, attach the catheter to the tubing (as shown below).

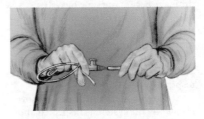

- With your nondominant hand, set the suction pressure according to facility policy. Typically, the pressure is set between 80 and 120 mm Hg. Higher pressures do not enhance secretion removal and may cause traumatic injury. Occlude the suction port to assess suction pressure (as shown below).

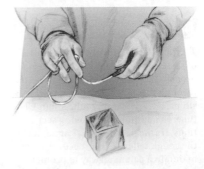

- Dip the tip of the catheter in the saline solution to lubricate the outside of the catheter and reduce tissue trauma during insertion.
- With the catheter tip in the sterile solution, occlude the control valve with the thumb of your nondominant hand. Suction a small amount of solution to lubricate the inside of the catheter, facilitating the passage of secretions through it (as shown below).

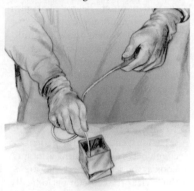

- For nasal insertion of the catheter, lubricate the tip of the catheter with the sterile water-soluble lubricant to reduce tissue trauma during insertion.
- If the patient is not intubated or is intubated but is not receiving a supplemental oxygen source or aerosol, instruct him or her to take three to six deep breaths to help minimize or prevent hypoxia during suctioning.
- If the patient is not intubated but is receiving oxygen, evaluate his or her need for preoxygenation. If indicated, instruct the patient to take three to six deep breaths while using his or her supplemental oxygen source. (If needed, the patient may continue to receive supplemental oxygen during suctioning by leaving his or her nasal cannula in one nostril or by keeping the oxygen mask over his or her mouth.)

- If the patient is being mechanically ventilated, preoxygenate him or her with a handheld resuscitation bag or the sigh mode on the ventilator. To use the resuscitation bag, set the oxygen flow meter at 15 L/minute, disconnect the patient from the ventilator, and deliver three to six breaths with the resuscitation bag (as shown below).

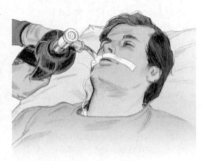

- If the patient is being maintained on PEEP, evaluate the need to use a resuscitation bag with a PEEP valve.
- To preoxygenate the patient using the ventilator, first adjust the FIO_2 and the V_T according to facility policy and patient need. Then use the sigh mode on the ventilator or manually deliver three to six breaths. If you have an assistant for the procedure, the assistant can manage the patient's oxygen needs while you perform the suctioning.

Nasotracheal insertion in a nonintubated patient

- Disconnect the oxygen from the patient, if applicable.
- Using your nondominant hand, raise the tip of the patient's nose to straighten the passageway and facilitate insertion of the catheter.
- Insert the catheter into the patient's nostril while you gently roll it between your fingers to help advance it through the turbinates.

- As the patient inhales, quickly advance the catheter as far as possible. To avoid oxygen loss and tissue trauma, do not apply suction during insertion.
- If the patient coughs as the catheter passes through the larynx, briefly hold the catheter still. Continue to advance the catheter when the patient inhales.

Nasotracheal insertion in an intubated patient

- If you are using a closed system, see *Closed tracheal suctioning.*
- Using your nonsterile hand, disconnect the patient from the ventilator.
- With your sterile hand, gently insert the suction catheter into the artificial airway (as shown below). Advance the catheter, without applying suction, until you meet resistance. If the patient coughs, pause briefly and then resume advancement.

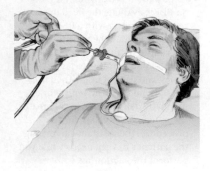

Suctioning the patient

- After inserting the catheter, apply suction intermittently by removing and replacing the thumb of your nondominant hand over the control valve. Simultaneously use your dominant hand to withdraw the catheter as you roll it between your thumb and forefinger. This rotating motion prevents the catheter from pulling tissue into the tube as it exits, thus avoiding tissue trauma. Never

suction for longer than 10 seconds at a time to prevent hypoxia.
- If the patient is intubated, use your nondominant hand to stabilize the tip of the ET tube as you withdraw the catheter to prevent accidental extubation or irritation of the mucous membranes.
- If applicable, resume oxygen delivery by reconnecting the source of oxygen or ventilation and hyperoxygenating the patient's lungs before you continue to prevent or relieve hypoxia.
- Observe the patient and allow him or her to rest for a few minutes before the next suctioning. The timing of each suctioning and the length of each rest period depend on the patient's tolerance of the procedure and the absence of complications. To enhance the removal of secretions, encourage the patient to cough between suctioning attempts.
- Look at the secretions. If they are thick, clear the catheter periodically by dipping the tip in the saline solution and applying suction. Normally, sputum is watery and tends to be sticky. Tenacious or thick sputum usually indicates dehydration. Watch for color variations. Sputum that is white or translucent is normal, yellow indicates pus, green indicates retained secretions or *Pseudomonas* infection, brown usually indicates old blood, red indicates fresh blood, and a red currant jelly appearance indicates *Klebsiella* infection. When the sputum contains blood, note whether it is streaked or well mixed. Also, indicate how often blood appears in the sputum. If the patient's heart rate and rhythm are being monitored, observe him or her for arrhythmias. If they occur, stop suctioning and ventilate the patient.
- Patients who cannot mobilize secretions effectively may need to perform tracheal suctioning after discharge.

Closed tracheal suctioning

The closed tracheal suction system can ease removal of secretions and reduce patient complications. Consisting of a sterile suction catheter in a clear plastic sleeve, the system permits the patient to remain connected to the ventilator during suctioning.

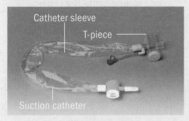

Catheter sleeve
T-piece
Suction catheter

As a result, the patient can maintain the tidal volume, oxygen concentration, and positive end-expiratory pressure delivered by the ventilator while being suctioned. In turn, this reduces the occurrence of suction-induced hypoxemia.

Another advantage of this system is a reduced risk of infection, even when the same catheter is used many times. Because the catheter remains in a protective sleeve, gloves are not required but are still recommended. The caregiver does not need to touch the catheter, and the ventilator circuit remains closed.

Implementation

To perform the procedure, gather a closed suction control valve, a T-piece to connect the artificial airway to the ventilator breathing circuit, and a catheter sleeve that encloses the catheter and has connections at each end for the control valve and the T-piece. Then follow these steps:

* Remove the closed suction system from its wrapping. Attach the control valve to the connecting tubing.
* Depress the thumb suction control valve and keep it depressed while setting the suction pressure to the desired level.
* Connect the T-piece to the ventilator breathing circuit, making sure that the irrigation port is closed. Then connect

the T-piece to the patient's endotracheal or tracheostomy tube (as shown below).

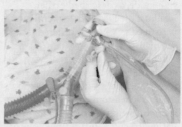

* Use one hand to keep the T-piece parallel to the patient's chin and use the thumb and index finger of the other hand to advance the catheter through the tube and into the patient's tracheobronchial tree (as shown below). You may need to retract the catheter sleeve gently as you advance the catheter.

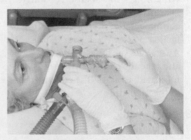

* While continuing to hold the T-piece and control valve, apply intermittent suction and withdraw the catheter until it reaches its fully extended length in the sleeve. Repeat the procedure as necessary.
* After you have finished suctioning, flush the catheter by maintaining suction while slowly introducing normal saline solution or sterile water into the irrigation port.
* Place the thumb control valve in the OFF position.
* Dispose and replace the suction equipment and supplies according to facility policy.
* Remove your gloves and wash your hands.
* Change the closed suction system every 24 hours to minimize the risk of infection.

After suctioning

- After suctioning, hyperoxygenate the patient who is being maintained on a ventilator using the handheld resuscitation bag or the ventilator's sigh mode, as described earlier.
- Readjust the FIO_2 and, for ventilated patients, the V_T to the ordered settings.
- After suctioning the lower airway, assess the patient's need for upper airway suctioning. If the cuff of the ET or tracheostomy tube is inflated, suction the upper airway before deflating the cuff with a syringe. Always change the catheter and sterile glove before resuctioning the lower airway to avoid introducing microorganisms into the lower airway.
- Discard the gloves and catheter in the waterproof trash bag. Clear the connecting tubing by aspirating the remaining saline solution or water. Discard and replace the suction equipment and supplies according to facility policy. Wash your hands.
- Auscultate the lungs bilaterally and take the patient's vital signs, if indicated, to assess the effectiveness of the procedure.

Special considerations

- Raising the patient's nose into the sniffing position helps to align the larynx and pharynx and may facilitate passage of the catheter during nasotracheal suctioning. If the patient's condition permits, have an assistant extend the patient's head and neck above his or her shoulders. The patient's lower jaw may need to be moved up and forward. If the patient is responsive, ask him or her to stick out his or her tongue so that he or she does not swallow the catheter during insertion.
- During suctioning, the catheter typically is advanced as far as the mainstem bronchi. However, because of the tracheobronchial anatomy, the catheter tends to enter the right mainstem bronchus instead of the left. Using an angled catheter (such as a coudé) may help you to guide the catheter into the left mainstem bronchus. Rotating the patient's head to the right seems to have a limited effect.
- Studies show that instilling normal saline solution into the trachea before suctioning may stimulate the patient's cough but does not liquefy secretions. Keeping the patient adequately hydrated and using bronchial hygiene techniques seem to have a greater effect on mobilizing secretions.
- In addition to the closed tracheal method, oxygen insufflation offers a new approach to suctioning. This method uses a double-lumen catheter that allows oxygen insufflation during suctioning.
- Do not allow the collection container on the suction machine to become more than three-quarters full to avoid damaging the machine.
- Assess the patient for complications. Because oxygen is removed along with secretions, the patient may have hypoxemia and dyspnea. In addition, anxiety may alter respiratory patterns. Cardiac arrhythmias can result from hypoxia and stimulation of the vagus nerve in the tracheobronchial tree. Tracheal or bronchial trauma can result from traumatic or prolonged suctioning.
- Patients with compromised cardiovascular or pulmonary status are at risk for hypoxemia, arrhythmias, hypertension, or hypotension. Patients with a history of nasopharyngeal bleeding, those who are taking an anticoagulant, those who recently have undergone a tracheostomy, and those who have a blood dyscrasia are at increased risk for bleeding because of suctioning.

- Use caution when suctioning patients who have increased ICP because suction may further increase pressure.
- If the patient has laryngospasm or bronchospasm (rare complications) during suctioning, disconnect the suction catheter from the connecting tubing and allow the catheter to act as an airway. Discuss with the patient's health care provider the use of a bronchodilator or lidocaine to reduce the risk of this complication.

Documentation

Record the date and time of the procedure; the technique used; the reason for suctioning; the amount, color, consistency, and odor (if any) of the secretions; any complications and the nursing action taken; and the patient's response to the procedure.

Transfusion of blood and blood products

Whole blood transfusion replenishes the volume and the oxygen-carrying capacity of the circulatory system by increasing the mass of circulating RBCs. Transfusion of packed RBCs, from which 80% of the plasma has been removed, restores only the oxygen-carrying capacity. After plasma is removed, the resulting component has a hematocrit of 65% to 80% and a usual volume of 300 to 350 ml. (Whole blood without the plasma removed has a hematocrit of about 38%.) Each unit of whole blood or RBCs contains enough hemoglobin to raise the hemoglobin level in an average-sized adult 1 g/L, or by 3%. Both types of transfusion treat decreased hemoglobin levels and hematocrit. Whole blood is rarely used and only when decreased levels result from hemorrhage; packed RBCs, the most commonly transfused, are used when

depressed levels accompany normal blood volume to avoid possible fluid and circulatory overload. (See *Transfusing blood and selected components*, pages 404 to 409.) Whole blood and packed RBCs contain cellular debris and require in-line filtration during administration. (Washed packed RBCs, commonly used for patients who were previously sensitized to transfusions, are rinsed with a special solution that removes white blood cells and platelets, thus decreasing the chance of a transfusion reaction.)

ALERT

Depending on facility policy, two licensed professionals need to identify the patient and blood products at the patient's bedside before administering a transfusion to prevent errors and a potentially fatal reaction.

ALERT

If the patient is a Jehovah's Witness, a transfusion requires special written permission.

Equipment and preparation

Blood administration set (170- to 260-micron filter and tubing with drip chamber for blood, or combined set) • I.V. pole • gloves • gown • face shield • whole blood or packed RBCs • 250 ml of normal saline solution • venipuncture equipment, if needed (should include 20G or larger catheter) • optional: ice bag and warm compresses

(Text continues on page 408.)

Transfusing blood and selected components

Blood component	Indications
Packed red blood cells (RBCs)	
Same RBC mass as whole blood but with 80% of the plasma removed *Volume: 250 ml*	• Inadequate circulating red cell mass • Symptomatic deficiency of oxygen-carrying capacity • Symptomatic chronic anemia • Hemoglobin <7 g/dl or hematocrit <21% • Sickle cell disease (red cell exchange)
Whole blood	
Complete (pure) blood *Volume: 500 ml*	• Massive blood loss • Deficiency of oxygen-carrying capability and volume expansion
White blood cells (WBCs or leukocytes)	
Whole blood with all of the RBCs and about 80% of the supernatant plasma removed *Volume: usually 150 ml*	• Sepsis unresponsive to antibiotics (especially if patient has positive blood cultures or a persistent fever >101° F [38.3° C]) and granulocytopenia (granulocyte count usually <500/μl)
Leukocyte-poor RBCs	
Same as packed RBCs, with about 95% of the leukocytes removed *Volume: 200 ml*	• Same as for packed RBCs • Prevention of febrile reactions from leukocyte antibodies • Immunocompromised patients

Compatibility	Nursing considerations
• Type A receives A or O. • Type B receives B or O. • Type AB receives AB, A, B, or O. • Type O receives O. • Rh match is necessary.	• Use a blood administration set to infuse blood within 4 hours. • Administer only with 0.9% normal saline solution. • An RBC transfusion is not appropriate for anemias treatable by nutritional or drug therapies.
• ABO identical: Type A receives A; type B receives B; type AB receives AB; type O receives O. • Rh match is necessary.	• Whole blood is seldom administered. • Use a blood administration set to infuse blood within 4 hours. • Administer only with 0.9% normal saline solution. • Closely monitor patient's volume status during administration for risk of volume overload.
• Same as for packed RBCs • Compatibility with human leukocyte antigen (HLA) is preferable but not necessary unless the patient is sensitized to HLA as a result of previous transfusions. • Rh match is necessary.	• Use a blood administration set to provide 1 unit daily for 5 days or until the infection resolves. • As prescribed, premedicate with diphenhydramine. • Because a WBC infusion induces fever and chills, administer an antipyretic if fever occurs. Do not discontinue the transfusion; instead, reduce the flow rate as ordered for patient comfort. • Agitate the container to prevent the WBCs from settling, thus preventing the delivery of a bolus infusion of WBCs.
• Same as for packed RBCs • Rh match is necessary.	• Use a blood administration set to infuse blood within 4 hours. • Other considerations are the same as those for packed RBCs.

(continued)

Transfusing blood and selected components *(continued)*

Blood component	Indications
Platelets	
Platelet sediment from RBCs or plasma *Volume: 35 to 50 ml/unit; 1 unit of platelets = 7 × 10^7 platelets*	• Bleeding resulting from critically decreased circulating platelet counts or functionally abnormal platelets • Prevention of bleeding caused by thrombocytopenia • Platelet count <50,000/μl before surgery or a major invasive procedure
Fresh frozen plasma (FFP)	
Uncoagulated plasma separated from RBCs and rich in coagulation factors V, VIII, and IX *Volume: 200 to 250 ml*	• Bleeding • Coagulation factor deficiencies • Warfarin reversal • Thrombotic thrombocytopenic purpura
Albumin 5% (buffered saline); albumin 25% (salt poor)	
A small plasma protein prepared by fractionating pooled plasma *Volume: 5% = 12.5 g/250 ml; 25% = 12.5 g/50 ml*	• Volume lost because of shock from burns, trauma, surgery, or infections • Hypoproteinemia (with or without edema)

Compatibility	Nursing considerations
• ABO identical when possible • Rh match is preferred.	• Use a filtered component drip administration set to infuse 100 ml over 15 minutes. • As prescribed, premedicate with antipyretics and antihistamines if the patient's history includes a platelet transfusion reaction. • Avoid administering platelets when the patient has a fever. • Prepare to draw blood for a platelet count as ordered, 1 hour after the platelet transfusion, to determine the increments for platelet transfusion. • Keep in mind that the health care provider seldom orders a platelet transfusion for conditions in which platelet destruction is accelerated, such as idiopathic thrombocytopenic purpura and drug-induced thrombocytopenia.
• ABO is required. • Rh match is not required.	• Use a straight-line I.V. set and administer the infusion rapidly. • Keep in mind that large-volume transfusions of FFP may require correction for hypocalcemia because citric acid in FFP binds calcium.
• Unnecessary	• Use the administration set supplied by the manufacturer, with the rate and volume dictated by the patient's condition and response. • Remember that reactions to albumin (fever, chills, nausea) are rare. • Avoid mixing albumin with protein hydrolysates and alcohol solutions. • Consider delivering albumin as a volume expander until the laboratory completes crossmatching for a whole blood transfusion. • Keep in mind that albumin is contraindicated in severe anemia and administered cautiously in cardiac and pulmonary disease because heart failure may result from circulatory overload.

(continued)

Transfusing blood and selected components *(continued)*

Blood component	Indications
Cryoprecipitate	
Insoluble portion of plasma recovered from FFP containing fibrinogen, factor VIII:c, factor VIII: vwf, factor XIII, and fibronectin *Volume: about 30 ml (freeze-dried)*	• Bleeding associated with hypofibrinogenemia or dysfibrinogenemia • Significant factor XIII deficiency (prevention or treatment)
Immunoglobulin (Ig)	
Processed human plasma from multiple donors that contains 95% IgG, <2.5% IgA, and a fraction of IgM	• Primary immune deficiencies • Secondary immune deficiencies • Kawasaki syndrome • Idiopathic thrombocytopenia purpura • Neurologic disorders (Guillain-Barré's syndrome, dermatomyositis, myasthenia gravis)

Straight-line and Y-type blood administration sets are commonly used. Although filters come in both mesh and microaggregate types, the latter is preferred especially when transfusing multiple units of blood. Highly effective leukocyte removal filters are available for use when transfusing blood and packed RBCs. The use of these filters can postpone sensitization to transfusion therapy.

Administer packed RBCs with a Y-type set. Using a straight-line set forces you to piggyback the tubing so that you can stop the transfusion, if necessary, but still keep the vein open. Piggybacking increases the chance that harmful microorganisms will enter the tubing as you are connecting the blood line to the established line.

Multiple-lead tubing minimizes the risk of contamination, especially when multiple units of blood are transfused. (A straight-line set would require multiple piggybacking.) A Y-type set gives you the option of adding normal saline solution to packed cells—decreasing their viscosity—if the patient can tolerate the added fluid volume.

Avoid obtaining either whole blood or packed RBCs until you are ready to begin the transfusion. Prepare the equipment when you are ready to start the infusion.

Implementation

• Verify the written order in the patient's medical record. Confirm that the order and the medical record are

Compatibility	Nursing considerations
• ABO compatible. • Rh compatibility is not required.	• Use a blood administration set. • Add 0.9% normal saline solution to each bag of cryoprecipitate as needed to facilitate transfusion. • Cryoprecipitate must be administered within 6 hours of thawing. • Before administering, check lab study results to confirm a deficiency of one of the specific clotting factors in cryoprecipitate. • Patients with hemophilia A or von Willebrand's disease should only be treated with cryoprecipitate when appropriate factor VIII concentrates are not available.
• ABO compatibility and Rh match are unnecessary.	• Use the administration set supplied by the manufacturer. • Reconstitute the lyophilized powder with 0.9% sodium chloride injection, 5% dextrose, or sterile water. • Administer at the minimal concentration available and at the slowest practical rate.

labeled with the patient's name and identification number.

- Confirm the patient's identity using two patient identifiers.
- Explain the procedure to the patient. Make sure that he or she has signed an informed consent form before any blood is transfused.
- Record the patient's baseline vital signs.
- If the patient does not have an I.V. line in place, perform a venipuncture, using a catheter with a diameter of 20G or larger. Avoid using an existing line if the needle or catheter lumen is smaller than 20G. CVADs may also be used for transfusion therapy.
- Obtain whole blood or packed RBCs from the blood bank within 30 minutes of the transfusion start time. Check the expiration date on the blood bag and observe the bag for abnormal color, RBC clumping, gas bubbles, and extraneous material. Return outdated or abnormal blood to the blood bank.
- Compare the name and identification number on the patient's wristband with the information on the label of the blood bag. Check the blood bag identification number, the ABO blood group, and Rh compatibility. Compare the patient's blood bank identification number, if present, with the number on the blood bag. Identification of blood and blood products is performed at the patient's bedside by two licensed professionals, according to facility policy.

- Put on gloves, a gown, and a face shield. Use a Y-type set and close all of the clamps on the set. Insert the spike of the line that you are using for the normal saline solution into the bag of saline solution. Open the port on the blood bag and insert the spike of the line that you are using to administer the blood or cellular component into the port. Hang the bag of normal saline solution and blood or cellular component on the I.V. pole, open the clamp on the line of saline solution, and squeeze the drip chamber until it is half full. Remove the adapter cover at the tip of the blood administration set, open the main flow clamp, and prime the tubing with saline solution.

- If you are administering packed RBCs with a Y-type set, you can add saline solution to the bag to dilute the cells by closing the clamp between the patient and the drip chamber and opening the clamp from the blood. Lower the blood bag below the saline container and let 30 to 50 ml of saline solution flow into the packed cells. Close the clamp to the blood bag, rehang the bag, rotate it gently to mix the cells and saline solution, and close the clamp to the saline container.

- Attach the prepared blood administration set to the venipuncture device and flush it with normal saline solution. Close the clamp to the saline solution and open the clamp between the blood bag and the patient. Adjust the flow rate to no greater than 5 ml/minute for the first 15 minutes of the transfusion so that you can observe the patient for a possible transfusion reaction.

- If signs of a transfusion reaction develop, record the patient's vital signs and stop the transfusion. Infuse saline solution at a moderately slow infusion rate and notify the health care provider at once. If no signs of a reaction appear within 15 minutes, adjust the flow clamp to the ordered infusion rate. A unit of RBCs may be given over 1 to 4 hours, as ordered.

- Recheck vital signs, including temperature, every 15 minutes for the first 30 minutes after beginning the transfusion and then according to facility policy.

- After completing the transfusion, put on gloves and remove and discard the used infusion equipment. Reconnect the original I.V. fluid, if necessary, or discontinue the I.V. infusion.

- Return the empty blood bag to the blood bank. Discard the tubing and filter.

- Record the patient's vital signs.

Special considerations

- Although some microaggregate filters can be used for up to 10 units of blood, replace the filter and tubing if more than 1 hour elapses between transfusions. When administering multiple units of blood under pressure, use a blood warmer to avoid hypothermia. Blood components may be warmed to no more than 107.6° F (42° C).

- For rapid blood replacement, you may need to use a pressure bag. Excessive pressure may develop, leading to broken blood vessels and extravasation, with hematoma and hemolysis of the infusing RBCs.

- If the transfusion stops, take the following steps, as needed:
  - Check that the I.V. container is at least 3' (0.9 m) above the level of the I.V. site.
  - Make sure that the flow clamp is open and that the blood completely covers the filter. If it does not, squeeze the drip chamber until it does.
  - Gently rock the bag back and forth, agitating blood cells that may have settled.

- Untape the dressing over the I.V. site to check cannula placement. Reposition the cannula, if necessary.
- Flush the line with saline solution and restart the transfusion. Using a Y-type set, close the flow clamp to the patient and lower the blood bag. Open the saline clamp and allow some saline solution to flow into the blood bag. Rehang the blood bag, open the flow clamp to the patient, and reset the flow rate.
- If a hematoma develops at the I.V. site, stop the infusion immediately. Remove the I.V. cannula. Notify the health care provider and expect to place ice on the site intermittently for 8 hours and then apply warm compresses. Follow facility policy.
- If the blood bag empties before the next one arrives, administer normal saline solution slowly. If you are using a Y-type set, close the blood line clamp, open the saline clamp, and let the saline run slowly until the new blood arrives. Decrease the flow rate or clamp the line before attaching the new unit of blood.
- Despite improvements in cross-matching precautions, transfusion reactions can still occur. Unlike a transfusion reaction, an infectious disease that is transmitted during a transfusion may go undetected until days, weeks, or even months later, when it produces signs and symptoms. Measures to prevent disease transmission include laboratory testing of blood products and careful screening of potential donors, neither of which is guaranteed.
- Hepatitis C accounts for most cases of posttransfusion hepatitis. The tests that detect hepatitis B and hepatitis C can produce false-negative results and may allow some cases of hepatitis to go undetected.

- When testing for antibodies to HIV, remember that antibodies do not appear until 6 to 12 weeks after exposure. According to the American Association of Blood Banks, the estimated risk of acquiring HIV from a single transfusion of blood products varies from 1 in 40,000 to 1 in 153,000.
- Many blood banks screen blood for cytomegalovirus (CMV). Blood with CMV is especially dangerous for an immunosuppressed, seronegative patient. Blood banks also test blood for syphilis, but refrigerating blood virtually eliminates the risk of transfusion-related syphilis.
- Circulatory overload and hemolytic, allergic, febrile, and pyogenic reactions can result from any transfusion. Coagulation disturbances, citrate intoxication, hyperkalemia, acid-base imbalance, loss of 2,3-diphosphoglycerate, ammonia intoxication, and hypothermia can result from massive transfusion.

Documentation

Record the date and time of the transfusion, the type and amount of transfusion product, the patient's vital signs, your check of all identification data, and the patient's response. Document any transfusion reaction and treatment.

Tube feedings

Tube feedings involve delivery of a liquid feeding formula directly to the stomach (known as gastric gavage), duodenum, or jejunum. Gastric gavage is typically indicated for a patient who cannot eat normally because of dysphagia or oral or esophageal obstruction or injury. Gastric feedings may also be given to an unconscious or intubated patient or to a patient who is recovering from GI tract surgery and cannot ingest food orally.

Duodenal or jejunal feedings decrease the risk of aspiration because the formula bypasses the pylorus. Jejunal feedings result in reduced pancreatic stimulation; thus, the patient may require an elemental diet.

Patients usually receive gastric feedings on an intermittent schedule. For duodenal or jejunal feedings, most patients seem to better tolerate a continuous slow drip.

Liquid nutrient solutions come in various formulas for administration through an NG tube, a small-bore feeding tube, a gastrostomy or jejunostomy tube, a percutaneous endoscopic gastrostomy or jejunostomy tube, or a gastrostomy feeding button. Tube feeding is contraindicated in patients who have no bowel sounds or have a suspected intestinal obstruction.

Equipment and preparation

For gastric feedings

Feeding formula • 120 ml of water • gavage bag with tubing and flow regulator clamp • towel or linen-saver pad • 60-ml syringe or barrel syringe • pH test strip • optional: infusion controller and gavage bag tubing set (for continuous administration) and adapter to connect gavage tubing to feeding tube

For duodenal or jejunal feedings

Feeding formula • enteral administration set, containing gavage container, drip chamber, roller clamp or flow regulator, and tube connector • I.V. pole • 60-ml syringe with adapter tip • water • optional: volumetric pump administration set (for enteral infusion pump) and Y-connector

A bulb syringe or large catheter-tip syringe may be substituted for a gavage bag after the patient shows tolerance for a gravity drip infusion. The health care provider may order an infusion pump to ensure accurate delivery of the prescribed formula.

Refrigerate formulas that are prepared in the dietary department or pharmacy. Refrigerate commercial formulas only after they have been opened. Check the date on all formula containers. Discard expired commercial formula. Use powdered formula within 24 hours of mixing. Shake the container vigorously to mix the solution thoroughly.

Allow the formula to warm to room temperature before administering it. Cold formula can increase the chance of diarrhea. Never warm formula over direct heat or in a microwave. Heat may curdle the formula or change its chemical composition, and hot formula may injure the patient.

Pour 60 ml of water into the graduated container. After you close the flow clamp on the administration set, pour the appropriate amount of formula into the gavage bag. Hang no more than a 4- to 6-hour supply at one time to prevent bacterial growth.

Open the flow clamp on the administration set to remove air from the lines. This keeps air from entering the patient's stomach and causing distention and discomfort.

Implementation

- Confirm the patient's identity using at least two patient identifiers, provide privacy, and wash your hands.
- Tell the patient that he or she will receive nourishment through the tube and explain the procedure to him or her.
- If the patient has a nasal or an oral tube, cover his or her chest with a towel or linen-saver pad to protect him or her and the bed linens from spills.
- Assess the patient's abdomen for bowel sounds and distention.

Delivering a gastric feeding

- Elevate the bed to semi-Fowler's or high Fowler's position to prevent aspiration by gastroesophageal reflux and to promote digestion.

- To check the patency and position of the tube, remove the cap or plug from the feeding tube and use the syringe to aspirate stomach contents. Examine the aspirate and place a small amount on the pH test strip. Probability of gastric placement is increased if the aspirate has a typical gastric fluid appearance (grassy green, clear and colorless with mucous shreds, or brown) and the pH is ≤5.
- To assess gastric emptying, aspirate and measure the residual gastric contents. Hold feedings if the residual volume is greater than the predetermined amount specified in the health care provider's order (usually 50 to 100 ml). Reinstill any aspirate obtained.
- Connect the gavage bag tubing to the feeding tube. Depending on the type of tube used, you may need to use an adapter to connect the two.
- If you are using a bulb or catheter-tip syringe, remove the bulb or plunger. Attach the syringe to the pinched-off feeding tube to prevent excess air from entering the patient's stomach, causing distention. If you are using an infusion controller, thread the tube from the formula container through the controller, according to manufacturer directions. Blue food dye can be added to the feeding

to allow you to identify aspiration quickly. Purge the tubing of air and attach it to the feeding tube.
- Open the flow regulator clamp on the gavage bag tubing and adjust the flow rate, as appropriate. When using a bulb syringe, fill the syringe with formula and release the feeding tube to allow formula to flow through it. The height at which you hold the syringe determines the flow rate. When the syringe is three-quarters empty, pour more formula into it.
- To prevent air from entering the tube and the patient's stomach, never allow the syringe to empty completely. If you are using an infusion controller, set the flow rate according to manufacturer directions. Always administer a tube feeding slowly—typically 200 to 350 ml over a period of 15 to 30 minutes, depending on the patient's tolerance and the health care provider's order—to prevent sudden stomach distention, which can cause nausea, vomiting, cramps, or diarrhea.
- After administering the appropriate amount of formula, flush the tubing by adding about 60 ml of water to the gavage bag or bulb syringe or manually flush it with a barrel syringe. This maintains the patency of the tube by removing excess formula, which could occlude the tube.
- If you are administering a continuous feeding, flush the feeding tube every 4 hours to help prevent occlusion of the tube. Monitor gastric emptying every 4 hours.
- To discontinue gastric feeding (depending on the equipment you are using), close the regulator clamp on the gavage bag tubing, disconnect the syringe from the feeding tube, or turn off the infusion controller.
- Cover the end of the feeding tube with its plug or cap to prevent leakage and contamination.

- Leave the patient in semi-Fowler's or high Fowler's position for at least 30 minutes.
- Rinse all reusable equipment with warm water. Dry it and store it in a convenient place for the next feeding. Change the equipment every 24 hours or according to facility policy.

Delivering a duodenal or jejunal feeding

- Elevate the head of the bed and place the patient in low Fowler's position.
- Open the enteral administration set and hang the gavage container on the I.V. pole.
- If you are using a nasoduodenal tube, measure its length to check tube placement. You may not obtain any residual when you aspirate the tube.
- Open the roller clamp and regulate the flow to the desired rate. To regulate the rate with a volumetric infusion pump, follow manufacturer directions for setting up the equipment. Most patients receive small amounts initially, with volumes increasing gradually once tolerance is established.
- Flush the tube with water every 4 hours to maintain patency and provide hydration. A needle catheter jejunostomy tube may need to be flushed every 2 hours to prevent buildup of formula inside the tube. A Y-connector may be useful for frequent flushing. Attach the continuous feeding tube to the main port and use the side port for flushes.
- Change the equipment every 24 hours or according to facility policy.

Special considerations

- If the feeding solution does not initially flow through a bulb syringe, attach the bulb and squeeze it gently to start the flow. Then remove the bulb. Never use the bulb to force the formula through the tube.

- If the patient becomes nauseated or vomits, stop the feeding immediately. He or she may vomit if his or her stomach becomes distended because of overfeeding or delayed gastric emptying.
- To reduce oropharyngeal discomfort from the tube, allow the patient to brush his or her teeth or care for his or her dentures regularly and encourage frequent gargling. If the patient is unconscious, administer oral care swabs every 4 hours. Use petroleum jelly on dry, cracked lips.

 ALERT

Dry mucous membranes may indicate dehydration, which requires increased fluid intake. Clean the patient's nostrils with cotton-tipped applicators, apply lubricant along the mucosa, and assess the skin for signs of breakdown.

- During continuous feedings, assess the patient frequently for abdominal distention. Flush the tubing by adding about 50 ml of water to the gavage bag or bulb syringe. This maintains the patency of the tube by removing excess formula, which could occlude the tube.
- If the patient has diarrhea, give him or her small, frequent, less concentrated feedings or administer bolus feedings over a longer period. Also, make sure that the formula is not cold and that proper storage and sanitation practices have been followed. The loose stools associated with tube feedings make extra perineal skin care necessary. Giving paregoric, tincture of opium, or diphenoxylate hydrochloride may improve the condition. Changing to a formula with more fiber may eliminate liquid stools.

- If the patient becomes constipated, the health care provider may increase the fruit, vegetable, or sugar content of the formula. Assess the patient's hydration status because dehydration may produce constipation. Increase fluid intake, as needed. If the condition persists, administer an appropriate drug or enema, as ordered.
- Drugs can be administered through the feeding tube. Except for enteric-coated, time-released, or sustained-release medications, crush tablets or open and dilute capsules in water before administering them. Make sure that you flush the tubing afterward to ensure full instillation of medication. Some drugs may change the osmolarity of the feeding formula and cause diarrhea.
- Small-bore feeding tubes may kink, making instillation impossible. If you suspect this problem, try changing the patient's position or withdraw the tube a few inches and restart. Never use a guide wire to reposition the tube.
- Constantly monitor the flow rate of a blended or high-residue formula to determine if the formula is clogging the tubing as it settles. To prevent such clogging, squeeze the bag frequently to agitate the solution.
- Collect blood samples, as ordered. Hyperglycemia and diuresis may indicate an excessive carbohydrate level, which could lead to fatal hyperosmotic dehydration. Monitor blood glucose levels to assess glucose tolerance. (A serum glucose level of less than 170 mg/dl is considered stable.) Also monitor serum levels of electrolytes, blood urea nitrogen, and glucose as well as serum osmolality and other pertinent findings to determine the patient's response to therapy and assess his or her hydration status.

- Special pulmonary formulas are available for patients who are prone to carbon dioxide retention.
- Check the flow rate hourly to ensure correct infusion. (With an improvised administration set, use a time tape to record the rate because it is difficult to obtain precise readings from an irrigation container or enema bag.)
- For duodenal or jejunal feeding, most patients tolerate a continuous drip better than bolus feedings. Bolus feedings can cause such complications as hyperglycemia and diarrhea.
- Until the patient acquires a tolerance for the formula, you may need to dilute it to one-half or three-quarters strength to start and increase it gradually. Patients who are under stress or who are receiving a steroid may experience a pseudodiabetic state. Assess these patients frequently to determine the need for insulin.

 Patient Teaching Tip

Patient education for home tube feeding includes instructions on an infusion control device to maintain accuracy, use of the syringe or bag and tubing, care of the tube and insertion site, and formula mixing. Formula may be mixed in an electric blender according to package directions. Formula that is not used within 24 hours must be discarded. If the formula must hang longer than 8 hours, advise the patient or caregiver to use a gavage or pump administration set with an ice pouch to decrease the incidence of bacterial growth. Tell him or her to use a new bag daily. Teach family members which signs and symptoms to report to the health care provider or home care nurse as well as what measures to take in an emergency.

- Erosion of the esophageal, tracheal, nasal, and oropharyngeal mucosa can result if tubes are left in place for a long time. If possible, use smaller lumen tubes to prevent such irritation. Check facility policy regarding the frequency of changing feeding tubes to prevent complications.
- With the gastric route, frequent or large-volume feedings can cause bloating and retention. Dehydration, diarrhea, and vomiting can cause metabolic disturbances. Cramping and abdominal distention usually indicate intolerance.
- With the duodenal or jejunal route, clogging of the feeding tube is common. The patient may have metabolic, fluid, and electrolyte abnormalities, including hyperglycemia, hyperosmolar dehydration, coma, edema, hypernatremia, and essential fatty acid deficiency.
- The patient may also experience dumping syndrome in which a large amount of hyperosmotic solution in the duodenum causes excessive diffusion of fluid through the semipermeable membrane and results in diarrhea. In a patient with low serum albumin levels, these signs and symptoms may result from low oncotic pressure in the duodenal mucosa. (See *Managing tube feeding problems*.)

Documentation

On the intake and output sheet, record the date, volume of formula, and volume of water. In your notes, document the findings of abdominal assessment (including the tube exit site, if appropriate); the amount of residual gastric contents; verification of tube placement; the amount, type, and time of feeding; and verification of tube patency. Discuss the patient's tolerance of the feeding, including nausea, vomiting, cramping, diarrhea, and distention.

Note the result of blood and urine tests, hydration status, and any drugs given through the tube. Include the date and time of administration set changes, the oral and nasal hygiene performed, and the results of specimen collections.

Venipuncture

Performed to obtain a venous blood sample, venipuncture involves piercing a vein with a needle and collecting blood in a syringe or an evacuated tube. Typically, venipuncture is performed using the antecubital fossa (median cubital veins). If necessary, however, it can be performed on a vein in the wrist, the dorsum of the hand, or another accessible location.

Equipment and preparation

Disposable tourniquet • gloves • syringe or evacuated tubes and needle holder • chlorhexidine swab • 21G needle for the forearm or 23G needle for the wrist, hand, and ankle and for children and infants • color-coded collection tubes containing appropriate additives • labels • laboratory requests • laboratory transport bag • 2″ × 2″ gauze pads • adhesive bandage • optional: cold compresses

If you are using evacuated tubes, open the needle packet, attach the needle to its holder, and select the appropriate tubes. If you are using a syringe, attach the appropriate needle to it. Make sure that you choose a syringe that is large enough to hold all of the blood required for the test. Label all collection tubes with the patient's name and room number, the health care provider's name, and the date and time of collection.

Implementation

- Confirm the patient's identity using at least two patient identifiers.
- Wash your hands thoroughly and put on gloves.

Managing tube feeding problems

Complications	Interventions
Aspiration of gastric secretions	• Discontinue feeding immediately. • Perform tracheal suction of the aspirated contents, if possible. • Notify the health care provider. Prophylactic antibiotics and chest physiotherapy may be ordered. • Check tube placement before feeding to prevent complications.
Tube obstruction	• Flush the tube with warm water. If necessary, replace the tube. • Flush the tube with 50 ml of water after each feeding to remove excess sticky formula, which could occlude the tube. • When possible, use liquid forms of medications. Otherwise, and if not contraindicated, crush well.
Oral, nasal, or pharyngeal irritation or necrosis	• Provide frequent oral hygiene using mouthwash or lemon-glycerin swabs. Use petroleum jelly on cracked lips. • Change the position of the tube. If necessary, replace the tube.
Vomiting, bloating, diarrhea, or cramps	• Reduce the flow rate. • Administer metoclopramide to increase gastrointestinal (GI) motility. • Warm the formula to prevent GI distress. • For 30 minutes after feeding, position the patient on his or her right side with his or her head elevated to facilitate gastric emptying. • Notify the health care provider. He or she may want to reduce the amount of formula being given during each feeding.
Constipation	• Provide additional fluids if the patient can tolerate them. • Administer a bulk-forming laxative. • Increase the fruit, vegetable, or sugar content of the feeding.
Electrolyte imbalance	• Monitor serum electrolyte levels. • Notify the health care provider. He or she may want to adjust the formula content to correct the deficiency.
Hyperglycemia	• Monitor blood glucose levels. • Notify the health care provider of elevated levels. • Administer insulin, if ordered. • The health care provider may adjust the sugar content of the formula.

- Tell the patient that you are about to collect a blood sample and explain the procedure to ease anxiety. Ask if he or she has ever felt faint, sweaty, or nauseated when having blood drawn.
- If the patient is on bed rest, ask him or her to lie in a supine position, with head slightly elevated and arms at his or her sides. Ask the ambulatory patient to sit in a chair and to support his or her arm securely on an armrest or a table.
- Assess the patient's veins to determine the best puncture site. (See *Common venipuncture sites*.)

Observe the skin for the blue color of the vein or palpate the vein for a firm rebound sensation.
- Tie a tourniquet 2″ (5 cm) above the antecubital fossa. By impeding venous return to the heart while allowing arterial flow, a tourniquet produces venous dilation. If arterial perfusion remains adequate, you will be able to feel the radial pulse. (If the tourniquet does not dilate the vein, have the patient open and close his or her fist repeatedly.)
- Clean the venipuncture site with a chlorhexidine swab. Wipe vigorously in a side-to-side motion to avoid

Common venipuncture sites

The illustrations below show the anatomic locations of veins commonly used for venipuncture sites. The most commonly used sites are on the forearm, followed by those on the hand.

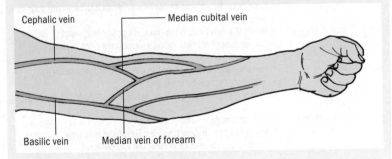

Cephalic vein — Median cubital vein

Basilic vein — Median vein of forearm

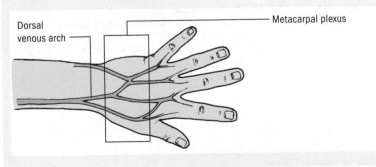

Dorsal venous arch — Metacarpal plexus

introducing potentially infectious skin flora into the vessel during the procedure. Allow the skin to dry before performing venipuncture.

- Immobilize the vein by pressing just below the venipuncture site with your thumb and drawing the skin taut.
- Position the needle holder or syringe with the needle bevel up and the shaft parallel to the path of the vein and at a 0- to 15-degree angle to the arm. Insert the needle into the vein. If you are using a syringe, venous blood will appear in the hub; withdraw the blood slowly, pulling the plunger of the syringe gently to create steady suction until you obtain the required sample. Pulling the plunger too forcibly may collapse the vein. If you are using a needle holder and an evacuated tube, grasp the holder securely to stabilize it in the vein and push down on the color-coded collection tube until the needle punctures the rubber stopper. Blood will flow into the tube automatically.
- Remove the tourniquet as soon as blood flows adequately to prevent stasis and hemoconcentration, which can impair test results. If the flow is sluggish, leave the tourniquet in place longer, but always remove it before withdrawing the needle.
- Continue to fill the required tubes, removing one and inserting another. Gently rotate each tube as you remove it to help mix the additive with the sample.
- After you have drawn the last sample, place a gauze pad over the puncture site and slowly and gently remove the needle from the vein. When using an evacuated tube, remove the last tube from the needle holder to release the vacuum before withdrawing the needle from the vein.

- Apply gentle dry pressure to the puncture site for 2 to 3 minutes or until bleeding stops. This prevents extravasation of blood into the surrounding tissue, which can cause a hematoma.
- After bleeding stops, apply an adhesive bandage.
- If you have used a syringe, transfer the sample to a collection tube. Place all specimen tubes inside the biohazard transport bag, being careful to avoid foaming, which can cause hemolysis.
- Check the venipuncture site to see if a hematoma has developed. If it has, apply cold compresses for the first 24 hours.
- Discard the tourniquet, syringes, needles, and used gloves in appropriate containers.
- Label all specimen tubes with the patient's name and identification number, date, and time of collection.
- Place all specimen tubes in a laboratory transport bag and send them to the laboratory with a properly completed request form.

Special considerations

- Several manufacturers make safety-engineered blood collection sets; their use is recommended to help prevent needle sticks.
- Never collect a venous sample from an arm that is already being used for I.V. therapy or blood administration because this may affect test results. Do not collect a venous sample from an infection site because this may introduce pathogens into the vascular system. Likewise, avoid collecting blood from edematous areas, arteriovenous shunts, and sites of previous hematomas or vascular injury.
- If the patient has a clotting disorder or is receiving anticoagulant therapy, maintain firm pressure on the venipuncture site until the bleeding stops to prevent hematoma formation.

- Avoid using veins in the patient's legs for venipuncture because this increases the risk of thrombophlebitis.
- Assess the patient for complications. A hematoma at the needle insertion site is the most common complication of venipuncture. Nerve compression injury and infection may result from poor technique.

Documentation

Record the date, time, and site of the venipuncture; the name of the test; the time that the sample was sent to the laboratory; the amount of blood collected; the size of the needle used; and any adverse reactions.

Selected references

American Association of Critical-Care Nurses. (2017). *AACN procedure manual of high acuity, progressive, and critical care* (7th ed.). St. Louis, MO: Elsevier.

American Heart Association. (2016). *Basic life support: Provider manual*. Dallas, TX: Author.

Good, V. S., & Kirkwood, P. L. (2018). *Advanced critical care nursing* (2nd ed.). St. Louis, MO: Elsevier.

Hinkle, J. L., & Cheever, K. H. (2018). *Brunner & Suddarth's textbook of medical-surgical nursing* (14th ed.). Philadelphia, PA: Wolters Kluwer.

Lewis, S. L., Bucher, L., Heitkemper, M. M., & Harding, M. M. (2017). *Medical-surgical nursing: Assessment and management of clinical problems* (10th ed.). St. Louis, MO: Elsevier.

Papadakis, M. A., & McPhee, S. J. (2019). *Current medical diagnosis and treatment* (58th ed.). New York, NY: McGraw-Hill.

7 Surgical Patient Care

Reviewing the techniques

Preoperative care

Assessing the preoperative patient

A thorough preoperative assessment is the foundation of good surgical care, providing a baseline for comparison throughout a patient's treatment and recovery. This assessment also helps to identify conditions that impair the patient's ability to tolerate the stress of surgery or to comply with postoperative routines. (See *Preoperative care for the bariatric surgery patient*, pages 423 and 424.)

Initial steps

Begin your preoperative assessment by focusing on problem areas suggested by the patient's history and on any body system that is directly affected by the surgical procedure:

- Note the patient's general appearance. Does the patient look healthy, well nourished, or does he or she appear ill?
- Record the patient's height, weight, and vital signs. Compare his or her blood pressure bilaterally, using a cuff that is two-thirds the length of the patient's arm. Document his or her position during this procedure.
- In most cases, the patient is admitted on the morning of surgery, so baseline vital signs are extremely important. Compare these values with prehospital data, if available.
- For an inpatient, measure his or her vital signs at least every 8 hours or as ordered throughout the preoperative period. Use these measurements to establish a baseline. Document any drug or food allergies.

Systematic examination

Examine the patient thoroughly from head to toe, using these procedures as a guide.

Head and neck

- Check the patient's scalp for lesions or a parasitic infection.
- Check the jugular veins for distention.
- Note the color of the sclerae; a yellowish color suggests jaundice; a red-pink color suggests bacterial infection.
- Evert the lower eyelid and note the color of the conjunctiva. Pale tissue suggests anemia.
- Check the nose and throat for signs of respiratory tract infection.
- Assess the mouth for sores, ulcerations, or bleeding of the tongue, gums, or cheeks. Check for loose teeth, caps, partial plates, or dentures. Check the lips for bluish or gray color, which may suggest cyanosis.
- Check the neck for stiffness or cervical node enlargement.

Neurologic system

- Assess the patient's level of consciousness. Note whether the pupils are uniform in size and shape.
- Assess the patient's gross and fine motor movements.
- Inform the health care provider of any behavioral changes (for example, from lethargy to agitation). Such changes may indicate increased intracranial pressure.
- Look for neurologic abnormalities such as slurred speech. If you know or suspect that the patient has a problem, conduct a complete neurologic examination.

Extremities and skin

- Look for changes in skin color or temperature that suggest impaired circulation. Check for cyanotic nail beds and clubbing of the fingers.
- Note any skin lesions.
- Assess skin turgor for signs of dehydration.

Preoperative care for the bariatric surgery patient

Bariatric surgery serves as a last resort in the treatment of morbid obesity. Such surgery requires significant preoperative assessment and care.

Three types of bariatric surgery are performed:

- *Restrictive surgery* decreases the size of the stomach, limiting how much the patient can eat, and slowing stomach emptying.
- *Malabsorptive surgery* bypasses 7 to 9′ feet (2.1 m to 2.7 m) of small intestine, leaving only 1.5′ of intestine for absorbing nutrients.
- *Combined restrictive and malabsorptive surgery* both decreases the patient's stomach size and bypasses much of the small intestine; however, combined surgery may give the patient symptoms of dumping syndrome.

Although all three types of surgery may be performed either laparoscopically or as open surgery, most are now performed laparoscopically because of the decreased pain, fewer wound complications, shorter hospital stays, and faster recovery time associated with laparoscopic procedures.

Selecting patients

In 1991, the National Institutes of Health established guidelines for the surgical treatment of obesity. To be a candidate for surgery, the patient must be:

- 100 lb overweight *or* have a body mass index (BMI) greater than or equal to 40 kg/m^2 *or* have a BMI greater than 35 kg/m^2 accompanied by obesity-related medical conditions
- able to demonstrate a failure to lose weight with a supervised diet and exercise program
- evaluated by an experienced bariatric surgeon.

Many bariatric surgery programs also have their own, additional criteria that encourage patient responsibility and lower the risks of surgery. Many programs will not accept a patient as a candidate if he or she cannot ambulate a short distance or is on continuous oxygen therapy.

Examples of additional criteria a patient must meet include:

- quitting smoking if the patient smokes
- losing at least 10% of the patient's current weight if the patient is at his or her heaviest weight to lower the risk of postoperative complications
- agreeing to use two forms of birth control for the first 18 to 24 months after surgery if the patient is a woman of child-bearing age because pregnancy requires increasing caloric intake and limits weight loss.

Preoperative evaluation

To help determine if a patient is a candidate for bariatric surgery, psychological and nutritional counseling should take place. A psychologist will discuss the patient's previous efforts to lose weight as well as factors that contributed to the patient's success or failure. The psychologist will also assess the patient's understanding of the surgery, including the risks and necessary lifestyle and dietary changes. The patient and psychologist should identify and deal with any potential or actual obstacles to successful weight loss. Developing the relationship before surgery will make it easier for the psychologist and patient to respond to any emotional stress that may develop after surgery. A dietitian will also obtain a nutritional history and assessment.

Depending on the patient's medical history, he or she may also need evaluation and surgical clearance from other medical specialists. He or she may need diagnostic tests as well, possibly including:

- a two-dimensional echocardiogram to determine cardiac function

(continued)

Preoperative care for the bariatric surgery patient *(continued)*

- a Persantine thallium stress test to detect underlying cardiovascular disease
- a sleep study to determine if the patient has sleep apnea
- an abdominal ultrasound to check for gallstones if the patient still has his or her gallbladder; if the patient does have gallstones, he or she may also have his or her gallbladder removed during surgery.

Patient teaching

Patient teaching should start preoperatively and continue after surgery. Topics should include:
- diet
- reading food labels
- vitamin and mineral supplements
- exercise
- realistic weight-loss expectations
- possible improvements in preexisting medical conditions.

- Check the extremities for edema. Ask the patient if his or her feet, ankles, or fingers ever swell.
- Note the distribution of hair on the patient's extremities. A line of demarcation of hair on the lower extremities may indicate poor peripheral circulation.
- Check all peripheral pulses (radial, pedal, femoral, and popliteal) bilaterally. Note any differences in their quality, rate, or rhythm.
- Mark pedal pulses for reference if the patient is having a lower extremity procedure or if positioning devices may be used on the lower extremities.

Respiratory system
- Document the patient's respiratory rate and pattern. A patient with questionable pulmonary status may require an alternative to inhalation anesthesia such as a spinal block.
- Assess the patient's breathing pattern. Check for asymmetrical chest expansion and the use of accessory muscles.
- Auscultate the anterior and posterior chest for breath sounds. Listen for normal, abnormal, and adventitious

sounds. Note dyspnea on exertion or resting.
- Ask the patient if he or she has a history of respiratory disorders, such as asthma or sleep apnea. If he or she reports sleep apnea, determine whether he or she uses a continuous positive airway pressure or bilevel positive airway pressure machine at home.
- Ask the patient whether he or she smokes. If he or she does, ask how many packs per day and whether there have been recent attempts to quit or cut down in anticipation of surgery. The health care provider should have advised him or her to stop smoking 4 to 6 weeks before surgery.

 Patient Teaching Tip

Although the immediate preoperative period is not the time to have a lengthy discussion about smoking cessation, information can be placed with the patient's belongings and discussed postoperatively.

Cardiovascular system

- Inspect the patient's chest for abnormal pulsations. Auscultate at the fifth intercostal space over the left midclavicular line. If you cannot hear an apical pulse, ask the patient to turn onto his or her left side; this movement may cause the heart to shift closer to the chest wall. Note the rate and quality of the apical pulse.
- Auscultate heart sounds. If you hear thrills, suspect mitral valve regurgitation or stenosis. Murmurs that you hear on the right side of the heart are more likely to change with respiration than those you hear on the left side.
- Palpate the chest to find the point of maximal impulse.

GI system

- Note the contour and symmetry of the abdomen. Check for distention.
- Note the position and color of the umbilicus. Look for herniation.
- Auscultate bowel sounds in each quadrant. Ask the patient if his or her bowel movements are regular. Note the date of the patient's last bowel movement.
- Percuss the abdomen for air and fluid.
- Palpate the abdomen for softness, firmness, and bladder height. Note tenderness.
- Assess the six *f*'s: fat, fluids, flatus, feces, fetus (if the patient is pregnant), and fibroid tissue (or any unusual mass).

Genitourinary system

- Ask the patient about pain, burning, or bleeding during urination.
- Ask about urinary frequency and incontinence. Can he or she empty his or her bladder completely? Does he or she awaken at night to urinate?

- If indicated, monitor urine output and try to correlate excess or deficient output with the blood urea nitrogen or creatinine levels. If urine output falls, first assess the patency of the catheter and urinary drainage system, if applicable. Compare intake and output over the last several days as well as daily weight measurements.
- Note any discharge or odor from the patient's genitalia.
- If the patient is female, ask when her last menstrual period occurred and find out whether her cycle is regular. Also ask if she could be pregnant. If pregnancy is suspected, suggest that a pregnancy test be ordered.

Psychological status

- Set aside time to allow the patient to discuss his or her feelings about the impending surgery. This step is important because depression and anxiety can significantly affect recovery. Offer the patient the option of seeing a member of the clergy.
- Expect the patient to exhibit some anxiety. If the patient seems inappropriately relaxed or unconcerned, consider whether he or she is suppressing any fears. A patient who suppresses fears may cope poorly with surgical stress, and it is important to encourage him or her to seek support from family or friends. If possible, allow the patient's family and friends to visit preoperatively. Also, include them in your nursing care plan.

Teaching the preoperative patient

Your teaching can help the patient to cope with the physical and psychological stress of surgery. Because of the rising number of shorter hospital stays and same-day surgeries, preadmission and preoperative teachings have become more important than ever.

Explaining preoperative measures

Include in your teaching strategy an evaluation of the patient's understanding of his or her upcoming surgery so that you can correct misconceptions. Plan the teaching to be brief because time is limited. Use the following teaching tips as a guide:

- Urge the patient to read the surgical consent form carefully and to ask questions of the surgeon before signing the form.
- Explain that the results of chest X-rays, a complete blood count, urine studies, an electrocardiogram, and other preoperative tests will determine whether the patient is ready for surgery.
- Discuss the rationale behind hair removal, if ordered—that is, to prevent infection of the surgical wound by cleaning the skin of microorganisms found in body hair.
- Stress the importance of withholding food and fluids for a specified time before surgery.

ALERT

Tell the patient to avoid taking aspirin and nonsteroidal anti-inflammatory drugs for several days before surgery because these drugs increase the risk of bleeding.

- Inform the patient that after completing all preoperative routines, including dressing in a surgical cap and gown, he or she will receive preanesthetic medication. Tell the patient that this medication will help him or her to relax, although he or she probably will not fall asleep.
- Tell the patient that an I.V. line will be inserted either before or after he or she goes into the operating room.
- Help the patient to deal with fears about anesthesia. Assure the patient that the anesthesiologist will monitor his or her condition throughout surgery and provide the right amount of anesthetic. In most cases, an anesthesiologist will meet with the patient before hospitalization or on the morning of surgery.
- Show the patient's family where they can wait during the operation. If they want to visit the patient preoperatively, tell them to arrive 2 hours before surgery is scheduled.

AGE ALERT

When the patient is a child, you can help make the surgical experience less threatening by using therapeutic play. Follow these guidelines:

- Allow the parent or designee to remain with the child as much as possible. Some facilities allow the parent to accompany the child into the operating room.
- Allow the child to bring a familiar toy or comfort object that can accompany him or her while in the operating room and the postanesthesia care unit.
- Allow the child to choose play articles.
- Provide materials specific to the child's experiences, such as a nasogastric tube, a syringe, or bandages.
- Allow the child to participate in unstructured play.
- Provide supervision to prevent accidental injury.

Previewing operating room procedures

Educate the patient on operating room procedures:

- Warn the patient that of the probability of waiting a short time in the holding area, a special area designated for use by patients who are awaiting surgery, to allow the anesthetic to take effect. Explain that the health care providers and nurses will wear surgical attire and will observe him or her closely.
- Explain to the patient about being repeatedly asked his or her name, the name of his or her surgeon, and the type of surgery he or she is having. Reassure the patient that this is a safety precaution used at most facilities.
- When discussing transfer procedures and techniques, describe sensations that the patient will experience. Advise the patient that he or she will be taken to the operating room on a stretcher and then transferred from the stretcher to the operating table. For safety, he or she will be strapped securely to the table. The nurses in the operating room will check vital signs frequently.
- Tell the patient that the operating room may feel cold and that electrodes may be placed on the chest to monitor heart rate during surgery.
- Explain to the patient that a blood pressure cuff will be placed on his or her arm and a clip placed on one of his or her fingers to monitor blood pressure and oxygen levels.
- Describe the drowsy, floating sensation that occurs as the anesthetic takes effect and the importance of relaxing when this occurs.

Getting ready for recovery

Prepare the patient for stay in the postanesthesia care unit (PACU). Briefly describe the sensations that the patient will experience when the anesthetic wears off. Tell him or her that the PACU nurse will call his or her name and then ask him or her to answer questions and follow simple commands such as wiggling his or her toes. The patient may feel pain at the surgical site, but medications can be given to minimize the pain.

- Describe the oxygen delivery device, such as the nasal cannula, that he or she will need after surgery.
- Tell the patient that after recovery from the anesthesia, he or she will return to his or her room and be able to see his or her family, but he or she will probably feel drowsy.
- Tell the patient that you will be taking his or her blood pressure and pulse frequently, so he or she will not be alarmed by these routine procedures.
- Reduce the patient's anxiety about postoperative pain by discussing the pain-control measures you will be using. Explain that the health care provider will order pain medication to be given according to the patient's needs.

 Patient Teaching Tip

Teach the patient how to use the 0 to 10 pain scale to rate his or her pain (with 0 indicating no pain and 10 describing unbearable pain). Tell the patient to describe pain in terms of its quality and location. Encourage the patient to let you know as soon as he or she feels pain, instead of waiting until it becomes intense.

- Discuss the type of medication that the patient will receive, including how it works and the route of administration that will be used. Describe other measures you will take to relieve pain and promote comfort, such as positioning, diversionary activities, and splinting.
- Teach the patient coughing exercises, unless the patient is scheduled for neurosurgery or eye surgery. If he or she is scheduled for chest or abdominal surgery, teach him or her how to

splint the incision before coughing. Instruct the patient to take a slow, deep breath and then to breathe out through the mouth. Tell him or her to take a second breath in the same manner. Next, tell him or her to take a third deep breath and hold it. He or she should then cough two or three times to clear his or her breathing passages. Have him or her take three to five normal breaths, exhaling slowly and relaxing after each breath.

- Teach the patient how to perform deep-breathing exercises. Instruct the patient to lie on his or her back in a comfortable position, with one hand placed on the chest and the other hand placed over the upper abdomen. Instruct the patient to exhale normally, close his or her mouth, and inhale deeply through the nose. His or her chest should not expand. Ask the patient to hold his or her breath and slowly count to five. Next, ask him or her to purse the lips and exhale completely through the mouth, without letting the cheeks expand. Tell the patient to repeat the exercise 5 to 10 times.
- Teach the patient the techniques of early mobility and ambulation.
- Explain that postoperative exercises help to prevent complications, such as atelectasis, thrombophlebitis, constipation, and loss of muscle tone. Explain to the patient that he or she may need to wear leg wraps, called sequential compression devices, until he or she is ambulatory. These devices compress the calf muscles to simulate walking.
- Demonstrate how to use an incentive spirometer and have the patient perform a return demonstration. Explain that this device will provide feedback when he or she is performing deep-breathing exercises. Explain how simple leg exercises, such as alternately contracting the calf muscles, will prevent venous pooling after surgery.

(Text continues on page 432.)

Identifying hazardous drugs

Some drugs may cause hazardous complications or interactions during or after surgery. Always review the patient's medication record carefully before he or she undergoes surgery. Use this chart to identify common drugs that can be hazardous to the patient undergoing surgery.

Drug	Possible effect
Antianxiety drugs	
diazepam Valium	• Excessive sedation • Preoperative or postoperative nausea and vomiting • Local tissue irritation (with I.V. administration)
hydroxyzine hydrochloride Vistaril	• Drowsiness and dry mouth
midazolam hydrochloride	• Respiratory depression (with high doses)

Identifying hazardous drugs *(continued)*

Drug	Possible effect
Antiarrhythmics	
All types	• Laryngospasm • Intensified cardiac depression and reduced cardiac output
procainamide	• Prolonged or enhanced effects of neuromuscular blockers • Hypotension
propranolol Inderal	• Prolonged or enhanced effects of neuromuscular blockers • Depressed myocardial function • Hypotension • Laryngospasm
Antibiotics	
All types	• Masked symptoms of infection
Aminoglycosides amikacin, gentamicin, kanamycin, neomycin, streptomycin, tobramycin	• Increased risk of neuromuscular blockade and respiratory paralysis
erythromycin Erythrocin, E-Mycin	• Prolonged action of opiates
Anticholinergics	
atropine sulfate	• Excessive dryness of the mouth, tachycardia, flushing, and decreased sweating • Increased intraocular pressure (IOP), blurred vision, and dilated pupils • Urine retention • Agitation and delirium (in elderly patients)
glycopyrrolate Robinul	• Excessive dryness of the mouth, tachycardia, flushing, and decreased sweating • Increased IOP, blurred vision, and dilated pupils • Urine retention
scopolamine bromide	• Excessive dryness of the mouth, tachycardia, and flushing • Increased IOP, blurred vision, and dilated pupils • Urine retention • Excessive drowsiness • Agitation and delirium (in elderly patients)

(continued)

Identifying hazardous drugs *(continued)*

Drug	Possible effect
Anticoagulants	
heparin sodium warfarin Coumadin	• Increased risk of hemorrhage
Anticonvulsants	
magnesium sulfate	• Increased risk of neuromuscular blockade
Antidiabetics	
insulin	• Increased insulin requirement during stress and healing • Decreased insulin requirement during fasting
Antihypertensives	
All types	• Worsened hypotension
Central nervous system depressants	
Alcohol, sedative hypnotics	• If given with general anesthetics, increased risk of respiratory depression, apnea, or hypotension
Corticosteroids	
betamethasone, cortisone, dexamethasone, hydrocortisone, methylprednisolone, prednisolone, prednisone, triamcinolone	• Delayed wound healing • Risk of acute adrenal insufficiency • Increased risk of infection • Masked symptoms of infection • Increased risk of hemorrhage
Diuretics	
furosemide Lasix Potassium-wasting diuretics	• If given with certain anesthetics, increased risk of hypotension • Increased risk of complications associated with hypokalemia
Histamine-2 receptor antagonists	
cimetidine Tagamet ranitidine Zantac	• Decreased clearance of all drugs, especially diazepam, lidocaine, and propranolol

Identifying hazardous drugs (continued)

Drug	Possible effect
Myotics	
demecarium, echothiophate, isoflurophate	• If given with succinylcholine, increased risk of neuromuscular blockade, cardiovascular collapse, prolonged respiratory depression, or apnea (Effects may occur up to a few months after the patient stops taking the drug.)
Nonsteroidal anti-inflammatory drugs	
celecoxib, ibuprofen, meloxicam, naproxen, rofecoxib	• Increased risk of bleeding or hemorrhage
Opiates	
All types	• If given with certain I.V. anesthetics (such as midazolam, propofol, thiopental, and droperidol), increased risk of respiratory depression, apnea, or hypotension
Opioids	
meperidine hydrochloride Demerol morphine	• Depressed respiration, circulation, and gastric motility • Dizziness, tachycardia, and sweating • Hypotension, restlessness, and excitement • Preoperative or postoperative nausea and vomiting
Sedative-hypnotics	
pentobarbital sodium Nembutal	• Confusion or excitement, especially in elderly patients or patients with severe pain
Thyroid hormones	
All types	• If given with ketamine, increased risk of hypertension and tachycardia
Tranquilizers	
promethazine hydrochloride Phenergan	• Postoperative hypotension

Reviewing care on the day of surgery

Early on the day of surgery, follow these procedures:

- Verify that the patient has had nothing by mouth since midnight.
- Verify that the patient took all prescribed medications as instructed.
- Make sure the patient has not taken any medications that have been prohibited, such as aspirin.
- Make sure that the diagnostic test results appear on the chart.
- Verify that all documentation, including informed consent, has been signed and completed.
- Ask the patient to remove jewelry, makeup, and nail polish, if applicable; to shower with antimicrobial soap, if ordered; and to perform mouth care.
- Instruct the patient to remove dentures or partial plates. Note on the chart whether he or she has dental crowns, caps, or braces. Also instruct him or her to remove contact lenses, glasses, prostheses, and hearing aids, if applicable. Policies for the removal of hearing aids vary among health care facilities. Some facilities allow the patient to leave in the hearing aid if it helps him or her to follow instructions. Document whether the patient is wearing a hearing aid into the operating room.
- Tell the patient to void and to put on a surgical cap and gown.
- Take and record the patient's vital signs.
- Reassure the patient and answer any last-minute questions he or she may have.
- Give preoperative medication, if ordered.

Preparing the bowel for surgery

The extent of bowel preparation depends on the type and site of surgery. For example, a patient who is scheduled for several days of postoperative bed rest and has not had a recent bowel movement may receive a mild laxative or an enema. However, a patient who is scheduled for gastrointestinal (GI), pelvic, perianal, or rectal surgery will undergo more extensive preparation.

Preoperative enemas or an osmotic cathartic solution, such as magnesium citrate, may help to empty the intestine, thereby minimizing injury to the colon and improving visualization of the operative site.

Expect to perform extensive preparation for the patient undergoing elective colon surgery. During surgical opening of the colon, escaping bacteria may invade the adjacent tissue, leading to infection. Perform a mechanical preparation and administer antimicrobials, as ordered. Mechanical bowel preparation removes gross stool; oral antimicrobials suppress potent microflora without encouraging resistant strains.

If enemas are ordered to clear the bowel, and the third enema still has not removed all the stool, notify the health care provider. Repeated enemas may cause fluid and electrolyte imbalances.

 AGE ALERT

The elderly patient who is allowed nothing by mouth and has not received I.V. fluids is at increased risk for fluid and electrolyte imbalances.

Preparing the skin for surgery

Before surgery, the patient's skin must be as free from microorganisms as possible to reduce the risk of infection at the incision site.

Hair removal should be done as close as possible to the time of surgery, such as while the patient is in the holding area and should be performed with a clipper.

(Text continues on page 440.)

Reviewing common neuromuscular blockers

Drug	Adverse effects	Special considerations
Nondepolarizing neuromuscular blockers		
atracurium besylate	• Slight hypotension in a few patients	• Acts for 20 to 30 minutes • May cause slight histamine release • Does not accumulate with repeated doses • Is useful for a patient with underlying hepatic, renal, or cardiac disease
pancuronium bromide	• Tachycardia • Transient rash and a burning sensation at the injection site	• Acts for 35 to 45 minutes • Is five times more potent than curare • Does not cause ganglion blockage, so it usually does not lead to hypotension • Has a vagolytic action that increases heart rate
vecuronium bromide	• Minimal and transient cardiovascular effects • Weakness or paralysis of the skeletal muscles; respiratory insufficiency; respiratory paralysis; prolonged, dose-related apnea	• Acts for 25 to 40 minutes • Is probably metabolized mostly in the liver • Has a short duration of action and causes fewer cardiovascular effects than other nondepolarizing neuromuscular blockers
Depolarizing neuromuscular blockers		
succinylcholine chloride Anectine, Quelicin	• Respiratory depression • Bradycardia • Excessive salivation • Hypotension • Arrhythmias • Tachycardia • Hypertension • Increased intraocular and intragastric pressure • Fasciculations • Muscle pain • Malignant hyperthermia	• Acts for 5 to 10 minutes • Is metabolized mostly in the plasma by pseudocholinesterase; therefore, it is contraindicated in the patient with a deficiency of plasma cholinesterase as a result of a genetic variant defect, liver disease, uremia, or malnutrition • Is used cautiously in patients with glaucoma or penetrating wounds of the eye; those undergoing eye surgery; those with burns, severe trauma, spinal cord injuries, or muscular dystrophy; and those with cardiovascular, hepatic, pulmonary, metabolic, or renal disorders; may cause sudden hyperkalemia and consequent cardiac arrest • Can cause pregnant patients who also receive magnesium sulfate to experience increased neuromuscular blockade because of decreased pseudocholinesterase levels

Reviewing common general anesthetics

Drug	Indications	Advantages
Inhalation agents		
nitrous oxide	• Maintains anesthesia • May provide an adjunct for inducing general anesthesia	• Has little effect on heart rate, myocardial contractility, respiration, blood pressure, liver, kidneys, or metabolism in the absence of hypoxia • Produces excellent analgesia • Allows for rapid induction and recovery • Does not increase capillary bleeding • Does not sensitize the myocardium to epinephrine
halothane	• Maintains general anesthesia	• Is easy to administer • Allows for rapid, smooth induction and recovery • Has a relatively pleasant odor and is nonirritating • Decreases salivary and bronchial secretions • Causes bronchodilation • Easily suppresses pharyngeal and laryngeal reflexes
enflurane Ethrane	• Maintains anesthesia • Occasionally used to induce anesthesia	• Allows for rapid induction and recovery • Is nonirritating and eliminates secretions • Causes bronchodilation • Provides good muscle relaxation • Allows cardiac rhythm to remain stable
isoflurane Forane	• Maintains general anesthesia • Occasionally used to induce general anesthesia	• Allows for rapid induction and recovery • Causes bronchodilation • Provides excellent muscle relaxation • Allows for an extremely stable cardiac rhythm

Disadvantages	Nursing interventions
• Excessive amounts may cause hypoxia. • Does not relax muscles (Procedures requiring muscular relaxation require the addition of a neuromuscular blocker.) • Soluble gas can diffuse into air-containing cavities, such as the chest or bowel.	• Monitor the patient for signs of hypoxia. (Always give with oxygen to prevent hypoxia.)
• May cause myocardial depression, leading to arrhythmias • Sensitizes the heart to the action of catecholamine • May cause circulatory or respiratory depression, depending on the dose • Has no analgesic property	• Watch for arrhythmias, hypotension, and respiratory depression. • Monitor the patient for a decrease in body temperature; he or she may shiver after prolonged use. Shivering increases oxygen consumption.
• Causes myocardial depression • Lowers the seizure threshold • Increases hypotension as the depth of anesthesia increases • May cause shivering during recovery • May cause circulatory or respiratory depression, depending on the dose • May increase intracranial pressure	• Monitor the patient for decreased heart and respiratory rates and hypotension. • Watch for shivering, which increases oxygen consumption.
• May cause circulatory or respiratory depression, depending on the dose • Potentiates the action of nondepolarizing muscle relaxants • May cause shivering • Tends to lower blood pressure as the depth of anesthesia increases; pulse remains somewhat elevated	• Watch for respiratory depression and hypotension. • Watch for shivering, which increases oxygen consumption.

(continued)

Reviewing common general anesthetics *(continued)*

Drug	Indications	Advantages
Inhalation agents (continued)		
desflurane Suprane	• Induces and maintains general anesthesia	• Can use decreased doses for neuromuscular blockers • Increased doses for maintenance anesthesia may produce dose-dependent hypotension.
sevoflurane Ultane	• Induces and maintains general anesthesia in adults and children	• Nonpungent odor • No respiratory irritability • Suitable for use with mask induction
I.V. barbiturates		
thiopental sodium	• Used primarily to induce general anesthesia	• Promotes rapid, smooth, and pleasant induction and quick recovery • Rarely causes complications • Does not sensitize the autonomic tissues of the heart to catecholamines
I.V. benzodiazepines		
diazepam Valium	• Induces general anesthesia • Provides amnesia during balanced anesthesia	• Minimally affects the cardiovascular system • Acts as a potent anticonvulsant • Produces amnesia
midazolam hydrochloride	• Induces general anesthesia • Provides amnesia during balanced anesthesia	• Minimally affects the cardiovascular system • Acts as a potent anticonvulsant • Produces amnesia

Disadvantages	Nursing interventions
• May increase heart rate • Respiratory irritant effect is more likely in an adult during induction of anesthesia via mask • Not recommended for induction of general anesthesia in infants or children because of high incidence of laryngospasm or other adverse respiratory effects (After anesthesia is induced and tracheal intubation is achieved, it can be used for maintenance anesthesia.) • Not indicated for patients with coronary artery disease or for those who will be adversely affected by increases in heart rate	• Monitor the patient's vital signs, especially heart rate and blood pressure. • Watch for shivering, which increases oxygen consumption.
• Dose-related cardiac depressant	• Monitor the patient's vital signs. • Watch for shivering, which increases oxygen consumption.
• Is associated with airway obstruction, respiratory depression, and laryngospasm, possibly leading to hypoxia • Does not provide muscle relaxation and produces little analgesia • May cause cardiovascular depression, especially in hypovolemic or debilitated patients	• Watch for signs and symptoms of hypoxia, airway obstruction, and cardiovascular and respiratory depression.
• May cause irritation when injected into a peripheral vein • Has a long elimination half-life	• Monitor the patient's vital signs, respiratory rate, and volume.
• Can cause respiratory depression	• Monitor the patient's vital signs, especially respiratory rate and volume.

(continued)

Reviewing common general anesthetics *(continued)*

Drug	Indications	Advantages
I.V. nonbarbiturates		
propofol Diprivan	• Used for induction and maintenance of anesthesia; particularly useful for short procedures and outpatient surgery	• Allows for rapid, smooth induction • Permits rapid awakening and recovery • Causes less vomiting than other anesthetics
dexmedetomidine Precedex	• Alpha$_2$-agonist, sedative with analgesic properties. Controls stress, anxiety, and pain, by facilitating patient comfort, compliance, and comprehension.	• Homeostatic cardiovascular reflexes maintained • Short duration of action • Does not cause respiratory depression • Decrease amount of inhalation anesthetics and opioids needed.
ketamine hydrochloride Ketalar	• Produces a dissociative state of consciousness; induces anesthesia when a barbiturate is contraindicated; sole anesthetic agent for short diagnostic and surgical procedures that do not require relaxation of the skeletal muscles	• Produces rapid anesthesia and profound analgesia • Does not irritate the veins or tissues • Maintains a patent airway without endotracheal intubation because it suppresses laryngeal and pharyngeal reflexes
I.V. tranquilizers		
droperidol Inapsine	• Used preoperatively and during induction and maintenance of anesthesia as an adjunct to general or regional anesthesia	• Allows for rapid, smooth induction and recovery • Produces sleepiness and mental detachment for several hours
Opioids		
fentanyl citrate Sublimaze	• Used preoperatively for minor and major surgery, urologic procedures, and gastroscopy; also used as an adjunct to regional anesthesia and to induce and maintain general anesthesia	• Promotes rapid, smooth induction and recovery • Does not cause histamine release • Minimally affects the cardiovascular system • Can be reversed by a opioid antagonist (naloxone)

Disadvantages	Nursing interventions
• Can cause hypotension • Can cause pain if injected into small veins • May cause clonic or myoclonic movements on emergence • May interact with benzodiazepines, increasing the effects of propofol • Does not cause profound analgesia	• Monitor the patient for hypotension. • Prepare the patient for rapid emergence.
• May cause significant bradycardia and hypotension • There may be symptoms of nervousness, agitation, headaches, and a rapid increase in blood pressure when the infusion is discontinued.	• Monitor for bradycardia and hypotension. • If necessary stop infusing drug and increase fluid infusion. • May need to administer anticholinergic for persistent bradycardia
• May cause unpleasant dreams, hallucinations, and delirium during recovery • Increases heart rate, blood pressure, and intraocular pressure • Preserves muscle tone, leading to poor relaxation during surgery	• Protect the patient from visual, tactile, and auditory stimuli during recovery. • Monitor the patient's vital signs.
• May cause hypotension because it is a peripheral vasodilator • Contraindicated in patients with known or suspected prolonged QT interval	• Monitor the patient for increased pulse rate, hypotension, and prolonged QT interval.
• May cause respiratory depression, euphoria, bradycardia, bronchoconstriction, nausea, vomiting, and miosis • May cause rigidity of the skeletal muscles and chest wall	• Observe the patient for respiratory depression. • Watch for nausea and vomiting. If vomiting occurs, position the patient to prevent aspiration. • Monitor the patient's blood pressure. • Decrease postoperative opioids to one-third or one-fourth the usual dose.

Postoperative care

Monitoring the postoperative patient

The goal of monitoring the postoperative patient is to minimize complications through early detection and prompt treatment. (See *Postoperative care for the bariatric surgery patient*, pages 441 and 442.)

Equipment

Thermometer • watch with a second hand • stethoscope • sphygmomanometer or automated blood pressure machine • postoperative flowchart or other documentation tool

Implementation

- Obtain the patient's record from the nurse in the PACU.
- Transfer the patient from the PACU stretcher to the bed. Position him or her properly. Keep transfer movements smooth to minimize pain and complications.
- If the patient has had orthopedic surgery, have a coworker move the affected extremity as you transfer the patient.
- If the patient is in skeletal traction, have a coworker move the weights as you and another coworker transfer the patient.
- Ensure the patient's comfort and raise the side rails of the bed to ensure safety.
- Assess the patient's level of consciousness.
- Monitor the patient's respiratory status by assessing the airway. Note the breathing rate and depth; auscultate breath sounds. If ordered, administer oxygen and initiate oximetry.
- Monitor the patient's postoperative pulse rate, which should be within 20% of the preoperative rate.
- Compare the patient's postoperative blood pressure with his or her preoperative blood pressure. It should be within 20% of the preoperative level unless the patient had a hypotensive episode during surgery.
- Assess the patient's ability to wiggle his or her toes. Assess the level of sensation if he or she received spinal anesthesia.
- Assess the patient's body temperature. If it is lower than 95.6° F (35.3° C), apply blankets and notify the health care provider. Lowered body temperature causes shivering, which increases the body's consumption of oxygen and may strain the heart's normal function.
- Assess the patient's infusion sites for redness, pain, swelling, and drainage.
- Assess the surgical wound dressings. If they are soiled, assess the drainage and outline the soiled area. Note the date and time of assessment on the dressing. Check the soiled area often; if it enlarges, reinforce the dressing and alert the health care provider.
- Note the presence and condition of drains and tubes. Note the color, type, odor, and amount of drainage as well as any sediment. Make sure that all drains are properly connected and free from kinks and obstructions.
- If the patient had vascular or orthopedic surgery, assess the appropriate extremities. Notify the health care provider of abnormalities. Make sure that any special positioning requirements, such as no hip adduction, are clearly posted for all patient caregivers to see.
- As the patient recovers from anesthesia, monitor his or her respiratory and cardiovascular status closely. Watch for airway obstruction and hypoventilation caused by laryngospasm. Also watch for sedation, which can lead to hypoxemia.

Postoperative care for the bariatric surgery patient

Postoperative care plays a crucial role in recovery from bariatric surgery. Following surgery, the patient is typically transferred to a medical-surgical unit. Once there, the patient typically needs extra attention because obesity leaves little reserve to cope with postoperative complications. Specialized materials that may be needed for such care include bariatric equipment and transfer aid devices, larger gowns, extra-large blood pressure cuffs, appropriately sized bed and support surfaces, and floor-mounted toilets.

Postoperative care focuses on preventing cardiovascular complications, particularly venous thromboembolism; providing respiratory care; meeting nutritional and hydration needs; and caring for the patient's skin.

Cardiovascular care

Because obesity increases intra-abdominal pressure, the patient recovering from bariatric surgery is at increased risk for venous thromboembolism; anesthesia during surgery may add to that risk by further increasing abdominal pressure. Other factors that increase the risk include immobility after surgery and venous stasis.

Postoperative care can help prevent the development of a pulmonary embolus—a life-threatening postoperative complication—and deep venous thromboembolism of the lower extremities. If the patient is at particular risk, he or she may also have an inferior vena cava filter placed before surgery.

Specific postoperative measures include:
- early ambulation
- use of sequential compression devices
- use of compression stockings
- prophylaxis with anticoagulants.

Respiratory care

In the morbidly obese patient, abdominal adipose tissue raises the diaphragm, which prevents its full movement when the patient breathes and leads to the collapse of the alveoli in the base of the lungs. This decrease in lung movement leads to the retention of carbon dioxide. As a result, the patient may feel sleepy, become apneic for short periods, and develop hypoxemia. Anesthetics during surgery and pain medication postoperatively may worsen these conditions, making postoperative respiratory care even more important.

Postoperative measures to prevent such respiratory complications as atelectasis or pneumonia include:
- elevating the head of the bed to 30 to 45 degrees
- promoting coughing and deep-breathing exercises
- providing incentive spirometry, as ordered
- encouraging early ambulation
- using continuous positive airway pressure or bilevel positive airway pressure (for the patient with a history of sleep apnea who uses one of these interventions at home).

Nutrition and hydration

Before receiving any fluids or food postoperatively, the bariatric surgery patient must undergo a limited upper gastrointestinal X-ray to look for any anastomotic leak or obstruction. If the test is negative, the patient can begin drinking water and advance to a liquid or pureed diet for the first 2 weeks after surgery. He or she can progress to soft foods 1 month after surgery, and after 6 months, he or she can begin to eat foods of normal texture. For the first 3 to 6 months, the patient must eat at specified times because he or she will not feel hungry.

The main goal at each of these stages is to take in sufficient protein. Once the patient can tolerate 3 to 4 oz (85 to 113 g) of protein-rich foods at a meal, he or she should add fruits and vegetables to his or her diet. The dietary goal is a minimum of 2 oz (60 g) of protein daily.

(continued)

Postoperative care for the bariatric surgery patient (continued)

Because the gastric pouch is swollen and stiff for the first month after surgery, the patient can drink only small sips of liquid, increasing the risk of dehydration. The patient may only be able to drink an average of 1 oz (28 ml) of liquid over 15 minutes. This restriction may make it physically impossible for the patient to meet the goal of 64 oz (2 L) of liquid daily.

Nausea, an early sign of dehydration, may cause the patient to drink even less, further complicating the situation. To combat this, the patient should be encouraged to "drink through" the nausea. If he or she can do that, the nausea should subside and he or she may be able to drink enough to prevent dehydration. If he or she cannot maintain adequate hydration on his or her own after discharge, he or she may need to go to an outpatient clinic to receive I.V. fluids.

Skin care

The obese patient has many skin folds, which can harbor moisture and microorganisms. As a result, the patient recovering from bariatric surgery is at higher risk for skin breakdown. The poor blood supply to adipose tissue may also lead to poor wound healing.

Preventive measures include:
- inspecting the skin every 8 hours (more frequently if needed), with special attention paid to areas of increased pressure and skin folds
- frequent turning (at least every 2 hours)
- early ambulation
- positioning of catheters and drainage tubes so that they do not become trapped in skin folds
- not using powders.

- Encourage coughing and deep-breathing exercises, unless the patient had nasal, ophthalmic, or neurologic surgery.
- Administer postoperative medications, as ordered.
- Remove all fluids from the patient's bedside until he or she is alert enough to eat and drink. Before giving liquids, assess his or her gag reflex.

Special considerations
- If the patient had epidural anesthesia or a postoperative continuous epidural opioid, monitor his or her respiratory status closely. The respiratory rate and quality, along with oxygen saturation levels, should be assessed every hour for at least the first 24 hours.

Preventing postoperative complications

After surgery, take these steps to avoid complications.

Turn and reposition the patient

Turning and repositioning the patient every 2 hours promote circulation, thereby reducing the risk of skin breakdown, especially over bony prominences. When the patient is in a lateral recumbent position, tuck pillows under bony prominences to reduce friction and promote comfort. Each time you turn him or her, inspect the skin carefully to detect redness or other signs of breakdown.

Turning and repositioning may be contraindicated in some cases, such as the patient who underwent neurologic or musculoskeletal surgery that requires postoperative immobilization.

Encourage coughing and deep breathing

Deep breathing promotes lung expansion, which helps to clear anesthetics from the body. Coughing and deep breathing also lower the risk of pulmonary and fat emboli and of hypostatic pneumonia associated with the buildup of secretions in the airways.

Encourage the patient to perform deep-breathing exercises at least every 2 hours and to cough. Show the patient how to splint the incision with his or her hands or a pillow to reduce pain. Also show him or her how to use an incentive spirometer. Because deep breathing does not increase intracranial pressure, it is safe to do after most neurosurgical procedures.

Monitor nutrition and fluids

Adequate nutrition and fluid intake are essential to ensure proper hydration, promote healing, and provide the energy needed to accommodate the increased basal metabolism associated with surgery. If the patient has a protein deficiency or compromised immune function preoperatively, expect to deliver supplemental protein by parenteral nutrition to promote healing. If the patient has renal failure, this treatment is contraindicated because his or her inability to break down protein could lead to dangerously high blood nitrogen levels.

Promote exercise and ambulation

Early postoperative exercise and ambulation can significantly reduce the risk of thromboembolism and improve ventilation. To encourage compliance, assess the patient's pain level before these activities and administer analgesics, as ordered.

Perform passive range-of-motion exercises to prevent joint contractures and muscle atrophy and promote circulation. These exercises can also help you to assess the patient's strength and tolerance.

Before encouraging ambulation, ask the patient to dangle his or her legs over the side of the bed and perform deep-breathing exercises. How well a

patient tolerates this step is commonly a key predictor of out-of-bed tolerance.

Begin ambulation by helping the patient to walk a few feet from the bed to a sturdy chair. Then have him or her gradually progress each day from ambulating in the room to ambulating in the hallway, with or without assistance, as necessary. Document the frequency of ambulation and the patient's tolerance, including the use of an analgesic.

Managing postoperative complications

Despite your best efforts, complications can occur. By knowing how to recognize and manage them, you can limit their effects.

The following is a list of complications. Some complications are more likely to produce acute changes, whereas others produce symptoms slowly. Also, some complications occur in the immediate postoperative period, and others are more prominent 2 or 3 days after surgery.

Abdominal distention, paralytic ileus, and constipation

Sluggish peristalsis and paralytic ileus usually last for 24 to 72 hours after surgery and cause abdominal distention. Paralytic ileus occurs whenever autonomic innervation of the GI tract is disrupted. Causes include intraoperative manipulation of the intestinal organs, hypokalemia, wound infection, and the use of codeine, morphine, or atropine. Postoperative constipation usually stems from colonic ileus caused by diminished GI motility and impaired perception of rectal fullness.

Assessment
• To detect abdominal distention, monitor the patient's abdominal girth and ask the patient if he or she feels bloated.
• To assess the patient for paralytic ileus, auscultate for bowel sounds in

all four quadrants. Notify the health care provider of decreased or absent bowel sounds.

- Monitor abdominal distention and the passage of flatus or stool.
- Ask the patient about feelings of nausea or abdominal fullness.

Interventions

- To treat abdominal distention, encourage ambulation and give nothing by mouth until bowel sounds return.
- Insert a rectal or nasogastric (NG) tube, as ordered. Keep the NG tube patent and functioning properly.
- To treat paralytic ileus, encourage ambulation and administer medications, as ordered. If it does not resolve within 24 to 48 hours, insert an NG tube, as ordered. Keep the NG tube patent and functioning properly.
- To treat constipation, encourage ambulation and administer a stool softener, laxative, or nonnarcotic analgesic, as ordered.

Atelectasis and pneumonia

After surgery, atelectasis may occur as a result of hypoventilation and excessive retained secretions. This provides a medium for bacterial growth and sets the stage for stasis pneumonia.

Assessment

- To detect atelectasis, auscultate for diminished or absent breath sounds over the affected area and note dullness on percussion.
- Assess the patient for decreased chest expansion; mediastinal shift toward the side of collapse; fever; restlessness or confusion; worsening dyspnea; and elevated blood pressure, pulse rate, and respiratory rate.
- To detect pneumonia, watch for sudden onset of shaking chills with high fever and headache.

- Auscultate for diminished breath sounds or for telltale crackles over the affected area of the lung.
- Assess the patient for dyspnea, tachypnea, sharp chest pain exacerbated by inspiration, productive cough with pinkish or rust-colored sputum, and cyanosis with hypoxemia that is confirmed by arterial blood gas measurement.
- Chest X-rays show patchy infiltrates or areas of consolidation.

Interventions

- Encourage the patient to perform deep-breathing exercises and cough every hour while awake.

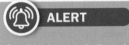

ALERT

Coughing is contraindicated in the patient who underwent neurosurgery or eye surgery.

- Demonstrate how to use an incentive spirometer.
- As ordered, perform chest physiotherapy, give an antibiotic, and administer humidified air or oxygen.
- Reposition the patient every 2 hours. Elevate the head of the bed.

Hypovolemia

A total blood volume loss of 15% to 25% may result from blood loss and severe dehydration, third-space fluid sequestration (as in burns, peritonitis, intestinal obstruction, or acute pancreatitis), and fluid loss (as in excessive vomiting or diarrhea).

Assessment

- Check for hypotension and a rapid, weak pulse.
- Note cool, clammy, and perhaps, mottled skin.

- Check for rapid, shallow respirations.
- Assess the patient for oliguria or anuria and lethargy.

Interventions

- To increase blood pressure, administer an I.V. crystalloid, such as normal saline solution or lactated Ringer's solution.
- To restore urine output and fluid volume, give a colloid, such as plasma, albumin, or dextran.

Pericarditis

Pericarditis is an acute or chronic inflammation of the pericardium—the fibroserous sac that envelops, supports, and protects the heart. After surgery, pericarditis may result from bacterial, fungal, or viral infection or from postcardiac injury that leaves the pericardium intact but causes blood to leak into the pericardial cavity.

Assessment

- To detect pericarditis, assess the patient for sharp, sudden pain that starts over the sternum and radiates to the neck, shoulders, back, and arms.
- Ask the patient to take a deep breath and then to sit up and lean forward. Pericardial pain is commonly pleuritic, increasing with deep inspiration and decreasing when the patient sits up and leans forward. You also may hear a pericardial friction rub.

Interventions

- Keep the patient on complete bed rest in an upright position.
- Provide an analgesic and oxygen, as ordered.
- Assess the patient's pain in relation to respiration and body position to distinguish pericardial pain from pain related to myocardial ischemia.
- Monitor the patient for signs of cardiac compression or cardiac tamponade. Signs include decreased blood pressure, increased central

venous pressure, and paradoxical pulse. Because cardiac tamponade requires immediate treatment, keep a pericardiocentesis set at the patient's bedside whenever pericardial effusion is suspected.

Postoperative psychosis

Mental aberrations typically stem from physiologic causes (cerebral anoxia, fluid and electrolyte imbalance, malnutrition, and such drugs as tranquilizers, sedatives, and opioids). However, psychological causes (fear, pain, and disorientation) can also contribute.

Assessment

- Assess the patient's mental status and compare it with the preoperative baseline.

Interventions

- Reorient the patient frequently to time, place, and person. Call the patient by his or her preferred name and encourage him or her to move about.
- Provide clean eyeglasses and a working hearing aid, if appropriate. Use sedatives and restraints only if needed.

Septicemia and septic shock

Septicemia may stem from a break in asepsis during surgery or wound care or from peritonitis (as in ruptured appendix or ectopic pregnancy). The most common cause of postoperative septicemia is *Escherichia coli.* Septic shock occurs when bacteria release endotoxins into the bloodstream, decreasing vascular resistance and causing dramatic hypotension.

Assessment

- To detect septicemia, check for fever, chills, rash, abdominal distention, prostration, pain, headache, nausea, and diarrhea.
- Early indicators of septic shock include fever and chills; warm, dry, flushed skin; slightly altered mental

status; increased pulse and respiratory rates; decreased or normal blood pressure; and reduced urine output.

- Late indicators include pale, moist, cold skin as well as decreased mental status, pulse and respiratory rates, blood pressure, and urine output.

Interventions

- To treat septicemia, obtain a urine specimen and blood and wound samples for culture and sensitivity tests.
- Administer an antibiotic, if ordered.
- Monitor the patient's vital signs and level of consciousness.
- To treat septic shock, administer an I.V. antibiotic, if ordered.
- Monitor serum peak and trough levels.
- Give I.V. fluids and blood or blood products to restore circulating blood volume.

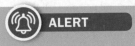

ALERT

Keep in mind that prompt identification and intervention is the key to helping the patient survive septicemia and septic shock.

Thrombophlebitis and pulmonary embolism

Postoperative venous stasis associated with immobility may lead to thrombophlebitis—an inflammation of a vein, usually in the leg, accompanied by formation of a clot. If a clot breaks away, it may become lodged in the lung, causing a pulmonary embolism.

Assessment

- To detect thrombophlebitis, ask the high-risk patient about leg pain, functional impairment, and edema.
- Inspect the patient's legs from feet to groin and record calf circumference. Note engorgement of the cavity behind the medial malleolus and increased temperature in the affected leg. Identify areas of cordlike venous segments.
- To detect a pulmonary embolism, assess the patient for sudden anginal or pleuritic chest pain; dyspnea; rapid, shallow respirations; cyanosis; restlessness; and possibly a thready pulse.
- Auscultate for fine to coarse crackles over the affected lung.

Interventions

- To treat thrombophlebitis, elevate the affected leg and apply warm compresses.
- Administer medications, as ordered.
- Monitor laboratory values, such as prothrombin and partial thromboplastin times, daily.
- To treat a pulmonary embolism, administer oxygen and medications, as ordered. Elevate the head of the bed.

Urine retention

The patient may not be able to void spontaneously within 12 hours after surgery. Urine retention is usually transient and reversible.

Assessment

- Monitor the patient's intake and output.
- Assess the patient for bladder distention above the level of the symphysis pubis as well as for discomfort and pain. Note restlessness, anxiety, diaphoresis, and hypertension.

Interventions

- To treat urine retention, help the patient to ambulate as soon as possible after surgery, unless contraindicated.
- Assist the patient to a normal voiding position and, if possible, leave him or her alone.
- Turn the water on so that the patient can hear it and pour warm water over the perineum.
- If these interventions are not successful, prepare the patient for urinary catheterization.

Wound infection

The most common wound complication, wound infection is also a major factor in wound dehiscence. Complete dehiscence leads to evisceration.

Assessment

- To detect infection, assess surgical wounds for increased tenderness, deep pain, and edema, especially from the third to the fifth day after the operation.
- Monitor the patient for increased pulse rate and temperature and an elevated white blood cell count.
- Note a temperature pattern of spikes in the afternoon or evening, with a return to normal by morning.

Interventions

- As ordered, obtain a wound culture and sensitivity test, administer antibiotics, and irrigate the wound with an appropriate solution, if ordered.
- Monitor wound drainage.

Caring for surgical wounds

Proper care of surgical wounds helps to prevent infection, protects the skin from maceration and excoriation, allows removal and measurement of wound drainage, and promotes patient comfort. When a surgical incision is closed primarily, it is covered with a sterile dressing for 24 to 48 hours. After 48 hours, the incision can be covered by a dressing or left open to air.

Managing a draining wound involves two techniques: dressing and pouching. Dressing is indicated when drainage does not compromise the integrity of the skin. Lightly seeping wounds with drains and wounds with minimal purulent drainage can usually be managed with packing and gauze dressings. Surgical incisions that are left open at the skin level for a few days before closure by the health care provider (delayed primary closure) are managed by packing with a sterile dressing. Incisions that are left open to heal by primary intention are packed with sterile moist gauze and covered with a sterile dressing.

Wounds that drain more than 100 ml in 24 hours and those with excoriating drainage require pouching.

Equipment and preparation

Waterproof trash bag or trash can • clean gloves • sterile gloves • gown, if indicated • sterile 4″ × 4″ gauze pads • abdominal bandage dressing pads, if needed • sterile cotton-tipped applicators • topical medication or ointment, if ordered • prescribed cleaning agent, if ordered • sterile container • adhesive or other tape • soap and water • optional: skin protectant, acetone-free adhesive remover or baby oil, sterile normal saline solution, a graduated container, and Montgomery straps or a T-binder

For a wound with a drain
Precut sterile 4″ × 4″ gauze pads • adhesive tape

For pouching
Pouch with or without a drainage port • skin protectant • sterile gauze pad

Determine the type of dressing needed and assemble all equipment in the patient's room. Check the expiration date on each sterile package and inspect the package for tears. Place the trash bag or trash can so that you can avoid carrying articles across the sterile field or the wound when disposing of them.

Implementation

- Check the health care provider's order for wound care instructions. Some health care providers prefer to not use cleaning agents on surgical incisions unless the area is soiled.
- Note the location of drains to avoid dislodging them during the procedure.

- Explain the procedure to the patient and position him or her properly. Expose only the wound site.
- Wash your hands. Put on a gown, if necessary, and clean gloves.

Removing the old dressing

- Hold the skin and pull the tape or dressing toward the wound. This protects newly formed tissue. Use acetone-free adhesive remover or baby oil, if needed. Do not apply solvents to the incision.
- Remove the soiled dressing. If needed, loosen gauze with sterile normal saline solution.
- Check the dressing to determine the amount, type, color, and odor of drainage. Discard the dressing and gloves in the waterproof trash bag.
- If ordered, obtain a wound culture.

Caring for the wound or incision

- Establish a sterile field for equipment and supplies. Squeeze the needed amount of ordered ointment onto the sterile field. Pour the ordered cleaning agent into a sterile container. Put on sterile gloves.
- If you are not using prepackaged swabs, saturate sterile gauze pads with the prescribed cleaning agent. Avoid using cotton balls because they may shed particles in the wound.
- Squeeze excess solution from the pad or swab. Wipe once from the top to the bottom of the incision and then discard the pad or swab. With a second pad, wipe from top to bottom in a vertical path next to the incision and then discard the pad.
- Continue to work outward from the incision in lines running parallel to it. Always wipe from the clean area toward the less-clean area. Use each pad or swab for only one stroke. Use sterile cotton-tipped applicators to clean tight-fitting wire sutures, deep wounds, or wounds with pockets.

- If the patient has a surgical drain, clean the surface of the drain last. Clean the surrounding skin by wiping in half or full circles from the drain site outward.
- Clean to at least 1″ (2.5 cm) beyond the new dressing or 2″ (5 cm) beyond the incision.
- Check for signs of infection, dehiscence, or evisceration. If you observe such signs or if the patient reports pain, notify the health care provider.
- Wash the surrounding skin with soap and water and pat dry. Apply prescribed topical medication and a skin protectant, if warranted.
- Pack an open wound with sterile moist gauze using the wet-to-damp method. Avoid using cotton-lined gauze pads.

Apply a fresh gauze dressing

- Place a sterile 4″ × 4″ gauze pad at the center of the wound and move the pad outward to the edges of the wound site. Extend the gauze at least 1″ beyond the incision in each direction. Use enough sterile dressings to absorb all of the drainage until the next dressing change.
- When the dressing is in place, remove and discard the gloves. Secure the dressing with strips of tape, a T-binder, or Montgomery straps.
- For a patient who recently underwent surgery or a patient with complications, check the dressing every 30 minutes or as ordered. If the wound is healing properly, check it at least every 8 hours.

Dressing a wound with a drain

- Use a precut sterile 4″ × 4″ gauze pad.
- Place the pad close to the skin around the drain so that the tubing fits into the slit. Press a second pad around the drain from the opposite direction to encircle the tubing.

- Layer as many uncut sterile pads around the tubing as needed to absorb the drainage. Secure the dressing with tape, a T-binder, or Montgomery straps.

Pouching a wound

- To create a pouch, measure the wound and cut an opening in the facing of the collection pouch that is ⅛" (0.3 cm) larger than the wound.
- Make sure that the surrounding skin is clean and dry. Apply a skin protectant.
- Make sure that the drainage port at the bottom of the pouch is closed. Press the contoured pouch opening around the wound, beginning at its lower edge.
- To empty the pouch, put on gloves, insert the bottom half of the pouch into a graduated container, and open the drainage port. Note the color, consistency, odor, and amount of fluid.
- Wipe the bottom of the pouch and the drainage port with a sterile gauze pad and reseal the port. Change the pouch if it leaks or comes loose.

Special considerations

- Because many health care providers prefer to change the first postoperative dressing, avoid changing it unless ordered. If you have no such order and drainage is seeping through the dressing, reinforce the dressing with fresh sterile gauze. To prevent bacterial growth, do not leave a reinforced dressing in place for longer than 24 hours. Immediately replace a dressing that becomes wet from the outside.
- Consider all dressings and drains infectious.
- If the patient has two wounds in the same area, cover each separately with layers of sterile 4" × 4" gauze pads. Then cover both sites with an abdominal bandage dressing pad secured to the skin with tape.

Draining closed wounds

Inserted during surgery, a closed-wound drain promotes healing and prevents swelling by suctioning sero-sanguineous fluid at the wound site. By removing this fluid, the drain helps to reduce the risk of infection and skin breakdown and the number of dressing changes.

A closed-wound drain consists of perforated tubing connected to a portable vacuum unit. The distal end of the tubing lies within the wound and usually leaves the body from a site other than the primary suture line to preserve the integrity of the surgical wound. The tubing exit site is treated as an additional surgical wound; the drain is usually sutured to the skin. The drain may be left in place for longer than 1 week to accommodate heavy drainage.

Equipment

Graduated cylinder • sterile laboratory container, if needed • alcohol pad • sterile gloves • clean gloves • sterile gauze pads • antiseptic cleaning agent • prepackaged antimicrobial swabs • waterproof trash bag or trash can

Implementation

- Check the health care provider's order and assess the patient's condition. Explain the procedure to the patient. Provide privacy. Wash your hands and put on clean gloves.
- Unclip the vacuum unit. Using aseptic technique, remove the spout plug to release the vacuum.
- Empty the contents of the unit into a graduated cylinder. Note the amount and appearance of the drainage. If ordered, empty the drainage into a sterile laboratory container and send it to the laboratory for diagnostic testing.
- Maintaining aseptic technique, clean the spout and plug it with an alcohol pad.

- To reestablish the vacuum that creates the suction power of the drain, fully compress the vacuum unit. Keep the unit compressed as you replace the spout plug.
- Check the patency of the equipment. Make sure that the tubing has no twists, kinks, or leaks. The drainage system must be airtight to work properly. Keep the vacuum unit compressed when you release manual pressure; rapid reinflation indicates an air leak. If this occurs, recompress the unit and secure the spout plug.

Patient Teaching Tip

If you anticipate that the patient will be discharged with the drain, teach the patient how to empty and reconstitute the drain at each session.

- Secure the vacuum unit to the patient's bedding or, if he or she is ambulatory, to his or her gown. Fasten it below the level of the wound to promote drainage. To prevent possible dislodgment, do not apply tension on the drainage tubing. Remove and discard gloves and wash your hands thoroughly.
- Put on the sterile gloves. Check for signs of pulling or tearing of the sutures and for swelling or infection of the surrounding skin. Gently clean the sutures with an antimicrobial swab or with sterile gauze pads soaked in an antiseptic cleaning agent.
- Properly dispose of drainage, solutions, and the waterproof trash bag, and clean or dispose of soiled equipment and supplies.

Special considerations
- Empty the system and measure the contents once during each shift if drainage has accumulated; do so more often if drainage is excessive.
- If the patient has more than one closed drain, number the drains so that you can record the amount of drainage from each site.

 ALERT

Do not mistake chest tubes for closed-wound drains. The vacuum of a chest tube should never be released.

Managing dehiscence and evisceration

Occasionally, the edges of a wound may not join, or they may separate after they seem to be healing normally. This abnormality, called wound dehiscence, may lead to a more serious complication known as evisceration, in which a portion of the viscera protrudes through the incision. In turn, this can lead to peritonitis and septic shock.

Equipment

Two sterile towels • 1 L of sterile normal saline solution • sterile irrigation set, including a basin, a solution container, and a 50-ml catheter-tip syringe • several large abdominal dressings • sterile waterproof drape • linen-saver pads • sterile gloves

For the patient who will return to the operating room
I.V. administration set and I.V. fluids • NG intubation equipment • sedative, as ordered • suction apparatus

Implementation

- Tell the patient to stay in bed. If possible, stay with him or her while someone else notifies the health care provider and collects the equipment.
- Place a linen-saver pad under the patient and create a sterile field. Place the basin, solution container, and 50-ml syringe on the sterile field.
- Open the bottle of sterile normal saline solution and pour 400 ml into the solution container and 200 ml into the basin.
- Place several large abdominal dressings on the sterile field. Wearing sterile gloves, place one or two dressings into the basin.
- Place the moistened dressings over the exposed viscera. Cover with sterile towels and a sterile waterproof drape.
- Keep the dressings moist by gently moistening them with the saline solution frequently. If the viscera appear dusky or black, notify the health care provider immediately. Interrupted blood supply may cause a protruding organ to become ischemic and necrotic.
- Keep the patient on strict bed rest in low Fowler's position (elevated no more than 20 degrees), with his or her knees flexed.
- Monitor the patient's vital signs every 15 minutes to detect shock. Prepare him or her to return to the operating room.
- Prepare for insertion of an NG tube and an I.V. line, if ordered. Connect the NG tube to the suction apparatus. NG intubation may make the patient gag, causing further evisceration. For this reason, the tube may be inserted in the operating room.
- Administer a preoperative sedative, as ordered.

Special considerations

- To help prevent dehiscence and evisceration, inspect the incision with each dressing change.

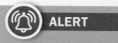 **ALERT**

By the fifth to the ninth postoperative day, teach the patient to feel for a healing ridge, which forms directly under the suture line. The lack of a healing ridge may indicate that the patient is at risk for dehiscence and evisceration.

- Treat early signs of infection immediately. Make sure that the bandages are not so tight that they limit the blood supply to the wound.
- If the patient has weak abdominal walls, apply an abdominal binder. Encourage a high-risk patient to splint his or her abdomen with a pillow during straining, coughing, or sneezing.
- If a postoperative patient detects a sudden gush of pinkish serous drainage on his or her wound dressing, inspect the incision for dehiscence. If the wound seems to be separating slowly and evisceration has not developed, place the patient in a supine position and call the health care provider.

Planning for discharge

Begin planning for discharge during your first contact with the patient. The initial nursing history and preoperative assessment as well as subsequent assessments can provide useful information.

Recognizing potential problems early will help your discharge plan to succeed. Assess the strengths and limitations of the patient and his or her family. Consider physiologic factors (such as the patient's general physical and functional abilities, current medications, and general nutritional status), psychological factors (such as self-concept, motivation, and learning abilities), and social factors (such as the duration of care needed, the types of services available, and the family's involvement in the patient's care).

Medication

Explain the purpose of the drug therapy, the duration of the regimen, the proper dosages and routes, any special instructions, and potential adverse effects as well as when to notify the health care provider. Try to establish a medication schedule that fits the patient's lifestyle.

Diet

Discuss dietary restrictions with the patient and, if appropriate, the person who will prepare his or her meals. Assess the patient's usual dietary intake. If appropriate, discuss how much the diet will cost and how the patient's dietary restrictions may affect other family members. Refer the patient to a dietitian, if appropriate.

Activity

After surgery, the patient may be advised not to lift heavy objects. Restrictions usually last 4 to 6 weeks after surgery. Discuss how these limitations will affect his or her daily routine. Let the patient know when to work, drive, and resume sexual activity. If the patient seems unlikely to comply, discuss compromises.

Home care procedures

Use nontechnical language and include caregivers when teaching about home care. After the patient watches you demonstrate a procedure, have him or her repeat the demonstration.

Explain to the patient that he or she may not need to use the same equipment that was used in the facility; discuss what is available at home. If the patient needs to rent or purchase equipment, such as a hospital bed or walker, arrange for delivery before discharge.

Wound care

Teach the patient how to change the wound dressing. Tell the patient to keep the incision clean and dry and teach proper hand-washing technique. Specify whether and when to begin to shower or bathe. If necessary, tell him or her where he or she can obtain the ordered wound-dressing supplies.

Potential complications

Teach the patient to recognize wound infection and other potential complications. Provide written instructions about reportable signs and symptoms, such as bleeding or discharge from the incision and acute pain. Advise the patient to call the health care provider with any questions.

Return appointments

Stress the importance of scheduling and keeping follow-up appointments and make sure that the patient has the health care provider's office telephone number. If the patient has no transportation, refer him or her to an appropriate community resource.

Referrals

Reassess whether the patient needs referral to a home care agency or another community resource. Discuss with the family how they will handle the patient's return home. In some facilities, a home care coordinator or discharge planning nurse is responsible for making referrals.

Selected references

Lippincott nursing procedures (8th ed.). (2019). Philadelphia, PA: Wolters Kluwer.

Nettina, S. (2019). *Lippincott manual of nursing practice* (11th ed.). Philadelphia, PA: Wolters Kluwer.

Odom-Forren, J. (2013). *Drain's perianesthesia nursing: A critical care approach* (6th ed.). St. Louis, MO: Saunders.

8

Pain Management

Assessing pain and using medications

Differentiating acute and chronic pain

Acute pain may cause certain physiologic and behavioral changes that nurses may not observe in a patient with chronic pain.

Type of pain	Physiologic evidence	Behavioral evidence
Acute	• Increased respirations • Increased pulse • Increased blood pressure • Dilated pupils • Diaphoresis	• Restlessness • Distraction • Worry • Distress
Chronic	• Normal respirations, pulse, blood pressure, and pupil size • No diaphoresis	• Reduced or absent physical activity • Despair or depression • Hopelessness

Pain is a unique experience for all individuals, with unique qualities and characteristics. Pain is no longer considered the fifth vital sign by many organizations and accrediting bodies. Nurses in all settings play a unique role in pain management, as experts in assessment, administration, and patient education regarding pain. Achieving adequate pain control depends on effectively assessing, treating, and monitoring pain. To provide the best care possible, nurses must work with health care providers and other members of the health care team to develop an individualized pain management program for each patient.

The physiology of pain is poorly understood; however, at its simplest, pain has a sensory component and a reaction component. The sensory component involves an electrical impulse that travels to the central nervous system via nerve cells called nociceptors, where it is perceived as pain. The response to this perception is the reaction component. Pain also manifests differently according to each patient's beliefs, culture, and age.

Pain affects individuals of every age, sex, race, and socioeconomic class. It is the primary reason that patients seek health care.

AGE ALERT

Older adults may have altered metabolism and excretion and experience the effects of analgesics differently from younger patients due to the effects of aging organs on the pharmacokinetic process. Older adults may be prescribed a greater number of drugs, both prescription and over the counter. This can contribute to more challenges in pain management for these patients.

AGE ALERT

Children may have altered metabolism and excretion and experience the effects of drugs differently from adults and may experience the effects of analgesics differently. As nurses, it is imperative to ensure safe dosages for the smallest patients to avoid medication-related adverse effects.

During the course of an illness, a patient may experience acute pain, chronic pain, or both.

Acute pain results from tissue damage from injury, trauma, surgery, or disease. It varies in intensity from mild to severe and is short in duration. Normal healing from acute pain is expected. Chronic pain is pain that has lasted 6 months or longer and is ongoing. It can be further differentiated as cancer pain and noncancer pain. Examples of noncancer pain are soft tissue injuries and osteoarthritis. (See *Differentiating acute and chronic pain*, page 454.)

Pain assessment

It is important for the nurse to have good pain assessment skills. Nurses must use a systematic method of assessing patients' pain, with every attempt to be as accurate and descriptive as possible. The PQRST method is an easy mnemonic to help nurses assess all aspects of pain. (See *PQRST: The alphabet of pain assessment*, page 456.) The most valid assessment of pain comes from the patient's own reports of his or her pain.

Many pain assessment tools are available. Most institutions use standardized pain assessment tools to ensure that everyone on the health care team is speaking the same language when addressing the patient's pain.

The most common pain assessment tools used by clinicians are the numeric rating scale (NRS), the FACES scale, and the visual analog scale (VAS). Each of these comes with advantages and disadvantages. The NRS asks the patient to rate his or her pain on a scale of 0 to 10, with 0 being no pain and 10 being the most pain imaginable. This is easily done at the bedside with no equipment necessary. However, patients must possess the cognitive and verbal skills to answer the question about quantifying their pain. This can be difficult for adults with cognitive or verbal disabilities or for children. The FACES scale consists of six cartoon faces depicting different levels of pain—from a smiling face (no pain) to a frowning and tearful face (most pain). Patients are asked to choose the face that best describes their pain. The method of pain assessment requires the nurse to have the FACES scale printed but can easily be obtained from most institutions. It is easy to perform at the bedside and is appropriate to use on adults as well as children older than 3 years. The VAS is a 10-cm line with the words "no pain" at one end and the words "worst possible pain" at the other. Patients are asked to place a mark on the line that best describes their pain. This is an easy assessment to do at the bedside; however, it requires patients to have cognitive and visual acuities to perform the task of marking the line. It may be inappropriate for children as well. (See *Visual analog scale*, page 456.)

Patients who cannot communicate about their pain are at increased risk for having untreated or undertreated pain. Pain assessment tools have been developed for these specific patient populations, such as the Facial expression, Leg movement, Activity, Crying, and Consolability (FLACC) scale for use in young children, the Pain Assessment in Advanced Dementia (PAINAD) for use in adults with dementia, and the Critical Care Pain Observation Tool (CPOT) for use in individuals in critical care areas. Nurses have less data to validate their assessments in these types of patients. The patient may exhibit many physiologic and psychological responses to pain, and the nurse should monitor for these during a pain assessment. (See *Pain behavior checklist*, page 457.)

(Text continues on page 458.)

PQRST: The alphabet of pain assessment

Use the PQRST mnemonic device to obtain more information about the patient's pain. Asking these questions elicits important details about his or her pain.

Provocative or palliative

Ask the patient:
- What provokes or worsens your pain?
- What relieves your pain or causes it to subside?

Quality or quantity

Ask the patient:
- What does the pain feel like? Encourage descriptors such as aching, intense, burning, or cramping.
- Are you having pain right now? If so, is it more or less severe than usual?
- To what degree does pain affect your normal activities?
- Do you have other symptoms along with the pain, such as nausea and vomiting?

Region and radiation

Ask the patient:
- Where is your pain?
- Does the pain radiate to other parts of your body?

Severity

Ask the patient:
- How severe is your pain? How would you rate it on a scale of 0 to 10, with 0 being no pain and 10 being the worst pain imaginable?
- How would you describe the intensity of your pain at its best? At its worst? Right now?

Timing

Ask the patient:
- When did your pain begin?
- At what time of day is your pain best? At what time of day is your pain worst?
- Is the onset sudden or gradual?
- Is the pain constant or intermittent?

Visual analog scale

To use the visual analog scale, ask the patient to place a mark on the scale to indicate his or her current level of pain, as shown here.

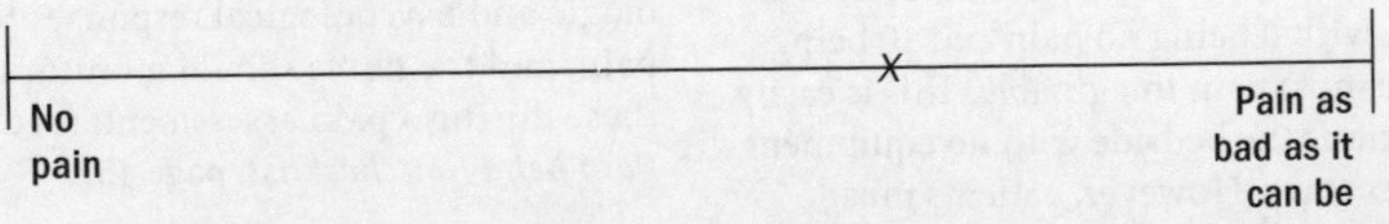

No
pain

Pain as
bad as it
can be

Numeric rating scale

A numeric rating scale can help the patient to quantify pain. To use this scale, ask the patient to choose a number from 0 (indicating no pain) to 10 (indicating the worst pain imaginable) to reflect his or her current level of pain. The patient can either circle the number on the scale or state the number that best describes the pain.

No pain 0 1 2 3 4 5 6 7 8 9 10 **Pain as bad as it can be**

Wong-Baker FACES pain rating scale

A child or an adult with language difficulties may not be able to express the pain he or she is feeling. In such instances, you can use the pain intensity scale below. To use this scale, ask the patient to choose the face that best represents the severity of his or her pain on a scale from 0 to 10.

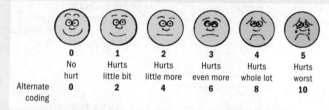

	0	1	2	3	4	5
	No hurt	Hurts little bit	Hurts little more	Hurts even more	Hurts whole lot	Hurts worst
Alternate coding	0	2	4	6	8	10

From Hockenberry, M. J., & Wilson, D. (2009). *Wong's essentials of pediatric nursing* (8th ed.). St. Louis, MO: Mosby. Used with permission. Copyright Mosby.

Pain behavior checklist

A pain behavior is something that a patient uses to communicate pain, distress, or suffering. Nurses may use this checklist to assist the patient as they assess his or her pain.

- Grimacing
- Moaning
- Sighing
- Clenching the teeth
- Holding or supporting the painful body area
- Sitting rigidly
- Frequently shifting posture or position
- Moving in a guarded or protective manner
- Moving very slowly
- Limping

- Using a cane, cervical collar, or another prosthetic device
- Walking with an abnormal gait
- Requesting help with walking
- Stopping frequently while walking
- Lying down during the day
- Avoiding physical activity
- Being irritable
- Asking such questions as, "Why did this happen to me?"
- Asking to be relieved from tasks or activities
- Taking medication

Pharmacologic pain management

Two classes of medications are commonly used for pain management:

- Nonopioids
- Opioids

Nonopioids are the first choice for managing mild pain. They decrease pain by inhibiting inflammation at the injury site. Nonopioids may be added to opioids and other medications for more comprehensive pain control. Examples of nonopioids are:

- acetaminophen
- nonsteroidal anti-inflammatory drugs (NSAIDS)
- salicylates such as aspirin.

Opioids are a class of medication used for managing moderate to severe

Pain management drugs

Drug	Indications	Adverse effects
Medications used for mild to moderate pain		
acetaminophen Tylenol, Ofirmev (I.V.), Acephen	• Mild pain • Fever	• Severe liver damage • Renal damage • Neutropenia, leukopenia, pancytopenia, thrombocytopenia • Hypoglycemia
aspirin ASA, Ascriptin, Bufferin	• Mild pain • Fever • Transient ischemic attacks and thromboembolic disorders • Treatment or reduction of the risk of myocardial infarction (MI) in the patient with previous MI or unstable angina • Pericarditis after acute MI • Prevention of reocclusion in coronary revascularization procedures • Stent implantation	• Tinnitus, hearing loss • Nausea, gastrointestinal (GI) distress, occult bleeding, dyspepsia, GI bleeding • Acute renal insufficiency • Leukopenia, thrombocytopenia, prolonged bleeding time • Liver dysfunction, hepatitis • Rash • Hypersensitivity reactions (anaphylaxis, asthma), Reye's syndrome (especially in children less than 18 years old), angioedema

pain. Opioids work by blocking the release of neurotransmitters that are involved in transmitting pain signals to the brain. This reduces the patient's perception of pain and produces sedation. Opioids may also decrease the action of prostaglandins, which occur because of inflammation.

Some of the most common pain management agents are discussed here. The World Health Organization (WHO) has developed a stepwise approach to pain management for pain that is associated with cancer. It has been suggested that this same stepped approach to cancer pain management be used in the treatment of acute noncancer pain as well. (See *Pain management drugs*, pages 458 to 465.)

Special considerations

- Use cautiously in patients with a history of chronic alcohol abuse because hepatotoxicity has occurred after therapeutic doses. Also use cautiously in patients with hepatic or cardiovascular disease, impaired renal function, or viral infection.
- Know the patient's total daily acetaminophen intake, especially if he or she is taking other prescribed drugs containing the compound such as Percocet. Toxicity can occur.
- Monitor the prothrombin time (PT) and international normalized ratio values in patients who are receiving oral anticoagulants (e.g., warfarin) and long-term acetaminophen therapy.

- Contraindicated in patients with glucose-6-phosphate dehydrogenase deficiency or bleeding disorders, such as hemophilia, von Willebrand's disease, or telangiectasia; also contraindicated in patients with nonsteroidal anti-inflammatory drug (NSAID)-induced sensitivity reactions
- Use cautiously in patients with GI lesions, impaired renal function, hypoprothrombinemia, vitamin K deficiency, thrombotic thrombocytopenic purpura, or hepatic impairment.
- Use cautiously in patients with a history of GI disease (especially peptic ulcer disease), increased risk of GI bleeding, or decreased renal function.
- Do not give oral or rectal aspirin products to children or teenagers because of the risk of developing Reye's syndrome.
- Give 8 oz (237 ml) of water or milk with salicylates to ensure passage into the stomach. Have the patient sit up for 15 to 30 minutes after taking salicylates to prevent lodging in the esophagus.
- Monitor the patient's vital signs frequently, especially temperature.
- Salicylates may mask the signs and symptoms of acute infection (fever, myalgia, and erythema); carefully evaluate patients who are at risk for infection, such as those with diabetes.
- Monitor the complete blood count, platelet count, PT, blood urea nitrogen level, serum creatinine level, and the results of liver function studies periodically during salicylate therapy to detect abnormalities.
- Assess the patient for signs and symptoms of hemorrhage, such as petechiae; bruising; coffee ground vomitus; and black, tarry stools.

(continued)

Pain management drugs *(continued)*

Drug	Indications	Adverse effects

Medications used for mild to moderate pain (continued)

ibuprofen
Advil, Motrin,
Motrin IB, Nuprin,
Caldolor (I.V.)

- Osteoarthritis and rheumatoid arthritis, gout
- Mild to moderate pain, headache, backache, minor aches associated with the common cold
- Fever reduction
- Dysmenorrhea

- GI effects: dyspepsia, heartburn, nausea
- Acute renal failure
- Neutropenia, pancytopenia, thrombocytopenia, aplastic anemia, leukopenia, agranulocytosis
- Bronchospasm
- Stevens-Johnson syndrome

Medications used to treat moderate to severe pain

ketorolac tromethamine
Toradol

- Short-term management of severe, acute pain
- Short-term management of moderately severe, acute pain when switching from parenteral to oral administration

- Drowsiness, sedation, dizziness, headache
- Arrhythmias
- Nausea, dyspepsia, GI pain
- Renal failure
- Thrombocytopenia

codeine phosphate, codeine sulfate

- Mild to moderate pain
- Nonproductive cough

- Respiratory depression
- Sedation, clouded sensorium, euphoria, dizziness, light-headedness
- Hypotension, bradycardia
- Nausea, vomiting, constipation, dry mouth, ileus
- Urine retention
- Diaphoresis

Special considerations

- Black box warning: contraindicated for treatment of pain in patients undergoing coronary artery bypass graft (CABG) surgery
- Contraindicated in patients who have the syndrome of nasal polyps, angioedema, and bronchospastic reaction to aspirin or other NSAIDs; contraindicated during the last trimester of pregnancy because it may cause problems with the fetus or complications during delivery
- Use cautiously in patients with impaired renal or hepatic function, GI disorders, peptic ulcer disease, cardiac decompensation, hypertension, or coagulation defects. Because chewable tablets contain aspartame, use cautiously in patients with phenylketonuria.
- Monitor auditory and ophthalmic functions periodically during ibuprofen therapy.
- Observe the patient for possible fluid retention.
- Patients older than age 60 may be more susceptible to the toxic effects of ibuprofen, especially adverse GI reactions. Use the lowest possible effective dose. The effect of the drug on renal prostaglandins may cause fluid retention and edema, a significant drawback for elderly patients, especially those with heart failure.

- Contraindicated in patients with active peptic ulcer disease, recent GI bleeding or perforation, advanced renal impairment, risk of renal impairment as a result of volume depletion, suspected or confirmed cerebrovascular bleeding, hemorrhagic diathesis, incomplete hemostasis, or an increased risk of bleeding
- Use cautiously in patients with impaired renal or hepatic function.
- The combined duration of ketorolac therapy (I.M., I.V., oral) should not exceed 5 days. Oral use is only for continuation of I.V. or I.M. therapy.

- Use cautiously in elderly or debilitated patients and in those with impaired renal or hepatic function, head injuries, increased intracranial pressure (ICP), increased cerebrospinal fluid (CSF) pressure, hypothyroidism, Addison's disease, acute alcoholism, central nervous system (CNS) depression, bronchial asthma, chronic obstructive pulmonary disease (COPD), respiratory depression, or shock.
- Because the safe use of codeine in pregnancy has not been established, it should not be given to pregnant women unless the potential benefits outweigh the possible hazards.
- Do not mix with other solutions because codeine phosphate is incompatible with many drugs.
- Patients who become physically dependent on the drug may experience acute withdrawal syndrome if given an opioid antagonist.
- The drug may delay gastric emptying, increase biliary tract pressure resulting from contraction of the sphincter of Oddi, and interfere with hepatobiliary imaging studies.

(continued)

Pain management drugs (continued)

Drug	Indications	Adverse effects
Medications used to treat moderate to severe pain (continued)		
hydrocodone* Vicodin, Lortab, Norco	• Mild to moderate pain	• Light-headedness, dizziness, sedation, nausea • Respiratory depression • Constipation • Urinary retention • Impaired judgment • Lethargy • Skin rash
oxycodone OxyContin, Roxicodone	• Moderate to severe pain	• Respiratory depression, apnea, respiratory arrest • Hypotension, bradycardia, shock, cardiac arrest • Nausea, vomiting, constipation, ileus, dry mouth, biliary tract spasms, anorexia • Urine retention • Seizures (with large doses), dizziness, nightmares (with long-acting oral forms), light-headedness • Thrombocytopenia • Diaphoresis, edema • Physical dependence, decreased libido
Medications used to treat severe pain		
morphine Astramorph-PF, Avinza, Duramorph, Infumorph, Kadian, MS Contin, Oramorph SR	• Severe pain • Severe, chronic pain related to cancer • Preoperative sedation and adjunct to anesthesia • Postoperative analgesia • Control of pain caused by acute MI • Control of angina pain • Adjunctive treatment of acute pulmonary edema	• Respiratory depression, apnea, respiratory arrest • Hypotension, bradycardia, shock, cardiac arrest • Nausea, vomiting, constipation, ileus, dry mouth, biliary tract spasms, anorexia • Urine retention • Seizures (with large doses), dizziness, nightmares (with long-acting oral forms), light-headedness • Thrombocytopenia • Diaphoresis, edema • Physical dependence, decreased libido

Special considerations

- This is one of the most commonly prescribed drugs in the United States.
- Hydrocodone is an schedule II drug.
- All patients taking hydrocodone should be evaluated for signs of abuse and addiction because dependence can occur even at normal doses.
- Can cause additive CNS depression if taken with other CNS depressants, like alcohol, benzodiazepines, and skeletal muscle relaxants
- Contraindicated in head injuries
- Elderly patients may have an increased sensitivity to hydrocodone products.
- Patients should be educated about impaired judgment and should be discouraged from driving or operating heavy machinery while on hydrocodone.

- Black box warning: Use of extended release oxycodone products may result in fatal respiratory depression.
- Deaths have resulted from its inappropriate use through diversion.
- Can cause additive CNS depression if taken with other CNS depressants like alcohol, benzodiazepines, and skeletal muscle relaxants
- Contraindicated in head injuries
- Elderly patients may have an increased sensitivity to oxycodone products.
- Patients should be educated about impaired judgment and should be discouraged from driving or operating heavy machinery while taking oxycodone.

- Contraindicated in patients with conditions that would preclude administration of opioids by the I.V. route, such as acute bronchial asthma and upper airway obstruction
- Use cautiously in elderly or debilitated patients and in those with head injury, increased ICP, seizures, pulmonary disease, benign prostatic hyperplasia, hepatic or renal disease, acute abdominal conditions, hypothyroidism, Addison's disease, or urethral strictures.
- Long-term therapy in patients with advanced renal disease may lead to toxicity because of accumulation of the active metabolite.
- Taper gradually when stopping therapy to avoid withdrawal symptoms.

(continued)

Pain management drugs *(continued)*

Drug	Indications	Adverse effects
Medications used to treat severe pain (continued)		
hydromorphone hydrochloride Dilaudid	• Moderate to severe pain • Cough	• Respiratory depression, bronchospasm • Sedation, somnolence, clouded sensorium, dizziness, euphoria • Hypotension, bradycardia • Nausea, vomiting, constipation • Urine retention
fentanyl citrate Sublimaze; fentanyl transdermal system (Duragesic-12, Duragesic-25, Duragesic-50, Duragesic-75, Duragesic-100)	• Preoperative analgesic • Adjunct to general anesthetic; low-dose regimen for minor procedures; moderate-dose regimen for major procedures; high-dose regimen for complicated procedures • Postoperative analgesic • Management of chronic pain in the patient who cannot be managed by lesser means • Management of breakthrough cancer pain	• Respiratory depression, apnea • Sedation, somnolence, clouded sensorium, confusion, asthenia • Arrhythmias • Nausea, vomiting, constipation, dry mouth • Urine retention

*Available only as a combination with acetaminophen.

Selected nonopioid analgesic combination products

Many common analgesics are combinations of two or more generic drugs. This table lists the components of common nonopioid analgesics.

Trade name	Generic drugs
Anacin, P-A-C Analgesic Tablets	• aspirin 400 mg • caffeine 32 mg

Special considerations

- Contraindicated in patients with intracranial lesions caused by increased ICP and whenever ventilator function is depressed, such as in status asthmaticus, COPD, cor pulmonale, emphysema, and kyphoscoliosis
- Use cautiously in elderly or debilitated patients and in those with hepatic or renal disease, Addison's disease, hypothyroidism, benign prostatic hyperplasia, or urethral strictures.
- For a better analgesic effect, give the drug before the patient has intense pain.
- Give by direct injection over no less than 2 minutes and monitor the patient constantly. Keep resuscitation equipment available. Respiratory depression and hypotension can occur with I.V. administration.
- Drug may worsen or mask gallbladder pain. Increased biliary tract pressure resulting from contraction of the sphincter of Oddi may interfere with hepatobiliary imaging studies.
- May be harmful to fetus and may cause addiction or withdrawal symptoms in a newborn. Women taking the drug should not breastfeed because the drug is excreted in breast milk.

- Use cautiously in elderly or debilitated patients and in those with head injuries; increased CSF pressure; COPD; decreased respiratory reserve; compromised respirations; arrhythmias; or hepatic, renal, or cardiac disease.
- Safety and efficacy in children younger than 2 years of age and in pregnant women has not been established.
- Give an anticholinergic, such as atropine or glycopyrrolate, to minimize the possible bradycardic effect of fentanyl.
- Gradually adjust the dosage in patients using the transdermal system. Reaching steady-state levels of a new dose may take up to 6 days; delay dose adjustment until after at least two applications.
- When reducing opiate therapy or switching to a different analgesic, expect to withdraw the transdermal system gradually. Because the serum level of fentanyl decreases very gradually after removal, give half of the equianalgesic dose of the new analgesic 12 to 18 hours after removal.
- Fentanyl Citrate Injection is a schedule II controlled substance that can produce drug dependence and has the potential for abuse.

Selected nonopioid analgesic combination products *(continued)*

Trade name	Generic drugs
Ascriptin, Magnaprin	• aspirin 325 mg • magnesium hydroxide 50 mg • aluminum hydroxide 50 mg • calcium carbonate 50 mg

(continued)

Selected nonopioid analgesic combination products *(continued)*

Trade name	Generic drugs
Ascriptin A/D, Magnaprin Arthritis Strength Caplets	• aspirin 325 mg • magnesium hydroxide 75 mg • aluminum hydroxide 75 mg • calcium carbonate 75 mg
Aspirin Free Anacin PM, Extra Strength Tylenol PM, Sominex Pain Relief	• acetaminophen 500 mg • diphenhydramine 25 mg
Esgic-Plus	• acetaminophen 500 mg • caffeine 40 mg • butalbital 50 mg
Excedrin Extra Strength, Excedrin Migraine	• aspirin 250 mg • acetaminophen 250 mg • caffeine 65 mg
Excedrin PM Caplets	• acetaminophen 500 mg • diphenhydramine citrate 38 mg
Fiorinal*, Fiortal*	• aspirin 325 mg • caffeine 40 mg • butalbital 50 mg
Sinutab Regular†	• acetaminophen 325 mg • chlorpheniramine 2 mg • pseudoephedrine hydrochloride 30 mg
Tecnal†	• aspirin 330 mg • caffeine 40 mg • butalbital 50 mg
Vanquish	• aspirin 227 mg • acetaminophen 194 mg • caffeine 33 mg • aluminum hydroxide 25 mg • magnesium hydroxide 50 mg

*Controlled substance schedule III.
†Available in Canada only.

Selected opioid analgesic combination products

Many common analgesics are combinations of two or more generic drugs. This table lists the components of common opioid analgesics and their controlled substance schedule classification.

Trade name	Controlled substance schedule	Generic drugs
Aceta with Codeine	III	• acetaminophen 300 mg • codeine phosphate 30 mg
Anexsia 7.5/650, Lorcet Plus	III	• acetaminophen 650 mg • hydrocodone bitartrate 7.5 mg
Capital with Codeine, Tylenol with Codeine Elixir	V	• acetaminophen 120 mg • codeine phosphate 12 mg/5 ml
Darvocet-N 50	IV	• acetaminophen 325 mg • propoxyphene napsylate 50 mg
Darvocet-N 100, Propacet 100	IV	• acetaminophen 650 mg • propoxyphene napsylate 100 mg
Empirin with Codeine No. 3	III	• aspirin 325 mg • codeine phosphate 30 mg
Empirin with Codeine No. 4	III	• aspirin 325 mg • codeine phosphate 60 mg
Fioricet with Codeine	III	• acetaminophen 325 mg • butalbital 50 mg • caffeine 40 mg • codeine phosphate 30 mg
Fiorinal with Codeine	III	• aspirin 325 mg • butalbital 50 mg • caffeine 40 mg • codeine phosphate 30 mg
Lorcet 10/650	III	• acetaminophen 650 mg • hydrocodone bitartrate 10 mg
Lortab 2.5/500	III	• acetaminophen 500 mg • hydrocodone bitartrate 2.5 mg

(continued)

Selected opioid analgesic combination products *(continued)*

Trade name	Controlled substance schedule	Generic drugs
Lortab 5/500	III	• acetaminophen 500 mg • hydrocodone bitartrate 5 mg
Lortab 7.5/500	III	• acetaminophen 500 mg • hydrocodone bitartrate 7.5 mg
Percocet 5/325	II	• acetaminophen 325 mg • oxycodone hydrochloride 5 mg
Percodan-Demi	II	• aspirin 325 mg • oxycodone hydrochloride 2.25 mg • oxycodone terephthalate 0.19 mg
Percodan, Roxiprin	II	• aspirin 325 mg • oxycodone hydrochloride 4.5 mg • oxycodone terephthalate 0.38 mg
Roxicet	II	• acetaminophen 325 mg • oxycodone hydrochloride 5 mg
Roxicet 5/500, Roxilox	II	• acetaminophen 500 mg • oxycodone hydrochloride 5 mg
Roxicet Oral Solution	II	• acetaminophen 325 mg • oxycodone hydrochloride 5 mg/5 ml
Talacen	IV	• acetaminophen 650 mg • pentazocine hydrochloride 25 mg
Talwin Compound	IV	• aspirin 325 mg • pentazocine hydrochloride 12.5 mg
Tylenol with Codeine No. 2	III	• acetaminophen 300 mg • codeine phosphate 15 mg
Tylenol with Codeine No. 3	III	• acetaminophen 300 mg • codeine phosphate 30 mg
Tylenol with Codeine No. 4	III	• acetaminophen 300 mg • codeine phosphate 60 mg

Selected opioid analgesic combination products *(continued)*

Trade name	Controlled substance schedule	Generic drugs
Tylox	II	• acetaminophen 500 mg • oxycodone hydrochloride 5 mg
Vicodin, Zydone	III	• acetaminophen 500 mg • hydrocodone bitartrate 5 mg
Vicodin ES	III	• acetaminophen 750 mg • hydrocodone bitartrate 7.5 mg

Selected references

Baker, D. W. (2017). *The Joint Commission's pain standards: Origins and evolutions*. Oakbrook Terrace, IL: The Joint Commission.

Blondell, R. D., Azadfard, M., & Wisniewski, A. M. (2013). Pharmacologic therapy for acute pain. *American Family Physician, 87*(11), 766–772. Retrieved from https://www.aafp.org/afp/2013/0601/p766.pdf

Drew, D. (2018). Pain management. In J. L. Hinkle & K. H. Cheever (Eds.), *Brunner and Suddarth's textbook of medical surgical nursing* (pp. 224–250). Philadelphia, PA: Wolters Kluwer.

Frandsen, G. (2018). Pharmacology and the care of adults and geriatric patients. In G. Frandsen & S. S. Pennington (Eds.), *Abrams' clinical drug therapy: Rationales for nursing practice* (11th ed., pp. 76–88). Philadelphia, PA: Wolters Kluwer.

Manworren, R. C. B. (2015). Multimodal pain management and the future of a personalized medicine approach to pain. *AORN Journal, 101*(3), 308–318. doi:10.1016/j.aorn.2014.12.009

McCaffery, M., Herr, K., & Pasero, C. (2011). Assessment. In C. Pasero & M. McCaffery (Eds.), *Pain assessment and pharmacologic management*. St. Louis, MO: Mosby.

World Health Organization. (2018). *WHO's cancer pain ladder for adults*. Retrieved from http://www.who.int/cancer/palliative/painladder/en/

9

Pressure Ulcers and Traumatic Wound Care

Preventing, staging, and treating wounds

Pressure ulcer care

Pressure ulcers result when pressure exceeding normal capillary closure pressure impairs circulation over a period of time, depriving tissues of oxygen and nutrients. This process damages skin and underlying structures.

Risk factors for pressure ulcers include compromised mobility, sensory deficits, poor skin perfusion, malnutrition, fecal and/or urinary incontinence, friction, and shearing forces.

Most pressure ulcers develop over bony prominences, where friction and shearing combine with pressure to damage skin and underlying tissues. Common sites include the sacrum, coccyx, ischial tuberosities, and greater trochanters. Other common sites include the vertebrae, scapulae, elbows, knees, and heels in bedridden and relatively immobile patients. (See *Pressure points: Common sites for ulcers.*)

Successful treatment of pressure ulcers involves relieving pressure, improving mobility, and improving nutritional status. The effectiveness and duration of the treatment depend on the characteristics of the pressure ulcer as well as other contributing factors. (See *Staging pressure ulcers*, pages 472 and 473.)

Ideally, prevention is the key to avoiding extensive therapy. Preventive measures include ensuring adequate nourishment and mobility to relieve pressure and promote circulation.

(Text continues on page 474.)

Pressure points: Common sites for ulcers

Ulcers may develop at pressure points, which are shown in these illustrations. To help prevent ulcers, emphasize the importance of repositioning the patient frequently and checking the skin carefully for changes.

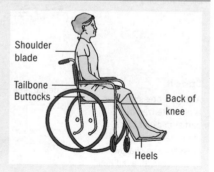

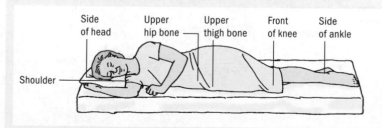

Staging pressure ulcers

The pressure ulcer staging system described here reflects the anatomic depth of exposed tissue. The presence of slough or eschar in the wound bed render the wound unstageable (see below).

Suspected deep tissue injury

Deep tissue injury (DTI) is typically characterized by a purple or maroon localized area of intact skin or a blood-filled blister caused by damage of underlying soft tissue from pressure or shear. DTI may be preceded by tissue that is painful, firm, mushy, boggy, or a different temperature compared to adjacent tissues.

Stage I

A stage I pressure ulcer is characterized by a localized area of intact skin with nonblanchable redness, typically over a bony prominence. Darkly pigmented skin may not have visible erythema or blanching, but the coloration of affected tissues may differ from the surrounding area.

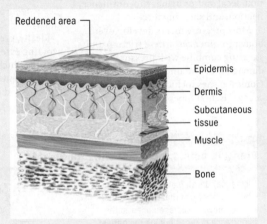

Stage II

A stage II pressure ulcer is characterized by partial-thickness loss of the dermis, which presents as a shallow open ulcer with a red-pink wound bed; slough is not present. It may also present as an intact or ruptured serum-filled blister.

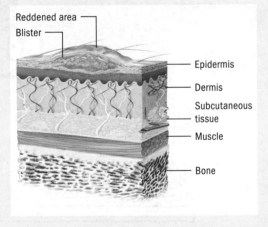

Stage III

A stage III pressure ulcer is characterized by full-thickness tissue loss. Subcutaneous fat may be visible. Undermining and tunneling may be present. Slough may be present but does not obscure the depth of tissue loss, which can vary by anatomic location.

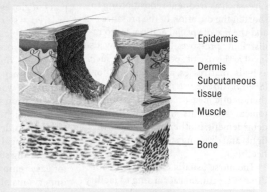

Epidermis

Dermis

Subcutaneous tissue

Muscle

Bone

Stage IV

A stage IV pressure ulcer is characterized by full-thickness tissue loss with exposed bone, tendon, or muscle. Undermining and tunneling are common. Slough or eschar may be present on some parts of the wound bed but does not obscure depth of tissue loss, which can vary by anatomical location.

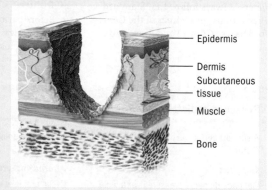

Epidermis

Dermis

Subcutaneous tissue

Muscle

Bone

Unstageable

An unstageable ulcer is characterized by full-thickness tissue loss in which the base of the ulcer in the wound bed is covered by slough and/or eschar. Stage cannot be determined until enough slough and/or eschar is removed to expose the base of the wound and its true depth.

When a pressure ulcer develops despite preventive efforts, treatment includes methods to decrease pressure, such as frequent repositioning to shorten the duration of the pressure and the use of special equipment to redistribute pressure. Treatment may also involve the use of special devices, such as beds, mattresses, and chair cushions. (See *Pressure redistribution.*) Other therapeutic measures include using topical treatments, wound cleansing, debridement, biotherapy, therapeutic light, and dressings to support wound healing.

The nurse usually performs or coordinates treatments according to facility policy. The procedures described here address cleaning and dressing pressure ulcers. Always follow the "Standard Precautions" guidelines of the Centers for Disease Control and Prevention.

Equipment and preparation

Hypoallergenic tape or elastic netting • piston-type irrigating system • two pairs of gloves • cleaning solution, as ordered • sterile 4″ × 4″ gauze pads • selected topical dressing (moist saline gauze, hydrocolloid, transparent, alginate, foam, or hydrogel) • linen-saver pads • impervious plastic trash bag • disposable wound-measuring device • sterile cotton swabs

Assemble the equipment at the patient's bedside. Cut the tape into strips for securing dressings. Loosen the lids on cleaning solutions and medications for easy removal. Make sure that the impervious plastic trash bag is within reach.

Implementation

- Before performing any dressing change, wash your hands and review the principles of standard precautions.

Pressure redistribution

A support surface is designed to redistribute pressure by managing tissue loads and other factors.

Gel pads

Gel pads disperse pressure over a wide surface area.

Foam pads

Foam pads, available in a variety of permeability, cushion skin and minimize pressure; some types of foam conform to the body shape in proportion to the applied weight.

Low-air-loss beds

The surface of low-air-loss beds consists of inflated air cushions that assist in managing the heat and humidity of the skin.

Alternating-pressure mattress

Cyclic changes in the air distribution allow for loading and unloading of pressure.

Air-fluidized beds

A fluidlike state is obtained by forcing air through beads in the bed, reducing pressure and friction.

Mechanical devices

Mechanical lifting devices prevent friction and shearing by lifting the patient, whereas slide sheets or mats prevent friction and shearing by optimizing glide.

Foot cradle

A foot cradle lifts the bed linens to relieve pressure over the feet.

Cleaning the pressure ulcer

- Provide privacy and explain the procedure to the patient to alleviate his or her fears and promote cooperation.
- Position the patient in a way that maximizes comfort while allowing easy access to the pressure ulcer site.
- Cover the bed linens with a linen-saver pad to prevent soiling.
- If irrigating the wound, open the irrigation solution container and the piston syringe. Carefully pour solution into an irrigation container to avoid splashing. (The container may be clean or sterile, depending on facility policy.) Put the piston syringe into the opening provided in the irrigation container.
- Open the packages of supplies.
- Put on gloves to remove the old dressing and expose the pressure ulcer. Discard the soiled dressing in the impervious plastic trash bag to avoid contaminating the sterile field and spreading infection.
- Assess the condition of the skin and the ulcer. Note the character of the wound bed and the surrounding skin.
- Using the piston syringe, irrigate the pressure ulcer to remove necrotic debris and help to decrease bacteria in the wound.
- Apply cleaning solution to 4″ × 4″ gauze. Clean the wound from least contaminated area to most contaminated area. For pressure wounds, clean in concentric circles from the inside of the wound toward the outside. Use a clean gauze for each wiping motion.
- Pat the wound dry with 4″ × 4″ gauze.
- Remove and discard the soiled gloves and put on a fresh pair.
- Inspect the wound. Note the color, amount, and odor of drainage and necrotic debris. (See *Tailoring wound care to wound color.*) Measure the

Tailoring wound care to wound color

You can promote healing by keeping the wound moist, clean, and free from debris. For open wounds, you can use wound color to guide the specific management approach that will aid healing.

Wound color	Management technique
Red	• Cover the wound while keeping it moist and clean and protect it from trauma. • Using a transparent dressing, a hydrogel, foam, or hydrocolloid dressing may help to insulate and protect partial-thickness wounds.
Yellow	• Clean the wound and remove the yellow layer. • Consider hydrotherapy with whirlpool or pulsatile lavage. • Cover the wound with a moisture-retentive dressing, such as a hydrogel or foam dressing. A moist gauze dressing with or without a debriding enzyme may also be considered.
Black	• Debride the wound as ordered using a topical enzyme product, conservative sharp debridement, or hydrotherapy with whirlpool or pulsatile lavage. • Do not debride noninfected heel ulcers or wounds with an inadequate blood supply.

perimeter of the wound with the disposable wound-measuring device.

- Insert a sterile cotton swab, foam-tipped swab, or a gloved finger into the wound to assess wound tunneling or undermining. Tunneling usually signals extension of the wound along fascial planes. Gauge the depth of the tunnel by determining how far you can insert the swab or your finger.
- Next, reassess the condition of the skin and the ulcer. Note the character of the clean wound bed and the surrounding skin.
- If you observe adherent necrotic material, notify a wound care specialist or a health care provider to ensure that appropriate debridement is performed.
- Prepare to apply the selected topical dressing. Directions for application of topical moist saline gauze, hydrocolloid, transparent, alginate, foam,

and hydrogel dressings follow. For other dressings or topical agents, follow facility protocol or the manufacturer's instructions. (See *Wound care dressings*.)

Applying a moist saline gauze dressing

- Moisten the gauze dressing with normal saline solution. Squeeze out excess fluid.
- Gently place the dressing over the surface of the ulcer. To separate surfaces within the wound, gently place a dressing between opposing wound surfaces. Do not pack the gauze too tightly.
- Apply a barrier to protect the surrounding skin from moisture.
- Change the dressing often enough to keep the wound moist. (See *Choosing a wound dressing*.)

Wound care dressings

Some dressings absorb moisture from a wound bed, whereas others add moisture. Use the chart below to quickly determine the category of dressing that is appropriate for the patient.

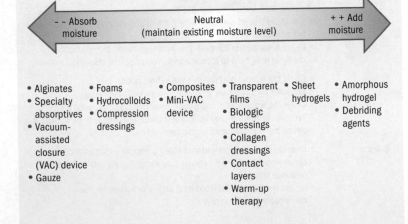

Moisture scale

- - Absorb moisture   Neutral (maintain existing moisture level)   + + Add moisture

• Alginates	• Foams	• Composites	• Transparent films	• Sheet hydrogels	• Amorphous hydrogel
• Specialty absorptives	• Hydrocolloids	• Mini-VAC device	• Biologic dressings		• Debriding agents
• Vacuum-assisted closure (VAC) device	• Compression dressings		• Collagen dressings		
• Gauze			• Contact layers		
			• Warm-up therapy		

Choosing a wound dressing

Use the information below to determine the type of dressing that is appropriate for the patient.

Gauze dressings

Made of absorptive cotton or synthetic fabric, gauze dressings are permeable to water, water vapor, and oxygen and may be impregnated with hydrogel or another agent. When uncertain about which type of dressing to use, a gauze dressing moistened with saline solution may be applied until a wound specialist recommends definitive treatment.

Hydrocolloid dressings

Hydrocolloid dressings are adhesive, moldable wafers made of a carbohydrate-based material. They usually have waterproof backings. These dressings are impermeable to oxygen, water, and water vapor, and most have some absorptive properties.

Transparent film dressings

Transparent film dressings are clear, adherent, and nonabsorptive. These polymer-based dressings are permeable to oxygen and water vapor but not to water. Their transparency allows inspection of the wound. They cannot absorb drainage and are often used on partial-thickness wounds with minimal exudate.

Alginate dressings

Made from seaweed, alginate dressings are nonwoven, absorptive dressings that are available as soft, white sterile pads or ropes. They absorb excessive exudate and may be used on infected wounds. As exudate is absorbed, these dressings turn into a gel that keeps the wound bed moist and promotes healing. When exudate is no longer excessive, switch to another type of dressing.

Foam dressings

Foam dressings are spongelike polymer dressings that may be impregnated or coated with other materials. They are somewhat absorptive and may be adherent. These dressings promote moist wound healing and are useful when a nonadherent surface is desired.

Hydrogel dressings

Water based and nonadherent, hydrogel dressings are polymer-based dressings that have some absorptive properties. They are available as a gel in a tube, as flexible sheets, and as saturated gauze packing strips. These are often used when the wound needs moisture.

Applying a hydrocolloid dressing

- Choose a clean, dry, presized dressing. If one is unavailable, cut a dressing to overlap the pressure ulcer by about 1″ (2.5 cm). Remove the dressing from its package, pull the release paper from the adherent side of the dressing and apply the dressing to the wound, being careful to smooth out wrinkles and avoiding stretching the dressing.
- If the edges of the dressing need to be secured with hypoallergenic tape, apply a skin protectant to the intact skin around the ulcer. After the area dries, tape the dressing to the skin. Avoid using tension or pressure when applying the tape.
- Remove the gloves and discard them in the impervious plastic trash bag. Dispose of refuse according to facility policy and wash your hands.
- Change a hydrocolloid dressing every 2 to 7 days and as necessary (for example, patient complains of pain, the dressing no longer adheres, dressing becomes soiled).

Applying a transparent dressing

- Select a dressing to overlap the ulcer by 1″ to 2″ (2.5 to 5 cm).
- Gently lay the dressing over the ulcer. To prevent shearing force, do not stretch the dressing. Press firmly on the edges of the dressing to promote adherence.
- Change the dressing every 3 to 5 days, depending on the amount of drainage.

Applying an alginate dressing

- Apply the alginate dressing to the surface of the ulcer. Cover the area with a secondary dressing (such as gauze pads or transparent film), as ordered. Secure the dressing with hypoallergenic tape or elastic netting.
- If the wound is draining heavily, change the dressing once or twice daily for the first 3 to 5 days. As the drainage decreases, change the dressing less frequently—every 2 to 4 days, or as ordered. When the drainage stops or the wound bed looks dry, use of an alginate dressing should be discontinued.

Applying a foam dressing

- Gently lay the foam dressing over the ulcer.
- Use hypoallergenic tape, elastic netting, or gauze to hold the dressing in place.
- Change the dressing when the foam no longer absorbs the exudate.

Applying a hydrogel dressing

- Apply a moderate amount of gel to the wound bed.
- Cover the area with a secondary dressing (gauze or transparent film).
- Change the dressing daily or as needed to keep the wound bed moist.
- If the selected dressing comes in sheet form, cut the dressing to match the wound base to avoid the surrounding skin becoming macerated.

- Hydrogel dressings also come as prepackaged, saturated gauze for wounds that require "dead space" to be filled. Follow the manufacturer's directions for these dressings.

Preventing pressure ulcers

- Turn and reposition the patient frequently, unless contraindicated. For a patient unable to self-reposition, use a pressure-redistributing device, such as a specialized mattress or padding for chairs and other mobility devices. As appropriate, implement active or passive range-of-motion exercises to relieve pressure and promote circulation. These exercises can often be combined with bathing to save time, if applicable.
- When turning the patient, lift rather than slide to reduce friction and shear. Use a specialized sheet or mobility device and get assistance from coworkers if necessary. (See *Preventing skin tears*.)
- Use pillows to position the patient and improve comfort.
- Avoid placing the patient directly on the trochanter. Instead, place on the side at about a 30-degree angle.
- Except for brief periods, avoid raising the head of the bed more than 30 degrees to prevent shearing forces.
- Direct the patient confined to a chair or wheelchair to shift weight every 15 minutes to redistribute pressure. For example, a paraplegic patient may shift weight by doing push-ups in the wheelchair. Some patients may benefit from shifting weight to one buttock for 60 seconds and then repeating the procedure on the other side.
- Adjust or pad appliances, casts, or splints, as needed, to ensure proper fit and to avoid increased pressure and impaired circulation.
- As the patient's condition permits, recommend a diet that includes

Preventing skin tears

As aging occurs, the skin becomes more prone to tearing. Taking appropriate precautions reduce risk to patients.
  Prevent skin tears by:

- using proper techniques for lifting, positioning, transferring, and turning the patient to reduce or eliminate friction and/or shear
- using pillows or cushions to support the patient's arms and legs
- encouraging the patient to wear long-sleeved shirts and long pants, as weather permits

- using nonadhering or minimally adherent dressings, such as paper tape, and using a skin barrier wipe before applying adherent dressings
- removing tape carefully
- using protective coverings or wraps, such as a stockinette or soft gauze, to protect areas of skin where the risk of tearing is high
- encouraging the patient to avoid sudden or sharp movements that can pull the skin and possibly cause a skin tear
- applying moisturizing lotion twice daily to areas at risk.

---

adequate calories, protein, and vitamins. Dietary therapy may involve nutrition consultation and the use of dietary supplements, enteral feeding, or total parenteral nutrition.

- If the patient is incontinent, clean and dry the soiled skin and apply a protective moisture barrier to prevent skin maceration.
- Make sure that the patient, family, and caregivers learn strategies for preventing and treating pressure ulcers, understand the importance of wound care and the choices that are available, the rationales for treatment, and their own role in shaping the patient's care plan.

Special considerations

- Avoid using elbow or heel protectors that fasten with a single narrow strap because the strap may impair neurovascular function in the involved hand, arm, or foot.
- Avoid using artificial sheepskin because it does not adequately reduce or redistribute pressure.
- Repair of stage III and IV ulcers may require surgical intervention (for example, direct closure, skin grafting,

flaps) depending on the patient's condition and needs.

- Infection may cause foul-smelling drainage, persistent pain, severe erythema, induration, and elevated localized skin and body temperatures. Advancing wound infection can lead to cellulitis or septicemia.

Documentation

Record the date and time of initial and subsequent treatments. Note the specific treatment used as well as the preventive strategies implemented. Document the location and size (length, width, and depth) of the pressure ulcer; the color and appearance of the wound bed; the amount, odor, color, and consistency of drainage; and the condition of the surrounding skin. Reassess pressure ulcers at least weekly.

  Update the care plan, as needed. Note any change in the condition or size of the pressure ulcer and any elevation of skin temperature in the clinical record. Document when the provider was notified of pertinent abnormal observations. Record the patient's temperature at least daily to allow easy assessment of body temperature patterns.

Traumatic wound care

Traumatic wounds include abrasions, lacerations, bites, and penetrating wounds. In an abrasion, the skin is scraped, resulting in a partial loss of the skin surface. In a laceration, a tear in the skin results from a sharp object or from blunt force trauma and can cause jagged, irregular edges. The severity of a laceration depends on its size, depth, and location. Bite wounds may be caused by humans or by animals. A penetrating wound can occur when an object, such as a knife or glass fragment, penetrates the skin and can result in damage to surrounding bone and soft tissues.

Implementation

- Administer pain medication, if ordered.
- Wash your hands and apply appropriate protective equipment.
- For a description of the specific care of a traumatic wound, see *Caring for a traumatic wound.*

Special considerations

- When irrigating a traumatic wound, avoid using more than 8 psi of pressure. High-pressure irrigation can seriously interfere with healing and allow bacteria to infiltrate the tissue.
- Avoid cleaning a traumatic wound with alcohol, which causes pain and tissue dehydration. Avoid using antiseptics for wound cleaning because they can impede healing.
- Observe the patient for signs and symptoms of infection, such as warm, red skin at the site or purulent discharge.
- Observe all dressings. If edema is present, adjust the dressing to avoid impairing circulation to the area.

Documentation

Document the date and time of the procedure, the size and condition of the wound, medication administration, specific wound care measures taken, and patient teaching provided.

Caring for a traumatic wound

When treating a patient with a traumatic wound, begin by assessing the ABCs: airway, breathing, and circulation. Move on to the wound itself only after the ABCs are stable. Here are the basic steps to follow in caring for each type of traumatic wound.

Abrasion

- Flush the area of the abrasion with normal saline solution or a wound cleaning solution.
- Use a sterile 4″ × 4″ gauze pad moistened with normal saline solution to remove any debris, such as dirt or gravel. Gently rub toward the entry point to work contaminants back out the way they entered.
- Wounds that are extremely dirty may require scrubbing with a surgical brush. Be as gentle as possible because this process is painful for the patient.

- Allow a small wound to dry and form a scab. Cover a larger wound with a nonadherent pad or petroleum gauze and a light dressing.

Laceration

- Moisten a sterile 4″ × 4″ gauze pad with normal saline solution or a wound cleaning solution. Gently clean the wound, beginning at the center and working out to approximately 2″ (5 cm) beyond the edge of the wound. When the pad becomes soiled, discard it and use a new one. Continue until the wound appears clean.

Caring for a traumatic wound *(continued)*

- If necessary, irrigate the wound with a 60-ml catheter-tip syringe and normal saline solution.
- Assist the provider in suturing the wound, if necessary, or apply commercially available sterile strips of porous tape if suturing is not needed.
- Apply a dry sterile dressing over the wound to absorb drainage and help prevent bacterial contamination.

Bite

- Irrigate the wound with copious amounts of normal saline solution. Do not immerse or soak the wound because this may allow bacteria to float back into the tissue.
- Clean the wound with sterile 4″ × 4″ gauze pads and wound cleanser.
- Assist with debridement, if ordered.
- Apply a loose dressing. If the bite is located on an extremity, elevate the area to reduce swelling.

- For animal bites, ask the patient about the animal that bit him or her to determine whether there may be a risk of rabies. Administer tetanus vaccines and human rabies immune globulin and vaccines, as needed.

Penetrating wound

- Minor puncture wounds may be allowed to bleed for a few minutes before cleaning, whereas a larger puncture wound may require irrigation.
- If the wound contains an embedded foreign object, such as a shard of glass or metal, stabilize the object until the provider can remove it. When the object is removed and bleeding is controlled, clean the wound as you would a laceration.
- Cover the wound with a dry dressing.

Selected references

Calianno, C. (2015). Wound assessment and monitoring. In P. A. Slachta (Ed.), *Wound care made incredibly easy!* (3rd ed., pp. 27–51). Philadelphia, PA: Wolters Kluwer.

Hinkle, J. L., & Cheever, K. H. (2014). Principles and practices of rehabilitation. In *Brunner & Suddarth's textbook of medical-surgical nursing* (13th ed., pp. 153–181). Philadelphia, PA: Wolters Kluwer.

McLaughlin, K. (2015). Basic wound care procedures. In P. A. Slachta (Ed.), *Wound care made incredibly easy!* (3rd ed., pp. 52–71). Philadelphia, PA: Wolters Kluwer.

Scardillo, J. (2015). Acute wounds. In P. A. Slachta (Ed.), *Wound care made incredibly easy!* (3rd ed., pp. 72–100). Philadelphia, PA: Wolters Kluwer.

The Healthcare Infection Control Practices Advisory Committee (HICPAC) of the Centers for Disease Control and Prevention (CDC) has developed guidelines for isolation precautions in hospitals. These guidelines have two levels of precautions:

- standard precautions
- transmission-based precautions, which are further divided into airborne precautions, droplet precautions, and contact precautions.

Standard precautions

Standard precautions are designed to decrease the risk of transmission of microorganisms from recognized and unrecognized sources of infection. The CDC defines standard precautions as the minimum precautionary infection preventive practices in any health care setting that patient care is delivered. These precautions include hand hygiene using personal protective equipment, sterile instruments, clean and disinfected surfaces, and sharp safety.

HICPAC and the CDC define these materials as infectious, and standard precautions must be observed:

- blood
- body fluids, secretions, and excretions (except sweat)
- nonintact skin
- mucous membranes.

Standard precautions combine the major features of universal precautions, which were developed specifically to reduce the transmission of blood-borne pathogens, such as HIV and hepatitis B virus (HBV), and body substance isolation, which was developed to decrease the risk of transmission of pathogens from moist body surfaces. Because standard precautions reduce the risk of transmission of blood-borne and other pathogens, many patients with diseases or conditions that previously required category- or disease-specific isolation precautions now require only standard precautions.

Implementation

- Handwashing should be performed before and after contact with each patient; before moving from a contaminated area to a clean area of a patient; and immediately if the patient become contaminated with blood or body fluids, secretions, or excretions.
- Use nonantimicrobial soap for routine handwashing. If hands are not visibly soiled, an alcohol-based hand rub is preferred.
- Gloves should be worn if there is a possibility of contact with blood, specimens, tissue, body fluids, secretions, excretions, or contaminated surfaces or objects.
- Change your gloves between tasks and procedures performed on the same patient if you touch anything that might have a high concentration of microorganisms. Also change gloves between patient contacts to avoid cross contamination. Remove your gloves immediately after use and before touching noncontaminated areas, and wash your hands. Vinyl and nitrile gloves are available for anyone who is allergic to latex.
- Personal protective equipment should be used when there is a possibility of exposure to microorganism. For example, wear a gown, eye protection (goggles or glasses), and a mask during procedures (such as extubation, endoscopic procedures, and dialysis) that are likely to generate droplets of blood or body fluids, secretions, or excretions.
- Carefully handle used patient care equipment that is soiled with blood, body fluids, secretions, or excretions to prevent exposure to skin and mucous membranes,

contamination of clothing, and transfer of microorganisms to other patients and environments. Patient care equipment must be cleaned with a facility-approved disinfectant between patients. Discard disposable equipment appropriately.

- Make sure that procedures for routine care, cleaning, and disinfection of environmental surfaces and equipment are followed.
- Keep contaminated linens away from your body to prevent contamination and transfer of microorganisms. Place linens in properly labeled containers and make sure that the linens are transported and processed according to facility policy.
- Handle used needles and other sharps carefully. Do not bend them, break them, reinsert them into their original sheaths, or handle them unnecessarily. Immediately after use, discard them intact in an impervious disposal box. These measures reduce the risk of accidental injury and infection.
- Use sharps with safety features whenever available.
- Use mouthpieces, resuscitation bags, or other ventilation devices in place of mouth-to-mouth resuscitation whenever possible.
- Place the patient who cannot maintain appropriate hygiene or who contaminates the environment in a private room. Notify infection control personnel.
- If you have an exudative lesion, avoid direct patient contact until the condition has resolved and the employee health provider clears you.
- Because precautions cannot be specified for every clinical situation, use your judgment in individual cases. Refer to your facility's infection control manual or check with infection control personnel when you need more information.

- If occupational exposure to blood is likely, get vaccinated with the HBV vaccine series. As recommended by the CDC, health care workers should be advised to immediately report blood or body fluid exposures to occupation health service for evaluation and management.

Transmission-based precautions

According to the CDC, transmission-based precautions are considered the "second tier" of basic infection prevention when used in conjunction with standard precautions. Whenever a patient is known or suspected to be infected with highly contagious or epidemiologically important pathogens that are transmitted by air, droplet, or contact with dry skin or other contaminated surfaces, follow transmission-based precautions along with standard precautions. Examples of such pathogens include those that cause measles (air); influenza (droplet); and gastrointestinal (GI) tract, respiratory tract, skin, and wound infections (contact). In fact, transmission-based precautions replace all older categories of isolation. One or more types of transmission-based precautions may be combined and followed when a patient has a disease with multiple routes of transmission.

Airborne precautions

Along with standard precautions, follow these precautions:
- Place the patient in a private room that has monitored negative air pressure in relation to surrounding areas, 6 to 12 air exchanges per hour, and appropriate outdoor air discharge or high-efficiency filtration of room air. The room door should remain closed. If a private room is not available, consult with infection

control personnel. As an alternative, he or she may be placed in a room with a patient who has an active infection with the same microorganism.

- Wear respiratory protection, such as a surgical mask or an N95 respirator (for tuberculosis [TB]), when entering the room of a patient with a known or suspected respiratory tract infection. Persons immune to measles and varicella do not need to wear respiratory protection when entering the room of a patient with these illnesses.
- Limit patient transport and movement out of the room. If the patient must leave the room, have him or her wear a surgical mask.
- Susceptible health care personnel should be restricted from entering the patient's room. Personnel not immune to measles, chickenpox, or smallpox should be assigned to other patients.

Droplet precautions

In addition to standard precautions, follow these precautions:

- Place the patient in a private room. If a private room is not available, consult with infection control personnel. As an alternative, the patient may be placed in a room with a patient who has an active infection with the same microorganism. Special ventilation is not necessary.
- Wear a mask when working within 6' to 10' (1.8 to 3.0 m) of the infected patient and when you enter the room. For a patient with known TB, it is necessary to wear an N95 respirator.
- Instruct visitors to stay at least 3' (0.9 m) away from the infected patient.
- Limit movement of the patient from the room. If the patient must leave the room, have him or her wear a surgical mask.

N95 respirator

You are required to wear a mask, called a respirator, when caring for a patient with known or suspected infectious pulmonary TB. The specific type that the National Institute for Occupational Safety and Health and the Occupational Safety and Health Administration has approved for this purpose is the N95 respirator. This type of respirator effectively protects and screens the wearer from at least 95% of particles the size of the TB droplet nuclei, if the respirator fits correctly and there is minimal face seal leakage. Fit testing, which detects such leakage, is mandatory when a respirator is first given to an employee. Make sure you wash your hands before and after handling the mask.

Contact precautions

In addition to standard precautions, follow these precautions:

- Place the patient in a private room. If a private room is not available, consult with infection control personnel. As an alternative, he or she may be placed in a room with a patient who has an active infection with the same microorganism.
- Wear gloves whenever you enter the patient's room. Always change them after contact with infected material. Remove them before leaving the room. Wash your hands immediately with an antimicrobial soap or rub them with a waterless antiseptic. Then, avoid touching contaminated surfaces.
- Wear a gown when entering the patient's room if you think your clothing will have contact with him or her or anything in his or her room or if he or she has diarrhea or is incontinent. Remove the gown before leaving the room and wash your hands.
- Limit the patient's movement from the room and check with infection control personnel whenever he or she must leave it.

List of reportable diseases and infections

The Centers for Disease Control and Prevention (CDC), the Occupational Safety and Health Administration, the Joint Commission, and the American Hospital Association all require health care facilities to document and report certain diseases acquired in the community or in hospitals and other health care facilities.

Generally, the health care facility reports diseases to the appropriate local authorities. These authorities notify the state health department, which reports the diseases to the appropriate federal agency or national organization.

Here is the CDC's list of nationally notifiable infectious diseases for 2018. Each state also keeps a list of reportable diseases appropriate to its region.

- Anthrax
- Arboviral diseases, neuroinvasive and nonneuroinvasive
  - California serogroup virus diseases
  - Chikungunya virus disease
  - Eastern equine encephalitis virus disease
  - Powassan virus disease
  - St. Louis encephalitis disease
  - Western equine encephalitis virus disease
  - West Nile virus disease
- Babesiosis
- Botulism (foodborne, infant, wound, and other)
- Brucellosis
- Campylobacteriosis
- Cancer
- Carbapenemase-producing carbapenem-resistant Enterobacteriaceae (CP-CRE)
  - *Enterobacter* spp.
  - *Escherichia coli*
  - *Klebsiella* spp.
- Chancroid
- *Chlamydia trachomatis*, genital infection
- Cholera
- Coccidioidomycosis
- Congenital syphilis
  - Syphilitic stillbirth
- Cryptosporidiosis
- Cyclosporiasis
- Dengue virus infections
  - Dengue
  - Dengue-like illness
  - Severe dengue
- Diphtheria
- Ehrlichiosis/anaplasmosis
  - *Anaplasma phagocytophilum* infection
  - *Ehrlichia chaffeensis* infection
  - *Ehrlichia ewingii* infection
  - Undetermined human ehrlichiosis/anaplasmosis
- Foodborne disease outbreak
- Giardiasis
- Gonorrhea
- *Haemophilus influenzae*, invasive disease
- Hansen's disease (leprosy)
- *Hantavirus* infection, non-*Hantavirus* pulmonary syndrome
- *Hantavirus* pulmonary syndrome
- Hemolytic uremic syndrome, postdiarrheal
- Hepatitis (viral, acute) (hepatitis A acute, hepatitis B acute, hepatitis B perinatal infection, hepatitis C acute, hepatitis C perinatal infection)
- Hepatitis (viral, chronic) (hepatitis B chronic, hepatitis C chronic, hepatitis C virus infection [past or current])
- HIV (AIDS has been reclassified as HIV stage III.)
- Influenza-associated pediatric mortality
- Invasive pneumococcal disease
- *Legionella* infections (Legionnaires' disease)
- Leptospirosis
- Listeriosis
- Lyme disease
- Malaria
- Measles
- Meningococcal disease

List of reportable diseases and infections *(continued)*

- Mumps
- Novel influenza A virus infections
- Pertussis
- Plague
- Poliomyelitis (paralytic)
- Poliovirus infection, nonparalytic
- Psittacosis (ornithosis)
- Q fever (acute, chronic)
- Rabies (animal, human)
- Rubella (German measles) and congenital syndrome
- Salmonellosis
- Severe acute respiratory syndrome–associated coronavirus
- Shiga toxin–producing *E. coli*
- Shigellosis
- Silicosis
- Smallpox
- Spotted fever rickettsiosis
- Streptococcal toxic shock syndrome
- Syphilis congenital (primary, secondary, early nonprimary nonsecondary, and unknown duration or late)
- Tetanus
- Toxic shock syndrome (other than *Streptococcus* bacteria)

- Trichinellosis
- Tuberculosis
- Tularemia
- Typhoid fever
- Vancomycin-intermediate *Staphylococcus aureus* and vancomycin-resistant *S. aureus*
- Varicella
- Varicella (deaths only)
- Vibriosis
- Viral hemorrhagic fever
  - Crimean-Congo hemorrhagic fever virus
  - Ebola virus
  - Lassa virus
  - Lujo virus
  - Marburg virus
  - New World arenavirus—Guanarito, Junin, Machupo, and Sabia
- Yellow fever
- Zika virus disease and Zika virus infection
  - Zika virus disease (congenital and noncongenital disease), (congenital and noncongenital infection)

Basic procedures

Putting on and removing a gown

Handling isolation clothing properly is an important part of protecting yourself and avoiding contamination. Follow these steps when using a gown.

Implementation

- Put on the gown and wrap it around the back of your clothing.
- Tie the strings or fasten the snaps or pressure-sensitive tabs at the neck.
- Make sure that your clothing is completely covered and secure the gown at the waist. Put on your gloves.

- Because the outside surfaces of the barrier clothing are contaminated, keep your gloves on when taking the clothing off.
- First, untie the waist strings of the gown and then untie the neck straps. Grasp the outside of the gown at the back of the shoulders and pull it down over your arms, turning it inside out to contain pathogens as you remove it.
- Holding the gown well away from you, fold it inside out. Discard the gown in the laundry if it is cloth and in a trash container if it is paper. Wash your hands.

Hand hygiene and hand rubs

In 2018, the Centers for Disease Control and Prevention (CDC) updated its Guideline for Hand Hygiene in Healthcare Settings. Hand hygiene is a general term that refers to handwashing, antiseptic handwashing, antiseptic hand rubs, and surgical hand antisepsis.

Handwashing

Redefined by the CDC guideline, hand hygiene refers to cleaning the hands by either hand-washing (such as nonantimicrobial) soap and water. The use of an antiseptic agent (such as chlorhexidine, triclosan, or iodophor) to wash the hands is an antiseptic hand-wash. Handwashing is appropriate whenever the hands are soiled or contaminated with infectious material. Surgical personnel perform surgical hand antisepsis preoperatively to eliminate transient bacteria and reduce resident hand flora. When it involves a plain agent, handwashing is still the single most effective method for preventing the spread of infection.

Hand rubs

Hand hygiene also includes the use of rubs or hand sanitizers. An antiseptic hand rub involves applying an antiseptic, alcohol-containing product, which is designed to reduce the number of viable microorganisms on the skin, to all surfaces of the hands and rubbing until the product has dried (usually within 30 seconds). These products are also referred to as waterless antiseptic agents because no water is required. Alcohol hand rubs usually contain emollients to prevent skin drying and chapping. Hand rubs and sanitizers are appropriate for decontaminating the hands after minimal contamination has occurred.

Putting on and removing a mask

Wear a face mask to avoid inhaling airborne particles. Follow these steps when using a mask.

Implementation

- Wash your hands. Place the mask snugly over your nose and mouth. Secure the ear loops or tie the strings behind your head high enough so that the mask will not slip off.
- If the mask has a metal strip, squeeze it to fit your nose firmly but comfortably. If you wear eyeglasses, tuck the mask under their lower edge.
- To remove your mask, untie it, holding it by the strings, or slip the ear loops off the ears. Discard it in the trash container. (If the patient's disease is spread by airborne pathogens, consider removing the mask last.)

Removing contaminated gloves

To prevent the spread of pathogens from contaminated gloves to your skin, carefully follow these steps.

Implementation

- Using your nondominant hand, pinch the glove of the dominant hand near the top, as shown below. Do not allow the outer surface of the glove to buckle inward against your skin.

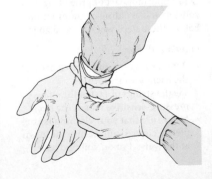

- Pull downward so that the glove turns inside out as it comes off, as shown below. Keep the glove from your dominant hand in your nondominant hand after removing it.

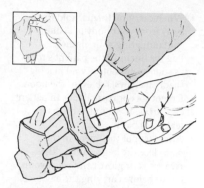

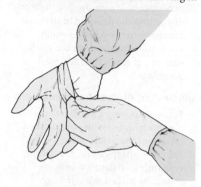

- Insert the first two fingers of your ungloved dominant hand under the edge of the nondominant glove, as shown below. Avoid touching the outer surface of the glove or folding it against the wrist of your nondominant hand.

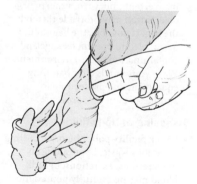

- Pull downward so that the glove turns inside out as it comes off, as shown at the top of the next column. Continue pulling until the glove completely encloses the glove from your dominant hand and has its uncontaminated inner surface facing out.

- Discard the gloves in the appropriate trash container and wash your hands.

Discarding contaminated equipment

To protect yourself and the patient from infection, observe precautions when disposing soiled linens or dressings, used disposable equipment, and contaminated reusable equipment. Have a biohazard container available, as needed, to dispose of contaminated waste.

Regulations for the disposal of contaminated waste vary from state to state and may change periodically. Follow facility policy for discarding contaminated waste.

Removing soiled linens

- All linens used in patient care settings are considered soiled. If you are handling visibly soiled linens, wearing gloves is recommended. If the bed linens are saturated with blood, feces, urine, or other body fluids, it is also recommended that you wear a gown.
- Handle linens as little as possible and with minimum agitation to prevent contaminating yourself. If certain areas of the linens are heavily soiled, fold the fabric so that the soiled areas are on the inside of the folds. Then roll or fold the linens together in one bundle.

- When carrying linens, hold them away from your body to avoid contaminating your clothes.
- Bag the linens in the patient's room as soon as possible. Avoid placing them on chairs, tables, or the floor. Do not sort or rinse linens in patient care areas. Place soiled linens in leakproof bags.
- After you put the linens in the bag, close the bag securely. Then remove your gloves and wash your hands before carrying the bag to its appropriate destination.

Disposing of soiled dressings

- Dispose all wound dressings in a way that confines and contains blood or body fluids. Avoid touching soiled areas on the dressing.
- Usually, you must wear nonsterile gloves to handle and remove soiled dressings. If the wound is large and draining, you will also need to wear a gown.

Large dressings

- Immediately after removing a large dressing, fold the dressing inward to enclose the soiled areas.
- Wrap the large dressing in the disposable linen-saver pad used during the dressing change.
- Dispose the dressing in a red-bagged biohazard container if the dressing is saturated with blood. Otherwise, it can be disposed in the regular trash container.
- Remove the gloves and wash your hands.

Small dressings

- When removing a small dressing, enclose it in the disposable glove that you used to remove it. Holding the dressing in your gloved hand, pull the glove off with the inside surface facing out to contain the dressing. Do not touch the dressing with your bare hands.
- After you have sealed the dressing inside the disposable glove, you may place it in a plastic bag prior to discarding the dressing in the trash container in the patient's room. Wash your hands; clean the work surfaces, if applicable; and wash hands again.

Discarding disposable equipment

- When disposing a sharp object that is contaminated with potentially infectious materials, place it in an approved sharps container. Other contaminated disposable items should be placed in a red-bagged biohazard container if they contain large amounts of blood. Items with small amounts of dried blood can be disposed in the regular trash container.
- When transporting a waste bag, hold it away from your body to prevent inadvertent injury from sharp objects that may protrude through the bag. If possible, the bag should be doubled to prevent leakage and contamination of the environment. Wash your hands after handling equipment and proceeding to another patient care area.

Disposing of body fluids

- Check facility policy before handling infectious waste. Large amounts of secretions, excretions, or bulk blood may be carefully poured into a sanitary sewer. Personal protective equipment should be worn when handling body fluids. If there is a potential for fluid splash, eye protection or splash guard is highly recommended.

Selected references

Centers for Disease Control and Prevention. (2013). *CDC guidance for evaluating health-care personnel for hepatitis B virus protection and for administering postexposure management.* Retrieved from https://www.cdc.gov/mmwr /preview/mmwrhtml/rr6210a1.htm

Centers for Disease Control and Prevention. (2017). *Transmission-based precautions.* Retrieved from https://www.cdc.gov /infectioncontrol/basics/transmission -based-precautions.html

Centers for Disease Control and Prevention. (2018a). *Hand hygiene in healthcare settings.* Retrieved from https://www.cdc .gov/handhygiene/index.html

Centers for Disease Control and Prevention. (2018b). *2018 National notifiable infectious diseases (historical).* Retrieved from https://www.cdc.gov/nndss /conditions/notifiable/2018/infectious -diseases/

Centers for Disease Control and Prevention. (2018c). *Standard precautions.* Retrieved from https://www.cdc.gov/oralhealth /infectioncontrol/summary-infection -prevention-Practices/standard -precautions.html

Siegel, J. D., Rhinehart, E., Jackson, M., & Chiarello, L. (2018). *2007 Guideline for isolation precautions: Preventing transmission of infectious agents in healthcare settings.* Retrieved from https://www.cdc .gov/infectioncontrol/guidelines /isolation/index.html

11

Troubleshooting

Spotting and correcting equipment problems

I.V. equipment

Peripheral I.V. lines

Signs and symptoms	Possible causes	Interventions
Local complications		
Phlebitis • Tenderness at the tip of and above the venipuncture device • Redness at the tip of the catheter and along the vein • Puffy area over the vein • Vein hard on palpation • Possible fever • Sluggish infusion rate	• Poor blood flow around the venipuncture device • Tip of the catheter located next to the vessel wall • Friction from movement of the catheter in the vein • Venipuncture device left in the vein too long • Clotting at the catheter tip (thrombophlebitis) • Drug or solution with a high or low pH or high osmolarity	• Remove the venipuncture device. • Apply warm soaks. Elevate the extremity if edema is present. • Notify the health care provider. Document the patient's condition and your interventions. *Prevention* • Restart the infusion according to facility policy, preferably in the other arm, using a larger vein for an irritating solution, or restart with a smaller gauge device to ensure adequate blood flow. • Tape the device securely to prevent motion. • Rotate the site at least every 96 hours and per facility policy.
Extravasation • Swelling at and above the I.V. site (may extend along the entire limb) • Discomfort, burning, or pain at the site (but may be painless) • Tight feeling at the site • Decreased skin temperature around the site • Blanching at the site • Continuing fluid infusion even when the vein is occluded (although the rate may decrease) • Slowed or stopped infusion • Blistering (a late sign)	• Venipuncture device dislodged from the vein or perforated vein • Vesicant in the tissue	• Remove the venipuncture device. Notify the health care provider and follow facility policy. • Monitor the patient's pulse and capillary refill time. • Restart the infusion in another limb. • Notify the health care provider. Document the patient's condition and your interventions. • Administer any possible antidote (these may alter the drug pH or DNA binding or neutralize or dilute the extravasated drug). • Elevate the limb. • Apply cold compresses. *Prevention* • Check the site often. • Do not obscure the area above the site with tape. • Teach the patient to observe the I.V. site and advise him or her to report pain or swelling.

(continued)

Peripheral I.V. lines (continued)

Signs and symptoms	Possible causes	Interventions
Local complications (continued)		
Catheter dislodgment • Catheter partially backed out of the vein • Solution infiltrating the tissue	• Loosened tape or tubing snagged in the bed linens, resulting in partial retraction of the catheter • Catheter pulled out by a confused patient	• Remove the I.V. catheter. *Prevention* • Tape the venipuncture device securely on insertion.
Occlusion • I.V. fluid that does not flow	• I.V. flow interrupted • Saline lock not flushed • Backflow of blood in the line when the patient walks • Line clamped too long	• Use a mild flush injection. Do not force it. If you are unsuccessful, reinsert the I.V. line. *Prevention* • Maintain the I.V. flow rate. • Flush the line before and after intermittent piggyback administration, according to facility policy. • Have the patient walk with his or her arm folded to his or her chest to reduce the risk of blood backflow.
Vein irritation or pain at the I.V. site • Pain during infusion • Possible blanching if vasospasm occurs • Red skin over the vein during infusion • Rapidly developing signs of phlebitis	• Solution with a high or low pH or high osmolarity, such as 40 mEq/L of potassium chloride, phenytoin, and some antibiotics (erythromycin, nafcillin, and vancomycin)	• Decrease the flow rate. • Try using an electronic flow device to achieve a steady flow. • Change the I.V. site. *Prevention* • Dilute the solutions before administration. For example, give antibiotics in a 250-ml solution rather than a 100-ml solution. • If long-term therapy with an irritating drug is planned, ask the health care provider to use a central I.V. line.

Peripheral I.V. lines (continued)

Signs and symptoms	Possible causes	Interventions

Local complications (continued)

Signs and symptoms	Possible causes	Interventions
Severed catheter • Leakage from the catheter shaft	• Catheter inadvertently cut by scissors • Reinsertion of the needle into the catheter	• If a broken part is visible, attempt to retrieve it. If you are unsuccessful, notify the health care provider. • If a portion of the catheter enters the bloodstream, place a tourniquet above the I.V. site to prevent progression of the broken part. Immediately notify the health care provider and radiology department. • Document the patient's condition and your interventions. *Prevention* • Do not use scissors around the I.V. site. • Never reinsert a needle into the catheter. • Remove an unsuccessfully inserted catheter and needle together.
Hematoma • Tenderness at the venipuncture site • Bruised area around the site	• Vein punctured through the opposite wall at the time of insertion • Leakage of blood into the tissue • Not applying pressure after I.V. discontinuation	• Remove the venipuncture device and restart the infusion in the opposite limb. • Apply pressure and cold compresses to the affected area. • Recheck the site for bleeding. • Document the patient's condition and your interventions. *Prevention* • Choose a vein that can accommodate the size of the venipuncture device. • Release the tourniquet as soon as a successful insertion is achieved.
Venous spasm • Pain along the vein • Sluggish flow rate when the clamp is completely open • Blanched skin over the vein	• Severe vein irritation as a result of irritating drugs or fluids • Administration of cold fluids or blood products • Very rapid flow rate (with fluids at room temperature)	• Apply warm soaks over the vein and surrounding area. • Decrease the flow rate. *Prevention* • Use a blood warmer for blood or packed red blood cells.

(continued)

Peripheral I.V. lines *(continued)*

Signs and symptoms	Possible causes	Interventions
Local complications (continued)		
Vasovagal reaction • Sudden collapse of the vein during venipuncture • Sudden pallor, sweating, faintness, dizziness, and nausea • Decreased blood pressure	• Vasospasm as a result of anxiety or pain	• Lower the head of the bed. • Have the patient take deep breaths. • Check the patient's vital signs. *Prevention* • To relieve the patient's anxiety, prepare him or her for the procedure. • Use a local anesthetic to prevent pain.
Thrombosis • Painful, reddened, and swollen vein • Sluggish or stopped I.V. flow	• Injury to the endothelial cells of the vein wall, allowing platelets to adhere and thrombi to form	• Remove the venipuncture device. Restart the infusion in the opposite limb, if possible. Notify the health care provider. • Apply warm soaks. • Watch for an I.V. therapy–related infection. *Prevention* • Use proper venipuncture techniques to reduce injury to the vein.
Thrombophlebitis • Severe discomfort at the site • Reddened, swollen, and hardened vein • Warmth at site	• Thrombosis and inflammation	• Follow the interventions for thrombosis. Notify the health care provider. • Apply warm, moist compress. *Prevention* • Check the site frequently. Remove the venipuncture device at the first sign of redness and tenderness.
Nerve, tendon, or ligament damage • Extreme pain (similar to electrical shock when the nerve is punctured), numbness, and muscle contraction • Delayed effects, including paralysis, numbness, and deformity	• Improper venipuncture technique, resulting in injury to the surrounding nerves, tendons, or ligaments • Tight taping or improper splinting with an arm board	• Stop the procedure. *Prevention* • Do not repeatedly penetrate tissues with the venipuncture device. • Do not apply excessive pressure when taping; do not encircle the limb with tape. • Pad the arm boards and the tape securing the arm boards, if possible.

Peripheral I.V. lines *(continued)*

Signs and symptoms	Possible causes	Interventions
Systemic complications		
Circulatory overload • Discomfort • Jugular vein distention • Respiratory distress • Increased blood pressure • Crackles • Increased difference between fluid intake and output • Weight gain • Edema	• Roller clamp loosened to allow run-on infusion • Flow rate too rapid • Miscalculation of fluid requirements	• Raise the head of the bed. • Administer oxygen, if needed. • Reduce the infusion rate to a keep-vein-open rate and notify the health care provider. • Give drugs as ordered. • Monitor vital signs. • Anticipate an order for diuretics for severe overload. *Prevention* • Use a pump, controller, or rate minder for an elderly or compromised patient. • Recheck calculations of the patient's fluid requirements. • Monitor the infusion frequently.
Systemic infection (septicemia or bacteremia) • Fever, chills, and malaise for no apparent reason • Contaminated I.V. site, usually with no visible signs of infection at the site	• Failure to maintain aseptic technique during insertion or site care • Severe phlebitis, causing organism growth • Poor taping that permits the venipuncture device to move, introducing organisms into the bloodstream • Prolonged indwelling time • Compromised immune system	• Notify the health care provider. • Administer medications, as prescribed. • Culture the site and the device. • Monitor the patient's vital signs. *Prevention* • Use scrupulous aseptic technique when handling solutions and tubing, inserting a venipuncture device, and discontinuing the infusion. • Secure all connections. • Change the I.V. solutions, tubing, and venipuncture device at the recommended times.
Speed shock • Flushed face, headache • Tightness in the chest • Irregular pulse • Syncope • Rapid hypertension • Shock • Cardiac arrest	• Too rapid injection of drug, causing plasma levels to become toxic • Improper administration of a bolus infusion (especially additives)	• Discontinue the infusion. • Begin an infusion of dextrose 5% in water at a keep-vein-open rate. • Notify the health care provider. *Prevention* • Check the infusion guidelines before giving a drug. • Dilute the drug with a compatible solution.

(continued)

Peripheral I.V. lines *(continued)*

Signs and symptoms	Possible causes	Interventions
Systemic complications (continued)		
Air embolism • Respiratory distress • Unequal breath sounds • Chest pain, dyspnea • Anxiety • Weak, rapid pulse • Increased central venous pressure • Decreased blood pressure • Altered consciousness	• Solution container empty • Tubing disconnected	• Discontinue the infusion. • Place the patient in left lateral Trendelenburg's position to allow air to enter the right atrium and disperse through the pulmonary artery. • Administer oxygen. • Notify the health care provider. • Have emergency equipment available. • Document the patient's condition and your interventions. *Prevention* • Purge the tubing of air completely before starting an infusion. • Use the air-detection device on the pump or an air-eliminating filter proximal to the I.V. site. • Secure all connections.
Allergic reaction • Itching • Watery eyes and nose • Bronchospasm • Wheezing • Urticarial rash • Anaphylactic reaction, which may occur within minutes (flushing, chills, anxiety, agitation, itching, palpitations, paresthesia, throbbing in the ears, wheezing, coughing, seizures, cardiac arrest)	• Allergens such as medications	• If a reaction occurs, stop the infusion immediately. • Maintain a patent airway. • Notify the health care provider. • Administer an antihistaminic corticosteroid and antipyretic medication(s), as ordered. • Give 0.2 to 0.5 ml of 1:1,000 aqueous epinephrine subcutaneously, as ordered. Repeat every 10 to 15 minutes as needed. *Prevention* • Obtain the patient's allergy history. Look for cross allergies. • Assist with test dosing. • Monitor the patient carefully during the first 15 minutes of administering of a new drug.

Central venous lines

Signs and symptoms	Possible causes	Interventions
Pneumothorax, hemothorax, chylothorax, hydrothorax • Chest pain • Dyspnea • Cyanosis • Decreased breath sounds on the affected side • With hemothorax, decreased hemoglobin levels because of blood pooling • Abnormal findings on chest X-ray • Apprehension	• Lung puncture by the catheter during insertion or exchange over a guide wire • Large blood vessel puncture with bleeding inside or outside the lung • Lymph node puncture with leakage of lymph fluid • Infusion of solution into the chest area through an infiltrated catheter	• Notify the health care provider and stop the infusion. • Remove the catheter or assist with removal, as ordered. • Administer oxygen, as ordered. • Set up and assist with chest tube insertion. • Document all interventions. *Prevention* • Position the patient head down with a rolled towel between his or her scapulae to dilate and expose the internal jugular or subclavian vein as much as possible during catheter insertion. • Assess the patient for early signs of fluid infiltration (swelling in the shoulder, neck, chest, and arm). • Ensure that the patient is immobilized and prepared for insertion. • Minimize the patient's activity after insertion, especially with a peripheral catheter.
Air embolism • Respiratory distress • Chest pain • Unequal breath sounds • Weak, rapid pulse • Increased central venous pressure • Decreased blood pressure • Churning murmur over the precordium • Alteration in consciousness or loss of consciousness • Anxiety	• Intake of air into the central venous system during catheter insertion or tubing changes or inadvertent opening, cutting, or breaking of the catheter	• Clamp the catheter immediately. • Place the patient in left lateral Trendelenburg's position so that air can enter the right atrium and pulmonary artery. Make sure that he or she remains in this position for 20 to 30 minutes. • Do not recommend Valsalva's maneuver because a large air intake worsens the condition. • Administer oxygen. • Notify the health care provider. • Document all interventions. *Prevention* • Purge all air from the tubing before hookup. • Teach the patient to perform Valsalva's maneuver during catheter insertion and tubing changes. • Use air-eliminating filters or an infusion device with air-detection capability. • Use luer-lock tubing, tape the connections, or use locking devices for all connections.

(continued)

Central venous lines *(continued)*

Signs and symptoms	Possible causes	Interventions
Thrombosis • Edema at the puncture site • Erythema • Ipsilateral swelling of the arm, neck, and face • Pain along the vein • Fever, malaise • Jugular vein distention	• Sluggish flow rate • Composition of the catheter material (Polyvinyl chloride catheters are more thrombogenic.) • Hematopoietic status of the patient • Infusion of irritating solutions • Repeated or long-term use of the same vein • Preexisting cardiovascular disease • Simultaneous administration of incompatible medications or inadequate flushing between administration of incompatible medications • Irritation of the vein during insertion of a central venous catheter • Improper location of catheter in the subclavian or brachiocephalic vein	• Notify the health care provider. • Stop the infusion. • Infuse a dose of heparin or a thrombolytic, if ordered. • Do not use the limb on the affected side for subsequent venipuncture. • Verify thrombosis with diagnostic studies. *Prevention* • Verify placement of the catheter tip in the superior vena cava (SVC) before using the catheter. If the tip is not in the SVC, the catheter should not be used.
Infection • Redness, warmth, tenderness, and swelling at the insertion or exit site • Possible exudate of purulent material • Local rash or pustules • Fever, chills, malaise • Leukocytosis • Nausea and vomiting • Elevated urine glucose level	• Failure to maintain aseptic technique during catheter insertion or care • Failure to comply with the dressing-change protocol • Wet or soiled dressing remaining on the site • Immunosuppression • Irritated suture line • Contaminated catheter or solution • Frequent opening of the catheter	• Monitor the patient's temperature and vital signs frequently. • Culture the site if drainage is present. • Redress the site using aseptic technique. • Use an antibiotic ointment locally, as needed. • Treat the patient systemically with an antibiotic or an antifungal, depending on the culture results and the health care provider's order. • Draw central and peripheral blood cultures; if the same organism appears in both, then the catheter is the primary source of infection and should be removed. *Staphylococcus epidermidis* is the most common organism. • If the cultures do not match but are positive, the catheter may be removed or the infection may be treated through the catheter. • Treat the patient with an antibiotic, as ordered.

Central venous lines *(continued)*

Signs and symptoms	Possible causes	Interventions
Infection *(continued)*		• If the catheter is removed, culture its tip. • Document all interventions. *Prevention* • Maintain sterile technique using sterile gloves, masks, and gowns, when appropriate. • Observe dressing-change protocols. • Teach the patient about restrictions on swimming, bathing, and other physical activities. • Change a wet or soiled dressing immediately. • Change the dressing more frequently if the catheter is located in the femoral area or near a tracheostomy. Perform tracheostomy care after catheter care. • Examine the solution for cloudiness and turbidity before infusing; check the fluid container for leaks. • Monitor the urine glucose level in the patient who is receiving total parenteral nutrition (TPN); if the level is greater than 2+, he or she may have early sepsis. • Use a 1.2-micron filter for three-in-one TPN solutions. • Change the catheter according to facility protocol. • Keep the system closed as much as possible.

Infusion control devices

When the alarm goes off, check for these problems.

Problems	Interventions
Air in the line	While setting up, make sure that all air is out of the line, including air trapped in Y-injection sites. Also, check that the connections are secure and that the container is filled properly. Withdraw any air from a piggyback port with a syringe or an air-eliminating filter. A wet-air detector may give a false reading.
Infusion completed	Reset the pump, as ordered, or discontinue the infusion. A slow keep-vein-open rate usually keeps the I.V. line patent if there is enough fluid.

(continued)

Infusion control devices *(continued)*

Problems	Interventions
Empty container	Check for adequate fluid levels in the I.V. container and have another container available before the last one runs out.
Low battery	Battery life varies; keep the machine plugged in on AC power as much as possible, especially while the patient is in bed. If the alarm goes off, plug in the machine immediately, or power may be lost for a while (usually a half hour to several hours).
Occlusion	Check that all clamps are open, look for kinked tubing, and check the patency of the venipuncture device.
Rate change	Check that the infusion control device displays the ordered rate. The patient or a family member may have tampered with the controls.
Open door	The door should be closed. It may not shut if the device is not set up properly (for example, if the cassette is not inserted all the way).
Malfunction	A mechanical failure usually must be handled by the biomedical engineering department or the manufacturer. Disconnect the infusion control device. Label it clearly with a sign that says DO NOT USE and indicate the specific problem.

I.V. flow rates

Problems and possible causes	Interventions
Flow rate too fast	
Clamp manipulated by the patient or a visitor	Instruct the patient not to touch the clamp and place tape over it. Administer the I.V. solution with an infusion pump or a controller, if necessary. Set the safety on the back of the pump.
Tubing disconnected from the catheter	Using alcohol, wipe the distal end of the tubing with luer-lock connections. Reinsert the end of the tubing firmly into the catheter hub and apply tape at the connection site.
Change in the patient's position	Use an infusion pump or a controller to ensure the correct flow rate.
Flow clamp drifting as a result of patient movement	Place tape below the clamp.

I.V. flow rates *(continued)*

Problems and possible causes	Interventions
Flow rate too slow	
Venous spasm after insertion	Apply warm soaks over the site.
Venous obstruction as a result of bending the patient's arm	Secure the I.V. line with a padded arm board, if necessary. Frequently check the patient's neurovascular status and monitor him or her according to facility policy.
Pressure change (as a result of decreased fluid in the bottle)	Readjust the flow rate.
Elevated blood pressure	Readjust the flow rate. Use an infusion pump or a controller to ensure the correct rate.
Cold solution	Allow the solution to warm to room temperature before hanging the bag.
Change in the viscosity of the solution from an added drug	Readjust the flow rate.
I.V. container that is too low or a patient's arm or leg that is too high	Hang the container higher or remind the patient to keep his or her arm below the level of his or her heart.
Excess tubing dangling below the insertion site	Replace the tubing with a shorter piece or tape the excess tubing to the I.V. pole below the flow clamp (making sure that the tubing is not kinked).
Venipuncture device that is too small	Remove the venipuncture device in use and insert a larger bore venipuncture device or use an infusion pump.
Infiltration or clotted venipuncture device	Remove the venipuncture device in use and insert a new one.
Kinked tubing	Check the tubing over its entire length and unkink it.
Tubing compressed at the clamped area	Massage or milk the tubing by pinching and wrapping it around a pencil four or five times. Then quickly pull the pencil out of the coiled tubing.

Infusion interruptions

When an infusion stops, assess the I.V. system systematically—from the patient to the fluid container—for potential trouble areas.

Check the I.V. site

Check for infiltration or phlebitis, which may slow or stop the flow rate.

Check for patency

Evaluate the I.V. device for patency and catheter-related complications, keeping in mind that several factors can affect it.

- Increased blood pressure may stop the I.V. flow if the patient's limb is flexed or is lying directly on the I.V. site. Reposition the limb as necessary.
- If the patient's arm is wrapped with tape, a tourniquet effect may reduce the I.V. flow rate. Taping the I.V. site too tightly can cause the same problem. Release or remove the tape and reapply it.
- Local edema or poor tissue perfusion as a result of disease can block the venous flow. Move the I.V. line to an unaffected site.
- Infusion of incompatible fluid or medication may cause a precipitate to form. This can block the I.V. tubing and venipuncture device and may even expose the patient to a life-threatening embolism. Always check the compatibility of all medications and the I.V. solution before administering them. Replace the venipuncture device if it is occluded.

Check the filter

Use filters with total parenteral nutrition (TPN) and medications that require filtering. Make sure that the in-line filter is the right size and type. TPN fluids are run through a 0.22- or 0.45-micron filter to eliminate air and microorganisms from the system. Use a 1.2-micron filter for lipid emulsion being infused as a separate solution.

If you use the wrong size or type of filter, the solution may not pass through it. For example, such drugs as amphotericin B and lymphocyte immune globulin (Atgam) consist of molecules that are too large to pass through a 0.22-micron filter; they rapidly block the filter and stop the I.V. flow. If necessary, replace the filter.

The interval between filter and tubing change depends on the manufacturer's instructions. They should be changed at least every 24 hours and with each new container of TPN solution, 12 hours for lipid emulsion.

Check the clamps

Make sure that the flow clamps are open. Check all clamps, including the roller clamp and any clamps on secondary sets such as a slide clamp on a filter. A roller clamp may become jammed if the roller is pushed up too far.

Check the tubing

Determine if the tubing is kinked or if the patient is lying on it. Also check whether the tubing remains crimped where a clamp was tightened around it. If so, gently squeeze the area between your fingers to round out the tubing to its original shape or change the tubing altogether.

Check the air vents

If you are using an evacuated glass container, you will need an air vent to make the I.V. solution flow. Insert one, as needed. On a volume-control set, the air vent is usually located at the top of the calibrated chamber. If the solution flow stops, check the patency of the vent and the position of the vent clamp. Follow the manufacturer's instructions to check the vent's patency.

Check the fluid level

Observe the fluid level in the
I.V. container. If the container is empty,
replace it, as ordered. If the solution is
cold, it may be causing venous spasm,
thus decreasing the flow rate. Applying
warm compresses can relieve venous
spasm and increase the flow rate. Make
sure that other solutions are given
at room temperature. Finally, check

to see if the spike at the end of the
administration set has been pushed far
enough into the container to allow the
solution to flow.

If you cannot identify the problem
with this series of checks, remove
the I.V. line and restart it at a different
site. Document the episode in the
patient's chart.

(Text continues on page 516.)

Implanted ports

Problems and possible causes	Interventions
Inability to flush the implanted port or withdraw blood	
• Kinked tubing or closed clamp	• Check the tubing or clamp.
• Incorrect needle placement • Needle not advanced through the septum	• Regain access to the device.
• Clot formation	• Assess the patency of the device by trying to flush the implanted port. • Notify the health care provider and obtain an order for a thrombolytic. • Teach the patient to recognize clot formation, to notify the health care provider if it occurs, and to avoid forcibly flushing the implanted port.
• Kinked catheter, catheter migration, port rotation	• Notify the health care provider immediately. • Tell the patient to notify the health care provider or home care nurse if he or she has difficulty using the implanted port.
Inability to palpate the implanted port	
• Deeply implanted port	• Note the portal chamber scar to locate the correct spot for palpation. • Use deep palpation to locate the implanted port. • Ask another nurse to locate the implanted port. If you cannot feel the port, do not attempt to access it. • Use a 1½" or 2" noncoring needle to gain access to the implanted port.

Cardiovascular monitors and devices

Blood pressure readings

Problems and possible causes	Interventions
False high reading	
Cuff that is too small	Make sure that the bladder of the cuff is 20% wider than the circumference of the arm or leg that is being used for measurement. Cuff bladder length should be 80% of the arm's circumference. Cuff bladder width should be at least 40% of the arm's circumference.
Cuff that is wrapped too loosely, reducing its effective width	Tighten the cuff.
Slow deflation of the cuff, causing venous congestion in the arm or leg	Never deflate the cuff more slowly than 2 mm Hg per heartbeat.
Tilted mercury column	Read pressures with the mercury column vertical.
Poorly timed measurement (after the patient has eaten, ambulated, appeared anxious, or flexed his or her arm muscles)	Postpone blood pressure measurement or help the patient to relax before taking pressure measurements.
False low reading	
Incorrect position of the arm or leg	Make sure that the arm or leg is level with the patient's heart.
Mercury column below eye level	Read the mercury column at eye level.
Failure to notice an auscultatory gap (Sound fades out for 10 to 15 mm Hg and then returns.)	Estimate the systolic pressure by palpation before measuring it. Then check this pressure against the measured pressure.
Inaudible low-volume sounds	Before reinflating the cuff, instruct the patient to raise his or her arm or leg to decrease venous pressure and amplify low-volume sounds. After you inflate the cuff, tell the patient to lower his or her arm or leg. Then deflate the cuff and listen. If you still do not detect low-volume sounds, use Doppler ultrasonography or chart the palpated systolic pressure according to facility policy.

Cardiac monitors

Problems and possible causes	Interventions
False high-rate alarm	
Monitor is interpreting large T waves as QRS complexes, which doubles the rate.	Reposition the electrodes to the lead where the QRS complexes are taller than the T waves.
Skeletal muscle activity	Place the electrodes away from major muscle masses.
False low-rate alarm	
Shift in the electrical axis caused by patient movement, making QRS complexes too small to register	Reapply the electrodes. Set the gain so that the height of the complex exceeds 1 mV.
Low amplitude of the QRS complex	Increase the gain.
Poor contact between the skin and electrodes	Reapply the electrodes.
Low amplitude	
Gain dial set too low	Increase the gain.
Poor contact between skin and electrodes, dried gel, broken or loose lead wires, poor connection between the patient and monitor, malfunctioning monitor, physiologic loss of amplitude of the QRS complex	Check the connections on all lead wires and the monitoring cable. Replace or reapply the electrodes as necessary.
Wandering baseline	
Poor electrode placement or poor skin contact	Reposition or replace the electrodes.
Movement of the thorax with respirations	Reposition the electrodes.
Artifact (waveform interference)	
Patient having seizures, chills, or anxiety	Notify the health care provider and treat the patient, as ordered. Keep the patient warm and reassure him or her.

(continued)

Cardiac monitors (continued)

Problems and possible causes	Interventions
Artifact (continued)	
Patient movement	Help the patient to relax.
Electrodes applied improperly	Check the electrodes and reapply them, if necessary. Make sure the patient's skin has been prepared properly.
Static electricity	Make sure that the cables do not have exposed connectors. Change static-causing clothing.
Electrical short circuit in the lead wires or cable	Replace the broken equipment. Use stress loops to apply the lead wires.
Interference from decreased room humidity	Regulate the humidity to 40%.
Broken lead wires or cable	
Tension on the lead wires as a result of repeated pulling	Replace and retape the lead wires, taping part of the wire into a loop. This absorbs tension that would otherwise tug at the ends of the wire.
Cables and lead wires cleaned with alcohol or acetone, causing brittleness	Clean the cable and the lead wires with soapy water. Do not let the ends of the cable get wet because an electric shock to the patient could occur. Replace the cable as necessary.
60-cycle interference (fuzzy baseline)	
Electrical interference from other equipment in the room	Attach the electrical equipment to a common ground, checking the plugs for loose prongs.
Patient's bed improperly grounded	Attach the bed ground to the room's common ground.
Skin excoriation under electrode	
Patient allergic to the electrode adhesive	Remove the electrodes and apply hypoallergenic electrodes.
Electrode remaining on the skin for too long	Remove the electrode, clean the site, and reapply the electrode at a new site.

Intra-aortic balloon pumps

When the patient undergoes intra-aortic balloon counterpulsation, you must respond to equipment problems immediately.

Problems and possible causes	Interventions
High gas leakage	
Balloon leakage or abrasion	Check for blood in the tubing. Stop pumping. Contact the health care provider to remove the balloon. The catheter should be removed within 30 minutes.
Condensation in the extension tubing, volume-limiter disk, or both	Remove the condensate from the tubing and the volume-limiter disk. Refill and resume pumping.
Kink in the balloon catheter or tubing	Check the catheter and tubing for kinks and loose connections. Refill and resume pumping.
Tachycardia (rapid flow of helium, causing insufficient fill pressure)	Change the wean control to 1:2 or operate in ON, or manual, mode. *Note*: Gas alarms are off in manual mode. Autopurge the balloon every 1 to 2 hours and monitor the balloon pressure waveform closely.
Malfunctioning or loose volume-limiter disk	Replace or tighten the volume-limiter disk. Refill, autopurge, and resume pumping.
System leak	Perform a leak test.
Balloon line block *(automatic mode only)*	
Kink in the balloon catheter or tubing	Check the catheter and tubing for kinks. Refill and resume pumping.
Balloon catheter not unfurled; sheath or balloon positioned too high	Contact the health care provider to verify placement; the balloon may need to be repositioned or inflated manually.
Condensation in the tubing, volume-limiter disk, or both	Remove the condensate from the tubing and volume-limiter disk. Refill, autopurge, and resume pumping.
Balloon too large for the aorta	Decrease the volume-control percentage by one notch.
Malfunctioning volume-limiter disk or incorrect volume-limiter disk size	Replace the volume-limiter disk. Refill, autopurge, and resume pumping.

(continued)

Intra-aortic balloon pumps *(continued)*

Problems and possible causes	Interventions
No electrocardiogram (ECG) trigger	
Inadequate signal	Adjust the ECG gain and change the lead or the trigger mode. Replace the lead.
Lead disconnected	Replace the lead.
Improper ECG input mode (skin or monitor) selected	Adjust the ECG input to the appropriate mode (skin or monitor). Apply new electrodes, as needed.
No arterial pressure trigger	
Arterial line damped	Flush the line.
Arterial line open to the atmosphere	Check the connections on the arterial pressure line.
Trigger mode change	
Trigger mode changed while pumping	Resume pumping.
Irregular heart rhythm	
Patient's rhythm is irregular (such as atrial fibrillation or ectopic beats).	Change to R or QRS sense, if necessary, to accommodate the irregular rhythm.
Erratic atrioventricular pacing	
Demand for paced rhythm occurs during atrioventricular sequential trigger mode.	Change to the pacer reject trigger or QRS sense.
Noisy ECG signal	
Malfunctioning leads	Replace the leads; check the ECG cable and electrodes.
Electrocautery in use	Switch to the arterial pressure trigger.
Internal trigger	
Trigger mode set on internal 80 beats/minute	Select an alternative trigger if the patient has a heartbeat or rhythm. *Caution:* Use an internal trigger only during cardiopulmonary bypass surgery or cardiac arrest.
Purge incomplete	
OFF button pressed during autopurge, interrupting the purge cycle	Initiate autopurge again or initiate pumping.

Intra-aortic balloon pumps *(continued)*

Problems and possible causes	Interventions
High fill pressure	
Malfunctioning volume-limiter disk	Replace the volume-limiter disk. Refill, autopurge, and resume pumping.
Occluded vent line or valve	Attempt to resume pumping. If this does not correct the problem, contact the manufacturer.
No balloon drive	
No volume-limiter disk	Insert the volume-limiter disk and lock it securely in place.
Tubing disconnected	Reconnect the tubing. Refill, autopurge, and pump.
Incorrect timing	
INFLATE and DEFLATE controls set improperly	Place the INFLATE and DEFLATE controls at set midpoints. Reassess the timing and readjust.
Low volume percentage	
Volume-control percentage not set on 100%	Assess the cause of the decreased volume and reset, if necessary.

Pacemakers

Life-threatening arrhythmias can result when the patient's pacemaker sends an impulse that is too weak to stimulate the heart (failure to capture). Furthermore, the pacemaker may not detect ventricular depolarization (failure to sense) or may not send an impulse at all (failure to fire). Below are rhythm strips that compare these problems with a normal wave strip as well as lists of possible causes and interventions.

Normal

The location of the spike is your first clue that the pacemaker is functioning normally.

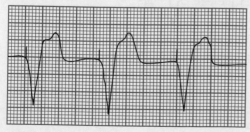

(continued)

Pacemakers *(continued)*

Failure to capture

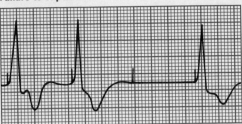

Causes
- Pacemaker output too low
- Catheter dislodged
- Loose connections

Interventions
- Increase the pacemaker output.
- Reposition the catheter.
- Secure all connections.

Failure to sense

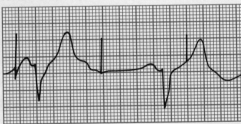

Causes
- Incorrect sensitivity setting

Interventions
- Adjust the sensitivity setting.

Failure to fire

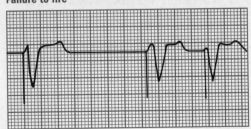

Causes
- Loose lead hookups
- Dead battery
- Malfunctioning pulse generator

Interventions
- Secure the lead hookups.
- Replace the battery.
- Replace the pulse generator.

Arterial lines

Problems	Possible causes	Interventions
Damped waveform Appearing as a small waveform with a slow rise in the anacrotic limb and a reduced or nonexistent dicrotic notch, a damped waveform may result from interference with the transmission of the physiologic signal to the transducer.	Air in the system	Check the system for air, paying particular attention to the tubing and the diaphragm of the transducer. If you find air, aspirate it or force it from the system through a stopcock port. Never flush a fluid that contains air bubbles into a patient.
	Loose connection	Check and tighten all connections.
	Clotted catheter tip	Attempt to aspirate the clot. If you are successful, flush the line. If you are unsuccessful, avoid flushing the line because you could dislodge the clot.
	Catheter tip resting against the arterial wall	Reposition the catheter by carefully rotating it or pulling it back slightly. Anticipate a possible change in the catheter placement site and assist, as appropriate.
	Kinked tubing	Unkink the tubing.
	Inadequately inflated pressure infuser bag	Inflate the pressure infuser bag to 300 mm Hg.
Drifting waveform Waveform floats above and below the baseline.	Temperature change in the flush solution	Allow the temperature of the flush solution to stabilize before the infusion.
	Kinked or compressed monitor cable	Check the cable and relieve the kink or compression.
Inability to flush the arterial line or to withdraw blood Activating the continuous flush device does not move the flush solution, and blood cannot be withdrawn from the stopcock.	Incorrectly positioned stopcocks	Reposition the stopcocks properly.
	Kinked tubing	Unkink the tubing.
	Inadequately inflated pressure infuser bag	Inflate the pressure infuser bag to 300 mm Hg.
	Clotted catheter tip	Attempt to aspirate the clot. If you are successful, flush the line. If you are unsuccessful, avoid flushing the line because you could dislodge the clot.

(continued)

Arterial lines (continued)

Problems	Possible causes	Interventions
Inability to flush the arterial line or to withdraw blood (continued)	Catheter tip resting against the arterial wall	Reposition the catheter insertion area and flush the catheter. Alternatively, reposition the catheter by carefully rotating it or pulling it back slightly.
	Position of the insertion area	Check the position of the insertion area and change it, as indicated. For radial and brachial arterial lines, use a padded arm board to immobilize the area according to facility policy. With a femoral arterial line, keep the head of the bed at a 45-degree angle or less to prevent the catheter from kinking.
Artifact Waveform tracings follow an erratic pattern or do not appear as a recognizable diagnostic pattern.	Electrical interference	Check the electrical equipment in the room.
	Patient movement	Ask the patient to lie quietly while you try to read the monitor.
	Catheter whip or fling (excessive movement of the catheter tip)	Shorten the tubing, if possible.
False high-pressure reading Arterial pressure exceeds the patient's normal pressure without a significant change in the baseline clinical findings. Before responding to this high-pressure reading, recheck the system to make sure that the reading is accurate.	Improper calibration	Recalibrate the system.
	Transducer positioned below the phlebostatic axis	Relevel the transducer with the phlebostatic axis.
	Catheter kinked	Unkink the catheter.
	Clotted catheter tip	Attempt to aspirate the clot. If you are successful, flush the line. If you are unsuccessful, avoid flushing the line because you could dislodge the clot.
	Catheter tip resting against the arterial line	Flush the catheter or reposition it by carefully rotating it or pulling it back slightly.
	I.V. tubing too long	Shorten the tubing by removing the extension tubing (if used) or replace the administration set with a set that has shorter tubing.
	Small air bubbles in the tubing close to the patient	Remove the air bubbles.

Arterial lines *(continued)*

Problems	Possible causes	Interventions
False low-pressure reading Arterial pressure drops below the patient's normal pressure without a significant change in the baseline clinical findings. Before responding to this low-pressure reading, recheck the system to ensure that the reading is accurate.	Improper calibration	Recalibrate the system.
	Transducer positioned above the level of the phlebostatic axis	Relevel the transducer with the phlebostatic axis.
	Loose connections	Check and tighten all connections.
	Catheter kinked	Unkink the catheter.
	Clotted catheter tip	Attempt to aspirate the clot. If you are successful, flush the line. If you are unsuccessful, avoid flushing the line because you could dislodge the clot.
	Catheter tip resting against the arterial line	Reposition the catheter insertion area and flush the catheter. Alternatively, reposition the catheter by carefully rotating it or pulling it back slightly.
	I.V. tubing too long	Shorten the tubing by removing the extension tubing (if used) or replace the administration set with a set that has shorter tubing.
	Large air bubble close to the transducer	Reprime the transducer.
No waveform No waveform appears on the monitor.	No power supply	Turn on the power.
	Loose connections	Check and tighten all connections.
	Stopcocks turned off to the patient	Position the stopcocks properly. Make sure that the transducer is open to the catheter.
	Transducer disconnected from the monitor module	Reconnect the transducer to the monitor module.
	Occluded catheter tip	Attempt to aspirate the clot. If you are successful, flush the line. If you are unsuccessful, avoid flushing the line because you could dislodge the clot.
	Catheter tip resting against the arterial wall	Flush the catheter or reposition it by carefully rotating it or pulling it back slightly.

Arterial line, accidental removal of

If the patient removes his or her arterial line, he or she is in danger of hypovolemic shock from blood loss. Here is what to do.

Stanching the blood flow

- Apply direct pressure to the insertion site immediately and send someone to call the health care provider. Maintain firm, direct pressure on the insertion site for 5 to 10 minutes to encourage clot formation because arterial blood flows under extremely high intravascular pressure.
- Check the patient's I.V. line and, if ordered, increase the flow rate temporarily to compensate for blood loss.

When the bleeding stops

- Apply a sterile pressure dressing.
- Reassess the patient's level of consciousness (LOC) and comfort and reassure him or her. Losing large quantities of blood may have significant psychological and physiologic effects.
- Estimate the amount of blood loss from what you see and from changes in the patient's blood pressure and heart rate.
- When the health care provider arrives, help him or her to reinsert the catheter, ensuring that the patient's arm is immobilized and that the tubing and catheter are secured.
- Withdraw blood for a complete blood count and arterial blood gas analysis, as ordered.

Ongoing care

- Closely monitor the patient's vital signs, LOC, skin color, temperature, and circulation to the extremity.
- Watch for further bleeding or hematoma.
- Decrease the I.V. flow rate to the previous level after the patient's condition has stabilized.

Respiratory monitors and devices

Pulse oximeters

To maintain a continuous display of arterial oxygen saturation levels, keep the monitoring site clean and dry. Make sure that the skin does not become irritated from the adhesives used to keep the disposable probes in place. You may need to change the site if this happens. Nondisposable probes that do not need tape can be used to replace disposable probes that irritate the skin.

Another common problem with pulse oximeters is failure to obtain a signal. If this happens, your first reaction should be to check the patient's vital signs. If they are sufficient to produce a signal, check for problems, including a poor connection, inadequate or intermittent blood flow to the site, and equipment malfunction.

Poor connection

Check to see if the sensors are aligned properly. Make sure that the wires are intact and fastened securely and that the pulse oximeter is connected to a power source.

Inadequate or intermittent blood flow to the site

Check the patient's pulse rate and capillary refill time and take corrective action if blood flow to the site is decreased. This may mean loosening restraints, removing tight-fitting clothing, taking off a blood pressure cuff, or checking arterial and I.V. lines. If none of these interventions works, you may need to find an alternate site. Finding a site with proper circulation may prove challenging in a patient who is receiving a vasoconstrictor. Use of a forehead sensor may be necessary.

Equipment malfunction

Remove the pulse oximeter from the patient, set the alarm limits at 90% and 100%, and try the instrument on yourself or another healthy person. This will tell you if the equipment is working correctly.

(Text continues on page 521.)

Sv̄o₂ monitors

During continuous mixed venous oxygen saturation (Sv̄o₂) monitoring, watch for signs of equipment malfunction so that you can distinguish them from changes in the patient's condition and respond appropriately. This chart identifies common problems, their causes, and nursing interventions.

Problems and possible causes	Interventions
Low-intensity alarm sounds	
Inadequate blood flow past the catheter tip	• Look for and straighten obvious kinks in the catheter. • Follow facility procedure to ensure distal lumen patency. • Check for a proper connection between the optical module and the computer.
Damaged fiber-optic filaments	• Replace the catheter.
Damped intensity	
Blood clot over the catheter tip	• Follow facility procedure to ensure distal lumen patency.
Wedging of the catheter tip	• Reposition the catheter.
Erratic intensity	
Blood clot over the catheter tip	• Follow facility procedure to ensure distal lumen patency.
Wedging of the catheter tip	• Reposition the catheter.
High-intensity alarm sounds	
Catheter tip pressing against the vessel wall	• Reposition the catheter and examine the pressure waveform to confirm the proper position.
Catheter floating distally into the wedge position	• Check the status of the balloon and confirm the proper position by examining the pressure waveform. • Reposition the catheter, as needed.

(continued)

Svo₂ monitors (continued)

Problems and possible causes	Interventions
LOW-LIGHT message	
Poor connection between the catheter and the optical module	• Disconnect the catheter from the optical module, close the lid, and place the optical module out of direct light. If the LOW-LIGHT message disappears, the problem is the catheter. Check the connection and reattach as needed.
Defective optical module	• Replace the optical module.
Poor connection between the optical module and the computer	• Check the connections and reconnect as needed. Turn off the computer for a few seconds and turn it back on. You will hear two beeps if the computer is functional and the connections are secure.
Damaged fiber-optic filaments	• Gently manipulate the catheter, particularly around the insertion site. If this does not solve the problem, replace the catheter.
CAL FAIL message	
Unsuccessful preinsertion calibration	• Verify correct attachment between the catheter and the optical module. Repeat calibration. • If the CAL FAIL message still appears, replace the optical module.
Dashes in oxygen saturation display	
Improper preinsertion calibration	• Verify correct attachment between the catheter and the optical module. Repeat calibration.
Malfunction of the optical module	• If dashes continue to appear, replace the optical module. Repeat calibration.
Catheter damage	• Gently manipulate the catheter. If the monitor does not compute a range, replace the catheter. Repeat calibration.
Improper positioning of the catheter tip	• Reposition the catheter.
Loss of electronic memory	• Determine the cause of the power loss and then repeat calibration.

Ventilators

Most ventilators have alarms to warn you of hazardous situations—for instance, when inspiratory pressure rises too high or drops too low. Use this chart to help you respond to a ventilator alarm quickly and effectively.

Problems and possible causes	Interventions
Low pressure	
Tube disconnected from the ventilator	Reconnect the tube to the ventilator.
Endotracheal (ET) tube displaced above the vocal cords or tracheostomy tube extubated	If extubation or displacement has occurred, open the patient's airway, ventilate the patient manually, and call the health care provider.
Leaking tidal volume from low cuff pressure (as a result of an underinflated or ruptured ET cuff or a leak in the cuff or one-way valve)	Listen for a whooshing sound (an air leak) around the tube and check the cuff pressure. If you cannot maintain pressure, the health care provider may insert a new tube.
Ventilator malfunction	Disconnect the patient from the ventilator and ventilate him or her manually, if necessary. Get another ventilator.
Leak in the ventilator circuitry (from a loose connection or a hole in the tubing, loss of a temperature-sensing device, or a cracked humidification container)	Make sure that all connections are intact. Check the humidification container and tubing for holes or leaks. Replace them, if necessary.
High pressure	
Increased airway pressure or decreased lung compliance as a result of worsening disease	Auscultate the lungs for evidence of increasing lung consolidation, barotrauma, or wheezing. Call the health care provider, if necessary.
Patient biting on the ET tube	If needed, insert a bite block.
Secretions in the airway	Suction the patient or have him or her cough.
Condensation in the large-bore tubing	Remove any condensation.
Intubation of the right mainstem bronchus	Check the position of the tube. If the position is incorrect, notify the health care provider. It will need to be repositioned.
Patient coughing, gagging, or trying to talk	If the patient is fighting the ventilator in any way, he or she may need a sedative or neuromuscular blocker. Administer the drug, as ordered.

(continued)

Ventilators *(continued)*

Problems and possible causes	Interventions
***High pressure** (continued)* Chest-wall resistance	Reposition the patient if his or her position limits chest expansion. If repositioning is ineffective, give him or her the prescribed analgesic.
Malfunctioning high-pressure relief valve	Have the faulty equipment replaced.
Bronchospasm, pneumothorax, or barotrauma	Assess the patient to determine the cause. Report the disorder to the health care provider and treat, as ordered.
Spirometer or low exhaled tidal volume, or low exhaled minute volume Power interruption	Check all electrical connections.
Loose connection or leak in the delivery system	Make sure that all connections in the delivery system are secure. Check for leaks.
Leaking cuff or inadequate cuff seal	Listen for a leak with a stethoscope. Reinflate the cuff according to facility policy. Replace the cuff, if necessary.
Leaking chest tube	Check all chest tube connections. Make sure that the water seal is intact and then notify the health care provider.
Increased airway resistance in a patient who is on a pressure-cycled ventilator	Auscultate the lungs for signs of airway obstruction, barotrauma, or lung consolidation.
Disconnected spirometer	Make sure that the spirometer is connected.
Any change that sets off high- or low-pressure alarms and prevents delivery of the full air volume	See the interventions for high- and low-pressure alarms.
Malfunctioning volume-measuring device	Alert the respiratory therapist to replace the device.
High respiratory rate Anxiety	Assess the patient to determine the cause. Dispel the patient's fears, if possible, and sedate him or her, if necessary. Establish an effective means of communication.
Pain	Position the patient comfortably. Administer a medication for pain, as ordered.
Secretions in the airway	Suction the patient.

Ventilators *(continued)*

Problems and possible causes	Interventions
Low positive end-expiratory pressure (PEEP)/continuous positive airway pressure	
Leak in the system	Make sure that all connections are secure. Check for holes in the tubing and replace it, if necessary.
Mechanical failure of the PEEP mechanism	Discontinue PEEP and call a respiratory therapist.

Endotracheal or tracheostomy tube, accidental removal of

If an endotracheal (ET) or tracheostomy tube is accidentally removed or if the patient deliberately removes it, immediately take these steps.

ET tube

- Remove any remaining part of the tube.
- Ventilate the patient using common resuscitation techniques or a hand-held resuscitation bag.
- Send someone to notify the health care provider.
- Restrain the patient according to facility policy if he or she extubated himself or herself.
- After the tube is reinserted, periodically check the position of the tube and the condition of the tape or the ET tube holder that is holding it. For a secure fit, anchor the tape from the nape of the patient's neck to and around the tube.

Tracheostomy tube

- Remove any remaining part of the tube.
- Keep the stoma open with a Kelly clamp and try to insert a new tube. If you cannot get the tube in, insert a suction catheter instead and thread the tube over the catheter.

- Call a code if you cannot establish an effective airway and you no longer detect a pulse. Then either ventilate with a face mask and resuscitation bag or remove the Kelly clamp to close the stoma and perform mouth-to-mouth resuscitation until the health care provider arrives. If air leaks from the stoma, cover it with an occlusive dressing.

 ALERT

Do not leave the patient alone until you have established that he or she has an effective airway and can breathe comfortably.

- When a new tracheostomy tube is in place and the patient can breathe more easily, give him or her supplemental humidified oxygen until he or she receives a full evaluation.
- Monitor the patient's vital signs, skin color, and LOC and, unless contraindicated, elevate the head of his or her bed.
- Obtain a chest X-ray, as ordered, to confirm tube placement.

Chest drains

Problems	Interventions
Patient rolls over on the drainage tubing, causing obstruction.	• Reposition the patient and remove any kinks in the tubing. • Auscultate for decreased breath sounds and percuss for dullness, which indicates fluid accumulation, or for hyperresonance, which indicates air accumulation.
Dependent loops in the tubing trap fluids and prevent effective drainage.	• Make sure that the chest drainage unit sits below the patient's chest level. If necessary, raise the bed slightly to increase gravity flow. Remove any kinks in the tubing. • Monitor the patient for decreased breath sounds and percuss for dullness.
No drainage appears in the collection chamber.	• If blood or other fluid is draining, suspect a clot or obstruction in the tubing. Gently milk the tubing to expel the obstruction, if facility policy permits. • Monitor the patient for lung tissue compression caused by accumulated pleural fluid.
Substantial increase in bloody drainage, indicating possible active bleeding or drainage of old blood	• Monitor the patient's vital signs. Look for an increased pulse rate, decreased blood pressure, and orthostatic changes that may indicate acute blood loss. • Measure the drainage every 15 to 30 minutes to determine if it is occurring continuously or in one gush as a result of position changes.
No bubbling in the suction-control chamber	• Check for obstructions in the tubing. Make sure that all the connections are tight. • Check that the suction apparatus is turned on. Increase the suction slowly until you see gentle bubbling.
Loud, vigorous bubbling in the suction-control chamber	• Turn down the suction source until bubbling is just visible.
Constant bubbling in the water-seal chamber	• Assess the chest drainage unit and the tubing for an air leak. • If an air leak is not noted in the external system, notify the health care provider immediately. Leaking and trapping of air in the pleural space can result in a tension pneumothorax.
Evaporation causes the water level in the suction-control chamber to drop below the desired level of -20 cm H_2O.	• Using a syringe and needle, add water or normal saline solution through a resealable diaphragm on the back of the suction-control chamber.
Patient has trouble breathing immediately after a special procedure; the chest drainage unit is improperly placed on the patient's bed, interfering with drainage.	• Raise the head of the bed and reposition the unit so that gravity promotes drainage. • Perform a quick respiratory assessment and take the patient's vital signs. Make sure that the water-seal and suction-control chambers contain enough water.

Chest drains *(continued)*

Problems	Interventions
As the bed lowers, the chest drainage unit is caught under the bed; the tubing comes apart and becomes contaminated.	• Do not clamp the chest tube because doing so could cause a tension pneumothorax. • Irrigate the tubing, using the sealed jar of sterile water or normal saline solution kept at the patient's bedside. • Insert the distal end of the chest tube into the jar of sterile fluid until the end of the tube is 2 to 4 cm below the top of the water. • Ask another nurse to obtain and set up a new closed chest drainage system. • Attach the chest tube to the new unit.

GI tubes

Nasoenteric-decompression tubes

If the patient's nasoenteric-decompression tube appears to be obstructed, notify the health care provider immediately. He or she may order these measures to restore patency quickly and efficiently:

• First, disconnect the tube from the suction source and irrigate it with normal saline solution. Use gravity flow to help clear the obstruction, unless ordered otherwise.

• If irrigation does not establish patency, the position of the tube against the gastric mucosa may be causing the obstruction. Gentle tugging may help. For a double-lumen tube, such as a Salem pump, irrigate the pigtail port (blue) with 10 to 30 cc of air to help move the tube away from the mucosa.

• Also check for proper functioning of the suction equipment
If these measures do not work, the tube may be kinked and may need additional manipulation. Before proceeding, follow these precautions:

• Never reposition or irrigate a nasoenteric-decompression tube (without a health care provider's order) in a patient who has had gastrointestinal (GI) surgery.

• Avoid manipulating a tube in a patient who had the tube inserted during surgery because you may disturb new sutures.

• Do not try to reposition the tube in a patient who was difficult to intubate (for example, because of an esophageal stricture).

T tubes

T tubes, which are typically inserted in the common bile duct after cholecystectomy, may become blocked by viscous bile or clots. Notify the health care provider and take these steps while you wait for him or her to arrive.

• Unclamp the T tube (if it was clamped before and after a meal) and connect the tube to a closed gravity-drainage system.

• Inspect the tube carefully to detect kinks or obstructions.

• Irrigate the tube with normal saline solution, if ordered, and prepare the patient for direct X-ray of the common bile duct (cholangiography). Briefly describe these measures to the patient to reduce his or her apprehension and promote his or her cooperation.

Total parenteral nutrition setups

Problems and possible causes	Interventions
Clotted catheter Interrupted flow rate, hypoglycemia, no blood return	• Reposition the patient on his or her side. Attempt to aspirate the clot. If the clot remains, use a thrombolytic, according to facility policy.
Dislodged catheter Catheter out of the vein, anterior chest pain, neck pain	• Place a sterile gauze pad on the site and apply pressure if the catheter is completely out. For partial displacement, call the health care provider. • Prepare the patient for an X-ray and repositioning with a guide wire or for removal and replacement.
Air embolism Chest pain, tachycardia, hypotension, fear, seizures, loss of consciousness, cardiac arrest	• Clamp the catheter. • Place the patient in Trendelenburg's position on his or her left side. Give oxygen, as ordered. • If cardiac arrest occurs, begin cardiopulmonary resuscitation.
Thrombosis Erythema, edema, or pain at the insertion site or along the vein; ipsilateral swelling of the arm, neck, and face; tachycardia	• Anticipate prompt removal of the catheter. • Administer heparin, as ordered. • Prepare for a venous flow study, as ordered.
Too rapid infusion Nausea, headache, lethargy, hyperglycemia	• Check the infusion rate. • Check the infusion pump.
Extravasation Swelling or pain around the insertion site	• Stop the infusion and assess the patient for cardiopulmonary abnormalities. • Obtain a chest X-ray, if needed.
Hyperglycemia Fatigue, restlessness, weakness, confusion	• Start insulin therapy, as ordered. • Slow the total parenteral nutrition (TPN) infusion rate, as ordered.

Total parenteral nutrition setups *(continued)*

Problems and possible causes	Interventions
Hypoglycemia	
Headache, sweating, dizziness, palpitations	• Give dextrose I.V. (10% as an infusion, 50% as an I.V. bolus), as ordered. • Avoid abrupt increases or decreases in the TPN flow rate; wean the patient from TPN slowly.
Cracked or broken tubing	
Fluid leakage	• Apply a padded hemostat above the break to prevent air from entering the line.
Sepsis	
Fever, chills, leukocytosis, positive blood cultures, glucose intolerance	• Remove the catheter and culture the tip. • Give the appropriate antibiotic.

Tube feedings

Problems	Interventions
Obstruction or clogging of the tube	• Flush the tube with warm water or cranberry juice. If necessary, replace the tube. • Enzyme declogging kit or mechanical declogging may be necessary • Flush the tube with 50 ml of water after each feeding or 30 ml of water every 2 hours if the patient is receiving continuous feeding, to remove excess sticky formula, which could occlude the tube. • Flush the tube with water before and after administering medication

(continued)

Tube feedings *(continued)*

Problems	Interventions
Aspiration of gastric secretions	• Discontinue the feeding immediately. • Perform tracheal suction of the aspirated contents, if possible. • Notify the health care provider who may order a prophylactic antibiotic or chest physiotherapy. • Check the tube placement before the feeding and elevate the head of the bed to prevent complications. • Avoid bolus feeding if the patient at risk for aspiration.
Nasal or pharyngeal irritation or necrosis	• Change the tube position. If necessary, replace the tube. • Provide frequent oral hygiene with mouthwash or lemon-glycerin swabs. Use petroleum jelly on cracked lips. • Use tube anchoring device.
Vomiting, bloating, diarrhea, or cramps	• Reduce the flow rate. • As ordered, administer metoclopramide to increase GI motility. • Warm the formula. • Position the patient on his right side, with his head elevated, for 30 minutes after the feeding to facilitate gastric emptying. • Notify the health care provider. He may reduce the amount of formula given during each feeding. • Check for residual feeding at least once a shift or according to facility policy.
Constipation	• Provide additional fluids if not contraindicated • Administer bulk forming laxative as ordered • Check if the patient is taking medication that may be causing constipation and review with the practitioner for the possibility of changing or stopping these meds.
Electrolyte imbalance	• Monitor electrolyte levels and notify the practitioner of any deficiencies.
Hyperglycemia	• Monitor blood glucose levels • Notify practitioner of elevated levels • Administer insulin as ordered.

Reprinted with permission from *Lippincott's nursing procedures* (8th ed.). (2019). Philadelphia, PA: Wolters Kluwer.

Neurologic monitors

Damped ICP waveforms

An intracranial pressure (ICP) waveform that looks like the one shown below signals a problem with the transducer or monitor. Check for obstruction of the line and determine if the transducer needs rebalancing.

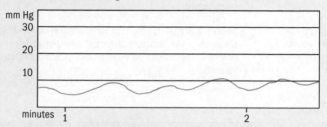

Problems	Interventions
Transducer or monitor needs recalibration.	• Turn the stopcock of the transducer off to the patient. • Open the stopcock to air and balance the transducer. • Recalibrate the transducer and monitor.
Air in the line	• Turn the stopcock off to the patient. • Using a syringe, flush the air out through an open stopcock port with sterile normal saline solution. *Note:* Never use heparin to flush the ICP line. You could accidentally inject some of the drug into the patient and cause bleeding. • Rebalance and recalibrate the transducer and monitor.
Loose connection in the line	• Check the tubing and stopcocks for moisture, which may indicate a loose connection. • Turn the stopcock off to the patient and then tighten all of the connections. • To prevent problems, make sure that the patient can turn his or her head without straining the tubing.
Disconnection in the line	• Turn the stopcock off to the patient immediately. (Rapid loss of cerebrospinal fluid through a ventricular catheter may allow the ICP to drop precipitously, causing a brain herniation.) • Replace the equipment using sterile technique to reduce risk of infection. Notify the health care provider of system integrity.

(continued)

Damped ICP waveforms *(continued)*

Problems	Interventions
Change in the patient's position	• Reposition the balancing port of the transducer level with Monro's foramen. • Rebalance and recalibrate the transducer and monitor. Always balance and recalibrate the transducer and monitor at least once every 4 hours and whenever the patient is repositioned.
Tubing, catheter, or screw occluded with blood or brain tissue	• Notify the health care provider. He or she may want to irrigate the screw or the catheter with a small amount (0.1 ml) of sterile normal saline solution. Never irrigate the screw or catheter yourself.

Bispectral index monitoring

Bispectral index monitoring requires the use of a monitor and cable connected to a sensor applied to the patient's forehead (as shown below). The sensor obtains information about the patient's electrical brain activity.

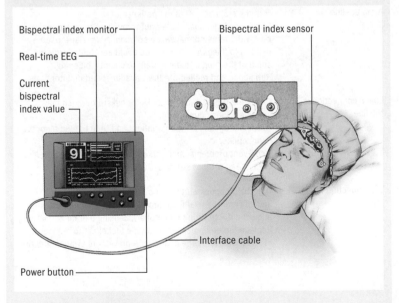

Bispectral index monitor

Real-time EEG

Current bispectral index value

Bispectral index sensor

91

Interface cable

Power button

Troubleshooting sensor problems

When initiating bispectral index monitoring, be aware that the monitor may display messages that indicate a problem. This chart highlights these messages and offers possible solutions.

Message	Possible solutions
High impedance message	Check sensor adhesion; reapply firm pressure to each of the numbered circles on the sensor for 5 seconds; if message continues, check the connection between the sensor and the monitor; if necessary, apply a new sensor.
Noise message	Remove possible pressure on the sensor; investigate possible large stimulus such as electrocautery.
Lead-off message	Check sensor for electrode displacement or lifting; reapply with firm pressure or, if necessary, apply a new sensor.

Selected references

Lippincott's nursing procedures (8th ed.). (2019). Philadelphia, PA: Wolters Kluwer.

Nettina, S. (2019). *Lippincott manual of nursing practice* (11th ed.). Philadelphia, PA: Wolters Kluwer.

Odom-Forren, J. (2013). *Drain's perianesthesia nursing: A critical care approach* (6th ed.). St. Louis, MO: Elsevier/Saunders.

12

Drug Administration

Reviewing the methods

Administration guidelines

Precautions for drug administration

Whenever you administer medication, observe these precautions to ensure that you are giving the right drug in the right dose to the right patient.

Check the order

Check the order on the patient's medication record against the health care provider's order.

Check the label

Check the label on the medication three times before administering it to a patient to ensure that you are administering the prescribed medication in the prescribed dose. Check it when you take the container from the shelf or drawer, right before pouring the medication into the medication cup or drawing it into the syringe, and before returning the container to the shelf or drawer. If you are administering a unit-dose medication, check the label for the third time immediately after pouring the medication and again before discarding the wrapper. Do not open a unit-dose medication until you are at the patient's bedside.

Confirm the patient's identity

Before giving the medication, confirm the patient's identity by checking two patient identifiers. Then make sure that you have the correct medication.

Explain the procedure to the patient and provide privacy.

Have a written order

Make sure that you have a written order for every medication that is to be given. If the order is verbal, make sure that the health care provider signs for it within the time specified by facility policy.

Give labeled medication

Do not give medication from a poorly labeled or unlabeled container. Furthermore, do not attempt to label drugs or reinforce drug labels yourself; a pharmacist must do that.

Monitor medication

Never give a medication that someone else has poured or prepared. Never allow your medication cart or tray out of your sight. Never return unwrapped or prepared medications to stock containers. Instead, dispose of them and notify the pharmacy.

Respond to the patient's questions

If the patient questions you about his or her medication or the dosage, check his or her medication record again. If the medication is correct, reassure him or her that it is correct. Make sure to tell him or her about changes in his or her medication or dosage. Instruct him or her, as appropriate, about possible adverse reactions and encourage him or her to report any that he or she experiences.

Monitor the patient's response to medication

To assess the patient's response to medication, be aware of his or her condition and what the drug's desired or expected effect should be. For example, if the patient is receiving an antiarrhythmic but continues to have premature ventricular contractions, tell the health care provider that the drug is not having the desired effect. Monitor the patient's condition carefully; changes such as weight loss or gain can affect the action of some drugs. Other factors, such as the patient's age, body build, gender, and emotional state, may also affect his or her response to drug therapy. Also, check the results of laboratory tests, which can indicate a therapeutic effect, an adverse effect, or a toxic level.

Monitor drug interactions

Because many patients receive more than one drug, it is important to understand drug interactions. A drug interaction is a change in drug absorption, distribution, metabolism, and excretion that may occur with or shortly after administration of another drug. A desirable interaction is used to help maintain an effective blood level or minimize or prevent adverse effects.

Some interactions, however, can have undesirable results, such as weakening a drug's desired effects or exaggerating its toxic ones. For example, a patient who smokes require larger doses of theophylline than a nonsmoking patient because cigarette smoke activates oxidative enzymes in the liver, increasing drug metabolism.

Watch for adverse effects

When you administer a drug, you must be able to recognize and identify adverse effects and toxic and allergic reactions. Some adverse effects are transient and subside as the patient develops a tolerance for the drug; others may require a change in therapy.

A toxic reaction to a drug can be acute, resulting from an excessive dose (an acetaminophen overdose, for instance), or chronic, resulting from progressive accumulation of the drug in the body. It can also result from impaired metabolism or excretion that results in elevated blood levels of a drug.

A drug allergy (hypersensitivity) results from an antigen-antibody reaction in a susceptible patient. Such a reaction can range from mild urticaria to potentially fatal anaphylaxis. Always check for known drug allergies before administering medications. In some instances, sensitivity tests may be performed before the first dose is given. For some patients, genetic testing for the detection of certain alleles can reveal increased risks for hypersensitivity

reactions. Be aware that a negative history does not rule out future allergic reactions. Other undesirable effects to watch for when administering drugs include idiosyncratic reactions and dependence.

Document carefully

Documenting all medications given to a patient provides a legal record of drugs the patient received during his or her stay in the facility. Medication administration involves documenting on a medication administration record (MAR) as well as in the nurse's notes. After administering a drug, document on the patient's Kardex or computer files the drug name, dosage, route and time of administration, and your signature and title. In the nurse's notes, include any assessment data that refer to the patient's response to the medication and any adverse effects of the medication.

If your facility documents medications digitally, make sure you enter each drug immediately after you give it. This gives all health care team members access to current medication information and is especially important if the system has no hard-copy backup.

Always write legibly. Use only acceptable abbreviations, and use them correctly. When in doubt as to how to abbreviate a term, spell it out. When documenting parenteral medications, be sure to include the injection site and the route used. After administering the first dose, sign your full name, licensure status, and identifying initials in the appropriate place on the MAR.

Topical administration

Topical drugs

Topical drugs, such as lotions and ointments, are applied directly to the patient's skin. They are commonly used for local, rather than systemic, effects. Typically, they must be applied two or three times per day to achieve a full therapeutic effect.

Equipment

Patient's medication record and chart • prescribed medication • sterile tongue blades • gloves • sterile 4″ × 4″ gauze pads • transparent semipermeable dressing • adhesive tape • solvent (such as cottonseed oil) • optional: cotton-tipped applicators, cotton gloves, or terry cloth scuffs

Implementation

- Verify the order on the patient's medication record by checking it against the health care provider's order. Check the patient's medication record for allergies.
- Confirm the patient's identity using two patient identifiers.
- Explain the procedure to the patient because, after discharge, he or she may have to apply the medication by himself or herself.
- Wash your hands to prevent cross-contamination and glove your dominant hand.
- Help the patient into a comfortable position and expose the area to be treated. Make sure that the skin or mucous membrane is intact (unless the medication has been ordered to treat a skin lesion). Application of medication to broken or abraded skin may cause unwanted systemic absorption and result in further irritation.
- If necessary, clean the skin of debris. You may need to change the glove if it becomes soiled.

To apply a paste, a cream, or an ointment

- Open the container. Place the cap upside down to avoid contaminating its inner surface.
- Remove a tongue blade from its sterile wrapper and cover one end of

it with medication from the tube or jar. Transfer the medication from the tongue blade to your gloved hand.
- Apply the medication to the affected area with long, smooth strokes that follow the direction of hair growth, as shown below.

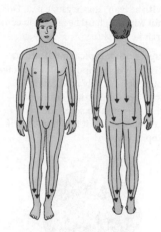

This technique avoids forcing medication into the hair follicles, which can cause irritation and lead to folliculitis.

- When applying medication to the patient's face, use a cotton-tipped applicator for small areas such as under the eyes. For larger areas, use a sterile gauze pad and follow the directions shown below.

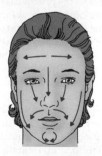

- To prevent contamination of the medication, use a new sterile tongue blade each time you remove medication from the container.

To remove an ointment

- Wash your hands and put on gloves. Then gently swab ointment from the patient's skin with a sterile 4″ × 4″ gauze pad saturated with a solvent such as cottonseed oil. Remove remaining oil by wiping the area with a clean, sterile gauze pad. Do not wipe too hard because you could irritate the skin.

To apply other topical medications

- To apply a shampoo, follow package directions. Apply medication with your fingertips, or instruct the patient to do so, as shown below. Massage it into the scalp, if appropriate.

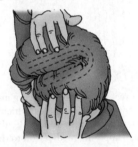

- To apply topical antifungal creams and nail lacquers, wash the affected area with soap and water. Apply cream and rub it gently into the nail beds. If the patient has athlete's foot, you can enhance absorption by applying the medication at night and covering the affected area with clean socks. Apply nail lacquers to the entire nail, starting at the nail bed. Allow the lacquer to dry thoroughly, which takes 5 to 10 minutes.
- To apply an aerosol spray, shake the container, if indicated, to mix the medication. Hold the container 6″ to 12″ (15 to 30.5 cm) from the skin or follow the manufacturer's recommendation. Spray the medication evenly over the treatment area to apply a thin film.
- To apply a powder, dry the skin surface and apply a thin layer of powder over the treatment area.
- To protect applied medications and prevent them from soiling the patient's clothes, tape a sterile gauze pad or a transparent semipermeable dressing over the treated area. If you are applying topical medication to his or her hands, cover them with cotton gloves; if you are applying medication to his or her feet, cover them with terry cloth scuffs.
- Assess the patient's skin for signs of irritation, allergic reaction, or breakdown.

Special considerations

- To prevent skin irritation from an accumulation of medication, remove residue from previous applications before each new application.
- Always wear gloves to prevent your skin from absorbing the medication.
- Never apply ointment to the eyelids or ear canal unless ordered. The ointment may congeal and occlude the tear duct or ear canal.
- Inspect the treated area frequently for adverse or allergic reactions.

Transdermal medications

Given through an adhesive patch or a measured dose of ointment applied to the skin, transdermal drugs deliver constant, controlled medication directly into the bloodstream for a prolonged systemic effect.

Medications that are available in transdermal form include nitroglycerin, which is used to control angina; scopolamine, which is used to treat motion sickness; estradiol, which is used for postmenopausal hormone replacement; clonidine, which is used to treat hypertension; nicotine, which is used for smoking cessation; fentanyl, which is used to control chronic pain; and estrogen and progesterone, which are used for hormonal birth control.

Nitroglycerin ointment dilates the coronary vessels for 4 hours; a patch can produce the same effect for as long as 24 hours.

The scopolamine patch can relieve motion sickness for as long as 72 hours. Transdermal estradiol and hormonal birth control last for up to 1 week; clonidine and nicotine, 24 hours; and fentanyl, up to 72 hours.

Equipment

Patient's medication record and chart • gloves • prescribed medication (patch or ointment) • application strip or measuring paper (for nitroglycerin ointment) • adhesive tape • optional: plastic wrap or semipermeable dressing (for nitroglycerin ointment)

Implementation

- Verify the order on the patient's medication record by checking it against the health care provider's order. Check the patient's medication record for allergies.
- Confirm the patient's identity using two patient identifiers.
- Wash your hands and put on gloves.
- Make sure that previously applied medication has been removed.
- Locate a new site for application, different from the previous site.

To apply transdermal ointment

- Place the prescribed amount of ointment on the application strip or measuring paper, taking care not to get any on your skin.
- Apply the strip to any dry, hairless area of the body. Do not rub the ointment into the skin.

- Tape the application strip and ointment to the skin. If desired, cover the application strip with plastic wrap and tape the wrap in place.

To apply a transdermal patch

- Open the package and remove the patch.
- Without touching the adhesive surface, remove the clear plastic backing.
- Apply the patch to a dry, hairless area—behind the ear, for example, as with scopolamine. Avoid areas that may cause uneven absorption, such as skin folds or scars, or irritated or damaged skin. Do not apply the patch below the elbow or knee.

After applying transdermal medications

- Instruct the patient to keep the area around the patch or ointment as dry as possible.
- Wash your hands immediately after applying the patch or ointment.

Special considerations

- Apply daily transdermal medications at the same time every day to ensure a continuous effect, but alternate the application sites to avoid skin irritation.
- Before applying nitroglycerin ointment, obtain the patient's baseline blood pressure. Obtain another blood pressure reading 5 minutes after applying the ointment. If the blood pressure has dropped significantly and the patient has a headache, notify the health care provider immediately. If the blood pressure has dropped but the patient has no symptoms, instruct him or her to lie still until the blood pressure returns to normal.
- Before reapplying nitroglycerin ointment, remove the plastic wrap, the

application strip, and any ointment remaining on the skin at the previous site.

- When applying a scopolamine patch, instruct the patient not to drive or operate machinery until his or her response to the drug has been determined.

- If the patient is using a clonidine patch, encourage him or her to check with his or her health care provider before using over-the-counter cough preparations. They may counteract the effects of clonidine.

Nitroglycerin ointment

Unlike most topical medications, nitroglycerin ointment is used for its transdermal systemic effect. It is used to dilate the arteries and veins, thus improving cardiac perfusion in a patient with cardiac ischemia or angina pectoris.

Nitroglycerin ointment is prescribed by the inch and comes with a rectangular piece of ruled paper to be used in applying the medication.

Equipment

Patient's medication record and chart • ointment • ruled paper • plastic wrap or transparent semipermeable dressing • adhesive tape • sphygmomanometer • optional: gloves

Implementation

- Verify the order on the patient's medication record by checking it against the health care provider's order. Check the patient's medication record for allergies.
- Confirm the patient's identity using two patient identifiers.
- Take a patient's baseline blood pressure for comparison with later readings.
- Wash your hands. Then put on gloves if you wish to avoid contact with the medication.

- Squeeze the prescribed amount of ointment onto the ruled paper, as shown below.

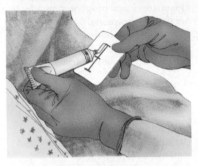

- After measuring the correct amount of ointment, tape the paper, with the drug side down, directly to the skin. Some health care facilities require you to use the paper to apply the medication to the patient's skin, usually on the chest or arm. Spread a thin layer of ointment over a 3″ (7.5-cm) area.

Special considerations

- For increased absorption, the health care provider may request that you cover the site with plastic wrap or transparent semipermeable dressing, as shown below.

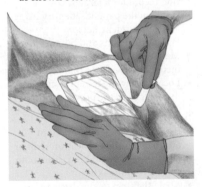

- After 5 minutes, record the patient's blood pressure. If it has dropped significantly and he or she has a headache (as a result of vasodilation of blood vessels in his or her head), notify the health care provider.

- If the patient's blood pressure has dropped but he or she has no adverse reactions, instruct him or her to lie still until it returns to normal.

Eye medications

Eye medications—drops or ointment—serve diagnostic and therapeutic purposes. During an eye examination, these medications can be used to anesthetize the eye, dilate the pupil, and stain the cornea to identify anomalies. Therapeutic uses include lubrication of the eye and treatment of such conditions as glaucoma and infections. Eye irrigation may be performed to remove foreign bodies, secretions, or harmful chemicals.

Equipment and preparation

Patient's medication record and chart • prescribed eye medication • sterile cotton balls • gloves • warm water or normal saline solution • sterile gauze pads • facial tissue • optional: ocular dressing

Make sure that the medication is labeled for ophthalmic use. Then check the expiration date. Remember to date the container after the first use.

Inspect ocular solutions for cloudiness, discoloration, and precipitation, but remember that some eye medications are suspensions and normally appear cloudy. Do not use a solution that appears abnormal.

Implementation

- Verify the order on the patient's medication record by checking it against the health care provider's order. Check the patient's medication record for allergies.
- Make sure that you know which eye to treat because different medications or doses may be ordered for each eye. Know that "OD" means right eye, "OS" means left eye, and "OU" means both eyes.
- Wash your hands and put on gloves.

- If the patient has an ocular dressing, remove it by pulling it down and away from his or her forehead. Avoid contaminating your hands.
- To remove exudate or meibomian gland secretions, clean around the eye with sterile cotton balls or sterile gauze pads moistened with warm water or normal saline solution. Have the patient close his or her eye and then gently wipe the eyelids from the inner to the outer canthus. Use a fresh cotton ball or gauze pad for each stroke.
- Have the patient sit or lie in the supine position. Instruct him or her to tilt his or her head back and toward his or her affected eye so that excess medication can flow away from the tear duct, minimizing systemic absorption through the nasal mucosa.
- Remove the dropper cap from the medication container and draw the medication into it.
- Before instilling eyedrops, instruct the patient to look up and away. This moves the cornea away from the lower lid and minimizes the risk of touching it with the dropper.

To instill eyedrops

- Steady the hand that is holding the dropper by resting it against the patient's forehead. With your other hand, pull down the lower lid of the affected eye and instill the drops in the conjunctival sac. Instruct patient to blink. Never instill eyedrops directly onto the eyeball.

 Patient Teaching Tip

When teaching an elderly patient how to instill eyedrops, keep in mind that he or she may have difficulty sensing drops in the eye. Suggest chilling the medication slightly to enhance the sensation.

To apply eye ointment

- Squeeze a small ribbon of medication on the edge of the conjunctival sac, from the inner to the outer canthus, as shown below. Cut off the ribbon by turning the tube.

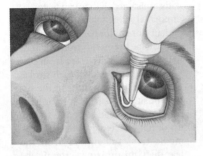

After instilling eyedrops or applying ointment

- Instruct the patient to close his or her eyes gently, without squeezing the lids shut. If you instilled drops, tell him or her to blink. If you applied ointment, tell him or her to roll his or her eyes behind closed lids to help to distribute the medication over the eyeball.
- Use a clean facial tissue to remove excess medication leaking from the eye. Use a fresh tissue for each eye to prevent cross-contamination.
- Apply a new ocular dressing, if necessary.
- Remove and discard gloves. Then wash your hands.

Special considerations

- When administering an eye medication that may be absorbed systemically, press your thumb on the inner canthus for 1 to 2 minutes after instillation while the patient closes his or her eyes.
- To maintain the sterility of the drug container, never touch the tip of the dropper or bottle to the eye area. Discard any solution that remains in the dropper before returning it to the bottle. If the dropper or bottle tip becomes contaminated, discard it and use another sterile dropper.

Eye medication disks

Small and flexible, an eye medication disk is an oval disk that can release medication (such as pilocarpine) in the eye for up to 1 week. Floating between the eyelids and the sclera, the disk stays in the eye while the patient sleeps and even during swimming and other athletic activities. The disk frees the patient from the need to remember to instill his or her eye medication. Moisture in the eye or the use of contact lenses does not adversely affect the disk.

Equipment

Patient's medication record and chart • prescribed eye medication • sterile gloves

Implementation

- Verify the order on the patient's medication record by checking it against the health care provider's order. Check the patient's medication record for allergies.
- Confirm the patient's identity using two patient identifiers.
- Make sure that you know which eye to treat because different medications or doses may be ordered for each eye.

To insert an eye medication disk

- Wash your hands and put on sterile gloves.
- Press your fingertip against the disk so that it sticks lengthwise across your fingertip.
- Gently pull the patient's lower eyelid away from the eye and place the disk in the conjunctival sac. The disk should lie horizontally, as shown

below, not vertically. The disk will adhere to the eye naturally.

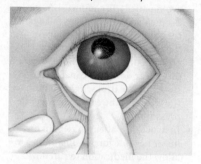

- Pull the lower eyelid out, up, and over the disk. Tell the patient to blink several times. If the disk is still visible, pull the lower lid out and over the disk again. Tell him or her that after the disk is in place, he or she can adjust its position by pressing his or her finger against his or her closed lid. Warn him or her not to rub his or her eye or move the disk across the cornea.
- If the disk falls out, rinse it in cool water and reinsert it. If the disk appears bent, replace it.
- If both eyes are being treated with medication disks, replace both disks at the same time.
- If the disk slips out of position repeatedly, reinsert it under the upper eyelid. To do this, gently lift and evert the upper eyelid and insert the disk in the conjunctival sac. Gently pull the lid back into position and tell the patient to blink several times. The more he or she uses the disk, the easier it should be for him or her to retain it. If not, notify the health care provider.

To remove an eye medication disk
- To remove the disk with one finger, put on sterile gloves and evert the lower eyelid to expose the disk. Use the forefinger of your other hand to slide the disk into the lid and out of the patient's eye. To use two fingers, evert the lower lid with one hand to

expose the disk. Then pinch it with the thumb and forefinger of your other hand and remove it.
- If the disk is located in the upper eyelid, apply long, circular strokes to the closed eyelid with your finger until you can see the disk in the corner of the eye. Then place your finger directly on the disk, move it to the lower sclera, and remove it as you would a disk located in the lower lid.

Special considerations
- If the patient will continue therapy with an eye medication disk after discharge, teach him or her to insert and remove it himself or herself. Ask him or her to demonstrate the techniques for you.
- Explain that mild reactions are common but should subside within the first 6 weeks of use. Foreign-body sensation in the eye, mild tearing, redness of the eye or eyelid, increased mucus discharge, and itchiness can occur. Blurred vision, stinging, swelling, and headaches can occur with pilocarpine, specifically. Tell the patient to report persistent or severe signs or symptoms.

Eardrops

Eardrops may be instilled to treat infection or inflammation, to soften cerumen for later removal, to produce local anesthesia, or to facilitate the removal of an insect trapped in the ear.

Equipment and preparation
Patient's medication record and chart • prescribed eardrops • light source • facial tissue or cotton-tipped applicator • optional: cotton ball, bowl of warm water

Warm the medication to body temperature in the bowl of warm water or carry it in your pocket for 30 minutes before administration. If necessary, test the temperature by placing a drop on your wrist. (If the medication is too hot, it may burn the patient's eardrum. Solution that is too hot or too cold may cause vertigo, nausea, and pain.) To avoid injuring the ear canal, check the dropper before use to make sure that it is not chipped or cracked.

Implementation

- Verify the order on the patient's medication record by checking it against the health care provider's order. Check the patient's medication record for allergies.
- Wash your hands.
- Confirm the patient's identity using two patient identifiers.
- Have the patient lie on the side opposite the affected ear.
- Straighten the patient's ear canal. For an adult, pull the auricle up and back.

AGE ALERT

For an infant or a child younger than age 3, gently pull the auricle down and back—the ear canal is straighter at this age.

- Using a light source, examine the ear canal for drainage. If you find any, clean the canal with a facial tissue or cotton-tipped applicator. Drainage can reduce the effectiveness of the medication.
- Compare the label on the eardrops with the order on the patient's medication record. Check the label again while drawing the medication into the dropper. Check the label for the final time before returning the eardrops to the shelf or drawer.
- To avoid damaging the ear canal with the dropper, gently rest the hand that is holding the dropper against the patient's head. Straighten

the patient's ear canal and instill the ordered number of drops. To avoid patient discomfort, aim the dropper so that the drops fall against the sides of the ear canal, not on the eardrum. Hold the ear canal in position until you see the medication disappear down the canal. After instilling the drops, lightly massage the tragus of the ear or apply gentle pressure.

- Instruct the patient to remain on his or her side for 5 to 10 minutes to allow the medication to run down into the ear canal.
- Tuck the cotton ball (if ordered) loosely into the opening of the ear canal to prevent the medication from leaking out. Be careful not to insert it too deeply into the canal because doing so would prevent drainage of secretions and increase pressure on the eardrum.
- Clean and dry the outer ear.
- If ordered, repeat the procedure in the other ear after 5 to 10 minutes.
- Help the patient into a comfortable position.
- Wash your hands.

Special considerations

- Some conditions make the normally tender ear canal even more sensitive, so be especially gentle when performing this procedure.
- To prevent injury to the eardrum when inserting a cotton-tipped applicator, make sure that the cotton tip always remains in view. After applying eardrops to soften cerumen, irrigate the ear, as ordered, to facilitate its removal.
- If the patient has vertigo, keep the side rails of his or her bed up, and assist him or her as necessary during the procedure. Move slowly and unhurriedly to avoid exacerbating his or her vertigo.
- If necessary, teach the patient to instill the eardrops correctly so that

he or she can continue treatment at home. Review the procedure, and let the patient try it himself or herself while you observe.

Nasal medications

Nasal medications may be instilled through drops, a spray (using an atomizer), or an aerosol (using a nebulizer). Nasal medications are commonly used to shrink swollen mucous membranes and to loosen secretions and provide drainage for treatment of nasal cavity or sinus infections. Most produce local rather than systemic effects. Nasal medications include vasoconstrictors, antiseptics, anesthetics, hormones, vaccines, and corticosteroids.

Equipment

Patient's medication record and chart • prescribed medication • emesis basin (for nose drops) • facial tissues • optional: pillow, piece of soft rubber or plastic tubing, gloves

Implementation

- Verify the order on the patient's medication record by checking it against the health care provider's order. Check the patient's medication record for allergies.
- Confirm the patient's identity using two patient identifiers.
- Wash your hands. Put on gloves, if necessary.
- Have the patient blow his or her nose to clear secretions and enhance drug absorption.

To instill nose drops

- Draw some medication into the dropper.
- To reach the ethmoidal and sphenoidal sinuses, have the patient lie on his or her back, with his or her neck hyperextended and his or her head tilted back over the edge of the bed. Support his or her head with one hand to prevent neck strain.

- To reach the maxillary and frontal sinuses, have the patient lie on his or her back, with his or her head toward the affected side and hanging slightly over the edge of the bed. Ask him or her to rotate his or her head laterally after hyperextension. Support his or her head with one hand to prevent neck strain.
- To relieve ordinary nasal congestion, help the patient into a reclining or supine position, with his or her head tilted slightly toward the affected side. Aim the dropper upward, toward the patient's eye, rather than downward, toward his or her ear.
- Insert the dropper about ⅓" (8 mm) into the nostril. Make sure that it does not touch the sides of the nostril to avoid contaminating the dropper or making the patient sneeze.

AGE ALERT

For a child or an uncooperative patient, place a short piece of soft tubing on the end of the dropper to avoid damaging the mucous membranes.

- Instill the prescribed number of drops, observing the patient for signs of discomfort.
- Keep the patient's head tilted back for at least 5 minutes. Have him or her breathe through his or her mouth to prevent the drops from leaking out and to allow time for the medication to work.
- Keep an emesis basin handy so that the patient can expectorate medication that flows into the oropharynx and mouth. Use facial tissues to wipe excess medication from the patient's face.

- Instruct the patient not to blow his or her nose for several minutes after instillation.
- Clean the dropper. Return the dropper to the bottle and close it tightly.

To use a nasal spray

- Have the patient sit upright, with his or her head erect.
- Remove the protective cap from the atomizer.
- Occlude one of the patient's nostrils, and insert the atomizer tip about ½″ (1.3 cm) into the open nostril. Position the tip straight up, toward the inner canthus of the eye.
- Depending on the drug, have the patient hold his or her breath or inhale. Squeeze the atomizer once quickly and firmly—just enough to coat the inside of the nose. Excessive force may propel the medication into the patient's sinuses and cause a headache. Repeat the procedure in the other nostril, as ordered.
- Tell the patient to keep his or her head tilted back for several minutes, to breathe slowly through his or her nose, and not to blow his or her nose to ensure that the medication has time to work.

To use a nasal aerosol

- Insert the medication cartridge according to the manufacturer's directions. Shake it well before each use and remove the protective cap.
- Hold the aerosol between your thumb and index finger, with the index finger on top of the cartridge.
- Tilt the patient's head back slightly, and carefully insert the adapter tip into one nostril. Depending on the medication, tell the patient to hold his or her breath or to inhale.
- Press your fingers together firmly to release one measured dose of medication.
- Shake the aerosol and repeat the procedure to instill medication into the other nostril.

- Remove the cartridge and wash the nasal adapter daily in lukewarm water. Allow the adapter to dry before reinserting the cartridge.
- Tell patient not to blow his or her nose for at least 2 minutes afterward.

Special consideration

- Calcitonin-Salmon (Miacalcin), a hormone used for osteoporosis, should be given in only one nostril daily, with the nostrils alternated each day. Be sure to document which nostril is used.

Vaginal medications

Vaginal medications include suppositories, creams, gels, ointments, and rings. These medications can be inserted as topical treatment for infection (particularly *Trichomonas vaginalis* and candidal vaginitis), inflammation or as a contraceptive. Suppositories melt when they come in contact with the warm vaginal mucosa, and their medication diffuses topically—as effectively as creams, gels, and ointments.

Vaginal medications usually come with a disposable applicator that allows placement of medication in the anterior and posterior fornices. Vaginal administration is most effective when the patient can remain lying down afterward to retain the medication. Apply a clean perineal pad if there is heavy drainage or if the patient is ambulatory. (The medication may melt and drain from the vagina by gravity.)

Equipment

Patient's medication record and chart • prescribed medication and applicator, if needed • gloves • water-soluble lubricant • cotton balls • soap and warm water • small sanitary pad

Implementation

- Verify the order on the patient's medication record by checking it against the health care provider's order. Check the patient's medication record for allergies.

- Confirm the patient's identity using two patient identifiers.
- Ask the patient to void.
- Wash your hands, explain the procedure to the patient, and provide privacy.
- Ask the patient if she would rather insert the medication herself. If so, provide appropriate instructions. If not, proceed with the following steps.
- Help her into the lithotomy position and expose only the perineum.

To insert a suppository

- Remove the suppository from the wrapper and lubricate it with a water-soluble lubricant.
- Put on gloves and expose the vagina by spreading the labia.
- If you see discharge, wash the area with several cotton balls soaked in warm, soapy water. Clean each side of the perineum and then the center using a fresh cotton ball for each stroke. While the labia are still separated, insert the suppository 3″ to 4″ (7.6 to 10 cm) into the vagina.

To insert an ointment, a cream, or a gel

- Fit the applicator to the tube of medication and gently squeeze the tube to fill the applicator with the prescribed amount of medication. Lubricate the applicator tip.
- Put on gloves and expose the vagina.
- Insert the applicator about 2″ (5 cm) into the patient's vagina and administer the medication by depressing the plunger on the applicator.
- Instruct the patient to remain in a supine position, with her knees flexed, for 5 to 10 minutes, to allow the medication to flow into the posterior fornix.

To insert a vaginal ring (NuvaRing)

- Choose an insertion position either lying, squatting, or standing with one leg up.

- Place the folded vaginal ring into the vagina and gently push it further up into the vagina using your index finger.
- Each ring is used for one cycle, this consist of 3 continuous weeks followed by a free week. The ring works by inhibiting ovulation and is 99.3% effective in protecting against pregnancy when used appropriately.

After vaginal insertion

- Wash the applicator with soap and warm water and store or discard it, as appropriate. Label it so that it will be used only for the same patient.
- Remove and discard your gloves.
- To prevent the medication from soiling the patient's clothing and bedding, provide a sanitary pad.
- Help the patient to return to a comfortable position and advise her to remain in bed as much as possible for the next several hours.
- Wash your hands thoroughly.

Special considerations

- Refrigerate vaginal suppositories that melt at room temperature.
- If possible, teach the patient how to insert vaginal medication. She may need to administer it herself after discharge. Give her a patient-teaching sheet if one is available.
- Instruct the patient not to wear a tampon after inserting vaginal medication because it will absorb the medication and decrease its effectiveness.

Respiratory administration

Handheld oropharyngeal inhalers

Handheld inhalers include the metered-dose inhaler, with or without a spacer; the turbo-inhaler; and the nasal inhaler. These devices deliver topical medications to the respiratory tract, producing local and systemic effects. The mucosal lining of the respiratory tract absorbs the inhalant almost immediately. Examples of inhalants are bronchodilators, which are used to improve airway patency and facilitate drainage of mucus, and mucolytics, which liquefy tenacious bronchial secretions.

Equipment

Patient's medication record and chart • metered-dose inhaler or turbo-inhaler • prescribed medications • normal saline solution • optional: spacer or extender

Implementation

- Verify the order on the patient's medication record by checking it against the health care provider's order. Check the patient's medication record for allergies.
- Confirm the patient's identity using two patient identifiers.

To use a metered-dose inhaler

- Shake the inhaler bottle. Remove the cap and insert the stem into the small hole on the flattened portion of the mouthpiece, as shown below.

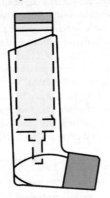

- If the metered-dose inhaler has a spacer built into the inhaler, pull the spacer away from the section holding the medication canister until it clicks into place.
- Have the patient exhale. Place the inhaler about 1″ (2.5 cm) in front of his or her open mouth.

- As you push the bottle down against the mouthpiece, instruct the patient to inhale slowly through his or her mouth and to continue inhaling until his or her lungs feel full. Compress the bottle against the mouthpiece only once.
- Remove the inhaler and tell the patient to hold his or her breath for several seconds. Then instruct him or her to exhale slowly through pursed lips to keep the distal bronchioles open, allowing increased absorption and diffusion of the drug.
- Have the patient gargle with tap water, if desired, to remove the medication from his or her mouth and the back of his or her throat.
- Have the patient wait 1 to 3 minutes before another inhalation is administered.
- Rinse the mouthpiece thoroughly with warm water to prevent the accumulation of residue.

To use a turbo-inhaler

- With the other hand, slide the sleeve away from the mouthpiece as far as possible, as shown below.

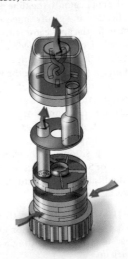

- Unscrew the tip of the mouthpiece by turning it counterclockwise.
- Press the colored portion of the medication capsule into the propeller stem of the mouthpiece. Screw the inhaler together again.
- Holding the inhaler with the mouthpiece at the bottom, slide the sleeve all the way down and then up again to puncture the capsule and release the medication. Do this only once.
- Have the patient exhale completely and tilt his or her head back. Instruct him or her to place the mouthpiece in his or her mouth, close his or her lips around it, and inhale once. Tell him or her to hold his or her breath for several seconds.
- Remove the inhaler from the patient's mouth and tell him or her to exhale as much air as possible.
- Repeat the procedure until all of the medication in the device has been inhaled.
- Have the patient gargle with normal saline solution, if desired.
- Discard the empty medication capsule. Rinse the inhaler with warm water at least once per week.

To use a nasal inhaler

- Have the patient clear his or her nostrils by blowing his or her nose
- Shake the medication cartridge and then insert it into the adaptor. (Before inserting a refill cartridge, remove the protective cap from the stem.)
- Remove the protective cap from the adapter tip.
- The patient should hold the inhaler with his or her index finger on top of the cartridge and his or her thumb under the nasal adapter. The adapter tip should point toward the patient.
- Have the patient tilt his or her head back and place the adapter tip into one nostril. He or she should occlude the other nostril with his or her finger.
- Instruct the patient to inhale gently as he or she presses the adapter and

the cartridge together to release a measured dose of medication. Follow the manufacturer's instructions; with some medications such as dexamethasone sodium phosphate, inhaling is not desirable.
- Tell the patient to remove the inhaler from his or her nostril and hold his or her breath for a few seconds.
- Have the patient exhale through his or her mouth.
- Have the patient shake the inhaler and repeat the procedure in the other nostril.

Special considerations

- Teach the patient how to use the inhaler so that he or she can continue treatments after discharge, if necessary. Explain that an overdose can cause the medication to lose its effectiveness. Tell him or her to record the date and time of each inhalation as well as his or her response.
- Some oral respiratory drugs can cause restlessness, palpitations, nervousness, other systemic effects, and hypersensitivity reactions, such as a rash, urticaria, and bronchospasm.
- If the patient has heart disease, use caution when administering an oral respiratory drug because it can potentiate coronary insufficiency, cardiac arrhythmias, or hypertension. If paradoxical bronchospasm occurs, discontinue the drug and call the health care provider.
- If the patient is using a bronchodilator and a steroid, have him or her use the bronchodilator first, wait 5 minutes and then use the corticosteroid.

Enteral administration

Oral drugs

Most drugs are administered orally because this route is usually the safest, most convenient, and least expensive. Drugs for oral administration are available in many forms, including tablets, enteric-coated tablets, capsules, syrups, elixirs, oils, liquids, suspensions, powders, and granules. Some require special preparation before administration, such as mixing with juice to make them more palatable.

Oral drugs are sometimes prescribed in higher dosages than their parenteral equivalents because, after absorption through the gastrointestinal (GI) system, the liver breaks them down before they reach the systemic circulation.

Equipment

Patient's medication record and chart • prescribed medication • optional: medication cup; appropriate vehicle (such as jelly or applesauce) for crushed pills commonly used with children or elderly patients, or juice, water, or milk for liquid medications; and crushing or cutting device

Implementation

- Verify the order on the patient's medication record by checking it against the health care provider's order. Check the patient's medication record for allergies.
- Confirm the patient's identity using two patient identifiers.
- Wash your hands.
- Assess the patient's condition, including his or her level of consciousness, ability to swallow, and vital signs, as needed. Changes in his or her condition may warrant withholding medication.
- Give the patient his or her medication and, as needed, liquid to aid swallowing, minimize adverse effects, or promote absorption. If appropriate, crush the medication to facilitate swallowing.
- Stay with the patient until he or she has swallowed the drug. If he or she seems confused or disoriented, check his or her mouth to make sure that he or she has swallowed

it. Return and reassess the patient's response within 1 hour after giving the medication.

Special considerations

- To avoid damaging or staining the patient's teeth, give acid or iron preparations through a straw. An unpleasant-tasting liquid can usually be made more palatable if taken through a straw because the liquid comes in contact with fewer taste buds.
- If the patient cannot swallow a whole tablet or capsule, ask the pharmacist if the drug is available in liquid form or if it can be administered by another route. If not, ask him or her if you can crush the tablet or open the capsule and mix it with food.

Drug delivery through a nasogastric tube or gastrostomy button

In addition to providing an alternate means of nourishment, a nasogastric (NG) tube allows direct instillation of medication into the GI system for the patient who cannot ingest it orally. A gastrostomy button, inserted into an established stoma, lies flush with the skin and receives a feeding tube.

Equipment and preparation

Patient's medication record and chart • prescribed medication • towel or linen-saver pad • 50- or 60-ml piston-type catheter-tip syringe • feeding tubing • two 4″ × 4″ gauze pads • pH test strip • gloves • diluent (juice, water, or a nutritional supplement) • cup for mixing medication and fluid • spoon • 50-ml cup of water • gastrostomy tube and funnel, if needed • optional: pill-crushing equipment, clamp (if not already attached to the tube)

Gather the equipment for use at the patient's bedside. Liquids should be at room temperature to avoid abdominal cramping. Make sure that the cup, syringe, spoon, and gauze are clean.

Implementation

- Verify the order on the patient's medication record by checking it against the health care provider's order. Check the patient's medication record for allergies.
- Confirm the patient's identity using two patient identifiers.

To give a drug through an NG tube

- Wash your hands and put on gloves.
- Unpin the tube from the patient's gown. To avoid soiling the sheets during the procedure, drape the patient's chest with a towel or linen-saver pad.
- Help the patient into Fowler's position, if his or her condition allows.
- After unclamping the tube, attach the catheter tip syringe and gently draw back on the piston of the syringe. Place a small amount of gastric contents on the pH test strip. The appearance of gastric contents and pH ≤5 implies that the tube is patent and in the stomach.
- If no gastric contents appear or if you meet resistance, the tube may be lying against the gastric mucosa. Withdraw the tube slightly or turn the patient to free it.
- Clamp the tube, detach the syringe, and lay the end of the tube on a 4″ × 4″ gauze pad.
- If the medication is in tablet form, crush it before mixing it with the diluent. (Make sure that the particles are small enough to pass through the eyes at the distal end of the tube.) Open the capsules and pour them into the diluent. Pour liquid medications into the diluent and stir well. Bring the liquid medication to room temperature. Cold liquids may cause patient discomfort.
- Reattach the syringe, without the piston, to the end of the tube. Holding the tube upright at a level slightly above the patient's nose, open the

clamp and pour in the medication slowly and steadily, as shown below.

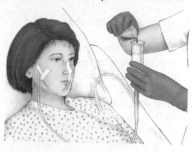

- To prevent air from entering the patient's stomach, hold the tube at a slight angle and add more medication before the syringe empties.
- If the medication flows smoothly, slowly give the entire dose. If it does not flow, it may be too thick. In this case, dilute it with water. If you suspect that the placement of the tube is inhibiting the flow, stop the procedure and reevaluate the placement.
- Watch the patient's reaction and stop administration immediately if he or she shows signs of discomfort.
- As the last of the medication flows out of the syringe, start to irrigate the tube by adding 30 to 50 ml of water (15 to 30 ml for a child). Irrigation clears medication from the tube and reduces the risk of clogging.
- When the water stops flowing, clamp the tube. Detach the syringe and discard it properly.
- Fasten the tube to the patient's gown and make sure that the patient is comfortable.
- Leave the patient in Fowler's position or on his or her right side, with his or her head partially elevated, for at least 30 minutes to facilitate flow and prevent esophageal reflux.

To give a drug through a gastrostomy button

- Help the patient into an upright position.

- Wash your hands. Put on gloves and open the safety plug on top of the device.
- Attach the feeding tube set to the button.
- Remove the piston from the catheter-tipped syringe and insert the tip into the distal end of the feeding tube.
- Pour the prescribed medication into the syringe and allow it to flow into the stomach.
- After instilling all of the medication, pour 30 to 50 ml of water into the syringe and allow it to flow through the tube.
- When all of the water has been delivered, remove the feeding tube and replace the safety plug. Keep the patient in semi-Fowler's position for 30 minutes after giving the medication.

Special considerations

- If you must give a tube feeding as well as instill medication, give the medication first to ensure that the patient receives it all. Do not give foods that interact adversely with the drug. Tube feedings must be withheld 2 hours before and 2 hours after phenytoin or warfarin administration.
- If residual stomach contents exceed 100 ml, withhold the medication and feeding and notify the health care provider. Excessive stomach contents may indicate intestinal obstruction or paralytic ileus.
- If the NG tube is on suction, turn it off for 20 to 30 minutes after giving the medication.
- Document the amount of water and medication given.

Buccal, sublingual, and translingual medications

Certain drugs are given buccally (between the patient's cheek and teeth) or sublingually (under the patient's tongue) to bypass the digestive tract and facilitate their absorption into the bloodstream.

Drugs that are given buccally include nitroglycerin and methyltestosterone. Drugs that are given sublingually include ergotamine tartrate, isosorbide, and nitroglycerin. Translingual drugs, which are sprayed onto the tongue, include nitrate preparations for patients with chronic angina. When using either administration method, observe the patient carefully to ensure that he or she does not swallow the drug or experience mucosal irritation.

Equipment

Patient's medication record and chart • prescribed medication • medication cup

Implementation

- Verify the order on the patient's medication record by checking it against the health care provider's order. Check the patient's medication record for allergies.
- Confirm the patient's identity using two patient identifiers.
- Wash your hands.
- For buccal administration, place the tablet in the patient's buccal pouch, between his or her cheek and teeth.
- For sublingual administration, place the tablet under the patient's tongue.
- Instruct the patient to keep the medication in place until it dissolves completely to ensure absorption.
- Caution the patient against chewing the tablet or touching it with his or her tongue to prevent accidental swallowing.
- For translingual administration, hold the medication canister vertically, with the valve head at the top, and then spray the orifice as close to the patient's mouth as possible.
- Spray the dose onto the patient's tongue by pressing firmly on the button. Have the patient wait 10 seconds before swallowing.

Special considerations

- Do not give liquids because some buccal tablets may take up to 1 hour to be absorbed.
- If the patient has angina, tell him or her to wet the nitroglycerin tablet with saliva and to keep it under his or her tongue until it is fully absorbed.

Rectal suppositories or ointment

A rectal suppository is a small, solid, medicated mass, usually cone-shaped, with a cocoa butter or glycerin base. It may be inserted to stimulate peristalsis and defecation or to relieve pain, vomiting, and local irritation. An ointment is a semisolid medication that is used to produce local effects. It may be applied externally to the anus or internally to the rectum.

Equipment and preparation

Patient's medication record and chart • rectal suppository or tube of ointment and ointment applicator • 4″ × 4″ gauze pads • gloves • water-soluble lubricant • optional: bedpan

Store rectal suppositories in the refrigerator until they are needed to prevent softening and possible decreased effectiveness of the medication. A softened suppository is difficult to handle and insert. To harden it again, hold the suppository (in its wrapper) under cold running water.

Implementation

- Verify the order on the patient's medication record by checking it against the health care provider's order. Check the patient's medication record for allergies.
- Confirm the patient's identity using two patient identifiers.
- Wash your hands.

To insert a rectal suppository

- Place the patient on his or her left side in Sims' position. Drape him or her with the bedcovers, exposing only the buttocks. Put on gloves. Unwrap the suppository and lubricate it with water-soluble lubricant.
- Lift the patient's upper buttock with your nondominant hand to expose the anus.
- Instruct the patient to take several deep breaths through his or her mouth to relax the anal sphincter and reduce anxiety during drug insertion.
- Using the index finger of your dominant hand, insert the suppository—tapered end first—about 3″ (7.6 cm) until you feel it pass the internal anal sphincter, as shown below.

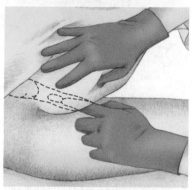

- Direct the tapered end of the suppository toward the side of the rectum so that it touches the membranes.
- Encourage the patient to lie quietly and, if applicable, to retain the suppository for the correct length of time. Press on the anus with a gauze pad, if necessary, until the urge to defecate passes.
- Discard the used equipment.

To apply an ointment

- Put on gloves.
- For external application, use gloves or a gauze pad to spread the medication over the anal area.
- For internal application, attach the applicator to the tube of ointment and coat the applicator with water-soluble lubricant.

- Expect to use about 1″ (2.5 cm) of ointment. To gauge how much pressure to use during application, try squeezing a small amount from the tube before you attach the applicator.
- Lift the patient's upper buttock with your nondominant hand to expose the anus.
- Tell the patient to take several deep breaths through his or her mouth to relax the anal sphincter and reduce discomfort during insertion. Then gently insert the applicator, directing it toward the umbilicus, as shown below.

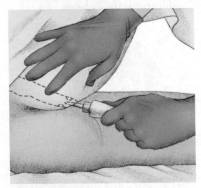

- Squeeze the tube to eject medication.
- Remove the applicator, and place a folded 4″ × 4″ gauze pad between the patient's buttocks to absorb excess ointment. Disassemble the tube and applicator. Recap the tube. Clean the applicator with soap and warm water. Remove and discard the gloves and wash your hands thoroughly.

Special considerations

- Because the intake of food and fluid stimulates peristalsis, a suppository for relieving constipation should be inserted about 30 minutes before mealtime to help soften the stool and facilitate defecation. A medicated retention suppository should be inserted between meals.
- Tell the patient not to expel the suppository. If he or she has difficulty retaining it, put him or her on a bedpan.

- Make sure that the patient's call button is handy, and watch for his or her signal because he or she may be unable to suppress the urge to defecate.
- Inform the patient that the suppository may discolor his or her next bowel movement.

Parenteral administration

Subcutaneous injection

A subcutaneous injection allows slower, more sustained drug administration than I.M. injection. Drugs and solutions for subcutaneous injections are injected through a relatively short needle, using meticulous sterile technique.

Equipment and preparation

Patient's medication record and chart • prescribed medication • needle of appropriate gauge and length • gloves • 1- to 3-ml syringe • alcohol pads • optional: antiseptic cleaner, filter needle, insulin syringe, insulin pump

Inspect the medication to make sure that it is not cloudy and does not contain precipitates.

Wash your hands. Select a needle of the proper gauge and length.

AGE ALERT

An average adult patient requires a 25G ⅝″ needle; an infant, a child, or an elderly or thin patient usually requires a 25G to 27G ½″ needle.

For single-dose ampules

Wrap a small gauze pad around the neck of the ampule. Always break away from your body. If desired, attach a filter needle and withdraw the medication. Tap the syringe to clear air from it. Cover the needle with the needle sheath. Before discarding the ampule, check the label against the patient's medication record. Discard the filter needle and the ampule. Attach the appropriate size and gauge needle to the syringe.

For single-dose or multidose vials
Reconstitute powdered drugs according to the instructions on the label. Clean the rubber stopper of the vial with an alcohol pad. Pull the plunger of the syringe back until the volume of air in the syringe equals the volume of drug to be withdrawn from the vial. Insert the needle into the vial. Inject the air, invert the vial, and keep the bevel tip of the needle below the level of the solution as you withdraw the prescribed amount of medication. Cover the needle with the needle sheath. Tap the syringe to clear air from it. Check the drug label against the patient's medication record.

Implementation

- Verify the order on the patient's medication record by checking it against the health care provider's order. Check the patient's medication record for allergies. Explain the purpose and action of the medication to the patient.
- Confirm the patient's identity using two patient identifiers.
- Select the injection site from those shown below, and tell the patient where you will be giving the injection.

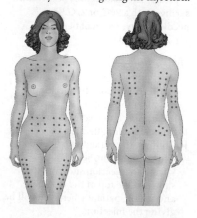

- Put on gloves. Position and drape the patient, if necessary.
- Clean the injection site with an alcohol pad. Loosen the protective needle cover. Use a firm, circular motion while moving outward from the injection site. Allow area to dry. Do not fan dry.
- With your nondominant hand, pinch the skin around the injection site firmly to elevate the subcutaneous tissue, forming a 1″ (2.5-cm) fat fold, as shown below.

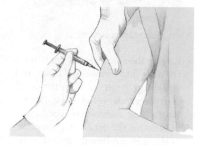

- Holding the syringe in your dominant hand (while pinching the skin around the injection site with the thumb and index finger of your nondominant hand), grip the needle sheath between the fourth and fifth fingers of your nondominant hand and pull back to uncover the needle. Do not touch the needle.
- Position the needle with its bevel up.
- Tell the patient that he or she will feel a prick as the needle is inserted. Insert the needle quickly in one motion at a 45- or 90-degree angle, as shown at the top of the next column, depending on the length of the needle, the medication, and the amount of subcutaneous tissue at the site. Some drugs, such as heparin, should always be injected at a 90-degree angle.

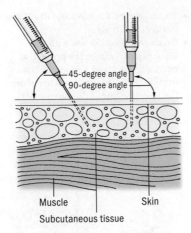

45-degree angle
90-degree angle

Muscle   Skin
Subcutaneous tissue

- Release the skin to avoid injecting the drug into compressed tissue and irritating the nerves. After the needle is in place, release the tissue. If you have a large skin fold, pinched up, ensure that the needle stays in place as the skin is released. Immediately move your nondominant hand to steady the lower end of the syringe. Slide your dominant hand to the end of the plunger. Avoid moving the syringe.
- If none appears, slowly inject the drug. If blood appears on aspiration, withdraw the needle, prepare another syringe, and repeat the procedure.
- After injection, remove the needle at the same angle used for insertion. Using a gauze pad/square, apply gentle pressure to the site after the needle is withdrawn. Do not massage the site.
- Remove the alcohol pad and check the injection site for bleeding or bruising.
- Dispose of injection equipment according to facility policy. Do not recap the needle.
- Assist patient to a position of comfort. Perform hand hygiene. Document the administration

of the medication immediately after administration. Evaluate the patient's response to the medication within an appropriate time frame for the particular medication.

Special considerations
- Do not aspirate for blood return when giving insulin or heparin. It is not necessary with insulin and may cause a hematoma with heparin.
- Repeated injections in the same site can cause lipodystrophy. A natural immune response, this complication can be minimized by rotating injection sites.

Intradermal injection

Used primarily for diagnostic purposes, as in allergy or tuberculin testing, an intradermal injection is administered in small amounts, usually 0.5 ml or less, into the outer layers of the skin. Because little systemic absorption takes place, this type of injection is used primarily to produce a local effect.

The ventral forearm is the most commonly used site because of its easy access and lack of hair.

Equipment
Patient's medication record and chart • prescribed medication • tuberculin syringe with a 26G or 27G ½" to ⅝" needle • gloves • alcohol pads • marking pen

Implementation
- Verify the order on the patient's medication record by checking it against the health care provider's order. Check the patient's medication record for allergies.
- Confirm the patient's identity using two patient identifiers.
- Locate an injection site from those shown at the top of the next page, and tell the patient where you will be giving the injection.

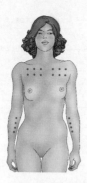
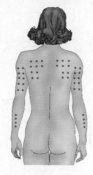

- Instruct the patient to sit up and to extend and support his or her arm on a flat surface, with the ventral forearm exposed.
- Wash your hands and put on gloves.
- With an alcohol pad, clean the surface of the ventral forearm about two or three fingerbreadths distal to the antecubital space. Make sure that the test site is free from hair and blemishes. Allow the skin to dry completely before administering the injection.
- While holding the patient's forearm in your hand, stretch the skin taut with your thumb.
- With your free hand, hold the needle at a 15-degree angle to the patient's arm, with its bevel up.
- Insert the needle about ⅛″ (3 mm) below the epidermis. Stop when the bevel tip of the needle is under the skin and inject the antigen slowly. You should feel some resistance as you do this, and a wheal should form as you inject the antigen, as shown below.

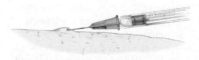

If no wheal forms, you have injected the antigen too deeply. Withdraw the needle and administer another

test dose at least 2″ (5 cm) from the first site.
- Withdraw the needle at the same angle at which it was inserted. Do not rub the site. This could irritate the underlying tissue, which may affect the test results.
- Circle each test site with a marking pen, and label each site according to the recall antigen given. Tell the patient to avoid washing off the circles until the test is completed.
- Dispose of needles and syringes according to facility policy.
- Remove and discard your gloves.
- Assess the patient's response to the skin testing in 24 to 48 hours.

Special considerations

- If the patient is hypersensitive to the test antigens, he or she can have a severe anaphylactic response. Be prepared to give an immediate epinephrine injection and other emergency resuscitation procedures. Be especially alert after giving a test dose of penicillin or tetanus antitoxin.

I.M. injection

An I.M. injection deposits medication deep into well-vascularized muscle for rapid systemic action and absorption of up to 5 ml.

Equipment and preparation

Patient's medication record and chart • prescribed medication • diluent or filter needle, if needed • 3- to 5-ml syringe • 20G to 25G 1″ to 3″ needle • gloves • alcohol pads • marking pen

The prescribed medication must be sterile. The needle may be packaged separately or already attached to the syringe. Needles used for I.M. injections are longer than subcutaneous needles because they reach deep into the muscle. Needle length also depends on the injection site, the patient's size, and the amount of subcutaneous fat covering the muscle.

Wipe the stopper of the vial with alcohol, and draw the prescribed amount of medication into the syringe.

Implementation

- Verify the order on the patient's medication record by checking it against the health care provider's order. Check the patient's medication record for allergies.
- Confirm the patient's identity using two patient identifiers.
- Provide privacy and explain the procedure to the patient.
- Wash your hands and select an appropriate injection site. Avoid any site that is inflamed, edematous, or irritated or that contains moles, birthmarks, scar tissue, or other lesions. The ventrogluteal muscle is the most common site, as shown below.

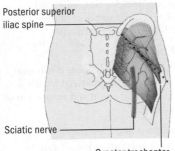

- *Note*: The dorsogluteal site. This site is no longer recommended for use for I.M. injections because it has been associated with damage to the sciatic nerve.
- I.M. injections into the deltoid muscle should be limited to 1 mL of solution, as shown at the top of the next column.

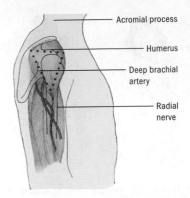

- The vastus lateralis muscle is usually used in children; the rectus femoris muscle may be used in infants, as shown below.

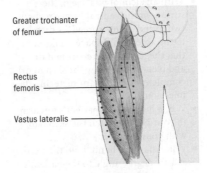

- Remember to rotate injection sites for the patient who requires repeated injections.
- Position and drape the patient appropriately.
- Loosen, but do not remove, the needle sheath.
- Clean the site by moving an alcohol pad in circles, increasing in diameter to about 2″ (5 cm). Allow the skin to dry; alcohol causes an unpleasant stinging sensation during injection.
- Put on gloves. With the thumb and index finger of your nondominant hand, gently stretch the skin, pulling it taut.
- With the syringe in your dominant hand, remove the needle sheath with the free fingers of your other hand.

- Position the syringe perpendicular to the skin surface and a couple of inches from the skin. Tell the patient that he or she will feel a prick. Then quickly and firmly thrust the needle into the muscle.
- Pull back slightly on the plunger to aspirate for blood. If none appears, inject the medication slowly and steadily to allow the muscle to distend gradually. You should feel little or no resistance. Gently, but quickly, remove the needle at a 90-degree angle.
- If blood appears, the needle is in a blood vessel. Withdraw it, prepare a fresh syringe, and inject the medication at another site.
- Using a gloved hand, apply gentle pressure to the site with a dry gauze. Do not massage the site.
- Inspect the site for bleeding or bruising. Apply pressure or ice, as necessary.
- Discard all equipment properly. Do not recap needles; put them in an appropriate biohazard container to avoid needle-stick injuries.

Special considerations

- Some drugs are dissolved in oil to slow absorption. Mix them well before use.
- Never inject into the gluteal muscles of a child who has been walking for less than 1 year.
- If the patient must have repeated injections, consider numbing the area with ice before cleaning it. If you must inject more than 5 ml, divide the solution and inject it at two sites.
- Urge the patient to relax the muscles to reduce pain and bleeding.
- I.M. injections can damage local muscle cells and elevate the serum creatine kinase level. This increase can be confused with the elevated levels caused by a myocardial infarction. Diagnostic tests can differentiate the two.

Z-track injection

The Z-track I.M. injection method prevents leakage, or tracking, into the subcutaneous tissue. Typically, it is used to administer drugs that irritate and discolor subcutaneous tissue—primarily iron preparations such as iron dextran. It may also be used in elderly patients who have decreased muscle mass. Lateral displacement of the skin during the injection helps to seal the drug in the muscle.

Equipment and preparation

Patient's medication record and chart • two 20G 1″ to 3″ needles • prescribed medication • gloves • 3- to 5-ml syringe • alcohol pad

Wash your hands. Make sure that the needle you are using is long enough to reach the muscle. As a rule of thumb, a 200-lb (91-kg) patient requires a 2″ needle; a 100-lb (45-kg) patient, a 1¼″ to 1½″ needle.

Attach one needle to the syringe and draw up the prescribed medication. Then draw 0.2 to 0.5 cc of air (depending on facility policy) into the syringe. Remove the first needle and attach the second to prevent tracking the medication through the subcutaneous tissue as the needle is inserted.

Implementation

- Verify the order on the patient's medication record by checking it against the health care provider's order. Check the patient's medication record for allergies.
- Confirm the patient's identity using two patient identifiers.
- Place the patient in the lateral position, exposing the gluteal muscle to be used as the injection site. The patient may also be placed in the prone position. Put on gloves.
- Clean an area on the upper outer quadrant of the patient's buttock with an alcohol pad.

- Displace the skin laterally by pulling it away from the injection site. To do so, place your finger on the skin surface and pull the skin and subcutaneous layers out of alignment with the underlying muscle. In doing so, the skin should move about 1″ (2.5 cm).
- Insert the needle at a 90-degree angle in the site where you initially placed your finger, as shown below.

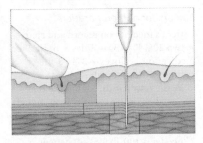

- Aspirate for blood return. If none appears, inject the drug slowly, followed by the air. Injecting air after the drug helps to clear the needle and prevents tracking the medication through subcutaneous tissues as the needle is withdrawn.
- Wait 10 seconds before withdrawing the needle to ensure dispersion of the medication.
- Withdraw the needle slowly. Release the displaced skin and subcutaneous tissues to seal the needle track, as shown below.

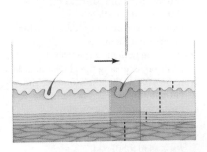

- Do not massage the injection site or allow the patient to wear a tight-fitting garment over the site because doing either could force the medication into subcutaneous tissue.
- Encourage the patient to walk or move about in bed to facilitate absorption of the drug from the injection site.
- Evaluate the patient's response to medication within an appropriate time frame. Assess the site, if possible, within 2 to 4 hours after administration.
- Discard the needles and syringe in an appropriate biohazard container. To avoid needle-stick injuries, do not recap the needles.
- Remove and discard your gloves.

Special considerations

- Never inject more than 5 ml of solution into a single site using the Z-track method. Alternate gluteal sites for repeat injections.
- If the patient is on bed rest, encourage active range-of-motion (ROM) exercises, or perform passive ROM exercises to facilitate absorption of the drug from the injection site.

Drug infusion through a secondary I.V. line

A secondary I.V. line is a complete I.V. set that is connected to the lower Y-port (secondary port) of a primary line instead of to the I.V. catheter or needle. It features an I.V. container, long tubing, and either a microdrip or macrodrip system. It can be used for continuous or intermittent drug infusion. When used continuously, it permits drug infusion and titration while the primary line maintains a constant total infusion rate.

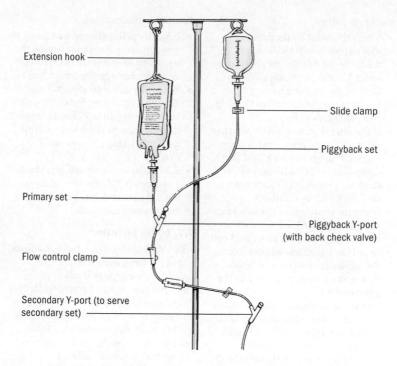

Extension hook

Slide clamp

Piggyback set

Primary set

Piggyback Y-port
(with back check valve)

Flow control clamp

Secondary Y-port (to serve
secondary set)

A secondary I.V. line, used only for intermittent drug administration, is called a piggyback set. In this case, the primary line maintains venous access between drug doses. A piggyback set includes a small I.V. container, short tubing, and usually a macrodrip system. It connects to the upper Y-port (piggyback port) of the primary line, as shown above.

Equipment and preparation
Patient's medication record and chart • prescribed I.V. medication • diluent, if necessary • prescribed I.V. solution • administration set with a secondary injection port • needleless adapter • alcohol pads • 1″ adhesive tape • time tape • labels • infusion pump • extension hook and solution for intermittent piggyback normal saline infusion

Wash your hands. Inspect the I.V. container for cracks, leaks, or contamination and check compatibility with the primary solution.

If necessary, add the drug to the secondary I.V. solution. To do so, remove any seals from the secondary container and wipe the main port with an alcohol pad. Inject the prescribed medication and agitate the solution to mix the medication. Label the I.V. mixture. Insert the administration set spike. Open the flow clamp and prime the line. Then close the flow clamp.

Some medications come in vials for hanging directly on an I.V. pole. In this case, inject the diluent directly into the medication vial. Then spike the vial, prime the tubing, and hang the set.

Implementation

- Verify the order on the patient's medication record by checking it against the health care provider's order. Check the patient's medication record for allergies.
- Confirm the patient's identity using two patient identifiers.
- If the drug is incompatible with the primary I.V. solution, replace the primary I.V. solution with a fluid that is compatible with both solutions, and flush the peripheral I.V. line before starting the drug infusion.
- Hang the container of the secondary set, and wipe the injection port of the primary line with an alcohol pad.
- Insert the needleless adapter from the secondary line into the injection port and tape it securely to the primary line.
- To run the container of the secondary set by itself, lower the container of the primary set with an extension hook. To run both containers simultaneously, place them at the same height.
- Open the slide clamp and adjust the drip rate. For continuous infusion, set the secondary solution to the desired drip rate and then adjust the primary solution to the desired total infusion rate.
- For intermittent infusion, wait until the secondary solution is completely infused and then adjust the primary drip rate, as required. If the tubing for the secondary solution is being reused, close the clamp on the tubing and follow facility policy: Either remove the needleless adapter and replace it with a new one, or leave it taped in the injection port and label it with the time that it was first used. Leave the empty container in place until you replace it with a new dose of medication at the prescribed time. If the tubing will not be reused, discard it appropriately with the I.V. container.

Special considerations

- If facility policy allows, use a pump for drug infusion. Put a time tape on the secondary container to help prevent an inaccurate administration rate.
- When reusing secondary tubing, change it according to facility policy, usually every 48 to 72 hours. Inspect the injection port for leakage with each use; change it more often, if needed.
- Except for lipids, do not piggyback a secondary I.V. line to a total parenteral nutrition line because of the risk of contamination.

I.V. bolus injection

The I.V. bolus injection method allows rapid I.V. drug administration to quickly achieve peak levels in the bloodstream. It may be used for drugs that cannot be given I.M. because they are toxic or for a patient with a reduced ability to absorb these drugs. This method may also be used to deliver drugs that cannot be diluted.

Bolus doses may be injected through an existing I.V. line or through an implanted port.

Equipment and preparation

Patient's medication record and chart • prescribed drug • needleless adapter and syringe • diluent, if necessary • antiseptic pad • alcohol pad • gloves • optional: second syringe (and needleless adaptor) filled with normal saline solution

Draw the drug into the syringe and dilute it, if necessary.

Implementation

- Verify the order on the patient's medication record by checking it against the health care provider's order. Check the patient's medication record for allergies.
- Confirm the patient's identity using two patient identifiers.
- Wash your hands and put on gloves.

To inject through an existing I.V. line
- Check the compatibility of the medication.
- Close the flow clamp, wipe the injection port with an antiseptic pad, and inject the drug as you would a direct injection.
- Open the flow clamp and readjust the flow rate.
- If the drug is incompatible with the I.V. solution, flush the line with normal saline solution before and after the injection.

To use an implanted port
- Wash your hands, put on gloves, and clean the site three times with an alcohol or antiseptic pad.
- Palpate for the septum, anchor the port between your thumb and the first two fingers of your nondominant hand, and give the injection.

Special considerations
- If the existing I.V. line is capped, making it an intermittent infusion device, verify the patency and placement of the device before injecting the medication. Flush the device with normal saline solution, administer the medication, and follow with the appropriate flush.
- Immediately report signs of acute allergic reaction or anaphylaxis. If extravasation occurs, stop the injection, estimate the amount of infiltration, and notify the health care provider.
- When giving diazepam or chlordiazepoxide, flush with normal saline solution to prevent precipitation.

Special administration

Epidural analgesics

When giving an epidural analgesic, the health care provider injects or infuses the drug into the epidural space, and thus into the cerebrospinal fluid, so that the medication can bypass the blood–brain barrier.

Epidural analgesia helps to manage pain, including postoperative pain.

Equipment and preparation
Patient's medication record and chart • prescribed epidural solutions • volume infusion device and epidural infusion tubing (depending on facility policy) • transparent dressing • epidural tray • label for epidural infusion line • silk tape • optional: monitoring equipment for blood pressure and pulse, apnea monitor, pulse oximeter

Make sure that the pharmacy has been notified of the medication order ahead of time because epidural solutions require special preparation.

Implementation
- Verify the order on the patient's medication record by checking it against the health care provider's order. Check the patient's medication record for allergies.
- Confirm the patient's identity using two patient identifiers.
- Tell the patient that he or she will feel some pain as the health care provider inserts the catheter.
- Put the patient on his or her side in the knee-chest position or have him or her sit on the edge of the bed and lean over a bedside table.
- After the catheter is in place, as shown at the top of the next page, prime the infusion device, confirm the medication and the infusion rate, and adjust the device.
- After the infusion tubing is connected to the epidural catheter, connect the tubing to the infusion pump. Tape all connection sites and apply a label that says EPIDURAL INFUSION.
- Tell the patient to report any pain. If pain occurs, the infusion rate may need to be increased.

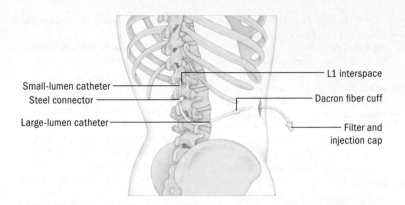

Small-lumen catheter
Steel connector
Large-lumen catheter
L1 interspace
Dacron fiber cuff
Filter and injection cap

- Change the dressing over the exit site every 24 to 48 hours or as specified.

Special considerations

- After starting the infusion, assess the patient's respiratory rate and blood pressure every 2 hours for 8 hours; every 4 hours for 8 hours; and then once per shift, unless ordered otherwise. Notify the health care provider if the respiratory rate is below 10 breaths/minute or if the systolic blood pressure is less than 90 mm Hg.
- Assess the patient's sedation level and mental status and the adequacy of pain relief every hour initially, and then every 2 to 4 hours, until adequate pain control is achieved.
- If the patient is receiving a local anesthetic, assess his or her lower extremity motor strength every 2 to 4 hours. If the patient has sensory and motor loss, large motor nerve fibers have been affected, and the dosage may need to be decreased.
- The patient should always have a peripheral I.V. line open to allow administration of emergency drugs. Have an opioid antidote, such as naloxone (Narcan), readily available.
- Do not give an analgesic by another route because such administration increases the risk of respiratory depression.

Selected references

Taylor, C., Lillis, C., & Lynn, P. (2015). *Fundamentals of nursing: The art and science of person-centered nursing care* (8th ed.). Philadelphia, PA: Wolters Kluwer.

Vallerand, A., & Sanoski, C. (2019). *Davis's drug guide for nurses* (16th ed.). Philadelphia, PA: F.A. Davis.

13

Dosage Calculation

Ensuring effective therapy

Calculating drug dosages

Reviewing ratios and proportions

A ratio is a mathematical expression of the relationship between two things. A proportion is a set of two equal ratios. A ratio may be expressed as a fraction, such as ⅓, or with a colon, such as 1:3. When ratios are expressed as fractions in a proportion, their cross products are equal.

Proportion

$$\frac{2}{4} \bowtie \frac{5}{10}$$

Cross products

$$2 \times 10 = 4 \times 5$$

When ratios are expressed using colons in a proportion, the product of the means equals the product of the extremes.

Proportion

means
↓   ↓
3 : 30 :: 4 : 40
↑ extremes ↑

Product of means and extremes

$$30 \times 4 = 3 \times 40$$

Whether fractions or ratios are used in a proportion, they must appear in the same order on both sides of the equal sign. When ratios are expressed as fractions, the units in the numerators must be the same and the units in the denominators must be the same (although they do not have to be the same as the units in the numerators).

$$\frac{mg}{kg} = \frac{mg}{kg}$$

If the ratios in a proportion are expressed with colons, the units of the first term on the left side of the equal sign must be the same as the units of the first term on the right side. In other words, the units of the mean on one side of the equal sign must match the units of the extreme on the other side, and vice versa.

$$mg : kg :: mg : kg$$

Tips for simplifying dosage calculations

Incorporate units of measure into the calculation

Incorporating units of measure into the dosage calculation helps to protect you from one of the most common errors made in dosage calculation—using the incorrect unit of measure. Keep in mind that the units of measure that appear in the numerator and denominator cancel each other out, leaving the correct unit of measure in the answer. The following example uses units of measure in calculating a drug with a usual dose of 4 mg/kg for a 55-kg patient.

1. State the problem as a proportion.

$$4 \text{ mg} : 1 \text{ kg} :: X : 55 \text{ kg}$$

2. Solve for *X* by applying the principle that the product of the means equals the product of the extremes.

$$1 \text{ kg} \times X = 4 \text{ mg} \times 55 \text{ kg}$$

3. Divide and cancel out the units of measure that appear in the numerator and denominator.

$$X = \frac{4 \text{ mg} \times 55 \text{ kg}}{1 \text{ kg}}$$

$$X = 220 \text{ mg}$$

Check the zeros and the decimal places

Suppose that you receive an order to administer 0.1 mg of epinephrine subcutaneously, but the only epinephrine on hand is a 1-ml ampule that contains 1 mg of epinephrine. To calculate the volume for injection, use the ratio-and-proportion method.

State the problem as a proportion.

1 mg : 1 ml :: 0.1 mg : X

Solve for X by applying the principle that the product of the means equals the product of the extremes.

1 ml × 0.1 mg = 1 mg × X

Divide and cancel out the units of measure that appear in both the numerator and the denominator, carefully checking the decimal placement.

$$\frac{1 \text{ ml} \times 0.1 \text{ mg}}{1 \text{ mg}} = X$$

0.1 ml = X

Recheck calculations that seem unusual

If, for example, your calculation indicates that you should administer 25 tablets, you have probably made an error. Carefully recheck any figures that seem unusual. If you still have doubts, review your calculations with another health care professional.

Determining the number of tablets to administer

Calculating the number of tablets to administer lends itself to the use of ratios and proportions. To perform the calculation, follow this process:
1. Set up the first ratio with the known tablet (tab) strength.
2. Set up the second ratio with the unknown quantity.
3. Use these ratios in a proportion.
4. Solve for X, applying the principle that the product of the means equals the product of the extremes.
    For example, suppose that a drug order calls for 100 mg of propranolol P.O. q.i.d., but only 40-mg tablets are available. To determine the number of tablets to administer, follow these steps:
1. Set up the first ratio with the known tablet (tab) strength.

40 mg : 1 tab

2. Set up the second ratio with the desired dose and the unknown number of tablets.

100 mg : X

3. Use these ratios in a proportion.

40 mg : 1 tab :: 100 mg : X

4. Solve for X by applying the principle that the product of the means equals the product of the extremes.

1 tab × 100 mg = 40 mg × X

$$\frac{1 \text{ tab} \times 100 \text{ mg}}{40 \text{ mg} \times X}$$

2½ tab = X

Determining the amount of liquid medication to administer

You can also use ratios and proportions to calculate the amount of liquid medication to administer. Simply follow the same four-step process used in determining the number of tablets to administer.

For example, suppose that a patient is to receive 750 mg of amoxicillin oral suspension. The label reads amoxicillin (amoxicillin trihydrate) 250 mg/5 ml. The bottle contains 100 ml. To determine how many milliliters of amoxicillin solution the patient should receive, follow these steps:
1. Set up the first ratio with the known strength of the liquid medication.

250 mg : 5 ml

2. Set up the second ratio with the desired dose and the unknown quantity.

750 mg : X

3. Use these ratios in a proportion.

250 mg : 5 ml :: 750 mg : X

4. Solve for X by applying the principle that the product of the means equals the product of the extremes.

5 ml × 750 mg = 250 mg × X

$$\frac{5 \text{ ml} \times 750 \text{ mg}}{250 \text{ mg}} = X$$

15 ml = X

Administering drugs available in varied concentrations

Because drugs, such as epinephrine, heparin, and allergy serums, are available in varied concentrations, you must consider the concentration of the drug when calculating a drug dosage. Otherwise, you could make a serious—even lethal—mistake. To avoid a dosage error, make sure that drug concentrations are part of the calculation.

For example, a drug order calls for 0.2 mg of epinephrine subcutaneously stat. The ampule is labeled as 1 ml of 1:1,000 epinephrine. Follow these steps to calculate the correct volume of drug to inject.

1. Determine the strength of the solution based on its unlabeled ratio.

   1:1,000 epinephrine = 1 g/1,000 ml

2. Set up a proportion with this information and the desired dose.

   1 g : 1,000 ml :: 0.2 mg : X

Before you can perform this calculation, however, you must convert grams to milligrams by using the conversion 1 g = 1,000 mg.

3. Restate the proportion with the converted units and solve for X.

   1,000 mg : 1,000 ml :: 0.2 mg : X

   1,000 ml × 0.2 mg = 1,000 mg × X

   $$\frac{1,000 \text{ ml} \times 0.2 \text{ mg}}{1,000 \text{ mg}} = X$$

   0.2 ml = X

Calculating I.V. drip and flow rates

To compute the drip and flow rates, set up a fraction with the volume of solution to be delivered over the prescribed duration. For example, if a patient is to receive 100 ml of solution within 1 hour, the fraction is:

$$\frac{100 \text{ ml}}{60 \text{ minutes}}$$

Next, multiply the fraction by the drip factor (the number of drops contained in 1 ml) to determine the drip rate (the number of drops per minute to be infused). The drip factor varies among I.V. sets and appears on the package containing the I.V. tubing administration set. Following the manufacturer's directions for the drip factor is crucial. Standard sets have drip factors of 10, 15, or 20 gtt/ml. A microdrip (minidrip) set has a drip factor of 60 gtt/ml.

Use the following equation to determine the drip rate:

$$\frac{\text{total ml}}{\text{total minutes}} \times \text{drip factor} = \text{gtt/minute}$$

The equation applies to solutions that are infused over many hours as well as to small-volume infusions such as those used for antibiotics, which are given for less than 1 hour.

You can modify the equation by first determining the number of milliliters to be infused over 1 hour (the flow rate). Then, divide the flow rate by 60 minutes. Next, multiply the result by the drip factor to determine the number of drops per minute. You will also use the flow rate when working with infusion pumps to set the number of milliliters to be delivered in 1 hour.

Quick calculations of drip rates

In addition to using the equation and its modified version, quicker computation methods are available. To administer solutions ordered at an hourly rate using a microdrip set, adjust the flow rate (ml/hour) to equal the drip rate (gtt/minute). Using the equation, divide the flow rate by 60 minutes and multiply the result by the drip factor, which also equals 60. Because the flow rate and the drip factor are equal, the two arithmetic operations cancel each other out. For example, if the flow rate is 125 ml/hour, the equation would be:

$$\frac{125 \text{ ml}}{60 \text{ minutes}} \times 60 = \text{drip rate (125)}$$

Instead of spending the time solving the equation, you can simply use the number assigned to the flow rate as the drip rate. For sets that deliver 15 gtt/ml, the flow rate divided by 4 equals the drip rate. For sets with a drip factor of 10, the flow rate divided by 6 equals the drip rate.

To determine how many micrograms of a drug are in a milliliter of solution, use the following equation:

$$\text{mcg/ml} = \text{mg/ml} \times 1{,}000$$

To express drip rates in micrograms per kilogram per minute (mcg/kg/minute), you must know the concentration of the solution (mcg/ml), the patient's weight (kg), and the infusion rate (ml/hour):

$$\text{mcg/kg/minute} = \frac{\text{mcg/ml} \times \text{ml/minute}}{\text{body weight (kg)}}$$

To find the milliliters per minute (ml/minute), divide the number of milliliters per hour (ml/hour) by 60.

You can also convert milliliters per hour (ml/hour) from a dosage given in micrograms per kilograms per minute (mcg/kg/minute) as follows:

$$\text{ml/hour} = \frac{\text{wt (kg)} \times \text{mcg/kg/minute}}{\text{mcg/ml}} \times 60$$

Dimensional analysis

Dimensional analysis (also known as factor analysis, or factor labeling) is an alternative method of solving mathematical problems. It eliminates the need to memorize formulas and requires only one equation to determine an answer. To compare the ratio-and-proportion method and dimensional analysis at a glance, read the following problem and solutions.

The physician prescribes 0.25 g of streptomycin sulfate I.M. The vial reads "2 ml = 1 g." How many milliliters should you administer?

Dimensional analysis

$$\frac{0.25 \text{ g}}{1} \times \frac{2 \text{ ml}}{1 \text{ g}} = 0.5 \text{ ml}$$

Ratio and proportion

$$1 \text{ g} : 2 \text{ ml} :: 0.25 \text{ g} : X$$

$$2 \text{ ml} \times 0.25 \text{ g} = 1 \text{ g} \times X$$

$$\frac{2 \text{ ml} \times 0.25 \,\cancel{g}}{1 \,\cancel{g}} = X$$

$$0.5 \text{ ml} = X$$

Dimensional analysis involves arranging a series of ratios, called factors, into a single fractional equation. Each factor, written as a fraction, consists of two quantities and their units of measurement that are related to each other in a given problem. For instance, if 1,000 ml of a drug should be administered over 8 hours, the relationship between 1,000 ml and 8 hours is expressed by the fraction.

$$\frac{1{,}000 \text{ ml}}{8 \text{ hours}}$$

When a problem includes a quantity and its unit of measurement that are unrelated to any other factor in the problem, they serve as the numerator of the fraction, and 1 (implied) becomes the denominator.

Some mathematical problems contain all of the information needed to identify the factors, set up the equation, and find the solution. Other problems require the use of a conversion factor. Conversion factors are equivalents (for example, 1 g = 1,000 mg) that can be memorized or obtained from a conversion chart. Because the two quantities and units of measurement are equivalent, they can serve as the numerator or the denominator. Thus, the conversion factor 1 g = 1,000 mg can be written in fraction form as:

$$\frac{1{,}000 \text{ mg}}{1 \text{ g}} \text{ or } \frac{1 \text{ g}}{1{,}000 \text{ mg}}$$

The factors given in the problem plus any conversion factors that are necessary to solve the problem are called knowns. The quantity of the answer, of course, is unknown. When setting up an equation in dimensional analysis, work backward, beginning with the unit of measurement of the answer. After plotting all of the knowns, find the solution by following this sequence:

1. Cancel similar quantities and units of measurement.
2. Multiply the numerators.
3. Multiply the denominators.
4. Divide the numerator by the denominator.

Mastering dimensional analysis can take practice, but you may find your efforts well rewarded. To understand more fully how dimensional analysis works, review the following problem and the steps taken to solve it.

The physician prescribes *X* grains (gr) of a drug. The pharmacy supplies the drug in 300-mg tablets (tab). How many tablets should you administer?

1. Write down the unit of measurement of the answer, followed by an "equal to" symbol (=).

$$\text{tab} =$$

2. Search the problem for the quantity with the same unit of measurement (if one does not exist, use a conversion factor); place this in the numerator and its related quantity and unit of measurement in the denominator.

$$\text{tab} = \frac{1 \text{ tab}}{300 \text{ mg}}$$

Separate the first factor from the next with a multiplication symbol (×).

$$\text{tab} = \frac{1 \text{ tab}}{300 \text{ mg}} \times$$

Place the unit of measurement of the denominator of the first factor in the numerator of the second factor. Search the problem for the quantity with the same unit of measurement (if there is

no common measurement, as in this example, use a conversion factor). Place this in the numerator and its related quantity and unit of measurement in the denominator; follow with a multiplication symbol. Repeat this step until all known factors are included in the equation.

$$\text{tab} = \frac{1 \text{ tab}}{300 \text{ mg}} \times \frac{60 \text{ mg}}{1 \text{ gr}} \times \frac{10 \text{ gr}}{1}$$

Alternatively, you can treat the equation as a large fraction, using these steps.

1. First, cancel similar units of measurement in the numerator and the denominator. What remains should be what you began with—the unit of measurement of the answer; if not, recheck your equation to find and correct the error.
2. Multiply the numerators and then the denominators.
3. Divide the numerator by the denominator.

$$\text{tab} = \frac{1 \text{ tab}}{300 \text{ mg}} \times \frac{60 \text{ mg}}{1 \text{ gr}} \times \frac{10 \text{ gr}}{1}$$

$$= \frac{60 \times 10 \text{ tab}}{300}$$

$$= \frac{600 \text{ tab}}{300}$$

$$= 2 \text{ tablets}$$

Administering drugs

Administering code drugs

Adenosine

Indicated for patients with paroxysmal supraventricular tachycardia, including that associated with accessory bypass tracts (Wolff-Parkinson-White's syndrome)

Dosage

Initially, give 6 mg I.V. as a rapid bolus over 1 to 3 seconds; if there is no response in 1 to 2 minutes, give 12 mg I.V. as a rapid bolus (12-mg dose may be given a second time if required).

Nursing considerations
- Adverse effects may include flushing or chest pain lasting 1 to 2 minutes.
- Flush immediately and rapidly with 20 ml of normal saline solution to ensure drug delivery.
- Monitor the cardiac rhythm to detect heart block and transient asystole.

Amiodarone

Indicated for recurrent hemodynamically unstable ventricular tachycardia and frequently recurring ventricular fibrillation

Dosage

Give 150 mg I.V. over the first 10 minutes (15 mg/minute [not to exceed 30 mg/minute]) and then 360 mg I.V. over the next 6 hours (1 mg/minute), followed by a maintenance infusion of 540 mg I.V. over the remaining 18 hours (0.5 mg/minute).

Nursing considerations
- Administer the drug through a central line whenever possible.
- Mix initial 150 mg dose in 100 ml dextrose 5% in water (D_5W); the

Estimating BSA in adults

Body surface area (BSA) is a critical component of the calculation of dosages for drugs (such as chemotherapeutic agents) that are extremely potent and must be given in precise amounts. The nomogram shown here lets you plot the patient's height and weight to determine the BSA. To estimate the BSA of an adult patient, place a straightedge from the patient's height in the left-hand column to his or her weight in the right-hand column. The intersection of this line with the center scale shows the BSA.

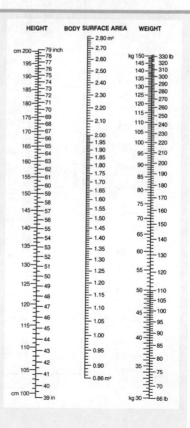

Reprinted with permission from Lentner, C. (1990). *Geigy scientific tables: Heart and circulation* (8th ed., Vol. 5, pp. 105). Basel, Switzerland: Ciba-Geigy. ©1990 by Novartis.

Estimating BSA in children

Pediatric drug dosages are calculated on the basis of body weight or body surface area (BSA). For an average-sized child, find the weight and the corresponding BSA in the box. Otherwise, to use the nomogram, place a straightedge on the correct height and weight points for the patient and note the point at which the line intersects on the scale. Do not use drug dosages based on BSA in premature or full-term neonates; instead, use body weight.

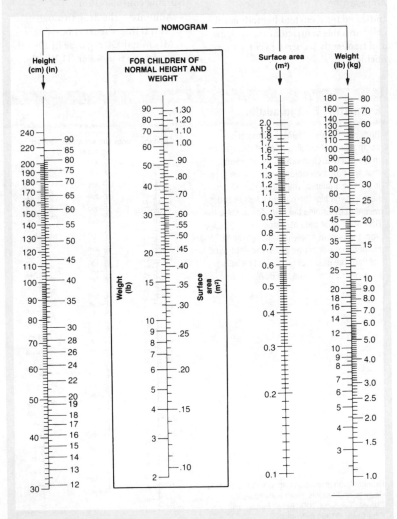

drug is incompatible with normal saline solution. Mix infusions to be administered over 2 hours or longer in glass or polyolefin bottles containing D_5W.

- Monitor the patient for hypotension, bradycardia, and arrhythmias.
- Must be delivered by volumetric infusion pump

Atropine

Indicated for symptomatic sinus bradycardia with hemodynamic compromise, atrioventricular (AV) block, pulseless electrical activity (PEA), and ventricular asystole

Dosage

For bradycardia or AV block, give 0.5 to 1 mg I.V. push, repeated every 3 to 5 minutes to a total dose of 0.04 mg/kg. A total dose of 2.5 mg (0.04 mg/kg) results in full vagal blockade in humans. For asystole or PEA, give 1 mg I.V. push; repeat in 3 to 5 minutes if asystole persists.

Nursing considerations

- Monitor the patient for paradoxical initial bradycardia, especially if he or she is receiving 0.4 to 0.6 mg.
- Monitor the patient's fluid intake and urine output.
- Watch for tachycardia.

Dobutamine

Indicated for inotropic support in short-term treatment of adults with cardiac decompensation caused by depressed contractility resulting from organic heart disease or surgery

Dosage

Give 0.5 to 1 mcg/kg/minute by I.V. infusion, titrating to an optimal dosage of 2 to 20 mcg/kg/minute.

Nursing considerations

- Watch for reflex peripheral vasodilation.
- Monitor the patient's heart rate closely; an increase of 10% or more may worsen myocardial ischemia.
- Avoid extravasation; give drug through a central venous catheter or a large peripheral vein. Use an infusion pump.

Dopamine

Indicated for patients with hypotension or bradycardia to treat shock, improve perfusion to vital organs, and increase cardiac output

Dosage

Initially, give 2 to 5 mcg/kg/minute, titrated until the desired response is achieved. Infusion may be increased by 1 to 4 mcg/kg/minute at 10- to 30-minute intervals.

Nursing considerations

- Drug effects vary with dosage. At 0.5 to 2 mcg/kg/minute, the drug dilates the renal and mesenteric vessels without increasing heart rate or blood pressure; at 2 to 10 mcg/kg/minute, it increases cardiac output without peripheral vasoconstriction; and at more than 10 mcg/kg/minute, it causes peripheral vasoconstriction.
- Use a central line or a large vein. Monitor for extravasation; if it occurs, stop the infusion immediately and call the physician.

Epinephrine

Indicated for the patient in cardiac arrest

Dosage

Give 1 mg I.V. or intraosseously repeated every 3 to 5 minutes, if necessary.

Nursing considerations

- If administering the drug by the I.V. or intraosseous route is not possible, the drug may be given endotracheally at 2 to 2.5 times the peripheral I.V. dose.
- Intracardiac injection is indicated only during open cardiac massage and if other routes are unavailable.

Lidocaine

Indicated for patients with ventricular tachycardia, ventricular ectopy, and ventricular fibrillation; prophylactic administration in patients with uncomplicated myocardial infarction is not recommended.

Dosage

Give 1 to 1.5 mg/kg I.V. bolus as a loading dose at 25 to 50 mg/minute; repeat the bolus dose every 3 to 5 minutes, until arrhythmias subside or adverse reactions develop, to a maximum of 3 mg/kg (300 mg over 1 hour); simultaneously, set up a continuous I.V. infusion at 1 to 4 mg/minute. (Dilute 1 g of lidocaine in 250 ml of D_5W for a 0.4% solution, or 4 mg/ml.)

Nursing considerations

- For an elderly patient, a patient weighing less than 110 lb (50 kg), or a patient with heart failure or hepatic disease, administer half of the bolus dose.
- Lidocaine improves the response to defibrillation when the patient is in ventricular fibrillation.

Magnesium sulfate

Indicated for the treatment of ventricular fibrillation, ventricular tachycardia, cardiac arrest associated with torsades de pointes, and torsades de pointes with pulses

Dosage

Give 1 to 2 g in 10 ml of D_5W administered I.V. or intraosseously over 5 to 20 minutes for cardiac arrest associated with torsades de pointes. Give 1 to 2 g in 50 to 100 ml of D_5W I.V. over 5 to 60 minutes and follow this with 0.5 to 1 g/hour I.V. for torsades de pointes with pulses.

Nursing considerations

- Monitor serum magnesium levels.
- Watch for respiratory depression and signs and symptoms of heart block.
- If hypotension develops, slow or stop the infusion.

Nitroglycerin

Indicated for patients with heart failure associated with myocardial infarction and for patients with unstable angina

Dosage

Give a 5 mcg/minute I.V. infusion initially, increasing by 5 mcg/minute every 3 to 5 minutes until a response occurs. If a 20 mcg/minute rate does not produce a response, increase the dosage by as much as 20 mcg/minute every 3 to 5 minutes. Up to 100 mcg/minute may be needed.

Nursing considerations

- Monitor the patient for hypotension, which could worsen myocardial ischemia.
- Because up to 80% of the drug binds to the plastic in normal I.V. administration sets, use the special I.V. tubing supplied by the manufacturer.
- Mix in glass bottles and avoid using I.V. filters. Use an infusion pump.

Nitroprusside

Indicated for the patient with heart failure or in hypertensive crisis

Dosage

Dissolve 50 mg in 2 to 3 ml of D_5W and then mix with 250 to 1,000 ml of D_5W, depending on the desired concentration. Begin the infusion at

0.3 mcg/kg/minute and titrate every few minutes to a maximum of 10 mcg/kg/minute.

Nursing considerations

- Wrap the container in opaque material to prevent deterioration of the drug.
- Monitor the patient's blood pressure every 5 minutes for 1 hour and every 15 minutes thereafter.
- Large doses given at fast infusion rates increase the risk of cyanide toxicity. Measure cyanide levels and monitor for acidosis. If a toxic reaction is suspected, start treatment without the test results.

Norepinephrine bitartrate

Indicated for the patient with severe hypotension or low total peripheral resistance

Dosage

Initially, give an 8 to 12 mcg/minute I.V. infusion. Titrate to maintain systolic blood pressure at 80 to 100 mm Hg in a previously normotensive patient. The average rate of maintenance infusion is 2 to 4 mcg/minute.

Nursing considerations

- Norepinephrine is contraindicated in the patient with hypovolemia.
- Monitor the patient's blood pressure with an intra-arterial line because measurements obtained with a standard cuff may be falsely low.
- Cardiac output may increase or decrease, depending on vascular resistance, left ventricular function, and reflux response.
- Avoid prolonged use; the drug may cause ischemia of vital organs.
- Use a central venous catheter or a large vein to minimize the risk of extravasation. If extravasation occurs, stop the infusion and call the physician.

Procainamide

Indicated for the patient with ventricular arrhythmias, such as premature ventricular contractions or tachycardia, when lidocaine is contraindicated or ineffective

Dosage

Give a loading dose infusion of 20 mg/minute, not to exceed a total dose of 500 mg, followed by a continuous infusion of 2 to 6 mg/minute.

Nursing considerations

- Lower the dosage, as ordered, for the patient with renal failure.
- Rapid infusion will cause acute hypotension. An infusion pump is required.
- Monitor electrocardiogram results carefully; if the QRS complex widens more than 50% or if the QT interval is prolonged, notify the physician and discontinue the infusion, as ordered.

Vasopressin

Indicated for the treatment of adult shock-refractory ventricular fibrillation, asystole, or PEA

Dosage

Give 40 units I.V., one time only.

Nursing considerations

- Use as an alternative to epinephrine.

Verapamil

Indicated for the patient with atrial fibrillation, atrial flutter, or multifocal atrial tachycardia; also used to help treat narrow QRS complex paroxysmal supraventricular tachycardia

Dosage

Give 2.5 to 5 mg I.V. over 2 minutes. Repeat dose of 5 to 10 mg every 15 to 30 minutes to a maximum dosage of 20 mg.

Nursing considerations

- Use cautiously and in lower doses for the patient receiving a beta blocker.
- Monitor the patient for hypotension, severe bradycardia, and heart failure.
- Because verapamil may decrease myocardial contractility, it can aggravate heart failure in the patient with severe left ventricular dysfunction.

A guide to equianalgesic doses

Opioid agonists

The standard opioid agonist dose, 10 mg of morphine I.M., is used to calculate equally effective (equianalgesic) doses of other opioid agonists. This method is useful when a patient must be switched from one opioid agonist to another

Infusion flow rates

The infusion flow rates are based on the concentrations shown at the top of each table. Be sure to check the label on the medication you are infusing to verify the correct infusion flow rate.

Epinephrine infusion rates

Mix 1 mg in 250 ml (4 mcg/ml).

Dose (mcg/minute)	Infusion rate (ml/hour)
1	15
2	30
3	45
4	60
5	75
6	90
7	105
8	120
9	135
10	150
15	225
20	300
25	375
30	450
35	525
40	600

Isoproterenol infusion rates

Mix 1 mg in 250 ml (4 mcg/ml).

Dose (mcg/minute)	Infusion rate (ml/hour)
0.5	8
1	15
2	30
3	45
4	60
5	75
6	90
7	105
8	120
9	135
10	150
15	225
20	300
25	375
30	450

Infusion flow rates (continued)

Nitroglycerin infusion rates

Determine the infusion rate in ml/hour using the ordered dose and the concentration of the drug solution.

Dose (mcg/minute)	25 mg/250 ml (100 mcg/ml)	50 mg/250 ml (200 mcg/ml)	100 mg/250 ml (400 mcg/ml)
5	3	2	1
10	6	3	2
20	12	6	3
30	18	9	5
40	24	12	6
50	30	15	8
60	36	18	9
70	42	21	10
80	48	24	12
90	54	27	14
100	60	30	15
150	90	45	23
200	120	60	30

Dobutamine infusion rates

Mix 250 mg in 250 ml of dextrose in 5% water (D_5W) (1,000 mcg/ml). Determine the infusion rate in ml/hour using the ordered dose and the patient's weight in pounds or kilograms.

Dose (mcg/kg/minute)	lb	88	99	110	121	132	143	154	165	176	187	198	209	220	231	242
	kg	40	45	50	55	60	65	70	75	80	85	90	95	100	105	110
2.5		6	7	8	8	9	10	11	11	12	13	14	14	15	16	17
5		12	14	15	17	18	20	21	23	24	26	27	29	30	32	33
7.5		18	20	23	25	27	29	32	34	36	38	41	43	45	47	50
10		24	27	30	33	36	39	42	45	48	51	54	57	60	63	66
12.5		30	34	38	41	45	49	53	56	60	64	68	71	75	79	83
15		36	41	45	50	54	59	63	68	72	77	81	86	90	95	99
20		48	54	60	66	72	78	84	90	96	102	108	114	120	126	132
25		60	68	75	83	90	98	105	113	120	128	135	143	150	158	165
30		72	81	90	99	108	117	126	135	144	153	162	171	180	189	198
35		84	95	105	116	126	137	147	158	168	179	189	200	210	221	231
40		96	108	120	132	144	156	168	180	192	204	216	228	240	252	264

(continued)

Infusion flow rates (continued)

Dopamine infusion rates

Mix 400 mg in 250 ml of D$_5$W (1,600 mcg/ml). Determine the infusion rate in ml/hour using the ordered dose and the patient's weight in pounds or kilograms.

Dose (mcg/kg/minute) lb kg	88 40	99 45	110 50	121 55	132 60	143 65	154 70	165 75	176 80	187 85	198 90	200 95	220 100	231 105
2.5	4	4	5	5	6	6	7	7	8	8	8	9	9	10
5	8	8	9	10	11	12	13	14	15	16	17	18	19	20
7.5	11	13	14	15	17	18	20	21	23	24	25	27	28	30
10	15	17	19	21	23	24	26	28	30	32	34	36	38	39
12.5	19	21	23	26	28	30	33	35	38	40	42	45	47	49
15	23	25	28	31	34	37	39	42	45	48	51	53	56	59
20	30	34	38	41	45	49	53	56	60	64	68	71	75	79
25	38	42	47	52	56	61	66	70	75	80	84	89	94	98
30	45	51	56	62	67	73	79	84	90	96	101	107	113	118
35	53	59	66	72	79	85	92	98	105	112	118	125	131	138
40	60	68	75	83	90	98	105	113	120	128	135	143	150	158
45	68	76	84	93	101	110	118	127	135	143	152	160	169	177
50	75	84	94	103	113	122	131	141	150	159	169	178	188	197

Nitroprusside infusion rates

Mix 50 mg in 250 ml of D$_5$W (200 mcg/ml). Determine the infusion rate in ml/hour using the ordered dose and the patient's weight in pounds or kilograms.

Dose (mcg/kg/minute) lb kg	88 40	99 45	110 50	121 55	132 60	143 65	154 70	165 75	176 80	187 85	198 90	209 95	220 100	231 105	242 110
0.3	4	4	5	5	5	6	6	7	7	8	8	9	9	9	10
0.5	6	7	8	8	9	10	11	11	12	13	14	14	15	16	17
1	12	14	15	17	18	20	21	23	24	26	27	29	30	32	33
1.5	18	20	23	25	27	29	32	34	36	38	41	43	45	47	50
2	24	27	30	33	36	39	42	45	48	51	54	57	60	63	66
3	36	41	45	50	54	59	63	68	72	77	81	86	90	95	99
4	48	54	60	66	72	78	84	90	96	102	108	114	120	126	132
5	60	68	75	83	90	98	105	113	120	128	135	143	150	158	165
6	72	81	90	99	108	117	126	135	144	153	162	171	180	189	198
7	84	95	105	116	126	137	147	158	168	179	189	200	210	221	231
8	96	108	120	132	144	156	168	180	192	204	216	228	240	252	264
9	108	122	135	149	162	176	189	203	216	230	243	257	270	284	297
10	120	135	150	165	180	195	210	225	240	255	270	285	300	315	330

with no change in dose effectiveness. This chart lists equianalgesic doses for selected opioid agonists.

Drug	Dose
codeine	120 mg P.O.
fentanyl	0.1 to 0.2 mg I.M.
hydromorphone	1.5 mg I.M.
meperidine	75 to 100 mg I.M.
methadone	8 to 10 mg I.M.
morphine	10 mg I.M.
oxymorphone	1 to 1.5 mg I.M.

Mixed opioid agonist-antagonists

This chart lists equianalgesic doses (based on the standard dose of 10 mg of morphine I.M.) for mixed opioid agonist-antagonists.

Drug	Dose
buprenorphine	0.3 mg I.M.
butorphanol	2 mg I.M.
dezocine	10 mg I.M.
morphine	10 mg I.M.
nalbuphine	10 mg I.M.
pentazocine	30 mg I.M.

Critical elements of medication teaching

As the patient becomes more responsible for his or her own care, it is important that you supply him or her with all of the information that he or she needs to comply with his or her treatment plan. Accurate written information is crucial for any patient, but it is especially important for young patients, elderly patients, and those with cognitive impairments. When preparing your written medication teaching plan, it is important to include these points:

* name, dosage, and action of the drug
* frequency and times of administration
* special instructions for storage and preparation
* drugs (including over-the-counter products) and foods (including additives) to avoid
* special comfort measures or safety precautions
* adverse effects and possible signs and symptoms of a toxic reaction
* warnings about discontinuing the medication.

Selected reference

Nursing 2019 drug handbook (39th ed.). (2019). Philadelphia, PA: Wolters Kluwer.

14

Drug Hazards

Recognizing and responding to them

Adverse or toxic drug reactions

Drug reactions and treatments

The key to successful treatment of toxic drug reactions is to identify the drug quickly and accurately and then immediately begin the appropriate treatment.

Identifying the most dangerous drugs

Almost any drug can cause an adverse reaction in some patients, but the following drugs cause about 90% of all reported reactions.

Anticoagulants
- Heparin
- Warfarin

Antimicrobials
- Cephalosporins
- Penicillins
- Sulfonamides

Bronchodilators
- Sympathomimetics
- Theophylline

Cardiac drugs
- Antihypertensives
- Digoxin
- Diuretics
- Quinidine

Central nervous system drugs
- Analgesics
- Anticonvulsants
- Neuroleptics
- Sedative-hypnotics

Diagnostic agents
- X-ray contrast media

Hormones
- Corticosteroids
- Estrogens
- Insulin

Reporting adverse drug reactions to the FDA

Drug manufacturers monitor adverse drug reactions (ADRs) and are required to report them to the U.S. Food and Drug Administration (FDA). That is the law.

The FDA also wants to hear from nurses whose patients have had serious reactions associated with drugs—especially drugs that have been on the market for 3 years or less. After all, you and your colleagues are the ones who are most likely to see the reactions, so you can give the best clinical descriptions. Unlike drug manufacturers, however, nurses are not required by law to make a report.

What constitutes a serious ADR? According to the FDA, it is one that:
- is life-threatening
- causes congenital anomaly/birth defect
- causes death
- leads to or prolongs hospitalization
- requires intervention that prevents permanent damage or impairment
- results in permanent or severe disability
- medical events that are important.

(Text continues on page 604.)

Managing toxic drug reactions

Toxic reactions and clinical effects	Interventions	Selected causative drugs
Anemia, aplastic • Bleeding from the mucous membranes, ecchymoses, petechiae • Fatigue, pallor, progressive weakness, shortness of breath, tachycardia (progresses to heart failure) • Fever, oral and rectal ulcers, sore throat without characteristic inflammation	• Discontinue the drug, if possible. • Order vigorous supportive care, including transfusions, neutropenic isolation, antibiotics, and oxygen. • Colony-stimulating factors may be given. • For severe cases, a bone marrow transplant may be needed.	• Antineoplastic agents • aspirin (long-term) • carbamazepine • chloramphenicol • penicillamine • Phenothiazines • propylthiouracil • phenytoin
Anemia, hemolytic • Chills, fever, back and abdominal pain (hemolytic crisis) • Jaundice, malaise, splenomegaly • Signs of shock	• Discontinue the drug. • Order supportive care, including transfusions and oxygen. • Consider obtaining a blood sample for Coombs test.	• Cephalosporins • ciprofloxacin • levodopa • methyldopa • phenazopyridine • quinidine • Sulfonamides
Bone marrow toxicity (agranulocytosis) • Enlarged lymph nodes, spleen, and tonsils • Septicemia, shock • Progressive fatigue and weakness followed by sudden, overwhelming infection with chills, fever, headache, and tachycardia • Pneumonia • Ulcers in the colon, mouth, and pharynx	• Discontinue the drug. • Begin antibiotic therapy while awaiting the results of blood culture and sensitivity tests. • Order supportive therapy, including neutropenic isolation, warm saline gargles, and oral hygiene.	• carbamazepine • chloramphenicol • clomipramine • clozapine • flucytosine • penicillamine • phenytoin • procainamide • propylthiouracil • Sulfonylureas
Bone marrow toxicity (thrombocytopenia) • Fatigue, weakness, lethargy, malaise • Hemorrhage, loss of consciousness, shortness of breath, tachycardia • Sudden onset of ecchymoses or petechiae; large, blood-filled bullae in the mouth	• Discontinue the drug or reduce the dosage. • Order corticosteroids and platelet transfusions. • Consider ordering platelet-stimulating factors. • Monitor the patient for signs of bleeding (bleeding gums, melena, hematuria, and hematemesis).	• floxuridine • flucytosine • ganciclovir • Gold salts • heparin • Interferons alfa-2a and alfa-2b • lymphocyte immune globulin • methotrexate • penicillamine

Managing toxic drug reactions *(continued)*

Toxic reactions and clinical effects	Interventions	Selected causative drugs
Bone marrow toxicity ***(thrombocytopenia)*** *(continued)*		• procarbazine • quinidine • quinine • Tetracyclines • valproic acid
Cardiomyopathy • Acute hypertensive reaction • Atrial and ventricular arrhythmias • Chest pain • Heart failure • Chronic cardiomyopathy • Pericarditis-myocarditis syndrome	• Discontinue the drug, if possible. • Closely monitor the patient who is receiving concurrent radiation therapy. • Institute cardiac monitoring at the earliest sign of problems. • If the patient is receiving doxorubicin, limit the cumulative dose to 550 mg/m^2 unless the cardioprotectant dexrazoxane is used concomitantly.	• cyclophosphamide • cytarabine • daunorubicin • doxorubicin • idarubicin • mitoxantrone
Dermatologic toxicity • May vary from phototoxicity to acneiform eruptions, alopecia, exfoliative dermatitis, lupus erythematosus-like reactions, and toxic epidermal necrolysis	• Discontinue the drug. • Topical antihistamines and analgesics may be ordered.	• Androgens • Barbiturates • Corticosteroids • Cephalosporins • Gold salts • hydralazine • Interferons • Iodides • Penicillins • pentamidine • Phenothiazines • procainamide • Psoralens • Quinolones • Sulfonamides • Sulfonylureas • Tetracyclines • Thiazides

(continued)

Managing toxic drug reactions *(continued)*

Toxic reactions and clinical effects	Interventions	Selected causative drugs
Hepatotoxicity • Abdominal pain, hepatomegaly • Abnormal levels of alanine aminotransferase, aspartate aminotransferase, serum bilirubin, and lactate dehydrogenase • Bleeding, low-grade fever, mental changes, weight loss • Dry skin, pruritus, rash • Jaundice	• Reduce the dosage or discontinue the drug. • Order monitoring of the patient's vital signs, blood levels, weight, intake and output, and fluids and electrolytes. • Promote rest. • Perform hemodialysis, if needed. • Order symptomatic care: vitamins A, B complex, D, and K; potassium for alkalosis; salt-poor albumin for fluid and electrolyte balance; neomycin for gastrointestinal flora; stomach aspiration for blood; reduced dietary protein; and lactulose for blood ammonia.	• amiodarone • asparaginase • carbamazepine • chlorpromazine • chlorpropamide • cytarabine • dantrolene • erythromycin estolate • ifosfamide • isoniazid • ketoconazole • leuprolide • methotrexate • methyldopa • mitoxantrone • niacin • phenobarbital • plicamycin • Quinolones • Statins • sulindac
Nephrotoxicity • Increased or decreased creatinine clearance • Blurred vision, dehydration (depending on the part of the kidney affected), edema, mild headache, pallor • Casts, albumin, or red or white blood cells in the urine • Dizziness, fatigue, irritability, slowed mental processes • Electrolyte imbalance • Elevated blood urea nitrogen level • Oliguria	• Reduce the dosage or discontinue the drug. • Perform hemodialysis, if needed. • Order monitoring of the patient's vital signs, weight changes, and urine volume. • Give symptomatic care: fluid restriction and loop diuretics to reduce fluid retention and I.V. solutions to correct an electrolyte imbalance.	• Aminoglycosides • amphotericin B • Cephalosporins • cisplatin • Contrast media • Corticosteroids • cyclosporine • furosemide • Gadolinium-based contrast agents • gallium • Gold salts (parenteral) • Nitrosoureas • Nonsteroidal anti-inflammatory drugs • penicillin

Managing toxic drug reactions *(continued)*

Toxic reactions and clinical effects	Interventions	Selected causative drugs
Nephrotoxicity *(continued)*		• pentamidine isethionate • plicamycin • vancomycin • Vasopressors or vasoconstrictors
Neurotoxicity • Akathisia • Bilateral or unilateral palsy • Muscle twitching, tremor • Paresthesia • Seizures • Stroke-like syndrome • Unsteady gait • Weakness	• Notify the physician as soon as changes appear. • Reduce the dosage or discontinue the drug. • Monitor the patient carefully for changes in his or her condition. • Order symptomatic care. Remain with the patient, reassure him or her, and protect him or her during seizures. Provide a quiet environment, draw the shades, and speak in soft tones. Maintain the airway and ventilate the patient as needed.	• Aminoglycosides • cisplatin • cytarabine • isoniazid • nitroprusside • polymyxin B injection • Vinca alkaloids
Ocular toxicity • Acute glaucoma • Blurred, colored, or flickering vision • Cataracts • Corneal deposits • Diplopia • Miosis • Mydriasis • Optic neuritis • Scotomata • Vision loss	• Notify the physician as soon as changes appear. • Discontinue the drug, if possible. (Some oculotoxic drugs that are used to treat serious conditions may be given again at a reduced dosage after the eyes are rested and have returned to near normal.) • Monitor the patient carefully for changes in symptoms. • Treat the effects symptomatically.	• amiodarone • Antibiotics such as chloramphenicol • Anticholinergics • Cardiac glycosides • chloroquine • clomiphene • Corticosteroids • cyclophosphamide • cytarabine • ethambutol • hydroxychloroquine • lithium carbonate • methotrexate • Phenothiazines • quinidine • quinine • rifampin • tamoxifen • Vinca alkaloids

(continued)

Managing toxic drug reactions *(continued)*

Toxic reactions and clinical effects	Interventions	Selected causative drugs
Ototoxicity • Ataxia • Hearing loss • Tinnitus • Vertigo	• Notify the physician as soon as changes appear. • Discontinue the drug or reduce the dosage. • Monitor the patient carefully for symptomatic changes.	• Aminoglycosides • Antibiotics, such as colistimethate sodium, erythromycin, gentamicin, kanamycin, and streptomycin • chloroquine • cisplatin • Loop diuretics • minocycline • quinidine • quinine • Salicylates • vancomycin
Pseudomembranous colitis • Abdominal pain • Colonic perforation • Fever • Hypotension • Severe dehydration • Shock • Sudden, copious diarrhea (watery or bloody)	• Discontinue the drug and order another antibiotic, such as vancomycin or metronidazole. • Maintain the fluid and electrolyte balance. • Check the serum electrolyte levels daily. If pseudomembranous colitis is mild, order an ion exchange resin. • Monitor the patient's vital signs and hydration status. • Immediately report signs of shock to the physician. • Observe the patient for signs of hypokalemia, especially malaise and weak, rapid, irregular pulse.	• Antibiotics

Dialyzable drugs

The amount of a drug removed by dialysis differs among patients and depends on several factors, including the patient's condition, the drug's properties, length of dialysis and dialysate used, rate of blood flow or dwell time, and purpose of dialysis. This table shows the effect of hemodialysis on selected drugs.

Drug	Level reduced by hemodialysis	Drug	Level reduced by hemodialysis
acebutolol	Yes	aztreonam	Yes
acetaminophen	Unknown	bivalirudin	Yes
acetazolamide	No	busulfan	Yes
acyclovir	Yes	captopril	Yes
allopurinol	Yes	carbamazepine	No
alprazolam	No	carbenicillin	Yes
amikacin	Yes	carboplatin	Yes
amiodarone	Unknown	carmustine	No
amitriptyline	No	cefadroxil	Yes
amlodipine	No	cefazolin	Yes
amoxicillin	Yes	cefepime	Yes (only by 68%)
amoxicillin and clavulanate potassium	Yes	cefotaxime	Yes
amphotericin B	Unknown	cefotetan	Yes (only by 20%)
ampicillin	Yes	cefoxitin	Yes
ampicillin and sulbactam sodium	Yes	cefpodoxime	Yes (only by 23%)
		ceftazidime	Yes
aprepitant	No	ceftriaxone	No
aspirin	Yes	cefuroxime	Yes
atenolol	Yes	cephalexin	Unknown
azathioprine	Yes	cephalothin	Yes

(continued)

Dialyzable drugs (continued)

Drug	Level reduced by hemodialysis	Drug	Level reduced by hemodialysis
chloral hydrate	Yes	doxazosin	No
chlorambucil	No	doxepin	No
chloramphenicol	Yes (very small amount)	doxorubicin	No
		doxycycline	No
chlordiazepoxide	No	enalapril	Yes
chloroquine	No	erythromycin	No
chlorpheniramine	No	ethacrynic acid	Unknown
chlorpromazine	No	ethambutol	Unknown
chlorthalidone	No	famciclovir	Yes
cimetidine	Yes	famotidine	No
cisplatin	No	flecainide	No
clindamycin	No	fluconazole	Yes (only by 50%)
clonazepam	No	fluorouracil	Yes
clonidine	No	fluoxetine	No
codeine	Unknown	foscarnet	Yes
colchicine	No	fosinopril	Yes (2% to 7%)
cyclophosphamide	Yes	furosemide	No
diazepam	No	gabapentin	Yes
diclofenac	Unknown	ganciclovir	Yes (50%)
didanosine	Yes (7% or less)	gemcitabine	Unknown
digoxin	No	gemfibrozil	Unknown
diltiazem	No	gemifloxacin	Yes (20% to 30%)
diphenhydramine	Unknown		
dipyridamole	Unknown	gentamicin	Yes (50%)

Dialyzable drugs *(continued)*

Drug	Level reduced by hemodialysis	Drug	Level reduced by hemodialysis
glipizide	Unknown	lisinopril	Yes
glyburide	Unknown	lithium	Yes
haloperidol	Unknown	lorazepam	Unknown
heparin	Unknown	meperidine	Unknown
hydralazine	Unknown	mercaptopurine	Unlikely
hydrochlorothiazide	Unknown	meropenem	Yes
hydroxyzine	Unknown	mesalamine	Unknown
ibuprofen	Unknown	methadone	No
imipenem and cilastatin	Yes	methotrexate	Yes
imipramine	No	methyldopa	Yes
indapamide	Unknown	methylprednisolone	Unknown
indomethacin	Unknown	metoclopramide	No
insulin	Unknown	metolazone	Unlikely
irbesartan	Unknown	metoprolol succinate	Yes
iron dextran	No	metronidazole	Yes
isoniazid	Yes	miconazole	Unknown
isosorbide mononitrate	Yes	midazolam	Unknown
		minocycline	No
ketoconazole	Unlikely	morphine	Yes
ketoprofen	Yes	nadolol	Yes
labetalol	No	nafcillin	No
levofloxacin	No	naproxen	No
lidocaine	No	nelfinavir	Unlikely

(continued)

Dialyzable drugs *(continued)*

Drug	Level reduced by hemodialysis	Drug	Level reduced by hemodialysis
nifedipine	Unlikely	quinapril	No
nitrofurantoin	Yes	quinidine	No
nitroglycerin	No	ranitidine	Yes
nitroprusside	Yes	rifampin	No
nortriptyline	No	salsalate	Yes
octreotide	Unknown	sertraline	Unknown
ofloxacin	No	sotalol	Yes
olanzapine	No	stavudine	Yes
omeprazole	Unlikely	sucralfate	Unknown
paroxetine	Unlikely	sulfamethoxazole	Yes
penicillin G	Yes	temazepam	Unknown
pentamidine	No	tobramycin	Yes
pentazocine	Unlikely	topiramate	Yes
phenytoin	Yes	triazolam	Unlikely
piperacillin	Yes	valacyclovir	Yes (33%)
piperacillin and tazobactam	Yes	valproic acid	Yes (20%)
		valsartan	No
prazosin	No	vancomycin	Yes but poorly dialyzable
prednisone	Unknown		
procainamide	Yes	verapamil	No
promethazine	No	warfarin	Unknown
propranolol	No	zolpidem	No

Drugs that should not be crushed

Many drug forms, such as slow-release, enteric-coated, encapsulated beads, wax-matrix, sublingual, and buccal forms, are designed to release their active ingredients over a certain period or at preset intervals after administration. The disruptions caused by crushing these drug forms can dramatically affect the absorption rate and increase the risk of adverse reactions.

Other reasons not to crush these drug forms include such considerations as taste, tissue irritation, and unusual formulation—for example, a capsule within a capsule, a liquid within a capsule, or a multiple-compressed tablet. Avoid crushing the following drugs, listed by brand name, for the reasons noted beside them.

Accutane (irritant)

AcipHex (delayed release)

Adalat CC (sustained release)

Aggrenox (extended release)

Allegra D (extended release)

Altocor (extended release)

Ambien CR (extended release)

Amnesteem (irritant)

Arthrotec (delayed release)

Asacol HD (delayed release)

Aspirin (enteric coated)

Augmentin XR (extended release)

Azulfidine EN-tabs (enteric coated)

Biaxin XL (extended release)

Bisacodyl (enteric coated)

Calan SR (sustained release)

Carbatrol (extended release)

Cardizem CD, LA, SR (slow release)

Cartia XT (extended release)

CellCept (teratogenic potential)

Chlor-Trimeton Allergy 8-hour and 12-hour (slow release)

Cipro XR (extended release)

Claritin-D 12-hour (slow release)

Claritin-D 24-hour (slow release)

Cleocin (taste)

Colace (liquid within a capsule)

Colazal (granules within capsules must reach the colon intact)

Colestid (protective coating)

Concerta (extended release)

Contac 12 Hour, Maximum Strength 12 Hour (slow release)

Cotazym-S (enteric coated)

Creon (enteric coated)

Cytovene (irritant)

Depakene (slow release, mucous membrane irritant)

Depakote (enteric coated)

Depakote ER (extended release)

Dexedrine Spansule (slow release)

Diamox Sequels (slow release)

Dilacor XR (extended release)

Dilatrate-SR (slow release)

Diltia XT (extended release)

Ditropan XL (slow release)

Dristan (protective coating)

Drixoral (slow release)

Dulcolax (enteric coated)

Ecotrin (enteric coated)

E.E.S. 400 Filmtab (enteric coated)

Effexor XR (extended release)

Emend (hard gelatin capsule)

E-Mycin (enteric coated)

Ery-Tab (enteric coated)

Erythromycin Base (enteric coated)

Feldene (mucous membrane irritant)

Feosol (enteric coated)

(continued)

Drugs that should not be crushed *(continued)*

Feratab (enteric coated)

FeverAll Children's Capsules, Sprinkle (taste)

Flomax (slow release)

Geocillin (taste)

Glucophage XR (extended release)

Glucotrol XL (slow release)

Glumetza (slow release)

ICAPS Plus (slow release)

ICAPS Time Release (slow release)

Imdur (slow release)

Inderal LA (slow release)

InnoPran XL (extended release)

Klor-Con (slow release)

Levbid (slow release)

Lithobid (slow release)

Macrobid (slow release)

Mestinon Timespans (slow release)

Metadate CD, ER (extended release)

Micro-K Extencaps (slow release)

MS Contin (slow release)

Mucinex (extended release)

Naprelan (slow release)

Nexium (sustained release)

Niaspan (extended release)

Nitrostat (sublingual)

Norpace CR (slow release)

OxyContin (slow release)

Pancreaze DR (delayed release)

Paxil CR (controlled release)

PCE (slow release)

Pentasa (controlled release)

Phazyme (slow release)

Phenytek (extended release)

Plendil (slow release)

Prevacid, Prevacid SoluTab (delayed release)

Prilosec (slow release)

Prilosec OTC (delayed release)

Procanbid (slow release)

Procardia (delayed absorption)

Procardia XL (slow release)

Propecia (women who are or who may become pregnant should not handle)

Proscar (women who are or who may become pregnant should not handle)

Protonix (delayed release)

Prozac Weekly (slow release)

Ritalin LA, SR (slow release)

Sinemet CR (slow release)

Slo-Niacin (slow release)

Slow FE (slow release)

Slow-Mag (slow release)

Sudafed 12 Hour (slow release)

Sular (extended release)

Tegretol XR (extended release)

Tessalon Perles (slow release)

Theo-24 (extended release)

Tiazac (sustained release)

Topamax (taste)

Toprol XL (extended release)

Uniphyl (slow release)

Verelan, Verelan PM (slow release)

Voltaren-XR (extended release)

Wellbutrin SR (sustained release)

Xanax XR (extended release)

Zomig-ZMT (delayed release)

Zyban (slow release)

Zyrtec-D 12 Hour (extended release)

Reversing anaphylaxis

Anaphylaxis—the sudden, extreme reaction to a foreign antigen—requires immediate treatment. Generally, the more rapid the onset of symptoms, the more severe the reaction. This table lists drugs that are useful in reversing anaphylactic reactions.

Drug	Action	Nursing considerations
Cimetidine (Tagamet) Severe anaphylaxis	• Competes with histamine for histamine-2 receptor sites • Treats urticaria	• Know that this drug is incompatible with aminophylline. • Reduce the dosage for patients with impaired renal or hepatic function.
Diphenhydramine (Benadryl)	• Competes with histamine for histamine$_1$-receptor sites • Prevents laryngeal edema • Controls localized itching	• Administer I.V. doses slowly to avoid hypotension. • Monitor the patient for hypotension and drowsiness. • Give fluids as needed. The drug causes dry mouth.
Epinephrine (Adrenalin) Severe anaphylaxis (drug of choice)	*Alpha-adrenergic effects* • Increases blood pressure • Reverses peripheral vasodilation and systemic hypotension • Considered the drug of choice for treating anaphylaxis • Decreases angioedema and urticaria • Improves coronary blood flow by raising diastolic pressure • Causes peripheral vasoconstriction	• Select a large vein for infusion. • Use an infusion controller to regulate the drip rate. • Check the patient's blood pressure and heart rate frequently. • Monitor the patient for arrhythmias. • Check the solution strength, dosage, and label before administration.
Severe anaphylaxis (drug of choice)	*Beta-adrenergic effects* • Causes bronchodilation • Causes positive inotropic and chronotropic cardiac activity • Decreases the synthesis and release of chemical mediators	• Watch for signs of extravasation at the infusion site. • Monitor the patient's intake and output. • Assess the color and temperature of the extremities.
Hydrocortisone (Solu-Cortef) Severe anaphylaxis	• The mechanism of action is not clearly defined. It inhibits multiple inflammatory cytokines. • Produces multiple glucocorticoid and mineralocorticoid effects	• Monitor the patient's weight, blood pressure, fluid and electrolyte balance, intake and output, and blood pressure closely. • Keep the patient on a prophylactic ulcer and antacid regimen. • Monitor glucose level.

Adverse reactions misinterpreted as age-related changes

In elderly patients, adverse drug reactions can easily be misinterpreted as the typical signs and symptoms of aging. This table shows common adverse reactions for common drug classifications and can help you avoid such misinterpretations.

Adverse reactions

Drug classifications	Agitation	Anxiety	Arrhythmias	Ataxia	Changes in appetite	Confusion	Constipation	Depression
Angiotensin-converting enzyme inhibitors								
Alpha₁ adrenergic blockers		•						•
Antianginals		•	•			•		
Antiarrhythmics			•			•	•	
Anticholinergics	•	•	•			•	•	•
Anticonvulsants	•		•	•		•	•	
Antidepressants, tricyclic	•	•	•	•	•	•	•	
Antidiabetics, oral								
Antihistamines						•	•	
Antilipemics							•	
Antiparkinsonians	•	•				•	•	•
Antipsychotics	•		•		•	•		•
Barbiturates	•	•	•			•		
Benzodiazepines	•			•		•	•	•
Beta-adrenergic blockers			•					•
Calcium channel blockers		•	•				•	
Corticosteroids	•					•		•
Diuretics						•		
Nonsteroidal anti-inflammatory drugs						•		
Opioids	•	•				•	•	•
Skeletal muscle relaxants	•	•		•		•		•
Thyroid hormones			•		•			

Difficulty breathing	Disorientation	Dizziness	Drowsiness	Edema	Fatigue	Hypotension	Insomnia	Memory loss	Muscle weakness	Restlessness	Sexual dysfunction	Tremors	Urinary dysfunction	Vision changes
		•			•	•								
		•	•	•	•	•					•			•
		•		•	•	•	•				•			•
•		•		•	•									
	•	•	•			•					•		•	•
•		•	•	•	•							•	•	•
•	•	•	•		•	•					•	•	•	•
		•	•		•									
	•	•	•		•							•	•	•
		•							•					•
	•	•	•	•		•	•				•		•	•
		•	•	•	•	•	•				•	•	•	•
•	•			•	•	•				•				
•	•	•	•		•		•	•	•			•	•	•
•		•			•	•					•			•
•		•		•	•	•								
				•			•		•					•
		•			•	•							•	
		•	•		•									•
•	•	•	•		•	•	•	•			•	•	•	•
		•	•		•	•	•					•		
							•					•		

Therapeutic drug monitoring guidelines

Drug	Laboratory test monitored	Therapeutic ranges of test
aminoglycoside antibiotics (amikacin, gentamicin, tobramycin)	Amikacin peak trough Gentamicin/tobramycin peak trough Creatinine	20 to 30 mcg/ml 1 to 8 mcg/ml 6 to 10 mcg/ml <2 mcg/ml 0.6 to 1.3 mg/dl
angiotensin-converting enzyme (ACE) inhibitors (benazepril, captopril, enalapril, enalaprilat, fosinopril, lisinopril, moexipril, quinapril, ramipril, trandolapril)	White blood cell count (WBC) with differential Creatinine BUN Potassium	***** Men: 0.9 to 1.3 mg/dl Women: 0.6 to 1.1 mg/dl 5 to 20 mg/dl 3.5 to 5 mEq/L
amphotericin B	Creatinine BUN Electrolytes (especially potassium and magnesium) Liver function Complete blood count (CBC)	Men: 0.9 to 1.3 mg/dl Women: 0.6 to 1.1 mg/dl 6 to 20 mg/dl Potassium: 3.5 to 5.2 mEq/L Magnesium: 1.3 to 2.2 mEq/L Sodium: 135 to 147 mEq/L Chloride: 95 to 110 mEq/L * *****
antibiotics	WBC with differential Cultures and sensitivities	*****
biguanides (metformin)	Creatinine Fasting glucose Glycosylated hemoglobin CBC	Men: 0.9 to 1.3 mg/dl Women: 0.6 to 1.1 mg/dl ≤100 mg/dl 5% to 7% of total hemoglobin *****
carbamazepine	Carbamazepine CBC with differential Liver function BUN Platelet count	4 to 12 mcg/ml ***** * 6 to 20 mg/dl 140 to 400 × 10^3/mm^3

Monitoring guidelines

Wait until the administration of the third dose to check drug levels. Obtain blood for peak level 30 minutes after I.V. infusion ends or 60 minutes after I.M. administration. For trough levels, draw blood just before the next dose. Dosage may need to be adjusted accordingly. Recheck after three doses. Monitor creatinine and blood urea nitrogen (BUN) levels and urine output for signs of decreasing renal function. Monitor urine for increased proteins, cells, and casts.

Monitor the WBC with differential before therapy, monthly during the first 3 to 6 months, and then periodically for the first year. Monitor renal function and potassium level periodically.

Monitor creatinine, BUN, and electrolyte levels at least daily at start of therapy and then as clinically indicated. Monitor blood counts and liver function test results regularly during therapy.

Results of specimen cultures and sensitivities will determine the cause of the infection and the best treatment. Monitor the WBC with differential weekly during therapy.

Check renal function and hematologic values before starting therapy and at least annually thereafter. If the patient has impaired renal function, do not use metformin because it may cause lactic acidosis. Monitor response to therapy by evaluating fasting glucose and glycosylated hemoglobin levels periodically. A patient's home monitoring of glucose levels helps monitor compliance and response.

Monitor blood counts and platelet count before therapy. Monitor closely during therapy. Liver function and BUN results should be checked before and periodically during therapy.

(continued)

Therapeutic drug monitoring guidelines *(continued)*

Drug	Laboratory test monitored	Therapeutic ranges of test
corticosteroids (cortisone, hydrocortisone, prednisone, prednisolone, triamcinolone, methylprednisolone, dexamethasone, betamethasone)	Electrolytes (especially potassium) Fasting glucose	Potassium: 3.5 to 5.2 mEq/L Magnesium: 1.8 to 2.6 mEq/L Sodium: 136 to 145 mEq/L Chloride: 96 to 106 mEq/L Calcium: 8.8 to 10.4 mg/dl ≤100 mg/dl
digoxin	Digoxin Digoxin in heart failure Electrolytes (especially potassium, magnesium, and calcium) Creatinine	0.8 to 2 ng/ml 0.5 to 0.9 ng/ml Potassium: 3.5 to 5.2 mEq/L Magnesium: 1.8 to 2.6 mEq/L Sodium: 136 to 145 mEq/L Chloride: 96 to 106 mEq/L Calcium: 8.8 to 10.4 mg/dl 0.6 to 1.3 mg/dl
diuretics	Electrolytes Creatinine BUN Uric acid Fasting glucose	Potassium: 3.5 to 5.2 mEq/L Magnesium: 1.8 to 2.6 mEq/L Sodium: 135 to 145 mEq/L Chloride: 96 to 106 mEq/L Calcium: 8.8 to 10.4 mg/dl 0.6 to 1.3 mg/dl 5 to 20 mg/dl 2 to 7 mg/dl ≤100 mg/dl
erythropoietin	Hematocrit Serum ferritin Transferrin saturation CBC with differential Platelet count	Women: 36% to 48% Men: 42% to 52% 18 to 270 mg/ml 250 to 425 mg/dl ***** 140 to 400 × 10^3/mm^3
ethosuximide	Ethosuximide Liver function CBC with differential	40 to 100 mcg/ml * *****

Monitoring guidelines

Monitor electrolyte and glucose levels regularly during long-term therapy.

Check digoxin levels just before the next dose or a minimum of 6 to 8 hours after the last dose. To monitor maintenance therapy, check drug levels at least 1 to 2 weeks after therapy is initiated or changed. Adjust therapy based on the entire clinical picture, not solely based on drug levels. Also, check electrolyte levels and renal function periodically during therapy.

To monitor fluid and electrolyte balance, perform baseline and periodic determinations of electrolyte, calcium, BUN, uric acid, and glucose levels.

After therapy is initiated or changed, monitor hematocrit twice weekly for 2 to 6 weeks until it is stabilized in the target range and a maintenance dose is determined. Monitor hematocrit regularly thereafter.

Check drug level 8 to 10 days after therapy is initiated or changed. Periodically monitor the CBC with differential and results of liver function tests and urinalysis.

(continued)

Therapeutic drug monitoring guidelines *(continued)*

Drug	Laboratory test monitored	Therapeutic ranges of test
gemfibrozil	Lipids	Total cholesterol: <200 mg/dl Low-density lipoprotein (LDL): <130 mg/dl High-density lipoprotein (HDL): ≥35 mg/dl Triglycerides: <150 mg/dl
	Liver function	*
	Serum glucose	≤100 mg/dl
	CBC	*****
	Creatine kinase (CK)	26 to 174 units/L
heparin (unfractionated)	Activated partial thromboplastin time (aPTT)	1.5 to 2 times control
	Hematocrit	*****
	Platelet count	140 to 400 × 10^3/mm^3
3-hydroxy-3- methylglutaryl-coenzyme A reductase inhibitors (atorvastatin, fluvastatin, lovastatin, pravastatin, rosuvastatin, simvastatin)	Lipids	Total cholesterol: <200 mg/dl LDL: <130 mg/dl HDL: ≥35 mg/dl Triglycerides: <150 mg/dl
	Liver function	*
insulin	Fasting glucose	≤100 mg/dl
	Glycosylated hemoglobin	5% to 7% of total hemoglobin
isotretinoin	Pregnancy test	Negative
	Liver function	*
	Lipids	Total cholesterol: <200 mg/dl LDL: <130 mg/dl HDL: ≥35 mg/dl Triglycerides: <150 mg/dl
	CBC with differential	*****
	Platelet count	140 to 400 × 10^3/mm^3
linezolid	CBC with differential	*****
	Cultures and sensitivities	
	Platelet count	150 to 450 × 10^3/mm^3
	Liver function	*
	Amylase	35 to 118 IU/L
	Lipase	10 to 150 units/L

Monitoring guidelines

Therapy is usually withdrawn after 3 months if response is inadequate. The patient must be fasting to measure triglyceride levels. Obtain blood counts and liver function tests during the first 12 months. Obtain CK for muscle pain or weakness.

When drug is given by continuous I.V. infusion, check partial thromboplastin time (PTT) every 4 hours and according to facility policy in the early stages of therapy and daily thereafter. Periodically during therapy, check platelet counts and hematocrit and test for occult blood in stool.

Perform liver function tests at baseline, 2 to 4 weeks after therapy is initiated or changed, and approximately every 6 months thereafter. If adequate response is not achieved within 6 weeks, consider changing therapy.

Monitor response to therapy by evaluating glucose and glycosylated hemoglobin levels. Glycosylated hemoglobin level is a good measure of long-term control. A patient's home monitoring of glucose levels helps measure compliance and response.

Use a serum or urine pregnancy test with a sensitivity of at least 25 mIU/ml. Perform one test before therapy and a second test during the first 5 days of the menstrual cycle before therapy begins or at least 11 days after the last unprotected act of sexual intercourse, whichever is later. Repeat pregnancy tests monthly. Obtain baseline liver function tests and lipid levels; repeat every 1 to 2 weeks until a response to treatment is established (usually 4 weeks).

Obtain a baseline CBC with differential and platelet count weekly during therapy. Monitor liver function test results and amylase and lipase levels during therapy.

(continued)

Therapeutic drug monitoring guidelines *(continued)*

Drug	Laboratory test monitored	Therapeutic ranges of test
lithium	Lithium	0.6 to 1.2 mEq/L
	Creatinine	Men: 0.9 to 1.3 mg/dl
		Women: 0.6 to 1.1 mg/dl
	CBC	*****
	Electrolytes (especially potassium and sodium)	Potassium: 3.5 to 5.2 mEq/L
		Magnesium: 1.8 to 2.6 mEq/L
		Sodium: 136 to 145 mEq/L
		Chloride: 96 to 106 mEq/L
	Fasting glucose	≤100 mg/dl
	Thyroid function tests	Thyroid-stimulating hormone
		(TSH): 0.45 to 4.5 microunits/ml
		T_3: 80 to 200 ng/dl
		T_4: 5.4 to 11.5 mcg/dl
methotrexate	Methotrexate	Normal elimination:
		~5 micromol/L 24 hours postdose
		~0.5 micromol/L 48 hours postdose
		<0.2 micromol/L 72 hours postdose
	CBC with differential	*****
	Platelet count	140 to 400 × 10^3/mm³
	Liver function	*
	Creatinine	Men: 0.9 to 1.3 mg/dl
		Women: 0.6 to 1.1 mg/dl
nonnucleoside reverse transcriptase inhibitors (nevirapine, delavirdine, efavirenz)	Liver function	*
	CBC with differential and platelets	*****
	Lipids (efavirenz)	Total cholesterol: <200 mg/dl
		LDL: <130 mg/dl
		HDL: ≥35 mg/dl
		Triglycerides: <150 mg/dl
	Amylase	25 to 125 IU/L
phenytoin	Phenytoin	10 to 20 mcg/ml
	CBC	*****
	Albumin	3.5 to 5.2 g/dl
potassium chloride	Potassium	3.5 to 5.2 mEq/L

Monitoring guidelines

Checking lithium levels is crucial to safe use of the drug. Obtain lithium levels immediately before the next dose. Monitor levels twice weekly until they are stable. Once at a steady state, levels should be checked weekly; when the patient is receiving the appropriate maintenance dose, levels should be checked every 2 to 3 months. Monitor creatinine, electrolyte, and fasting glucose levels; CBC; and thyroid function test results before therapy is initiated and periodically during therapy.

Monitor methotrexate levels according to the dosing protocol. Monitor the CBC with differential, platelet count, and liver and renal function test results more frequently when therapy is initiated or changed and when methotrexate levels may be elevated, such as when the patient is dehydrated.

Obtain baseline liver function tests and monitor results closely during the first 12 weeks of therapy. Continue to monitor them regularly during therapy. Check the CBC with differential and platelet count before therapy and periodically during therapy. Monitor lipid levels during efavirenz therapy. Monitor the amylase level during efavirenz and delavirdine therapy.

Monitor phenytoin levels immediately before the next dose and 7 to 10 days after therapy is initiated or changed. Obtain a CBC at baseline and monthly early in therapy. Watch for toxic effects at therapeutic levels. Adjust the measured level for hypoalbuminemia or renal impairment, which can increase free drug levels.

After oral replacement therapy is initiated, check the level weekly until it is stable and every 3 to 6 months thereafter.

(continued)

Therapeutic drug monitoring guidelines *(continued)*

Drug	Laboratory test monitored	Therapeutic ranges of test
procainamide	Procainamide N-acetylprocainamide (NAPA) CBC Liver function Antinuclear antibody (ANA) titer	4 to 8 mcg/ml (procainamide) 15 to 25 mcg/ml (combined procainamide and NAPA) ***** * Negative
protease inhibitors (amprenavir, indinavir, lopinavir, nelfinavir, ritonavir, saquinavir)	Fasting glucose Liver function CBC with differential Lipids Amylase CK	≤100 mg/dl * ***** Total cholesterol: <200 mg/dl LDL: <130 mg/dl HDL: ≥35 mg/dl Triglycerides: <150 mg/dL 25 to 125 IU/L 26 to 174 units/L
quinidine	Quinidine CBC Liver function Creatinine Electrolytes (especially potassium)	2 to 5 mcg/ml ***** * Men: 0.9 to 1.3 mg/dl Women: 0.6 to 1.1 mg/dl Potassium: 3.5 to 5.2 mEq/L Magnesium: 1.8 to 2.6 mEq/L Sodium: 136 to 145 mEq/L Chloride: 96 to 108 mEq/L
sulfonylureas	Fasting glucose Glycosylated hemoglobin	≤100 mg/dl 5% to 7% of total hemoglobin
theophylline	Theophylline	10 to 20 mcg/ml
thiazolidinediones (rosiglitazone, pioglitazone)	Fasting glucose Glycosylated hemoglobin Liver function	≤100 mg/dl 5% to 7% of total hemoglobin *

Monitoring guidelines

Measure procainamide levels 6 to 12 hours after a continuous infusion is started or immediately before the next oral dose. Combined (procainamide and NAPA) levels can be used as an index of toxicity in patients with renal impairment. Obtain a CBC, liver function tests, and ANA titer periodically during longer term therapy.

Obtain a baseline glucose level; liver function test results; a CBC with differential; and lipid, CK, and amylase levels. Monitor during therapy.

Obtain levels immediately before the next oral dose and 30 to 35 hours after therapy is initiated or changed. Obtain blood counts, liver and kidney function test results, and electrolyte levels periodically.

Monitor response to therapy by evaluating fasting glucose and glycosylated hemoglobin levels periodically. The patient should monitor glucose levels at home to help measure compliance and response.

Obtain theophylline levels immediately before the next dose of sustained-release oral drug and at least 2 days after therapy is initiated or changed.

Monitor response by evaluating fasting glucose and glycosylated hemoglobin levels. Obtain baseline liver function test results and repeat the tests periodically during therapy. Do not initiate therapy with pioglitazone or rosiglitazone if alanine aminotransferase is more than 2.5 × upper limits of normal.

(continued)

Therapeutic drug monitoring guidelines *(continued)*

Drug	Laboratory test monitored	Therapeutic ranges of test
thyroid hormone	Thyroid function tests	TSH: 0.45 to 5.4 microunits/ml T_3: 80 to 200 ng/dl T_4: 5.4 to 11.5 mcg/dl
valproate sodium, valproic acid, divalproex sodium	Valproic acid Liver function Ammonia PTT BUN Creatinine CBC with differential Platelet count Amylase	50 to 120 mcg/ml * 15 to 45 mcg/dl 11 to 13 seconds 8 to 25 mg/dl 0.6 to 1.3 mg/dl ***** 140 to 400 $\times$ 10^3/mm³ 25 to 125 units/L
vancomycin	Vancomycin Creatinine	20 to 40 mcg/ml (peak) 10 to 20 mcg/ml (trough) Men: 0.9 to 1.3 mg/dl Women: 0.6 to 1.3 mg/dl
warfarin	International normalized ratio (INR)	For acute myocardial infarction, atrial fibrillation, treatment of pulmonary embolism, prevention of systemic embolism, tissue heart valves, valvular heart disease, or prophylaxis or treatment of venous thrombosis: 2 to 3 For mechanical prosthetic valves or recurrent systemic embolism: 3 to 4.5

Note: For those areas marked with asterisks, the following values can be used:
Hemoglobin: women: 12 to 16 g/dl;
        men: 13 to 18 g/dl
Hematocrit: women: 37% to 48%;
        men: 42% to 52%
Red blood cell count: 4 to 5.5 $\times$ 10^6/mm³
WBC: 5 to 10 $\times$ 10^3/mm³

Differential: neutrophils: 45% to 74%
    Bands: 0% to 8%
    Lymphocytes: 16% to 45%
    Monocytes: 4% to 10%
    Eosinophils: 0% to 7%
    Basophils: 0% to 2%

Monitoring guidelines

Monitor thyroid function test results every 2 to 3 weeks until the appropriate maintenance dose is determined and annually thereafter.

Monitor liver function test results, ammonia level, coagulation test results, renal function test results, CBC, and platelet count at baseline and periodically during therapy. Monitor liver function test results closely during the first 6 months of therapy.

Check vancomycin levels with the third dose administered, at the earliest. Obtain peak levels 1.5 to 2.5 hours after a 1-hour infusion or when I.V. infusion is complete. Obtain trough levels within 1 hour of the next dose administered. Renal function can be used to adjust dosing and intervals.

Check INR daily, beginning 3 days after therapy is initiated. Continue checking it until the therapeutic goal is achieved and monitor it periodically thereafter. Also check levels 7 days after a change in the warfarin dose or concomitant, potentially interacting therapy.

For those areas marked with one asterisk, the following values can be used:
Alanine aminotransferase: 7 to 56 units/L
Aspartate aminotransferase: 5 to 40 units/L
Alkaline phosphatase: 17 to 142 units/L
Lactate dehydrogenase: 140 to 280 units/L
Gamma glutamyl transferase (GGT): <40 units/L
Total bilirubin: 0.2 to 1 mg/dl

The FDA also wants to know about drugs that do not produce a therapeutic response. It does not need to hear about inappropriate use of drugs, prescriber errors, or administration errors. However, the U.S. Pharmacopeia does want to know about medication errors—especially those caused by sound-alike or look-alike drug names. (See the pharmacist for more information.)

You can submit a report to the FDA even if you are not sure if a patient's reaction was serious or if you suspect—but do not know for certain—that a reaction is the result of a drug.

To file a report, use the MedWatch form, which should be available in the pharmacy or online. Fill out this form as completely as possible. Do not include the patient's name or social security number. You may use their initials, patient number, or some identifier that will allow you to identify the patient if the FDA requests follow-up information.

What The Joint Commission requires

To meet the standards set by The Joint Commission, a facility must have a program in place for reporting ADRs. The pharmacy and therapeutics committee at the facility is required to review "all significant untoward ADRs" to ensure quality patient care.

According to The Joint Commission, a "significant" reaction is one in which the:
- drug suspected of causing the reaction must be discontinued
- patient requires treatment with another drug, such as an antihistamine, a steroid, or epinephrine
- patient's hospital stay is prolonged—for example, because surgery had to be delayed or more diagnostic tests had to be done.

According to The Joint Commission, a "sentinel" event is one in which:
- death
- harm that is permanent

- harm that is severe but temporary and intervention required to sustain life.

Why is this type of reporting program important? First, the quality of care improves when you know which patients are at higher risk for an ADR and which drugs are most likely to cause these reactions. You will be more alert for the early signs and symptoms of problems, and you will be prepared to intervene promptly.

Second, the facility will make better use of its health care dollars because the lengthy stays and extra treatments associated with ADRs will be decreased.

Third, reducing drug-induced injuries will decrease the number of malpractice lawsuits brought against the facility and staff, saving time, money, and aggravation.

Managing I.V. extravasation

Extravasation is leakage of infused solution from a vein into the surrounding tissue caused by a needle puncturing the vessel wall or leakage around a venipuncture site. Extravasation causes local pain and itching, edema, blanching, and changes in skin temperature in the affected extremity. Know and follow the facility's policy for treating extravasation.

Extravasation of a small amount of isotonic fluid or nonirritating drug usually causes only minor discomfort. Treatment involves stopping the drug and providing routine comfort measures, such as the application of warm compresses. However, extravasation of some drugs can severely damage tissue through irritative, sclerotic, vesicant, corrosive, or vasoconstrictive action. In these cases, emergency measures must be taken to minimize tissue damage and necrosis, prevent the need for skin grafts or, rarely, avoid amputation.

Equipment and preparation

Three 25G ⅝″ needles • antidote for extravasated drug in an appropriate syringe • 5-ml syringe • three tuberculin syringes • alcohol pad or gauze pad soaked in antiseptic cleaning agent • 4″ × 4″ gauze pad • cold and warm compresses

Implementation

Facility policy dictates the procedures for extravasation treatment, which may include some or all of these steps:

- Stop the infusion and remove the I.V. needle unless you need the route to infiltrate the antidote. Carefully estimate the amount of extravasated solution and notify the health care provider.
- Disconnect the tubing from the I.V. needle. Attach the 5-ml syringe to the needle and try to withdraw 3 to 5 ml of blood to remove any medication or blood in the tubing or needle and to provide a path to the infiltrated tissues.
- Clean the area around the I.V. site with an alcohol pad or a 4″ × 4″ gauze pad soaked in an antiseptic agent. Then insert the needle of the empty tuberculin syringe into the subcutaneous tissue around the site and gently aspirate as much solution as possible from the tissue.
- Instill the prescribed antidote into the subcutaneous tissue around the site. Then, if ordered, slowly instill an anti-inflammatory drug subcutaneously to help reduce inflammation and edema.
- If ordered, instill the prescribed antidote through the I.V. needle.
- Apply cold compresses to the affected area for 24 hours or apply an ice pack for 20 minutes every 4 hours to cause vasoconstriction that may localize the drug and slow cell metabolism. After 24 hours, apply warm compresses and elevate the affected extremity to reduce discomfort and promote reabsorption of fluid. If the extravasated drug is a

vasoconstrictor, such as norepinephrine or metaraminol bitartrate, apply warm compresses only.
- Monitor the I.V. site continuously for signs of abscess, necrosis, or compartment syndrome.

Special considerations

- If you are administering a potentially tissue-damaging drug by I.V. bolus or push, first start an I.V. infusion, preferably with normal saline solution. Infuse a small amount of this solution and check for signs of infiltration before injecting the drug.
- Know the antidote (if any) for an I.V. drug that can cause tissue necrosis, in case extravasation occurs. Make sure that you are familiar with the facility policy for the administration of such drugs and their antidotes.
- Tell the patient to report discomfort at the I.V. site. During infusion, check the site frequently for signs of infiltration.

Drug overdoses

General guidelines

If the patient has signs of an acute toxic reaction, institute advanced life-support measures, as indicated. Administer the prescribed antidote, if available, and institute measures to block absorption and speed elimination of the drug. Consult with a regional poison control center for additional information about treating patients who ingested specific toxins. The steps below outline the management of an acute overdose of ingested systemic drugs.

Starting advanced life support

- Establish and maintain an airway. This is usually done by inserting an oropharyngeal or endotracheal airway.
- If the patient is not breathing, start ventilation with a bag valve mask until a mechanical ventilator is available. Check the pulse oximetry

Antidotes for extravasation

Antidote	Extravasated drug
Dexrazoxane (Totect)	• daunorubicin • doxorubicin • epirubicin • idarubicin
Hyaluronidase	• aminophylline • Calcium solutions • Contrast media • Dextrose solutions (concentrations of 10% or more) • nafcillin • Potassium solutions • Total parenteral nutrition solutions • vinblastine • vincristine • vindesine
Phentolamine	• dobutamine • dopamine • epinephrine • metaraminol bitartrate • norepinephrine

results or arterial blood gas levels, and administer oxygen as needed.

- Maintain circulation. Start an I.V. infusion and obtain laboratory specimens to check for toxic drug levels as well as electrolyte and glucose levels, as indicated. If the patient has hypotension, administer fluids and a vasopressor such as dopamine (Intropin). If the patient has hypertension, prepare to administer an antihypertensive (usually a beta-adrenergic blocker, if a catecholamine was ingested). Prepare to treat arrhythmias as indicated for the specific toxin.
- Protect the patient from injury and monitor him or her for seizures. Observe him or her and provide supportive care. Prepare to administer diazepam, lorazepam, or phenytoin.

Administering the antidote

The antidote is administered as soon as possible. Administer the prescribed antidote, which depends on the type of drug the patient has taken.

Blocking drug absorption

- Gastric emptying is effective up to 2 hours after drug ingestion. Two methods are used: syrup of ipecac for a conscious patient whose condition is not expected to deteriorate and gastric lavage for a comatose patient or one who does not respond to syrup of ipecac.
- Adsorption with activated charcoal is used in place of emesis or lavage, if the drug is well adsorbed by activated charcoal, or after emesis or lavage to adsorb coingestants, if the

primary toxin is not well adsorbed by activated charcoal.

- A cathartic may be given to speed transit of the poison through the gastrointestinal (GI) tract. Whole-bowel irrigation with a balanced polyethylene glycol and electrolyte solution may be ordered if the patient ingested a sustained-release product.

Speeding drug elimination

- Gastric dialysis uses timed doses of activated charcoal for 1 to 2 days. The charcoal binds to the drug, facilitating its removal in stools.
- Diuresis is effective for some drug overdoses. Forced diuresis uses furosemide and an osmotic diuretic, alkaline diuresis uses I.V. sodium bicarbonate, and acid diuresis uses oral or I.V. ascorbic acid or ammonium chloride.
- Peritoneal dialysis and hemodialysis are occasionally used for severe overdose.

Managing an acute toxic reaction

If the patient has signs of an acute toxic reaction, institute advanced life-support measures, as indicated. Administer the prescribed antidote, if available, and take steps to block absorption and speed elimination of the drug. Consult with a regional poison control center for information on how to treat ingestion of a specific toxin.

Acetaminophen overdose

In patients with acute overdose of acetaminophen, plasma levels of 300 mcg/ml 4 hours after ingestion or 50 mcg/ml 12 hours after ingestion are associated with hepatotoxicity. Signs and symptoms of overdose include cyanosis, anemia, jaundice, skin eruptions, fever, emesis, central nervous system (CNS) stimulation, delirium, and methemoglobinemia progressing to CNS depression, coma, vascular collapse,

seizures, and death. Acetaminophen poisoning develops in stages.

- Stage 1 (12 to 24 hours after ingestion): nausea, vomiting, diaphoresis, anorexia, and pallor
- Stage 2 (24 to 72 hours after ingestion): right upper quadrant abdominal pain, anorexia, nausea, vomiting; elevated liver function tests
- Stage 3 (72 to 96 hours after ingestion): peak hepatotoxicity; continued nausea, vomiting, abdominal pain; patient may become jaundiced and may develop encephalopathy, hypoglycemia, and cardiomyopathy.
- Stage 4 (7 to 8 days after ingestion): recovery

To treat acetaminophen toxicity, immediately induce emesis with syrup of ipecac if the patient is conscious or with gastric lavage if comatose or does not respond to syrup of ipecac. Administer activated charcoal via a nasogastric tube and give oral acetylcysteine. Monitor the patient's laboratory results and vital signs closely. Provide symptomatic and supportive measures, including respiratory support and correction of fluid and electrolyte imbalances.

Oral or I.V. acetylcysteine, a specific antidote for acetaminophen poisoning, is most effective if started within 8 to 10 hours after ingestion but can help if started as late as 24 hours after ingestion. Doses vomited within 1 hour of administration must be repeated. Remove charcoal by lavage before administering acetylcysteine because it may interfere with absorption of this antidote. Acetylcysteine minimizes hepatic injury by supplying sulfhydryl groups that bind with acetaminophen metabolites.

Hemodialysis may help to remove acetaminophen from the body, and cimetidine has been used investigationally to block the metabolism of acetaminophen to toxic intermediates. Determine plasma levels of acetaminophen at least 4 hours

(Text continues on page 611.)

Managing poisoning or overdose

Antidote and indications	Nursing considerations
acetylcysteine (Mucomyst, Mucosil, Parvolex) • Treatment of acetaminophen toxicity	• Use cautiously in an elderly or debilitated patient and in a patient with asthma or severe respiratory insufficiency. • Monitor patient receiving I.V. form for anaphylactoid reactions. • Do not use with activated charcoal. • Do not combine with amphotericin B, ampicillin, or erythromycin lactobionate. Administer separately. • Monitor acetaminophen levels 4 hours after ingestion to determine risk of hepatotoxicity.
activated charcoal (Actidose-Aqua, Liqui-Char) • Treatment of poisoning or overdose with most orally administered drugs, except caustic agents and hydrocarbons	• Do not give to a semiconscious or unconscious patient. • If possible, administer within 30 minutes of poisoning. • Do not give in or with ice cream, milk, or sherbet because these foods reduce the adsorption capacities of charcoal. • Repeat the dose if the patient vomits shortly after administration.
aminocaproic acid (Amicar) • Antidote for alteplase, anistreplase, streptokinase, or urokinase toxicity	• Dilute in compatible I.V. fluids. • Monitor the patient's coagulation studies, heart rhythm, and blood pressure. • Monitor patient for signs of clotting.
atropine sulfate • Antidote for cholinergic drugs and cholinesterase inhibitors	• Atropine sulfate is contraindicated in patients with glaucoma, myasthenia gravis, obstructive uropathy, or unstable cardiovascular status. • Monitor the patient's intake and output to assess for urine retention. • Monitor blood pressure, pulse, and renal function.
botulism antitoxin, trivalent equine • Treatment of botulism	• Obtain an accurate patient history of allergies, especially to horses, and of reactions to immunizations. • Test the patient for sensitivity (against a control of normal saline solution in the opposing extremity) before administration. Read the results after 5 to 30 minutes. A wheal indicates a positive reaction and patient desensitization is required. • Keep epinephrine 1:1,000 available in case of an allergic reaction. • Monitor vital signs during infusion.

Managing poisoning or overdose *(continued)*

Antidote and indications	Nursing considerations
deferoxamine mesylate (Desferal) • Adjunctive treatment of acute iron intoxication	• Do not administer the drug to a patient who has severe renal disease or anuria. • Monitor the patient for visual or auditory changes, angioedema, shock, and hypotension. • Keep epinephrine 1:1,000 available in case of an allergic reaction. • Use the I.M. route if possible. Use the I.V. route only when the patient is in shock. • Monitor the patient's intake and output carefully. Warn the patient that his or her urine may turn red. • Monitor vital signs.
digoxin immune Fab (ovine) (Digibind) • Treatment of potentially life-threatening digoxin or digitoxin intoxication	• Use the drug cautiously in a patient who is allergic to ovine proteins because it is derived from digoxin-specific antibody fragments obtained from immunized sheep. Perform a skin test before administering. • Use only for a patient who is in shock or cardiac arrest with ventricular arrhythmias, such as ventricular tachycardia or fibrillation; with progressive bradycardia, such as severe sinus bradycardia; or with second- or third-degree atrioventricular block if the patient is unresponsive to atropine. • Refrigerate powder for reconstitution. If possible, use the reconstituted drug immediately, although you may refrigerate it for up to 4 hours. • Drug interferes with immunoassay measurements of digoxin, resulting in misleading standard serum digoxin levels until the drug is cleared from the body (about 3 days). • Total serum digoxin levels may rise after administration of the drug, reflecting fat-bound (inactive) digoxin. • Monitor the patient's serum electrolytes and vital signs.
edetate calcium disodium (Calcium Disodium Versenate, Calcium EDTA) • Treatment of acute and chronic lead poisoning	• Do not give the drug to a patient who has severe renal disease or anuria. • Avoid using the I.V. route in a patient who has lead encephalopathy because intracranial pressure may increase; use the I.M. route. • Avoid rapid infusion; the I.M. route is preferred, especially for children. • If giving a high dose, give the drug with dimercaprol to avoid a toxic reaction. • Give plenty of fluids to facilitate the excretion of lead, except in patients with lead encephalopathy and increased intracranial pressure.

(continued)

Managing poisoning or overdose *(continued)*

Antidote and indications	Nursing considerations
edetate calcium disodium *(continued)*	• Before giving the drug, obtain baseline intake and output; urinalysis; blood urea nitrogen; and serum alkaline phosphatase, calcium, creatinine, and phosphorus levels. Then monitor these values on the first, third, and fifth days of treatment. Monitor the patient's electrocardiogram results periodically. • Monitor vital signs.
naloxone hydrochloride *(Narcan)* • Treatment of respiratory depression caused by opioids • Treatment of postoperative narcotic depression • Treatment of asphyxia neonatorum	• Use cautiously in a patient with cardiac irritability or opioid addiction. • Monitor the patient's respiratory depth and rate. Be prepared to provide oxygen, ventilation, and other resuscitative measures. • Respiratory rate increases within 2 minutes. • Duration of narcotic may exceed that of naloxone, causing the patient to relapse into respiratory depression. • Drug may be administered by continuous I.V. infusion to control the adverse effects of epidurally administered morphine. • An "overshoot" effect may occur in which the patient's respiratory rate after receiving the drug exceeds his or her rate before respiratory depression occurred. • Naloxone is the safest drug to use when the cause of respiratory depression is uncertain. • Naloxone is only effective for reversing respiratory depression caused by opioids and not for other drug-induced respiratory depression, including caused by benzodiazepines.
pralidoxime chloride *(Protopam Chloride)* • Antidote for organophosphate poisoning and cholinergic overdose	• Do not give to a patient poisoned with carbaryl (Sevin), a carbamate insecticide because it increases the toxic effects of carbaryl. • Use with caution in a patient with renal insufficiency, myasthenia gravis, asthma, pregnancy, or lactation. • Use in a hospitalized patient only and have respiratory and other supportive equipment available. • Administer the antidote as soon as possible after poisoning. • Before administering, suction secretions and make sure the airway is patent. • Give atropine along with pralidoxime for organophosphate poisoning. • If the patient's skin was exposed, remove the clothing and wash the skin and hair with sodium bicarbonate, soap, water, and alcohol as soon as possible. He or she may need a second washing. When washing the patient, wear protective gloves and clothes to avoid exposure.

Managing poisoning or overdose *(continued)*

Antidote and indications	Nursing considerations
pralidoxime chloride *(continued)*	• Observe the patient for 48 to 72 hours after the ingestion of poison. Delayed absorption may occur. Watch for signs of rapid weakening in a patient with myasthenia gravis who is being treated for an overdose of cholinergic drugs. The patient may pass quickly from cholinergic crisis to myasthenic crisis and require more cholinergic drugs to treat the myasthenia. Keep edrophonium available.
protamine sulfate • Treatment of heparin overdose	• Administer slowly to reduce adverse reactions. Have equipment available to treat shock. • Monitor the patient continuously and check the vital signs frequently. • Screen for heparin rebound and response to drug by monitoring coagulation studies.

after overdose occurs. If the levels indicate hepatotoxicity, perform liver function tests every 24 hours for at least 96 hours.

Analeptic overdose (amphetamines, cocaine)

Individual responses to overdose with analeptics vary widely. Toxic doses also vary, depending on the drug and the route of ingestion.

Signs and symptoms of overdose include restlessness, tremor, hyperreflexia, tachypnea, confusion, aggressiveness, hallucinations, and panic; fatigue and depression usually follow the excitement stage. Other effects include arrhythmias, shock, altered blood pressure, nausea, vomiting, diarrhea, and abdominal cramps; seizures and coma usually precede death.

Treat overdose symptomatically and supportively: If oral ingestion is recent (within 4 hours), use gastric lavage to empty the stomach and reduce further absorption. Follow with activated charcoal. Monitor the patient's vital signs and fluid and electrolyte balance. If the drug was smoked or injected, focus on enhancing drug elimination and providing

supportive care. Administer a sedative if needed. Urine acidification may enhance excretion. A saline cathartic (magnesium citrate) may hasten GI evacuation of unabsorbed sustained-release drug.

Anticholinergic overdose

Signs and symptoms of anticholinergic overdose include peripheral effects, such as dilated, nonreactive pupils; blurred vision; flushed, hot, dry skin; dry mucous membranes; dysphagia; decreased or absent bowel sounds; urine retention; hyperthermia; tachycardia; hypertension; and increased respiratory rate.

Treatment is primarily symptomatic and supportive, as needed. If the patient is alert, a single dose of activated charcoal is usually sufficient if ingestion was <1 hour. In severe cases, physostigmine may be administered to block central antimuscarinic effects. Give fluids as needed to treat shock. If urine retention occurs, catheterization may be necessary.

Anticoagulant overdose

Signs and symptoms of oral anticoagulant overdose vary with the severity of overdose. They may include internal or external bleeding and skin necrosis, but the most common sign is hematuria.

If the patient has an excessively prolonged prothrombin time, an elevated international normalized ratio, or minor bleeding, anticoagulant therapy must be stopped. In some cases, withholding one or two doses may be adequate. Other measures to control bleeding include oral or I.V. phytonadione (vitamin K_1) and, for severe hemorrhage, fresh frozen plasma or whole blood. Menadione (vitamin K_3) is not as effective. The use of phytonadione may interfere with subsequent oral anticoagulant therapy and may cause an anaphylactic reaction.

Antihistamine overdose

Drowsiness is the most common sign of antihistamine overdose. Seizures, coma, and respiratory depression may occur with severe overdose. Certain histamine antagonists, such as diphenhydramine, also block cholinergic receptors and produce modest anticholinergic signs and symptoms, such as dry mouth, flushed skin, fixed and dilated pupils, and GI symptoms, especially in children. Phenothiazine-type antihistamines such as promethazine also block dopamine receptors. The patient may have movement disorders that mimic Parkinson's disease. Children may also have CNS stimulation or seizures.

Treat the overdose with gastric lavage followed by activated charcoal. Syrup of ipecac usually is not recommended because acute dystonic reactions may increase the risk of aspiration. Also, phenothiazine-type antihistamines may have antiemetic effects. Treat hypotension with fluids or a vasopressor, and treat seizures with phenytoin or diazepam. Watch the patient for arrhythmias and provide treatment accordingly.

Barbiturate overdose

A barbiturate overdose can cause unsteady gait, slurred speech, sustained nystagmus, somnolence, confusion,

respiratory depression, pulmonary edema, areflexia, and coma. Typical shock syndrome with tachycardia and hypotension, jaundice, hypothermia followed by fever, and oliguria may occur.

To treat barbiturate overdose, maintain and support the patient's ventilation and pulmonary function as necessary; support cardiac function and circulation with a vasopressor and I.V. fluids, as needed. If the patient is conscious and the gag reflex is intact, induce emesis (if ingestion was recent). If emesis is contraindicated, perform gastric lavage while a cuffed endotracheal tube is in place to prevent aspiration. Then administer activated charcoal and a saline cathartic. Measure the patient's intake and output, vital signs, and laboratory parameters; maintain his or her body temperature. The patient should be rolled from side to side every 30 minutes to avoid pulmonary congestion.

Alkalinization of urine may help remove the drug from the body; hemodialysis may be useful in severe overdose.

Benzodiazepine overdose

Benzodiazepine overdose can produce somnolence, confusion, coma, hypoactive reflexes, dyspnea, labored breathing, hypotension, bradycardia, slurred speech, and unsteady gait or impaired coordination.

Treatment of overdose involves supporting the patient's blood pressure and respiration and monitoring vital signs until the effects of the drug subside. Mechanical ventilatory assistance via an endotracheal tube may be required to maintain a patent airway and support adequate oxygenation. Flumazenil, a specific benzodiazepine antagonist, may be useful. Use I.V. fluids or a vasopressor, such as dopamine and phenylephrine, to treat hypotension, as needed. If the patient is conscious and his or her gag reflex is intact, induce emesis (if ingestion was recent). If emesis is contraindicated, perform gastric lavage while a cuffed endotracheal tube is in place, to prevent aspiration. After emesis or lavage, administer activated charcoal with a cathartic as a single dose. Dialysis is of limited value.

CNS depressant overdose

Signs of CNS depressant overdose include prolonged coma, hypotension, hypothermia followed by fever, and inadequate ventilation, even without significant respiratory depression. Absence of pupillary reflexes, dilated pupils, loss of deep tendon reflexes, tonic muscle spasms, and apnea may also occur.

Treatment of overdose involves supporting the patient's respiratory and cardiovascular function; mechanical ventilation may be needed. Maintain adequate urine output with adequate hydration while avoiding pulmonary edema. Empty the gastric contents by inducing emesis. For lipid-soluble drugs such as glutethimide, charcoal, and resin hemoperfusion are effective in removing the drug; hemodialysis and peritoneal dialysis are of minimal value. Because glutethimide is stored in fat tissue, blood levels commonly show large fluctuations with worsening symptoms.

Digoxin overdose

Signs and symptoms of digoxin overdose are primarily related to the GI, cardiovascular, and CNS. Severe overdose may cause hyperkalemia, which may develop rapidly and result in life-threatening cardiac effects. Cardiac signs of digoxin toxicity may occur with or without other signs of toxic reaction and commonly precede other toxic effects. Because cardiotoxic effects can also occur with heart disease, determining whether these effects result from underlying heart disease or from digoxin toxicity may be difficult. Digoxin has caused almost every kind of arrhythmia; various combinations of arrhythmias may occur in the same patient. Patients with chronic digoxin toxicity commonly have ventricular arrhythmias, atrioventricular (AV) conduction disturbances, or both. Patients with digoxin-induced ventricular tachycardia have a high mortality rate because ventricular fibrillation or asystole may result.

Treatment should be based on the patient's signs and symptoms. If toxicity is suspected, the drug should be discontinued and serum levels of the drug obtained. Usually, the drug takes at least 6 hours to be distributed between plasma and tissue and to reach equilibrium; plasma levels obtained earlier may show higher levels of digoxin than those obtained after the drug has distributed into the tissues.

The first line of treatment is usually activated charcoal. Inducing emesis with ipecac syrup is not recommended. Gastric lavage may worsen arrhythmias; therefore, precaution should be taken. Cholestyramine may be useful for chronic toxicity.

Ventricular arrhythmias may be treated with I.V. potassium (replacement doses but not in patients with significant AV block), I.V. phenytoin, I.V. lidocaine, or I.V. propranolol. Refractory ventricular tachyarrhythmias may be controlled with overdrive pacing. Procainamide may be used for ventricular arrhythmias that do not respond to these treatments. For severe AV block, asystole, and hemodynamically significant sinus bradycardia, atropine restores a normal rate.

Administration of digoxin-specific antibody fragments (digoxin immune Fab [Digibind]) treats life-threatening digoxin toxicity. Each 40 mg of digoxin immune Fab binds about 0.6 mg of digoxin in the bloodstream. The complex is excreted in the urine, rapidly decreasing serum levels and, therefore, cardiac drug concentrations.

Iron supplement overdose

Iron supplements are a major source of poisoning, especially in small children. Signs and symptoms of poisoning result from the acute corrosive effects of iron on the GI mucosa as well as the adverse metabolic effects of iron overload. These signs and symptoms may occur within the first 10 minutes of ingestion or may be delayed for several hours. There are five stages of acute iron poisoning.

The first findings reflect acute GI irritation and include epigastric pain, nausea, and vomiting. The patient may have green diarrhea, followed by tarry stools and then melena. Hematemesis may be accompanied by drowsiness, lassitude, shock, and coma. Local erosion of the stomach and small intestine may further enhance the absorption of iron. If death does not occur in the first phase, the patient may appear to improve during the second phase. During the third phase, metabolic and cardiovascular complications may occur. This is the stage that death more frequently occurs. It is marked by CNS abnormalities, metabolic acidosis, hepatic dysfunction, renal failure, and bleeding diathesis. This phase may progress to circulatory failure, coma, and death. If the patient survives, the fourth phase consists of hepatic dysfunction and hypoglycemia may be seen. Stage five occurs several weeks after poisoning. There may be stomach or intestinal scarring that causes vomiting and abdominal cramping.

Patients who are vomiting, have diarrhea, leukocytosis, or hyperglycemia and have an abdominal X-ray that is positive for iron within 6 hours of ingestion are at risk for a serious toxic reaction. Perform gastric lavage within 1 hour with normal saline or polyethylene glycol electrolyte solution. Ipecac-induced emesis is not recommended.

Some clinicians add sodium bicarbonate to the lavage solution to convert ferrous iron to ferrous carbonate, which is poorly absorbed. Disodium phosphate has also been used; however, life-threatening hyperphosphatemia or hypocalcemia may develop in some children. Other possible treatments include administration of a saline cathartic, surgical removal of tablets, and chelation therapy with deferoxamine mesylate. Hemodialysis is of little value. Supportive treatment includes monitoring the acid-base balance, maintaining a patent airway, and controlling shock and dehydration with appropriate I.V. therapy.

NSAID overdose

Signs and symptoms of nonsteroidal anti-inflammatory drug (NSAID) overdose include dizziness, drowsiness, paresthesia, vomiting, nausea, abdominal pain, headache, sweating, nystagmus, apnea, and cyanosis.

Treatment for NSAID overdose involves supportive care. Syrup of ipecac is no longer recommended. To treat an ibuprofen overdose, gastric lavage is used. Administer activated charcoal via a nasogastric tube. Provide symptomatic and supportive measures, including respiratory support and correction of fluid and electrolyte imbalances. Monitor the patient's vital signs and the results of laboratory tests closely. Alkaline diuresis may enhance renal excretion. Dialysis is of minimal value because NSAIDs are strongly protein bound.

Opiate overdose

Rapid I.V. administration of opiates may result in overdose because of a 30-minute delay in the maximum CNS effect. The most common signs of morphine overdose are respiratory depression, with or without CNS depression and miosis (pinpoint pupils). Other acute toxic effects include hypotension, bradycardia, hypothermia, shock, apnea, cardiopulmonary arrest, circulatory collapse, pulmonary edema, and seizures.

To treat an acute overdose, establish adequate respiratory exchange via a patent airway and provide ventilation, as needed, and then administer an opioid antagonist (naloxone) to reverse respiratory depression. (Because the duration of action of morphine is longer than that of naloxone, repeated doses of naloxone are needed.) Naloxone is given only when clinically significant respiratory or cardiovascular depression is present. Monitor the patient's vital signs closely.

The method of choice is the use of activated charcoal. Administer activated charcoal via a nasogastric tube to remove the drug. This should be attempted as long as it is not contraindicated.

Provide symptomatic and supportive treatment (continued respiratory support and correction of fluid or electrolyte imbalances). Monitor the patient's vital signs, neurologic status, and laboratory test results closely.

Phenothiazine overdose

Phenothiazine overdose can cause CNS depression, which is characterized by deep sleep—from which the patient cannot be roused—and possible coma, hypotension or hypertension, extrapyramidal symptoms, abnormal involuntary muscle movements, agitation, seizures, arrhythmias, electrocardiogram changes, hypothermia or hyperthermia, and autonomic nervous system dysfunction.

Treatment is symptomatic and supportive; it includes maintaining vital signs, a patent airway, a stable body temperature, and fluid and electrolyte balance. Do not induce vomiting; phenothiazines inhibit the cough reflex, so aspiration may occur. Use gastric lavage and then activated charcoal and saline cathartics. Dialysis does not help. Regulate the patient's body temperature as needed. Treat hypotension with I.V. fluids. Do not give epinephrine. Treat seizures with parenteral diazepam or barbiturates, arrhythmias with parenteral phenytoin, and extrapyramidal reactions with benztropine or parenteral diphenhydramine.

Salicylate overdose

Signs and symptoms of salicylate overdose include metabolic acidosis with respiratory alkalosis, hyperpnea, and tachypnea as a result of increased production of carbon dioxide and direct stimulation of the respiratory center.

To treat the overdose, perform gastric lavage. Administer activated charcoal via a nasogastric tube. Provide symptomatic and supportive measures (respiratory support and correction of fluid and electrolyte imbalances). Closely monitor the patient's laboratory values and vital signs. Enhance renal excretion by administering sodium bicarbonate to alkalinize urine. Use a cooling blanket or sponging if the patient's rectal temperature is above 104° F (40° C). Hemodialysis is effective in removing aspirin but is used only with severe poisoning or in patients who are at risk for pulmonary edema.

Tricyclic antidepressant overdose

Tricyclic antidepressant overdose is often life-threatening, particularly when the drug is combined with alcohol. The onset of symptoms is usually seen within the first 2 hours of ingestion. Signs and symptoms include drowsiness, respiratory depression, coma, hypotension, urinary retention, blurred vision, tachycardia, and absent bowel sounds.

Treatment is symptomatic and supportive; it includes maintaining a patent airway, a stable body temperature, and fluid and electrolyte balance. Induce emesis if the patient is conscious; gastric lavage may be helpful. Dialysis is of little use. The treatment of choice for seizures is benzodiazepines. Do not give barbiturates; they may enhance CNS and respiratory depressant effects.

Interactions

Compatibility of drugs combined in a syringe

KEY
Y = compatible for at least 30 minutes
P = provisionally compatible; administer within 15 minutes
P(5) = provisionally compatible; administer within 5 minutes
N = not compatible
* = conflicting data
(A blank space indicates no available data.)

	atropine sulfate	butorphanol tartrate	chlorpromazine HCl	cimetidine HCl	codeine phosphate	dexamethasone sodium phosphate	dimenhydrinate	diphenhydramine HCl	droperidol	fentanyl citrate	glycopyrrolate	heparin Na	hydromorphone HCl	hydroxyzine HCl	meperidine HCl	metoclopramide HCl
atropine sulfate	■	Y	P	Y			P	P	P	P	Y	P(5)	Y	P*	P	P
butorphanol tartrate	Y	■	Y	Y			N	Y	Y	Y				Y	Y	Y
chlorpromazine HCl	P	Y	■	N			N	P	P	P	P	Y	N	Y	P	P
cimetidine HCl	Y	Y	N	■			Y	Y	Y	Y	Y	P(5)*	Y	Y	Y	
codeine phosphate					■		P(5)				Y			Y		
dexamethasone sodium phosphate						■	N*					N	N*			Y
dimenhydrinate	P	N	N		P(5)		■	P	P	P	N	P(5)*	Y	N	P	P
diphenhydramine HCl	P	Y	P	Y		N*	P	■	P	P	P	Y	Y	Y	P	P
droperidol	P	Y	P	Y			P	P	■	P	Y	N			P	P
fentanyl citrate	P	Y	P	Y			P	P	P	■		P(5)	Y	P	P	P
glycopyrrolate	Y		Y	Y	Y	N	N	Y	Y		■		Y	Y	Y	
heparin Na	P(5)		N	P(5)*			P*		N	P(5)		■	N		N	Y
hydromorphone HCl	Y		Y	N		N*	Y	Y		Y	Y	N	■	Y		
hydroxyzine HCl	P*	Y	P	P	Y		N	P	P	P	Y		Y	■	P	P
meperidine HCl	P	Y	P	Y			P	P	P	P	Y	N		P	■	P
metoclopramide HCl	P	Y	P			Y	P	Y	P	P		Y		P	P	■
midazolam HCl	Y	Y	Y	Y			N	Y	Y	Y	Y	N	Y	Y	Y	Y
morphine sulfate	P	Y	P	Y			P	P	P	P	Y	N*		P	N	P
nalbuphine HCl	Y			Y			N	Y	Y		Y			Y		
pentazocine lactate	P	Y	P	Y			P	P	P	P	N	N	Y	P	P	P
pentobarbital Na	P*	N	N	N			N	N	N	N	N			Y	N	N
perphenazine	Y	Y	Y	Y			Y	Y	Y	Y				Y	Y	P
phenobarbital Na												P(5)	N			
prochlorperazine edisylate	P	Y	P	Y			N	P	P	P	Y		N*	P	P	P
promazine HCl	P		P				N	P	P	P	Y			P	P	P
promethazine HCl	P	Y	P	Y			N	P	P	P	Y	N	Y	P	P	P
ranitidine HCl	Y		N*			Y	Y	Y		Y	Y		Y	N	Y	Y
scopolamine HBr	P	Y	P	Y			P	P	P	P	Y		Y	P	P	P
secobarbital Na				N									N			
sodium bicarbonate							N					N				N
thiethylperazine maleate		Y												Y		
thiopental Na			N				N	N				N				

midazolam HCl	morphine sulfate	nalbuphine HCl	pentazocine lactate	pentobarbital Na	perphenazine	phenobarbital Na	prochlorperazine edisylate	promazine HCl	promethazine HCl	ranitidine HCl	scopolamine HBr	secobarbital Na	sodium bicarbonate	thiethylperazine maleate	thiopental Na	
Y	P	Y	P	P*	Y		P	P	P	Y	P					atropine sulfate
Y	Y		Y	N	Y		Y		Y		Y			Y		butorphanol tartrate
Y	P		P	N	Y		P	P	P	N*	P				N	chlorpromazine HCl
Y	Y	Y	Y	N	Y		Y	Y	Y		Y	N				cimetidine HCl
																codeine phosphate
										Y						dexamethasone sodium phosphate
N	P	N	P	N	Y		N	N	N	Y	P				N	dimenhydrinate
Y	P	Y	P	N	Y		P	P	P	Y	P				N	diphenhydramine HCl
Y	P	Y	P	N	Y		P	P	P		P					droperidol
Y	P		P	N	Y		P	P	P	Y	P					fentanyl citrate
Y	Y	Y	N	N			Y	Y	Y	Y	Y	N	N		N	glycopyrrolate
N	N*		N			P(5)		N								heparin Na
Y		Y	Y		N	N*		Y	Y	Y				Y		hydromorphone HCl
Y	P	Y	P	N	Y		P	P	P	N	P					hydroxyzine HCl
Y	N		P	N	Y		P	P	P	Y	P					meperidine HCl
Y	P		P		P		P	P	P	Y	P		N			metoclopramide HCl
■	Y	Y		N	N		N	Y	Y	N	Y			Y		midazolam HCl
Y	■		P	N*	Y		P	P*	P*	Y	P				N	morphine sulfate
Y		■		N			Y		N*	Y	Y			Y		nalbuphine HCl
	P		■	N	Y		P*	P*	P*	Y	P					pentazocine lactate
N	N*	N	N	■			N	N	N	N	P		Y		Y	pentobarbital Na
N	Y		Y	N	■		Y		Y	Y	Y		N			perphenazine
						■				N						phenobarbital Na
N	P*	Y	P	N	Y		■	P	P	Y	P				N	prochlorperazine edisylate
Y	P		P*	N			P	■	P		P					promazine HCl
Y	P*	N*	P*	N	Y		P	P	■	Y	P				N	promethazine HCl
N	Y	Y	Y	N	Y	N	Y		Y	■	Y			Y		ranitidine HCl
Y	P	Y	P	P	Y		P	P	P	Y	■				Y	scopolamine HBr
												■				secobarbital Na
			Y										■		N	sodium bicarbonate
Y		Y		N							Y			■		thiethylperazine maleate
	N			Y			N		N		Y		N		■	thiopental Na

Drug combinations

Drugs can interact to produce undesirable, even hazardous, effects. These interactions can decrease therapeutic efficacy or cause a toxic reaction.

Drug-tobacco interactions

Smoking—or living and working in a smoke-filled environment—can affect a patient's drug therapy, especially if he or she is taking one of the drugs

(Text continues on page 622.)

Serious drug interactions

When administering these combinations, monitor the patient to prevent serious drug interactions.

Drug	Interacting drug	Possible effect
Aminoglycosides amikacin gentamicin kanamycin neomycin netilmicin streptomycin tobramycin	Parenteral cephalosporins	May enhance nephrotoxicity
	I.V. loop diuretics • bumetanide • ethacrynic acid • furosemide	May enhance ototoxicity; nephrotoxicity
Amphetamines amphetamine benzphetamine dextroamphetamine methamphetamine	Urine alkalinizers • potassium citrate • sodium acetate • sodium bicarbonate • sodium citrate • sodium lactate • tromethamine	Decreases urinary excretion of amphetamine; may increase amphetamine levels
Angiotensin-converting enzyme (ACE) inhibitors captopril enalapril lisinopril benazepril fosinopril ramipril quinapril	indomethacin Nonsteroidal anti-inflammatory drugs (NSAIDs)	Decreases or abolishes the effectiveness of the antihypertensive action of ACE inhibitors; risk of nephrotoxicity and hyperkalemia
Barbiturate anesthetics methohexital thiopental	Opiate analgesics	Enhances central nervous system and respiratory depression

Serious drug interactions (continued)

Drug	Interacting drug	Possible effect
Barbiturates butabarbital phenobarbital primidone secobarbital	valproic acid	Increases serum barbiturate levels; may decrease valproic acid levels; risk of central nervous system and respiratory depression
Beta-adrenergic blockers acebutolol atenolol betaxolol carteolol esmolol levobunolol metoprolol nadolol penbutolol pindolol propranolol timolol	verapamil	Enhances the pharmacologic effects of both beta-adrenergic blockers and verapamil; risk of hypotension and arrhythmias
carbamazepine	erythromycin	Increases the risk of carbamazepine toxicity
Cardiac glycosides	Loop and thiazide diuretics	Increases the risk of cardiac arrhythmias as a result of hypokalemia
	Thiazide-like diuretics	Increases the therapeutic or toxic effects
carmustine	cimetidine	Enhances the risk of bone marrow toxicity
ciprofloxacin	Antacids that contain magnesium or aluminum hydroxide, iron supplements, sucralfate, multivitamins that contain iron or zinc	Decreases plasma levels as well as the effectiveness of ciprofloxacin
clonidine	Beta-adrenergic blockers	Enhances rebound hypertension after rapid withdrawal of clonidine; risk of hypotension and arrhythmias
cyclosporine	carbamazepine, isoniazid, phenobarbital, phenytoin, rifabutin, rifampin	Reduces plasma levels of cyclosporine and may decrease immunosuppressant effect

(continued)

Serious drug interactions *(continued)*

Drug	Interacting drug	Possible effect
digoxin	amiodarone	Decreases the renal clearance of digoxin, which increases digoxin level
	quinidine	Elevates serum levels of digoxin; cardiac arrhythmias
	verapamil	Elevates serum levels of digoxin
dopamine	phenytoin	Hypertension, bradycardia, and cardiac arrest
epinephrine	Beta-adrenergic blockers	Increases systolic and diastolic pressures; causes a marked decrease in heart rate; may decrease antihypertensive agent efficacy
erythromycin	astemizole	Increases the risk of arrhythmia
	carbamazepine	Decreases carbamazepine clearance
	theophylline	Decreases hepatic clearance of theophylline
ethanol	disulfiram metronidazole	Causes an acute alcohol intolerance reaction
heparin	Salicylates NSAIDs	Enhances the risk of bleeding
lithium	Thiazide diuretics NSAIDs	Decreases the excretion of lithium
meperidine	Monoamine oxidase (MAO) inhibitors	Causes cardiovascular instability and increases toxic effects
methotrexate	probenecid	Decreases the elimination of methotrexate
	Salicylates	Increases the risk of methotrexate toxicity
MAO inhibitors	Amine-containing foods Anorexiants meperidine	Risk of hypertensive crisis
Potassium supplements	Potassium-sparing diuretics	Increases the risk of hyperkalemia

Serious drug interactions *(continued)*

Drug	Interacting drug	Possible effect
quinidine	amiodarone	Increases the risk of quinidine toxicity; cardiac arrhythmias
Sympathomimetics	MAO inhibitors	Increased the risk of hypertensive crisis
Tetracyclines	Antacids containing magnesium, aluminum, or bismuth salts Iron supplements	Decreases plasma levels as well as the effectiveness of tetracyclines
theophylline	carbamazepine	Reduces theophylline levels
	cimetidine	Increases theophylline levels
	ciprofloxacin	Increases theophylline levels
	erythromycin	Increases theophylline levels
	phenobarbital	Reduces theophylline levels
	rifampin	Reduces theophylline levels
warfarin	testosterone	May enhance bleeding caused by increased hypoprothrombinemia
	Barbiturates carbamazepine	Reduces the effectiveness of warfarin
	amiodarone Certain cephalosporins cimetidine clofibrate disulfiram erythromycin glucagon metronidazole quinidine quinine Salicylates	Increases the risk of bleeding
	griseofulvin	Decreases the pharmacologic effect
	rifampin trazodone	Decreases the risk of bleeding
	methimazole propylthiouracil	Changes in thyroid status

listed here. For a patient who is using any of these drugs, monitor plasma drug levels closely and watch for possible adverse reactions.

Ascorbic acid (vitamin C)

Possible effects

- Low serum levels of vitamin C
- Decreased oral absorption of vitamin C

Nursing considerations

- Tell the patient to increase his or her vitamin C intake.
- Encourage the patient to stop smoking.

Chlordiazepoxide hydrochloride, chlorpromazine hydrochloride, diazepam

Possible effects

- Increased drug metabolism, which results in reduced plasma levels
- Decreased sedative effects

Nursing considerations

- Teach the patient about the medication-tobacco interaction.
- Encourage patient to stop smoking.
- Watch for a decrease in the effectiveness of the drug.
- Adjust the patient's drug dosage, if ordered.

Propoxyphene hydrochloride

Possible effect

- Increased drug metabolism and diminished analgesic effects

Nursing considerations

- Watch for a decrease in the effectiveness of the drug.

Propranolol hydrochloride

Possible effects

- Increased metabolism, which decreases the effectiveness of the drug
- Reduced effectiveness of the drug (Smoking increases the heart rate, stimulates the release of catecholamine from the adrenal medulla, raises arterial blood pressure, and increases myocardial oxygen consumption.)

Nursing considerations

- Monitor the patient's blood pressure and heart rate.
- To reduce the interaction between the drug and tobacco, the physician may order a selective beta-adrenergic blocker such as atenolol.

Hormonal contraceptives that contain estrogen and progestogen

Possible effects

- Increased risk of adverse reactions, such as headache, dizziness, depression, changes in libido, migraine, hypertension, thromboembolism, pulmonary embolism, myocardial infarction, stroke, edema, worsening of astigmatism or myopia, nausea, vomiting, and gallbladder disease

Nursing considerations

- Inform the patient of increased risk of myocardial infarction and stroke.
- Suggest that the patient stop smoking or use a different birth control method.

Theophylline

Possible effects

- Increased metabolism of theophylline as a result of the induction of liver microsomal enzymes
- Lower plasma levels of theophylline

Nursing considerations

- Monitor plasma theophylline levels and watch for a decreased therapeutic effect.
- Increase the drug dosage, if ordered.

Selected drug-food interactions

acebutolol hydrochloride (Sectral): Food in general. *Slightly decreases drug absorption and peak levels.*

amiloride hydrochloride (Midamor): Potassium-rich diet. *May rapidly increase serum potassium levels.*

antihypertensives: Licorice. *Decreases the antihypertensive effect.*

bacampicillin hydrochloride (Spectrobid powder for oral suspension): Food in general. *Decreases drug absorption.*

buspirone hydrochloride (BuSpar): Food in general. *May decrease presystemic drug clearance.* Grapefruit juice. *May increase serum drug levels.*

caffeine (NoDoz): Caffeine-containing beverages and food. *May cause sleeplessness, irritability, nervousness, and rapid heartbeat.*

calcium glubionate (Neo-Calglucon syrup): Large quantities of bran, whole-grain cereals, dairy products, rhubarb, spinach. *Interferes with calcium absorption.*

captopril (Capoten): Food in general. Avoid eating large amounts of foods high in potassium. Patient should take 1 hour before meals. *Reduces drug absorption by 30% to 40%.*

cefuroxime axetil (Ceftin tablets): Food in general. *Increases drug absorption.*

demeclocycline hydrochloride (Declomycin): Dairy products, multivitamins, antacids, food in general. *Interferes with the absorption of oral forms of demeclocycline.*

dextroamphetamine sulfate (Dexedrine elixir): Fruit juice; caffeine-containing foods/beverages. Acidic juices should be taken 1 hour before or after taking medication. *Lowers blood drug levels and efficacy.*

dicumarol: Diet high in vitamin K. *Decreases prothrombin time.*

digoxin (Lanoxin tablets, Lanoxicaps): Food high in bran fiber. *May reduce the bioavailability of oral digoxin.* Food in general. *Slows the drug absorption rate.*

dyclonine hydrochloride (Dyclone 0.5% and 1% topical solutions, USP): Food in general. *Topical anesthesia may impair swallowing, enhancing the risk of aspiration; food should not be ingested for 60 minutes.*

erythromycin base (PCE Dispertab tablets): Food in general. Grapefruit juice. *Optimum blood levels are obtained on a fasting stomach; administration is preferable 30 minutes before or 2 hours after meals.*

estramustine phosphate sodium (Emcyt): Dairy products, calcium-rich foods. *Impairs drug absorption.*

etodolac (Lodine): Food in general. *Reduces peak levels by about 50% and increases the time to peak levels by 1.4 to 3.8 hours.*

etretinate (Tegison capsules): Dairy products, high-lipid diet. *Increases drug absorption.*

famotidine (Pepcid oral suspension): Food in general. *Slightly increases bioavailability.*

felodipine (Plendil): Grapefruit juice. *Increases bioavailability more than twofold.*

fenoprofen calcium (Nalfon Pulvules and tablets): Dairy products, food in general. *Delays and diminishes peak blood levels.*

ferrous sulfate (Feosol, Slow FE): Dairy products, eggs. Food in general. *Inhibits iron absorption.*

fluoroquinolone antibiotics, such as ciprofloxacin (Cipro), norfloxacin (Noroxin), ofloxacin (Floxin): Food in general (particularly dairy products).

May decrease the absorption of oral fluoroquinolones.

flurbiprofen (Ansaid): Food in general. *Alters the rate of absorption, but not the extent, of drug availability.*

fosinopril sodium (Monopril): Avoid moderately high or high potassium dietary intake. Do not use potassium supplements. Food in general. *May slow the rate, but not the extent, of drug absorption.*

glipizide (Glucotrol): Food in general. *Delays absorption by about 40 minutes. Give an immediate-release tablet about 30 minutes before meals.*

hydralazine hydrochloride (Apresoline tablets): Food in general. *Increases plasma levels.*

hydrochlorothiazide (Esidrix, HydroDIURIL): Food in general. *Enhances GI drug absorption.*

ibuprofen (Advil, Children's Advil suspension, Motrin, Nuprin, Children's Motrin suspension, Rufen): Food in general. *Reduces the rate, but not the extent, of absorption.*

isotretinoin (Accutane): Dairy products, food in general. *Increases the absorption of oral isotretinoin.*

isradipine (DynaCirc): Grapefruit and grapefruit juice. Food in general. *Significantly increases the time to peak levels by about 1 hour, with no effect on bioavailability.*

ketoprofen (Orudis capsules): Food in general. *Slows the absorption rate and delays and reduces peak levels.*

levodopa-carbidopa (Sinemet tablets): High-protein diet. *May impair levodopa absorption.* Food in general. *Increases the extent of availability and peak levels of sustained-release levodopa-carbidopa.*

levothyroxine sodium (Synthroid injection): Soybean formula (infants). *May cause excessive fecal loss.*

lidocaine hydrochloride (Xylocaine): Food in general. *Topical anesthesia may impair swallowing, enhancing the risk of aspiration; avoid ingestion of food for 60 minutes.*

liotrix (Thyrolar): Soybean formula (infants). *May cause excessive fecal loss.*

lovastatin (Mevacor): Grapefruit juice. *Increases serum levels.*

meclofenamate (Meclomen): Food in general. *Decreases the rate and extent of drug absorption.*

methenamine mandelate (Mandelamine granules): Food that raises urinary pH. *Reduces essential antibacterial activity.*

methotrexate sodium (Rheumatrex): Food in general. *Delays absorption and reduces peak levels of oral methotrexate sodium.*

minocycline hydrochloride (Minocin): Dairy products. *Slightly decreases peak plasma levels and delays them by 1 hour.*

misoprostol (Cytotec): Food in general. *Diminishes maximum plasma concentrations.*

monoamine oxidase (MAO) inhibitors, such as isocarboxazid (Marplan tablets), phenelzine sulfate (Nardil), or tranylcypromine sulfate (Parnate tablets); drugs that also inhibit MAO, such as amphetamines, furazolidone (Furoxone), isoniazid (Laniazid), or procarbazine (Matulane capsules): Anchovies, avocados, bananas, beans (broad, fava), beer (including alcohol-free and reduced-alcohol types), caviar, cheese (especially aged, strong, and unpasteurized types), chocolate, sour cream, canned figs, pickled herring, liver, liqueurs, meat extracts, meat prepared with tenderizers, raisins, sauerkraut, sherry, soy sauce, red wine, yeast extract, yogurt. *Can cause hypertensive crisis.*

nifedipine (Procardia XL tablets): Grapefruit juice. *May increase bioavailability and drug levels.*

nitrofurantoin (Macrodantin capsules): Food in general. *Increases drug bioavailability.*

pancrelipase (Cotazym capsules): Food in general. *Dissolves the protective enteric coating.*

pentoxifylline (Trental): Food in general. *Delays drug absorption but does not affect total absorption.*

phenytoin (Dilantin): Enteral tube feedings. *May interfere with the absorption of oral phenytoin. Enteral feedings should be stopped for 2 hours before and 2 hours after administration.*

polyethylene glycol electrolyte solution (GoLYTELY, NuLYTELY): Food in general. *For best results, no solid food should be eaten for 3 to 4 hours before the solution is consumed.*

propafenone hydrochloride (Rythmol): Food in general. *Increased peak blood levels and bioavailability in a single-dose study.*

propranolol hydrochloride (Inderal): Food in general. *May increase the bioavailability of oral propranolol.*

ramipril (Altace): Foods high in potassium. Avoid potassium supplements. Food in general. *Reduces the rate, but not the extent, of drug absorption.*

salsalate (Disalcid, Mono-Gesic, Salflex): Food that lowers urinary pH. *Decreases urinary excretion and increases plasma levels.* Food that raises urinary pH. *Increases renal clearance and urinary excretion of salicylic acid.*

selegiline hydrochloride (Eldepryl): Food with a high concentration of tyramine. *May precipitate hypertensive crisis if the daily dosage exceeds the recommended maximum.*

sodium fluoride (Luride): Dairy products. *Forms calcium fluoride, which is poorly absorbed.*

tetracycline hydrochloride (Achromycin V): Dairy products, food in general. *Interferes with the absorption of oral tetracycline.*

theophylline (Theo-24, Uniphyl): Caffeine-containing beverages, chocolate, cola. *Large quantities increase the adverse effects of theophylline.*

tolmetin sodium (Tolectin): Dairy products. *Decreases total tolmetin bioavailability by 16%.* Food in general. *Decreases total tolmetin bioavailability by 16% and reduces peak plasma levels by 50%.*

trazodone hydrochloride: Food in general. *May affect bioavailability, including the amount of drug absorbed and peak plasma levels.*

triazolam (Halcion): Grapefruit juice. *May increase serum levels.*

verapamil hydrochloride (Calan SR, Isoptin SR): Grapefruit juice. *Increases absorption.*

warfarin sodium (Coumadin, Panwarfin): Diet high in vitamin K. *Decreases prothrombin time.* Charcoal-broiled meats. *May decrease blood drug levels.*

Drug-alcohol interactions

Drug-alcohol interactions are more than just potentiated CNS depression. Combined with NSAIDs, alcohol is highly irritating to the stomach; combined with some diuretics and cardiac medications, it may cause a steep drop in blood pressure.

Compatibility of drugs with tube feedings

Some feeding formulas such as Ensure may break down chemically when combined with a drug such as Dimetapp Elixir. Increased formula viscosity, and a clogged tube, can occur as a result of giving Klorvess or Phenergan syrup with a feeding formula.

Drug preparations, such as ferrous sulfate or potassium chloride liquids, are incompatible with some formulas, causing clumping and other problems when mixed in a tube. Still other combinations may alter the bioavailability of some drugs, such as phenytoin.

To avoid problems with incompatibility, follow these guidelines:
• Never add a drug to a feeding formula container.
• Always check the compatibility of an ordered drug and the feeding formula before administering.
• Infuse 30 ml of water before and after giving a single drug dose through the tube.

• Flush the feeding tube with 5 ml of water between drug doses if you are giving more than one drug.
• Dilute highly concentrated liquids with 60 ml of water before administering them.
• Instill drugs in liquid form when possible. If you must crush a tablet, crush it into fine dust and dissolve it in warm water. (Never crush and liquefy enteric-coated tablets or timed-release capsules.)
• Time the intervals for drug and formula administration appropriately. You may need to withhold tube feeding and supply medication by mouth to an empty stomach or with food.

(Text continues on page 642.)

Effects of mixing drugs and alcohol

Drug	Effects
• Analgesics • Anxiolytics • Antidepressants • Antihistamines • Antipsychotics • Hypnotics	Deepened central nervous system (CNS) depression
• Monoamine oxidase inhibitors	Deepened CNS depression; possible hypertensive crisis with certain types of beer and wine that contain tyramine (Chianti, Alicante)
• Oral antidiabetics	Disulfiram-like effects (facial flushing, headache), especially with chlorpropamide; inadequate food intake may trigger increased antidiabetic activity.
• Cephalosporins • metronidazole • disulfiram	Facial flushing, headache

Drug interference with test results

Drugs can interfere with the results of blood or urine tests in two ways. A drug in a blood or urine specimen may interact with the chemicals used in the laboratory test, causing a false result. Alternatively, a drug may cause a physiologic change in the patient, resulting in an actual increase or decrease in the blood or urine level of the substance being tested. This chart identifies drugs that can cause these two types of interference in common blood and urine tests.

Test and drugs that cause chemical interference	Drugs that cause physiologic interference	
	Increase test values	*Decrease test values*
Alkaline phosphatase • albumin • Fluorides	• Anticonvulsants • Hepatotoxic drugs • ticlopidine	• clofibrate • Estrogens • prednisone • vitamin D
Ammonia, blood	• acetazolamide • ammonium chloride • asparaginase • Barbiturates • Diuretics, loop and thiazide • ethanol	• kanamycin, oral • lactulose • neomycin, oral • Potassium salts • Tetracyclines
Amylase, serum • Chloride salts • Fluorides	• asparaginase • Cholinergic agents • Contraceptives, hormonal • contrast media with iodine • Drugs that induce acute pancreatitis: azathioprine, corticosteroids, loop and thiazide diuretics • methyldopa • Opioids	• somatostatin • zidovudine
Aspartate aminotransferase • erythromycin • methyldopa	• Cholinergic agents • Hepatotoxic drugs • Opium alkaloids	• interferon • naltrexone • prednisone
Bilirubin, serum • ascorbic acid • dextran • epinephrine • pindolol • propranolol • levodopa • theophylline	• Hemolytic agents • Hepatotoxic drugs • methyldopa • rifampin	• Barbiturates • Sulfonamides • theophylline

(continued)

Drug interference with test results *(continued)*

Test and drugs that cause chemical interference	Drugs that cause physiologic interference	
	Increase test values	*Decrease test values*
Blood urea nitrogen • chloral hydrate • chloramphenicol • streptomycin	• Angiotensin-converting enzyme (ACE) inhibitors • Anabolic steroids • Nephrotoxic drugs • pentamidine	• amikacin • levodopa • streptomycin
Calcium, serum • aspirin • heparin • hydralazine • sulfisoxazole	• Calcium salts • Diuretics, loop and thiazide • lithium • Thyroid hormones • vitamin D • Anabolic steroids	• acetazolamide • Anticonvulsants • calcitonin • cisplatin • Contraceptives, hormonal • Corticosteroids • Laxatives • Magnesium salts • plicamycin
Chloride, serum	• acetazolamide • Androgens • Estrogens • Nonsteroidal anti-inflammatory drugs (NSAIDs)	• Corticosteroids • Diuretics, loop and thiazide • Laxatives
Cholesterol, serum • Androgens • aspirin • Corticosteroids • Nitrates • Phenothiazines • vitamin D	• alcohol • Beta-adrenergic blockers • Contraceptives, hormonal • Corticosteroids • cyclosporine • Diuretics, thiazide • Phenothiazines • Sulfonamides • ticlopidine	• Androgens • captopril • chlorpropamide • cholestyramine • clofibrate • colestipol • haloperidol • neomycin, oral
Creatine kinase	• aminocaproic acid • amphotericin B • chlorthalidone • ethanol (long-term use) • gemfibrozil	• aspirin • amikacin • calcium • prednisone

Drug interference with test results *(continued)*

Test and drugs that cause chemical interference	Drugs that cause physiologic interference	
	Increase test values	*Decrease test values*
Creatinine, serum • cefoxitin • cephalothin • flucytosine	• cimetidine • flucytosine • Nephrotoxic drugs	• amikacin • captopril • ibuprofen • prednisone
Glucose, serum • acetaminophen • ascorbic acid (urine) • Cephalosporins (urine)	• Antidepressants, tricyclic • Beta-adrenergic blockers • Corticosteroids • cyclosporine • dextrothyroxine • diazoxide • Diuretics, loop and thiazide • epinephrine • Estrogens • isoniazid • lithium • Phenothiazines • phenytoin • Salicylates • somatostatin	• acetaminophen • Anabolic steroids • clofibrate • disopyramide • ethanol • gemfibrozil • Monoamine oxidase inhibitors • pentamidine
Magnesium, serum	• lithium • Magnesium salts	• albuterol • Aminoglycosides • amphotericin B • Calcium salts • cisplatin • Cardiac glycosides • Diuretics, loop and thiazide • ethanol
Phosphates, serum	• Anabolic steroids • aspirin • vitamin D (excessive amounts)	• Antacids, phosphate-binding • lithium • mannitol

(continued)

Drug interference with test results *(continued)*

Test and drugs that cause chemical interference	Drugs that cause physiologic interference	
	Increase test values	*Decrease test values*
Potassium, serum	• aminocaproic acid • ACE inhibitors • Antineoplastics • cyclosporine • Diuretics, potassium-sparing • isoniazid • lithium • mannitol • succinylcholine	• Aminoglycosides • ammonium chloride • amphotericin B • Corticosteroids • Diuretics, potassium wasting • glucose • insulin • Laxatives • Penicillins, extended spectrum • Salicylates
Protein, serum	• Anabolic steroids • Corticosteroids • phenazopyridine	• Contraceptives, hormonal • Estrogens • Hepatotoxic drugs
Protein, urine • Aminoglycosides • Cephalosporins • contrast media • magnesium sulfate • miconazole • nafcillin • phenazopyridine • Sulfonamides • tolbutamide • tolmetin	• ACE inhibitors • Cephalosporins • contrast media with iodine • Corticosteroids • nafcillin • Nephrotoxic drugs • Sulfonamides	• Not applicable

Drug interference with test results *(continued)*

Test and drugs that cause chemical interference	Drugs that cause physiologic interference	
	Increase test values	*Decrease test values*
Prothrombin time	• Anticoagulants • asparaginase • aspirin • azathioprine • Certain cephalosporins • chloramphenicol • cholestyramine • colestipol • cyclophosphamide • Hepatotoxic drugs • propylthiouracil • quinidine • quinine • Sulfonamides	• Anabolic steroids • Contraceptives, hormonal • Estrogens • vitamin K
Sodium, serum	• carbamazepine • clonidine • diazoxide • Estrogens • guanabenz • guanadrel • guanethidine • methyldopa • NSAIDs	• ammonium chloride • carbamazepine • desmopressin • Diuretics • lithium • lypressin • vasopressin • vincristine
Uric acid, serum • ascorbic acid • caffeine • hydralazine • isoniazid • levodopa • theophylline	• acetazolamide • cisplatin • cyclosporine • diazoxide • Diuretics • epinephrine • ethambutol • ethanol • levodopa • niacin • phenytoin • propranolol • spironolactone	• acetohexamide • allopurinol • clofibrate • contrast media with iodine • diflunisal • Glucose infusions • guaifenesin • Phenothiazines • Salicylates (small doses) • Uricosuric agents

Drug-herb interactions

The use of herbs is becoming more prevalent. It is important to ask the patient if he or she is using any herbs. Certain herb and drug combinations have potential adverse effects. Monitor the patient closely and watch for possible effects.

Herb	Drug	Possible effect
alfalfa	warfarin	Increased risk of bleeding
	chlorpromazine	Increased photosensitivity
	Antidiabetic medications	Increased risk of hypoglycemia
	Hormonal contraceptives	Decreased effectiveness
aloe	Cardiac glycosides, antiarrhythmics	May lead to hypokalemia, which may potentiate cardiac glycosides and antiarrhythmics
	Thiazide diuretics, licorice, and other potassium-wasting drugs	Increases the effects of potassium wasting with thiazide diuretics and other potassium-wasting drugs
	Orally administered drugs	May decrease the absorption of drugs because gastrointestinal (GI) transit time is more rapid
basil	Antidiabetic medications	Increased risk of hypoglycemia
bee pollen	Antidiabetic medications	Increased risk of hyperglycemia
bilberry	Anticoagulants	Increased risk of bleeding
	Alcohol	Disulfiram-like reaction
black cohosh root	Sedatives, antihypertensives, anesthetics	Decrease blood pressure
	Immunosuppressants	Increased risk of fungal infection
capsicum	Antiplatelets, anticoagulants	Decreases platelet aggregation and increases fibrinolytic activity, prolonging bleeding time
	Nonsteroidal anti-inflammatory drugs (NSAIDs)	Stimulates GI secretions to help protect against NSAID-induced GI irritation

Drug-herb interactions (continued)

Herb	Drug	Possible effect
capsicum (continued)	Angiotensin-converting enzyme inhibitors	May cause cough
	theophylline	Increases the absorption of theophylline, possibly leading to higher serum levels or toxicity
	Monoamine oxidase (MAO) inhibitors	Decreases the effects of MAO inhibitors as a result of increased catecholamine secretion
	Central nervous system (CNS) depressants (such as opioids, benzodiazepines, or barbiturates)	Increases the sedative effect
	Histamine-2 (H_2) blockers, proton pump inhibitors	May decrease effectiveness because of increased acid secretion
chamomile	Drugs that require GI absorption	May delay drug absorption
	Anticoagulants	May enhance anticoagulant therapy and prolong bleeding time
	iron	May reduce iron absorption because of the tannic acid content
chondroitin	Anticoagulants	Increased risk of bleeding
echinacea	Immunosuppressants	May counteract immunosuppressant drugs
	Hepatotoxics	May increase hepatotoxicity with drugs that elevate liver enzyme levels
	warfarin	Increases bleeding time without an increased international normalized ratio (INR)
evening primrose	Anticonvulsants	Lowers the seizure threshold
feverfew	Antiplatelets, anticoagulants	May decrease platelet aggregation and increase fibrinolytic activity
	methysergide	May potentiate methysergide

(continued)

Drug-herb interactions *(continued)*

Herb	Drug	Possible effect
garlic	Antiplatelets, anticoagulants	Enhances platelet inhibition, leading to increased anticoagulation
	insulin, other drugs that cause hypoglycemia	May increase serum insulin levels, causing hypoglycemia, an additive effect with antidiabetics
	Antihypertensives	May increase hypotension
	Antihyperlipidemics	May have additive lipid-lowering properties
ginger	Chemotherapeutic drugs	May reduce nausea associated with chemotherapy
	H_2 blockers, proton pump inhibitors	May decrease effectiveness because of increased acid secretion by ginger
	Antiplatelets, anticoagulants	Inhibits platelet aggregation by antagonizing thromboxane synthase and enhancing prostacyclin, leading to prolonged bleeding time
	Calcium channel blockers	May increase calcium uptake by myocardium, leading to altered drug effects
	Antihypertensives	May antagonize the antihypertensive effect
ginkgo	Antiplatelets, anticoagulants	May enhance platelet inhibition, leading to increased anticoagulation
	Anticonvulsants	May decrease the effectiveness of anticonvulsants
	Drugs that lower the seizure threshold	May further reduce the seizure threshold
ginseng	Stimulants	May potentiate the stimulant effects
	warfarin	May antagonize warfarin, resulting in a decreased INR
	Antibiotics	May enhance the effects of some antibiotics (Siberian ginseng)

Drug-herb interactions (continued)

Herb	Drug	Possible effect
ginseng (continued)	Anticoagulants, antiplatelets	Decreases platelet adhesiveness
	digoxin	May falsely elevate digoxin levels
	MAO inhibitors	Potentiates the action of MAO inhibitors
	Hormones, anabolic steroids	May potentiate the effects of hormone and anabolic steroid therapies (Estrogenic effects of ginseng may cause vaginal bleeding and breast nodules.)
	alcohol	Increases alcohol clearance, possibly by increasing the activity of alcohol dehydrogenase
	furosemide	May decrease the diuretic effect of furosemide
	Antipsychotics	May stimulate CNS activity
goldenseal	Antidiabetic agents	May alter glucose regulation
	heparin	May counteract the anticoagulant effect of heparin
	Diuretics	Increases the diuretic effect
	H_2 blockers, proton pump inhibitors	May decrease effectiveness because of increased acid secretion by goldenseal
	General anesthetics	May potentiate the hypotensive action of general anesthetics
	CNS depressants (such as opioids, barbiturates, or benzodiazepines)	Increases the sedative effect
glucosamine	insulin and antidiabetic agents	Insulin and oral antidiabetic agents may be less effective
grapeseed	warfarin	Increases the effects and the INR as a result of the tocopherol content of grapeseed
green tea	warfarin	Decreases effectiveness as a result of the vitamin content of green tea

(continued)

Drug-herb interactions *(continued)*

Herb	Drug	Possible effect
hawthorn berry	digoxin	Causes an additive positive inotropic effect, with the potential for digoxin toxicity
kava	CNS stimulants or depressants	May interfere with CNS stimulant therapy
	Benzodiazepines	May result in coma-like states
	alcohol, other CNS depressants	Potentiates the depressant effect of alcohol and other CNS depressants
	levodopa	Decreases the effectiveness of levodopa
licorice	digoxin	Causes hypokalemia, which predisposes the patient to digoxin toxicity
	Hormonal contraceptives	Increases fluid retention and the potential for increased blood pressure as a result of fluid overload
	Corticosteroids	Causes additive and enhanced effects of corticosteroids
	spironolactone	Decreases the effects of spironolactone
melatonin	CNS depressants (such as opioids, barbiturates, or benzodiazepines)	Increases the sedative effect
milk thistle	Drugs that cause diarrhea	Increases bile secretion and commonly causes loose stools; may increase the effects of other drugs that commonly cause diarrhea; also causes liver membrane stabilization and antioxidant effects, leading to protection from liver damage from various hepatotoxic drugs, such as acetaminophen, phenytoin, ethanol, phenothiazines, and butyrophenones
nettle	Anticonvulsants	May increase sedative adverse effects and the risk of seizure
	Opioids, anxiolytics, hypnotics	May increase sedative adverse effects

Drug-herb interactions *(continued)*

Herb	Drug	Possible effect
nettle *(continued)*	warfarin	Decreases effectiveness as a result of the vitamin K content of the aerial parts of nettle
	iron	May reduce iron absorption because of the tannic acid content
passionflower	CNS depressants (such as opioids, barbiturates, or benzodiazepines)	Increases the sedative effect
St. John's wort	Selective serotonin reuptake inhibitors (SSRIs), MAO inhibitors, nefazodone, trazodone	Causes additive effects with SSRIs, MAO inhibitors, and other antidepressants, potentially leading to serotonin syndrome, especially when combined with SSRIs
	indinavir; HIV protease inhibitors (PIs); nonnucleoside reverse transcriptase inhibitors (NNRTIs)	Induces the cytochrome P450 metabolic pathway, which may decrease the therapeutic effects of drugs that use this pathway for metabolism (Use of St. John's wort and PIs or NNRTIs should be avoided because of the potential for subtherapeutic antiretroviral levels and insufficient virologic response that could lead to resistance or class cross-resistance.)
	Opioids, alcohol	Enhances the sedative effects of opioids and alcohol
	Photosensitizing drugs	Increases photosensitivity
	Sympathomimetic amines (such as pseudoephedrine)	Causes additive effects
	digoxin	May reduce serum digoxin concentrations, decreasing the therapeutic effects
	reserpine	Antagonizes the effects of reserpine
	Hormonal contraceptives	Increases breakthrough bleeding when taken with hormonal contraceptives; also decreases the effectiveness of the contraceptive

(continued)

Drug-herb interactions *(continued)*

Herb	Drug	Possible effect
St. John's wort *(continued)*	theophylline	May decrease serum theophylline levels, making the drug less effective
	Anesthetics	May prolong the effect of anesthetic drugs
	cyclosporine	Decreases cyclosporine levels to less than therapeutic levels, threatening the rejection of transplanted organs
	iron	May reduce iron absorption because of the tannic acid content
	warfarin	May alter the INR; reduces the effectiveness of anticoagulant, requiring increased dosage of the drug
valerian	Sedative hypnotics, CNS depressants	Enhances the effects of sedative hypnotic drugs
	alcohol	Increases sedation with alcohol (although this is debated)
	iron	May reduce iron absorption because of the tannic acid content

Monitoring patients using herbs

Altered laboratory values and changes in a patient's condition can help target your assessments and better meet the needs of a patient who uses herbs.

Herb	What to monitor	Explanation
aloe	• Serum electrolyte level • Weight pattern • Blood urea nitrogen (BUN) and creatinine levels • Heart rate • Blood pressure • Urinalysis	Aloe has cathartic properties that inhibit water and electrolyte reabsorption, which may lead to potassium depletion, weight loss, and diarrhea. Long-term use may lead to nephritis, albuminuria, hematuria, and cardiac disturbances.
capsicum	• Liver function • BUN and creatinine levels	Oral administration of capsicum may lead to gastroenteritis and hepatic or renal damage.
cat's claw	• Blood pressure • Lipid panel • Serum electrolyte level	Cat's claw may cause hypotension through inhibition of the sympathetic nervous system and its diuretic properties. It may also lower the cholesterol level.
chamomile (German, Roman)	• Menstrual changes • Pregnancy • Prothrombin time (PT) and partial thromboplastin time (PTT)	Chamomile may cause changes in the menstrual cycle and is a known teratogen in animals. It also enhances the effects of anticoagulants, making chamomile unsafe to use with these drugs.
echinacea	• Temperature	When echinacea is used parenterally, dose-dependent, short-term fever, nausea, and vomiting can occur.
evening primrose	• Pregnancy • Complete blood count (CBC) • Lipid profile	Evening primrose elevates plasma lipid levels and reduces platelet aggregation. It may increase the risk of pregnancy complications, including premature rupture of the membranes, the need for oxytocin augmentation, arrest of descent, and the need for vacuum extraction.
fennel	• Liver function • Blood pressure • Serum calcium level • Blood glucose level	Fennel contains trans-anethole and estragole. Trans-anethole has estrogenic activity, and estragole is a procarcinogen that can cause liver damage. Adverse effects include photodermatitis and allergic reactions, particularly in patients who are sensitive to carrots, celery, and mugwort.

(continued)

Monitoring patients using herbs *(continued)*

Herb	What to monitor	Explanation
feverfew	• CBC • Pregnancy • Sleep pattern	Feverfew may inhibit blood platelet aggregation and decrease neutrophil and platelet secretory activity. It can cause uterine contractions in full-term, pregnant women. Adverse effects include mouth ulceration, tongue irritation and inflammation, abdominal pain, indigestion, diarrhea, flatulence, nausea, and vomiting. Post-feverfew syndrome includes nervousness, headache, insomnia, joint pain, stiffness, and fatigue.
flaxseed	• Lipid panel • Blood pressure • Serum calcium level • Blood glucose level • Liver function	Flaxseed has weak estrogenic and antiestrogenic activity. It may reduce platelet aggregation and the serum cholesterol level. Oral administration with inadequate fluid intake can cause intestinal blockage.
garlic	• Blood pressure • Lipid panel • Blood glucose level • CBC • PT and PTT	Garlic is associated with hypotension, leukocytosis, inhibition of platelet aggregation, and decreased blood glucose and cholesterol levels. Postoperative bleeding and prolonged bleeding time can occur.
ginger	• Blood glucose level • Blood pressure • Heart rate • Respiratory rate • Lipid panel • Electrocardiogram	Ginger contains gingerols, which have positive inotropic properties. Adverse effects include platelet inhibition, hypoglycemia, hypotension, hypertension, and stimulation of respiratory centers. Overdoses cause central nervous system (CNS) depression and arrhythmias.
ginkgo	• Respiratory rate • Heart rate • PT and PTT	Consumption of ginkgo seed may cause difficulty breathing, weak pulse, seizures, loss of consciousness, and shock. Ginkgo leaf is associated with infertility as well as gastrointestinal (GI) upset, headache, dizziness, palpitations, restlessness, lack of muscle tone, weakness, bleeding, subdural hematoma, subarachnoid hemorrhage, and a bleeding iris.

Monitoring patients using herbs (continued)

Herb	What to monitor	Explanation
ginseng (American, Panax, Siberian)	• BUN and creatinine levels • Blood pressure • Serum electrolyte levels • Liver function • Serum calcium level • Blood glucose level • Heart rate • Sleep pattern • Menstrual changes • Weight pattern • PT, PTT, and international normalized ratio (INR)	Ginseng contains ginsenosides and eleutherosides that can affect blood pressure, CNS activity, platelet aggregation, and coagulation. Reduced glucose and glycosylated hemoglobin levels have also been reported. Adverse effects include drowsiness, mastalgia, vaginal bleeding, tachycardia, mania, cerebral arteritis, Stevens-Johnson syndrome, cholestatic hepatitis, amenorrhea, decreased appetite, diarrhea, edema, hyperpyrexia, pruritus, hypotension, palpitations, headache, vertigo, euphoria, and neonatal death.
goldenseal	• Respiratory rate • Heart rate • Blood pressure • Liver function • Mood pattern	Goldenseal contains berberine and hydrastine. Berberine improves bile secretion, increases coronary blood flow, and stimulates or inhibits cardiac activity. Hydrastine causes hypotension, hypertension, increased cardiac output, exaggerated reflexes, seizures, paralysis, and death as a result of respiratory failure. Other adverse effects include GI upset and constipation, excitatory states, hallucinations, delirium, nervousness, depression, dyspnea, and bradycardia.
kava	• Weight pattern • Lipid panel • CBC • Blood pressure • Liver function • Urinalysis • Mood changes	Kava contains arylethylene pyrone constituents that have CNS activity. It also has antianxiety effects. Long-term use may lead to weight loss, increased high-density lipoprotein cholesterol levels, hematuria, increased red blood cell count, decreased platelet count, decreased lymphocyte levels, reduced protein levels, and pulmonary hypertension.
milk thistle	• Liver function	Milk thistle contains flavonolignans, which have liver protective and antioxidant effects.

(continued)

Monitoring patients using herbs (continued)

Herb	What to monitor	Explanation
nettle	• Blood glucose level • Blood pressure • Weight pattern • BUN and creatinine levels • Serum electrolyte level • Heart rate • PT and INR	Nettle contains significant amounts of vitamin C, vitamin K, potassium, and calcium. Nettle may cause hyperglycemia, decreased blood pressure, decreased heart rate, weight loss, and diuretic effects.
passionflower	• Liver function • Amylase level • Lipase level	Passionflower may contain cyanogenic glycosides, which can cause liver and pancreas toxicity.
St. John's wort	• Vision • Menstrual changes • Excessive response to other medications administered concomitantly	St. John's wort may cause changes in menstrual bleeding and reduced fertility. Other adverse effects include GI upset, fatigue, dry mouth, dizziness, headache, delayed hypersensitivity, phototoxicity, and neuropathy. St. John's wort may also increase the risk of cataracts. St John's wort interferes with the metabolism of many drugs.
saw palmetto	• Liver function	Saw palmetto inhibits the conversion of testosterone to dihydrotestosterone and may inhibit growth factors. Adverse effects include cholestatic hepatitis, erectile or ejaculatory dysfunction, and altered libido.

Drug additives

Drugs with ethanol additives

Many oral liquid drug preparations contain ethanol, which produces a slight sedative effect but is not harmful to most patients and can in fact be beneficial. However, ingesting ethanol can be undesirable and even dangerous in some circumstances. The following list identifies generic drugs that commonly contain ethanol. (Note that some manufacturers of these drugs also produce ethanol-free [alcohol-free] formulations. Check with the pharmacist for more information.)

- acetaminophen, acetaminophen with codeine elixir
- bitolterol mesylate
- brompheniramine maleate elixir
- butabarbital sodium
- chlorpheniramine maleate elixir
- chlorpromazine hydrochloride
- clemastine fumarate
- co-trimoxazole
- cyproheptadine hydrochloride
- dexchlorpheniramine maleate

- dextroamphetamine sulfate
- diazepam
- diazoxide
- digoxin
- dihydroergotamine mesylate injection
- diphenhydramine hydrochloride
- epinephrine
- ergoloid mesylates
- esmolol hydrochloride
- ferrous sulfate elixirs
- fluphenazine hydrochloride
- hydromorphone hydrochloride cough syrup
- hyoscyamine sulfate
- indomethacin suspension
- isoproterenol hydrochloride
- methadone hydrochloride oral solution
- methyldopa suspension
- minocycline hydrochloride
- molindone hydrochloride
- nitroglycerin infusion
- nystatin
- opium alkaloids hydrochlorides
- oxycodone hydrochloride
- paramethadione
- pentobarbital sodium elixir, pentobarbital sodium injection
- perphenazine
- phenobarbital injection
- phenytoin sodium injection
- promethazine hydrochloride
- pyridostigmine bromide
- thioridazine hydrochloride

Drugs with sulfite additives

Used as a drug preservative, sulfites can cause allergic reactions in certain patients. The following list identifies generic drugs that commonly contain sulfites. (A pharmacist can provide definitive information on brand name drugs.)

- amikacin sulfate
- amrinone lactate
- atropine sulfate with meperidine hydrochloride
- bupivacaine hydrochloride and epinephrine 1:200,000

- chlorpromazine, chlorpromazine hydrochloride
- dexamethasone acetate, dexamethasone sodium phosphate
- dobutamine hydrochloride
- dopamine hydrochloride
- epinephrine, epinephrine bitartrate, epinephrine bitartrate with pilocarpine hydrochloride, epinephrine hydrochloride
- etidocaine hydrochloride with epinephrine bitartrate 1:200,000
- heparin calcium, heparin sodium
- hyoscyamine sulfate
- isoproterenol hydrochloride, isoproterenol sulfate
- lidocaine hydrochloride with epinephrine hydrochloride
- mafenide acetate
- methotrimeprazine hydrochloride
- orphenadrine citrate, orphenadrine hydrochloride
- oxycodone hydrochloride with acetaminophen
- theophylline
- thiethylperazine maleate
- tinzaparin sodium

Drugs with tartrazine additives

Also known as FD&C Yellow No. 5, tartrazine is a dye that is used as an additive in certain drugs. It can provoke a severe allergic reaction in some people, especially those who are also allergic to aspirin. However, not all dosage forms contain the dye. If you or the patient is concerned about tartrazine additives, consult with the pharmacist.

How aging increases the risk of drug hazards

The physiologic changes associated with aging make older adults more susceptible than younger adults to drug-induced illnesses, adverse effects, toxicity, and interactions. Other conditions that are common to older adults also increase the risk of these problems.

To help prevent these problems or detect them early, check the patient's history for the following risk factors when developing a teaching plan:

- altered mental status
- financial problems
- frail health
- history of allergies
- history of previous adverse effects
- multiple chronic illnesses
- female gender
- living alone
- polypharmacy or complex medication regimen
- poor nutritional status
- renal failure

- small frame
- treatment by several physicians.

Substance abuse

Acute toxic reactions

Treatment of substance abuse is a long-term process that is often beset with relapses. You must understand the signs and symptoms of a toxic reaction before you can take steps to help the patient recover from his or her addiction.

Managing acute toxicity

Substance	Signs and symptoms	Interventions
alcohol (ethanol) • Beer and wine • Distilled spirits • Other preparations, such as cough syrup, aftershave, or mouthwash	• Ataxia • Seizures • Coma • Hypothermia • Alcohol breath odor • Respiratory depression • Bradycardia or tachycardia • Hypotension • Nausea and vomiting	• Induce vomiting or perform gastric lavage if ingestion occurred in the previous 4 hours. Give activated charcoal and a saline cathartic. • Start I.V. fluid replacement and administer dextrose 5% in water, thiamine, B complex vitamins, and vitamin C to prevent dehydration and hypoglycemia and correct nutritional deficiencies. Monitor the magnesium level. • Pad the bed rails and apply cloth restraints to protect the patient from injury. • Give an anticonvulsant such as diazepam to control seizures. • Watch the patient for signs and symptoms of withdrawal, such as hallucinations and alcohol withdrawal delirium. If these occur, consider giving chlordiazepoxide or benzodiazepines. • Auscultate the patient's lungs frequently to detect crackles or rhonchi, which may indicate aspiration pneumonia. If you note these breath sounds, consider antibiotics. • Monitor the patient's neurologic status and vital signs every 15 minutes until his or her condition is stable. Assist with dialysis if his or her vital functions are severely depressed.

Managing acute toxicity *(continued)*

Substance	Signs and symptoms	Interventions
Amphetamines • Amphetamine sulfate (Benzedrine): bennies, greenies, cartwheels • Dextroamphetamine sulfate (Dexedrine): dexies, hearts, oranges • Methamphetamine: speed, meth, crystal	• Dilated reactive pupils • Altered mental status (from confusion to paranoia) • Hallucinations • Tremors and seizure activity • Hyperactive deep tendon reflexes • Exhaustion • Coma • Dry mouth • Shallow respirations • Tachycardia • Hypertension • Hyperthermia • Diaphoresis	• If the drug was taken orally, induce vomiting or perform gastric lavage; give activated charcoal and a sodium or magnesium sulfate cathartic. • Lower the patient's urine pH to 5 by adding ammonium chloride or ascorbic acid to his or her I.V. solution. • Force diuresis by giving the patient mannitol. • Give a short-acting barbiturate such as pentobarbital to control stimulant-induced seizures. • Place the patient in a protective environment, especially if he or she is paranoid or hallucinating, so he or she does not injure himself or herself or others. • Give haloperidol I.M. or I.V. to treat agitation or assaultive behavior. • Give an alpha-adrenergic blocker such as phentolamine for hypertension. • Watch the patient for cardiac arrhythmias. If these develop, consider propranolol or lidocaine to treat tachyarrhythmias or ventricular arrhythmias, respectively. • Treat hyperthermia with tepid sponge baths or a hypothermia blanket. • Provide a quiet environment to avoid overstimulation. • Be alert for signs and symptoms of withdrawal, such as abdominal tenderness, muscle aches, and long periods of sleep. • Observe suicide precautions, especially if the patient shows signs of withdrawal.

(continued)

Managing acute toxicity *(continued)*

Substance	Signs and symptoms	Interventions
Antipsychotics • Chlorpromazine (Thorazine) • Phenothiazines • Thioridazine (Mellaril)	• Constricted pupils • Photosensitivity • Extrapyramidal effects (dyskinesia, opisthotonos, muscle rigidity, ocular deviation) • Dry mouth • Decreased level of consciousness (LOC) • Decreased deep tendon reflexes • Seizures • Hypothermia or hyperthermia • Dysphagia • Respiratory depression • Hypotension • Tachycardia	• Expect to perform gastric lavage if the patient ingested the drug within the previous 6 hours. (Do not induce vomiting because phenothiazines have an antiemetic effect.) Consider activated charcoal and a cathartic. • Give diphenhydramine to treat extrapyramidal effects. • Give physostigmine salicylate to reverse anticholinergic effects in severe cases. • Replace fluids I.V. to correct hypotension; monitor the patient's vital signs often. • Monitor the patient's respiratory rate and give supplemental oxygen to treat respiratory depression. • Give an anticonvulsant such as diazepam or a short-acting barbiturate such as pentobarbital sodium to control seizures. • Keep the patient's room dark to avoid exacerbating photosensitivity.
Anxiolytic sedative-hypnotics • Benzodiazepines (Ativan, Valium, Librium, Xanax)	• Confusion • Drowsiness • Stupor • Decreased reflexes • Seizures • Coma • Shallow respirations • Hypotension	• Induce vomiting or perform gastric lavage; consider activated charcoal and a cathartic. • Give supplemental oxygen to correct hypoxia-induced seizures and insert an endotracheal tube, if necessary. • Replace fluids I.V. to correct hypotension; monitor the patient's vital signs often. • For benzodiazepine overdose or to reverse the effect of benzodiazepine-induced sedation or respiratory depression, give flumazenil (Romazicon).

Managing acute toxicity *(continued)*

Substance	Signs and symptoms	Interventions
Barbiturate sedative-hypnotics • Amobarbital sodium (Amytal): blue angels, blue devils, blue birds • Phenobarbital (Luminal): phennies, purple hearts, goofballs • Secobarbital sodium (Seconal): reds, red devils	• Poor pupillary reaction to light • Nystagmus • Depressed LOC (from confusion to coma) • Flaccid muscles and absent reflexes • Hyperthermia or hypothermia • Cyanosis • Respiratory depression • Hypotension • Blisters or bullous lesions	• Induce vomiting or perform gastric lavage if the patient ingested the drug within the previous 4 hours; consider activated charcoal and a saline cathartic. • Maintain the patient's blood pressure with I.V. fluid challenges and vasopressors. • If the patient took an overdose of phenobarbital, give him or her sodium bicarbonate I.V. to alkalinize his or her urine and speed elimination of the drug. • Maintain the patient's airway and monitor his or her respiratory status. • Apply a hyperthermia or hypothermia blanket to help return the patient's temperature to normal. • Prepare the patient for hemodialysis or hemoperfusion if the toxic reaction is severe. • Perform frequent neurologic assessments and check the patient's pulse rate, temperature, skin color, and reflexes often. • Notify the physician if you see signs of respiratory distress or pulmonary edema. • Watch the patient for signs and symptoms of withdrawal, such as hyperreflexia, tonic-clonic seizures, and hallucinations. Provide symptomatic relief of withdrawal symptoms. • Protect the patient from injuring himself or herself.

(continued)

Managing acute toxicity (continued)

Substance	Signs and symptoms	Interventions
Cocaine • Cocaine hydrochloride: crack, freebase	• Dilated pupils • Confusion • Alternating euphoria and apprehension • Hyperexcitability • Visual, auditory, and olfactory hallucinations • Spasms and seizures • Coma • Tachypnea • Hyperpnea • Pallor or cyanosis • Respiratory arrest • Tachycardia • Hypertension or hypotension • Fever • Nausea and vomiting • Abdominal pain • Perforated nasal septum or mouth sores	• Maintain the patient's airway and monitor his or her respiratory status. • Calm the patient by talking to him or her in a quiet room. • If the patient ingested cocaine, induce vomiting or perform gastric lavage; give activated charcoal followed by a saline cathartic. • Give the patient a tepid sponge bath and administer an antipyretic to reduce fever. • Monitor his or her blood pressure and heart rate. Expect to give propranolol for symptomatic tachycardia. • Administer an anticonvulsant such as diazepam to control seizures. • Scrape the inside of his or her nose to remove residual amounts of the drug. • Monitor the patient's cardiac rate and rhythm. Ventricular fibrillation and cardiac standstill can occur as a direct cardiotoxic result of cocaine ingestion. Defibrillate the patient and initiate cardiopulmonary resuscitation, if indicated.
Hallucinogens • Lysergic acid diethylamide (LSD): hawk, acid, sunshine • Mescaline (peyote): mese, cactus, big chief	• Dilated pupils • Intensified perceptions • Agitation and anxiety • Synesthesia • Impaired judgment • Hyperactive movement • Flashbacks • Hallucinations • Depersonalization • Moderately increased blood pressure • Increased heart rate • Fever	• Reorient the patient repeatedly to time, place, and person. • Place the patient in a protective environment. • Calm the patient by talking to him or her in a quiet room. • If the drug was taken orally, induce vomiting or perform gastric lavage; give activated charcoal and a cathartic. • Give diazepam I.V. to control seizures.

Managing acute toxicity (continued)

Substance	Signs and symptoms	Interventions
Opioids • Codeine • Heroin: junk, smack, H, snow • Hydromorphone hydrochloride (Dilaudid): D, lords • Morphine: Mort, M, monkey, Emma • Oxycodone (OxyContin): OCs, ox, and oxy	• Constricted pupils • Depressed LOC (although the patient is usually responsive to persistent verbal or tactile stimuli) • Seizures • Hypothermia • Slow, deep respirations • Hypotension • Bradycardia • Skin changes (pruritus, urticaria, flushing)	• Give naloxone until the depressant effects of the drug on the central nervous system are reversed. • Replace fluids I.M. to increase the circulatory volume. • Correct hypothermia by applying extra blankets; if the patient's body temperature does not increase, use a hyperthermia blanket. • Reorient the patient often. • Auscultate the lungs often for crackles, which may indicate pulmonary edema. Onset may be delayed. • Administer oxygen with a nasal cannula, a mask, or mechanical ventilation to correct hypoxemia caused by hypoventilation. • Monitor the patient's cardiac rate and rhythm. Be alert for atrial fibrillation, which should resolve when hypoxemia is corrected. • Watch the patient for signs of withdrawal, such as piloerection (gooseflesh), diaphoresis, and hyperactive bowel sounds. • Institute safety measures to prevent patient injury.

(continued)

Managing acute toxicity *(continued)*

Substance	Signs and symptoms	Interventions
phencyclidine (PCP) • Angel dust, peace pill, hog	• Blank stare • Nystagmus • Amnesia • Decreased awareness of surroundings • Recurrent coma • Violent behavior • Hyperactivity • Seizures • Gait ataxia • Muscle rigidity • Drooling • Hyperthermia • Hypertensive	• If the drug was taken orally, induce vomiting or perform gastric lavage; instill and remove activated charcoal repeatedly. • Acidify the patient's urine with ascorbic acid to increase excretion of the drug. • Expect to continue to acidify the urine for 2 weeks because signs and symptoms may recur when fat cells release PCP stores. • Give diazepam and haloperidol to control agitation or psychotic behavior. • Institute safety measures to protect the patient from injury. • Administer diazepam to control seizures. • Institute seizure precautions. • Provide a quiet environment and dimmed light. • Give propranolol for hypertension and tachycardia and give nitroprusside for severe hypertension. • Closely monitor the patient's urine output and the results of serial renal function tests. Rhabdomyolysis, myoglobinuria, and renal failure may occur in severe intoxication. • If renal failure develops, prepare the patient for hemodialysis.

Selected references

Bond, G. R., Caravati, E. M., Dart, R. C., Heard, K., Hoffman, R. S., Rumarck, B. H., & Snodgrass, W. R. (2015). *Guidelines for the management of acetaminophen overdose.* Retrieved from https://www.tylenolprofessional.com/sites/tylenol_hcp_us/files/acetaminphen_overdose_treatment_info.pdf

Drugs.com. (n.d.). *Isradipine.* Retrieved from https://www.drugs.com/mtm/isradipine.html

Farrell, S., & Defendi, G. (2018). *Acetaminophen toxicity.* Retrieved from https://emedicine.medscape.com/article/820200-overview

Lilley, L. L., Collins, S. R., & Snyder, J. S. (2017). *Pharmacology and the nursing process* (8th ed.). St. Louis, MO: Elsevier.

Nursing 2019 drug handbook. (39th ed.). (2019). Philadelphia, PA: Wolters Kluwer.

O'Malley, G. F., & O'Malley, R. (2018). *Iron poisoning.* Retrieved from https://www.merckmanuals.com/home/injuries-and-poisoning/poisoning/iron-poisoning

Patel, V., & James, A. (2017). *Digitalis toxicity treatment & management.*

Retrieved from https://emedicine
.medscape.com/article/154336-treatment

Ramnarine, M., & Amad, D. A. (2018).
*Anticholinergic toxicity treatment &
management*. Retrieved from https://
emedicine.medscape.com/article
/812644-treatment#d10

Rao, K. (n.d.). *Pharmacotherapy a patho-
physiologic approach*. Retrieved from
https://accesspharmacy.mhmedical.com
/content.aspx?bookid=689&Sectionid
=48811451#57525041

Spanierman, C. (2018). *Iron toxicity*.
Retrieved from https://emedicine
.medscape.com/article/815213
-overview

The Joint Commission. (2017). *Sentinel
event policies and procedures*. Retrieved
from https://www.jointcommission
.org/sentinel_event_policy_and
_procedures/

Tsai, V., & Silverberg, M. A. (2017). *Tricyclic
antidepressant toxicity*. Retrieved
from https://emedicine.medscape.com
/article/819204-overview

U.S. Food and Drug Administration. (2016).
What is a serious drug reaction?

Retrieved from https://www.fda.gov
/Safety/MedWatch/HowToReport
/ucm053087.htm

U.S. Food and Drug Administration. (2018).
*Instructions for completing form FDA
3500*. Retrieved from https://www.fda
.gov/Safety/MedWatch/HowToReport
/DownloadForms/ucm149236.htm

U.S. Food and Drug Administration. (n.d.).
MedWatch voluntary report. Retrieved
from https://www.accessdata.fda.gov
/scripts/medwatch/index.cfm?action
=professional.reporting1

WebMD. (2018). *Caffeine*. Retrieved from
https://www.webmd.com/vitamins/ai
/ingredientmono-979/caffeine

Weigand, T., & Vernetti, C. M. (2017).
*Nonsteroidal anti-inflammatory
drug (NSAID) toxicity*. Retrieved from
https://emedicine.medscape.com
/article/816117-overview

Web sites

Epocrates. (n.d.). https://www.epocrates.com/
Merck Manual: Professional Version. (n.d.).
https://www.merckmanuals.com
/professional

15

Complications

Spotting and correcting life-threatening conditions

Air embolism

Air embolism is the migration of a bolus of gas from the systemic circulation into the microvasculature. Obstruction occurs when the gas reaches the capillary system. Besides impairing blood flow, an air embolus causes a physiologic response as fibrin, platelets, and red blood cells congregate at the site of occlusion. This further restricts blood flow and contributes to an inflammatory vasospasm of the affected vessel.

Arterial air emboli may lodge in the small vessels that supply major organs or the peripheral circulation. Venous air emboli commonly occlude pulmonary blood flow; they may also obstruct arterial circulation if the patient has an intracardiac defect or a microvascular shunt between the arterioles and venules of the lungs.

Causes

A bolus of air may enter the bloodstream during positive-pressure ventilation if the patient has a lung tear or when air enters an artery or vein during insertion, maintenance, or removal of the arterial or venous line. Air emboli have also been associated with oral-vaginal sex, laser surgery, and pneumoperitoneum. They may also occur as a complication of needle biopsy or pregnancy. Air emboli also result from rapid decompression after underwater diving.

Venous air emboli may occur as a complication of surgery or blunt or penetrating trauma to the head, neck, chest, heart, or abdomen.

Signs and symptoms

The first sign of a venous air embolism may be cardiopulmonary collapse, especially in the presence of a rapid infusion of a large volume of air.

If the embolus moves into the arterial circulation, central nervous system (CNS) and cardiac symptoms may develop. The patient may have dyspnea, vertigo, anxiety, or a sense of impending doom. The patient may also experience a "gasp" reflex (cough, short exhalation, and prolonged inhalation).

Other signs include tachycardia, tachypnea, hypoxemia, and elevated central venous and pulmonary artery pressures. Electrocardiogram results show ST-segment changes that reflect ischemia. A transient churning heart murmur has been noted. Hypotension and decreased peripheral vascular resistance indicate progressive shock. Crepitus occasionally is palpable, and wheezes and crackles may be auscultated when pulmonary edema is present.

Treatment

The goal of treatment is to promote reabsorption of trapped air and mitigate life-threatening signs and symptoms. In the event of cardiac arrest, cardiopulmonary resuscitation (CPR) is initiated immediately. External cardiac massage improves circulation and may help break up large right ventricular bubbles, increasing blood flow to the pulmonary vasculature.

An air embolus may be removed through a central venous catheter or by needle aspiration. The size of the bubble may be reduced by administering 100% oxygen, which reduces the amount of nitrogen in the bubble, or by administering hyperbaric oxygen; the latter approach may also improve the patient's signs and symptoms by oxygenating ischemic tissue.

Nursing interventions

- Preventing air embolism is the key to nursing care. Make sure that all air is purged from catheters and I.V. lines before connecting them.
- Keep closed systems as airtight as possible; tape all tubing connections, use Luer Lok devices for all connections, fill tubings completely with solution, and use alarms that detect air on I.V. infusion pumps.

- Place the patient in Trendelenburg's position when inserting all central venous line catheters. Have the patient perform Valsalva's maneuver during catheter insertion and tubing changes.
- Position the patient on his or her left side in Trendelenburg's position so that air can enter the right atrium and be dispersed by the pulmonary artery.
- Initiate CPR immediately if cardiac collapse occurs.

Atelectasis

In atelectasis, alveolar clusters (lobules) or lung segments do not expand completely during respiration, causing all or part of the affected lung to collapse. This condition can be acute or chronic. Because the collapsed lung tissue is effectively isolated from gas exchange, unoxygenated blood is shunted and passes unchanged through these tissues, producing hypoxia.

Causes

Atelectasis can result from bronchial occlusion by mucus plugs—a problem for patients with chronic obstructive pulmonary disease, bronchiectasis, or cystic fibrosis. Atelectasis may also result from occlusion caused by foreign bodies, bronchogenic cancer, or inflammatory lung disease.

Other causes include idiopathic respiratory distress syndrome of the neonate, oxygen toxicity, and pulmonary edema.

External compression, which inhibits full lung expansion, or any condition that makes deep breathing painful may also cause atelectasis. Compression or pain may result from surgical incisions in the upper abdomen, rib fractures, pleuritic chest pain, tight chest dressings, or obesity (which elevates the diaphragm and reduces tidal volume).

Lung collapse or reduced expansion may accompany prolonged immobility or mechanical ventilation. CNS depression eliminates periodic sighing and predisposes the patient to progressive atelectasis.

Signs and symptoms

Clinical effects vary with the causes of lung collapse, the degree of hypoxia, and the underlying disease. If atelectasis affects a small area of the lung, symptoms may be minimal and transient; however, if atelectasis affects a large area, symptoms may be severe and may include dyspnea, tachypnea, tachycardia, anxiety, and pleuritic chest pain.

Inspection may show decreased movement of the chest wall, cyanosis, diaphoresis, and substernal or intercostal retractions. Palpation may show decreased fremitus and a mediastinal shift to the affected side. Percussion may show dullness or flatness over the lung fields. Auscultation may show crackles during the last part of inspiration and decreased (or absent) breath sounds with major lung involvement; auscultation may also disclose tachycardia.

A chest X-ray is the primary diagnostic tool. Other diagnostic tests include bronchoscopy to rule out an obstructing neoplasm or a foreign body; arterial blood gas (ABG) analysis to detect respiratory acidosis and hypoxemia resulting from atelectasis; and pulse oximetry, which may show deteriorating arterial oxygen saturation levels.

Treatment

Incentive spirometry, chest percussion, postural drainage, mucolytics, and frequent coughing and deep-breathing exercises may improve oxygenation. If these measures are unsuccessful, bronchoscopy may help to remove secretions. Humidity and a bronchodilator can improve mucociliary clearance and dilate the airways.

To minimize the risk of atelectasis after thoracic and abdominal surgery, the patient may require an analgesic to facilitate deep breathing. If the patient has atelectasis as a result of an obstructing neoplasm, he or she may need surgery or radiation therapy.

Nursing interventions

- Offer the patient reassurance and emotional support because he or she may be frightened by his or her limited ability to breathe.
- Encourage a patient who is recovering from surgery to perform coughing and deep-breathing exercises and incentive spirometry every 1 to 2 hours while splinting the incision. Encourage these procedures in any patient who is at increased risk for atelectasis.
- Assess the patient's breath sounds and respiratory status frequently. Report changes immediately; monitor pulse oximetry readings and ABG values for evidence of hypoxia.
- Gently reposition the patient often and help him or her walk as soon as possible. Administer adequate analgesics to control pain.
- If the patient is receiving mechanical ventilation, maintain the tidal volume at 10 to 15 cc/kg of body weight to ensure adequate lung expansion. Use the sigh mechanism on the ventilator, if appropriate, to increase the tidal volume intermittently at the rate of 10 to 15 sighs per hour.
- Humidify inspired air and encourage adequate fluid intake to mobilize secretions. Use postural drainage and chest percussion to remove secretions. Suction as needed.
- Administer sedatives cautiously. They depress respirations and the cough reflex and suppress sighs.

Bone marrow suppression

Bone marrow suppression is characterized by reduced numbers of hematopoietic (blood-forming) stem cells in the bone marrow. Impaired hematopoiesis leads to reduced numbers of peripheral blood leukocytes and neutrophils (neutropenia), thrombocytes (thrombocytopenia), and erythrocytes (anemia).

Causes

Many chemotherapeutic agents injure the rapidly proliferating stem cells. Other drugs, such as sulfa compounds, anticonvulsants, and immunosuppressants, also may suppress bone marrow.

Radiation to large marrow-bearing areas—such as the pelvis, ribs, spine, and sternum—may produce significant, permanent bone marrow damage. Bone marrow suppression and depressed peripheral blood cell counts occur in patients with tumor replacement of the bone marrow (leukemia, myeloma, or metastatic deposits from solid tumors). Additional causes of bone marrow suppression include autoimmune disorders; certain congenital disorders; and exposure to pesticides, benzene-containing solvents, and other toxins.

Signs and symptoms

Clinical effects of bone marrow suppression are related to its severity. A patient with neutropenia is at risk for infection from bacteria, viruses, or fungi and may have fever, chills, malaise, or other localized signs of infection.

Thrombocytopenia is associated with bleeding (especially from the gums and nose), bruising, petechiae, ecchymoses, hematuria, and, possibly, hematochezia. Spontaneous bleeding is likely to occur if the platelet count drops below 20,000/mm^3.

Signs and symptoms of anemia include fatigue, weakness, pallor, tachycardia, palpitations, dizziness, exertional dyspnea, and headache.

Treatment

Improved antimicrobial therapy has dramatically reduced the rates of morbidity and mortality in patients with neutropenia. Chemotherapy-induced neutropenia can be reduced by the use of myeloid growth factors (granulocyte colony-stimulating factor [filgrastim] or granulocyte-macrophage colony-stimulating factor [sargramostim]).

In patients with drug-induced thrombocytopenia, removal of the causative agents or proper treatment of the underlying cause (when possible) is essential. A corticosteroid, lithium carbonate, or folate may be used to increase platelet production. Platelet transfusions may be used to stop episodic abnormal bleeding caused by a low platelet count; however, if platelet destruction is caused by an immune disorder, platelet infusions may have only a minimal effect and may be reserved for life-threatening bleeding.

Recombinant erythropoietin may help improve anemia caused by chronic disease or renal dysfunction. Packed red blood cells and platelets are administered to support the patient until bone marrow function recovers.

Nursing interventions

See *Nursing interventions in bone marrow suppression.*

Nursing interventions in bone marrow suppression

This table summarizes the essential nursing interventions for patients who have anemia, neutropenia, or thrombocytopenia.

Conditions	Interventions
Anemia	
(Hemoglobin <14 g/dl in men and boys; <12 g/dl in women and girls) (Severe anemia, hemoglobin <8 g/dl)	• Monitor the patient's complete blood count (CBC) at least daily. • Monitor the patient for signs of inadequate oxygenation, such as pallor, tachypnea, and increased capillary refill time. • Teach the patient about nutritional supplementation (such as iron or folic acid). • Assess the patient for source of blood loss, if applicable. • Teach the patient energy conservation measures. • Teach the patient to avoid driving or participating in hazardous activities if he or she is dizzy. • Teach the patient to change positions slowly to avoid syncope and orthostatic hypotension. • Administer transfusions of packed red blood cells, as ordered. Monitor the patient for transfusion reactions. • Administer recombinant erythropoietin or other blood replacement alternatives, as ordered.

(continued)

Nursing interventions in bone marrow suppression *(continued)*

Conditions	Interventions
Neutropenia (Neutrophil count <1,500/mm^3) (Severe neutropenia, neutrophil count <500/mm^3)	• Monitor the patient's temperature and vital signs. Report fever >101° F (38° C). • Monitor the patient's CBC, differential, and blood chemistry results. • Assess the patient for localized signs of infection. • Assess the patient for symptoms of sepsis. • Obtain cultures of the patient's blood, urine, throat, sputum, and stool, as ordered. Obtain blood cultures if the patient has a temperature spike >101° F (38° C). • Avoid invasive procedures or rectal manipulation. • Avoid contact with persons with viral or bacterial infections. • Administer broad-spectrum antibiotics as indicated. • Explain to the patient or caregiver the rationale for the use of hematopoietic growth factors and demonstrate self-administration, if indicated. • Teach proper storage and precautions for hematopoietic growth factors. • Teach the patient to avoid fresh flowers and to refrain from eating raw fruits and vegetables.
Thrombocytopenia (Platelet count <100,000/mm^3) (Severe thrombocytopenia, platelet count <20,000/mm^3)	• Teach the patient to avoid injury and sharp objects. • Teach the patient to avoid straining and to avoid performing Valsalva's maneuver. • Avoid invasive procedures, such as I.M. injections, enemas, or suppositories. • Apply direct pressure for 5 minutes to needle puncture sites. • Assess the patient for signs of bleeding, increased petechiae, or increased bruising. • Monitor the patient for signs of internal bleeding (such as blood in the stool and hematuria) and signs and symptoms of intracranial bleeding (such as headache, restlessness, decreased level of consciousness, pupillary changes, and seizures). • Administer platelet transfusions, as ordered. • Monitor the patient for transfusion reactions. Check the posttransfusion platelet count.

Brain herniation

Brain herniation is caused by distortion and displacement of brain tissue through a natural opening in the intracranial cavity.

Five types of brain herniation syndrome occur: central, uncal, tonsillar, cingulate, and extracranial. Central herniation—also known as transtentorial herniation—is an upward or downward displacement of the temporal lobe and diencephalon through the tentorium. In uncal herniation, the inner part of the temporal lobe passes the tentorium and presses on the brain stem. In tonsillar herniation, the tonsils of the cerebellum pass down through the foramen magnum and press on the brain stem and spinal cord, possibly causing respiratory and cardiac dysfunction. Cingulate, or subfalcine, herniation involves displacement of the frontal lobe of the brain under the falx cerebri. Finally, in extracranial herniation, the brain is displaced through a cranial defect, such as a fracture or a craniotomy.

Causes

Brain herniation is caused by space-occupying lesions, cerebral edema as a result of trauma or stroke, or hydrocephalus. It can also be caused by excessive drainage of cerebrospinal fluid (CSF) from a ventricular catheter or lumbar puncture.

Signs and symptoms

Signs and symptoms vary with the type of herniation. General early signs include decreasing level of consciousness, pupillary abnormalities, impaired motor function, and impaired brain stem reflexes. Signs of central herniation include small, reactive pupils (early phase); roving eye movements with loss of upward gaze; intermittent agitation and drowsiness progressing

to stupor; contralateral hemiparesis; and Cheyne-Stokes respirations. Signs of transtentorial herniation include ipsilateral pupil dilation, paralysis of eye movements, restlessness progressing to loss of consciousness, contralateral hemiparesis, decorticate or decerebrate posturing, and bilateral Babinski's sign. Late in the syndrome, altered vital signs become evident, such as widening pulse pressure and bradycardia.

Treatment

If herniation is caused by a space-occupying lesion, such as a hematoma or tumor, surgical removal of the lesion will relieve the pressure and allow adjacent structures to resume their normal shape. If herniation is related to increased intracranial pressure (ICP) as a result of cerebral edema, treatment involves reducing the edema with an osmotic diuretic or a corticosteroid, CSF drainage, hyperventilation, and, in extreme cases, barbiturate therapy. Maintaining temperature control and a normal fluid balance is also important. In some situations, such as cerebral edema caused by traumatic injury, the patient may have an ICP monitor in place to help guide treatment.

Nursing interventions

- Adhere to facility policy.
- Perform a neurologic assessment at least hourly.
- Institute precautionary measures to decrease ICP, including elevating the head of the bed at 15 to 30 degrees to promote venous drainage. Place the patient in a neutral position, avoiding extreme hip and neck flexion.
- Institute seizure precautions and assess the patient frequently for signs of seizures.
- Monitor the patient's vital signs frequently to ensure adequate cerebral perfusion.

- If the patient underwent a craniotomy for a hematoma or tumor, provide postoperative craniotomy care.
- Observe the patient carefully for other postoperative complications, such as infection, thrombophlebitis, or diabetes insipidus.

Cardiac tamponade

In cardiac tamponade, a rapid, unchecked increase in intrapericardial pressure impairs diastolic filling of the heart. The increased pressure usually results from the accumulation of blood or fluid in the pericardial sac. If fluid accumulates rapidly, as little as 200 ml can create an emergency situation. Gradual accumulation of fluid, as in pericardial effusion associated with cancer, may not produce immediate signs and symptoms because the fibrous wall of the pericardial sac can stretch to accommodate as much as 1 to 2 L of fluid.

Causes

Cardiac tamponade may be idiopathic (Dressler's syndrome), or it may result from effusion (in lung cancer, bacterial infection, tuberculosis, lupus, and, rarely, acute rheumatic fever), hemorrhage as a result of trauma, hemorrhage from nontraumatic causes (with pericarditis), acute myocardial infarction, chronic renal failure during dialysis, drug reaction, or a connective tissue disorder.

Signs and symptoms

Cardiac tamponade classically produces increased venous pressure, with jugular vein distention, reduced arterial blood pressure, muffled heart sounds on auscultation, and paradoxical pulse (an abnormal inspiratory drop in systemic blood pressure greater than 10 mm Hg).

Cardiac tamponade may also cause dyspnea, diaphoresis, pallor or cyanosis, anxiety, tachycardia, narrowed pulse pressure, restlessness, and hepatomegaly, but the lung fields will be clear. The patient typically sits upright and leans forward.

Chest X-rays show a slightly widened mediastinum and an enlarged cardiac silhouette. Electrocardiography is performed to rule out other cardiac disorders. Pulmonary artery pressure monitoring detects increases in right atrial pressure, right ventricular diastolic pressure, and central venous pressure (CVP). Echocardiography records pericardial effusion with signs of right ventricular and atrial compression.

Treatment

The goal of treatment is to relieve intrapericardial pressure and cardiac compression by removing accumulated blood or fluid. Pericardiocentesis (needle aspiration of the pericardial cavity) or surgical creation of an opening dramatically improves systemic arterial pressure and cardiac output with the aspiration of as little as 25 ml of fluid.

In a patient with hypotension, trial volume loading with normal saline solution I.V. with albumin—and perhaps an inotropic drug such as dopamine—is necessary to maintain cardiac output. Depending on the cause of tamponade, additional treatment may be needed.

Nursing interventions

- Infuse I.V. solutions and inotropic drugs (such as dopamine), as ordered, to maintain the patient's blood pressure.
- Administer oxygen therapy as needed.
- Prepare the patient for pericardiocentesis, thoracotomy, or central venous line insertion, as indicated.
- Check for signs of increasing tamponade, increasing dyspnea, and arrhythmias.

- Watch for a decrease in CVP and a concomitant rise in blood pressure after treatment; these indicate relief of cardiac compression.
- Monitor the patient's respiratory status for signs of respiratory distress, such as severe tachypnea or changes in the level of consciousness.

Disseminated intravascular coagulation

Also known as consumption coagulopathy or defibrination syndrome, disseminated intravascular coagulation (DIC) complicates conditions that accelerate clotting—thereby causing small vessel occlusion, organ necrosis, depletion of circulating clotting factors and platelets, and activation of the fibrinolytic system—which can provoke severe hemorrhage.

Clotting in the microcirculation usually affects the kidneys and extremities but can occur in the brain, lungs, pituitary and adrenal glands, and gastrointestinal (GI) mucosa. Other conditions—such as vitamin K deficiency, hepatic disease, and anticoagulant therapy—can cause a similar hemorrhage.

Although usually acute, DIC may be chronic in patients with cancer. The prognosis depends on early detection and treatment, the severity of the hemorrhage, and treatment of the underlying condition.

Causes

DIC results when tissue factor, a lipoprotein that helps initiate blood coagulation, is introduced into the bloodstream as a result of pathologic states, such as infections, obstetric complications, neoplastic disease, and disorders that produce necrosis. Other causes include heatstroke, shock, poisonous snakebite, cirrhosis, fat embolism, incompatible blood transfusion, cardiac arrest, surgery requiring cardiopulmonary bypass, giant hemangioma, severe venous thrombosis, and purpura fulminans.

Signs and symptoms

The most significant sign of DIC is abnormal bleeding without an accompanying history of a hemorrhagic disorder. Principal signs of such bleeding include cutaneous oozing, petechiae, ecchymoses, and hematomas caused by bleeding into the skin. Bleeding at the sites of surgical or invasive procedures and from the GI tract are equally significant indications, as are acrocyanosis and signs of acute tubular necrosis.

Related signs and symptoms and other possible effects include nausea; vomiting; dyspnea; oliguria; seizures; coma; shock; failure of major organ systems; and severe muscle, back, and abdominal pain.

The following initial laboratory findings suggest a tentative diagnosis of DIC: decreased platelet count, reduced fibrinogen levels, prolonged prothrombin time, prolonged partial thromboplastin time, and increased fibrin degradation products.

Treatment

Successful management of DIC requires prompt recognition and adequate treatment of the underlying disorder. If the patient is not actively bleeding, supportive care alone may reverse DIC. However, active bleeding may require the administration of blood, fresh frozen plasma, platelets, or packed red blood cells.

Heparin therapy is controversial but is usually mandatory if thrombosis occurs. Drugs such as antithrombin III and gabexate are being considered for use as antithrombins to inhibit the clotting cascade.

Nursing interventions

- Administer prescribed analgesics for pain, as needed.
- Administer oxygen therapy, as ordered.
- To prevent clots from dislodging and causing fresh bleeding, do not rub these areas vigorously when washing. If bleeding occurs, use pressure, cold compresses, and topical hemostatic agents to control it.
- After giving an I.V. injection or removing a catheter or needle, apply pressure to the injection site for at least 10 minutes. Alert other staff members to the patient's tendency to hemorrhage. Limit venipunctures whenever possible.
- Protect the patient from injury. Enforce complete bed rest during bleeding episodes. If the patient is very agitated, pad the bed rails.
- Reposition the patient every 2 hours and provide meticulous skin care to prevent skin breakdown.
- If the patient cannot tolerate activity because of blood loss, provide frequent rest periods.
- Monitor the patient's intake and output hourly. Watch for transfusion reactions and signs of fluid overload.
- Weigh dressings and linens, and record drainage. Weigh the patient daily.
- Watch for bleeding from the GI and genitourinary tracts. If you suspect intra-abdominal bleeding, measure the patient's abdominal girth at least every 4 hours and observe him or her closely for signs of shock.
- Monitor the results of serial blood studies.
- Test all stools and urine for occult blood.
- Inform the family of the patient's progress and provide emotional support and encouragement.

Hyperglycemic crisis

Diabetic ketoacidosis (DKA) and hyperosmolar hyperglycemic non-ketotic syndrome (HHNS) are acute complications of hyperglycemic crisis that may occur in a patient with diabetes. Quick and effective treatment is required to prevent coma and possibly death. DKA usually occurs in patients with type 1 diabetes; DKA may be the first sign of previously unrecognized diabetes. HHNS usually occurs in patients with type 2 diabetes but may also occur in patients whose insulin tolerance is stressed and in those who have undergone certain therapeutic procedures, such as peritoneal dialysis, hemodialysis, total parenteral nutrition, or tube feedings.

Causes

Acute insulin deficiency (absolute in DKA; relative in HHNS) precipitates both conditions. Causes include illness, trauma, stress, infection, and failure to take insulin (only in a patient with DKA).

Signs and symptoms

Signs and symptoms of DKA and HHNS result primarily from extremely elevated blood glucose levels. They include fluid loss, dehydration, shock, coma, and, possibly, death. Acetone breath; dehydration; Kussmaul's respirations; and a weak, rapid pulse are evident in patients with DKA. Polyuria, thirst, neurologic abnormalities, and stupor are seen in patients with HHNS. The patient with DKA also shows evidence of metabolic acidosis. Acidosis may start a cycle that leads to additional breakdown of tissue, followed by more ketosis, more acidosis, and eventually shock, coma, and death.

Treatment

Both DKA and HHNS are treated with fluid and electrolyte replacement and supportive care. Normal or half-normal saline solution is given I.V. at 1 L/hour until blood pressure is stabilized and urine output reaches ≥50 ml/hour. Then regular insulin is started, initially as an I.V. bolus dose, followed by continuous infusion. The rate is adjusted until the patient's serum glucose levels decrease by 50 to 70 mg/dl/hour.

When renal blood flow and urine output are established, potassium is given I.V. If acidosis is severe (pH less than 7.1), sodium bicarbonate may also be infused.

Nursing interventions

- When you recognize the signs and symptoms of DKA or HHNS, notify the physician immediately and prepare the patient for transfer to the intensive care unit.
- Monitor the patient's vital signs; level of consciousness; intake and output; electrocardiogram results; and ABG, electrolyte, glucose, and osmolarity levels frequently, as ordered. Also check the patient's urine for ketones.
- Begin I.V. fluid replacement therapy as soon as possible. Monitor elderly and very young patients for indications of fluid overload.
- Expect to administer an injection of regular insulin immediately—either I.M. or I.V.—followed by a continuous I.V. insulin drip.
- Provide supportive care as indicated by the patient's condition.
- Prepare to administer potassium replacements, as ordered.

Hypoglycemia

Hypoglycemia, which is an abnormally low blood glucose level, can be dangerous. It occurs when glucose burns up too rapidly, when the glucose release rate falls behind tissue demands, or when too much insulin enters the bloodstream.

Hypoglycemia is classified as reactive or fasting. Reactive hypoglycemia is caused by a reaction to a meal or the administration of too much insulin. Fasting hypoglycemia causes discomfort during periods of abstinence from food (for example, in the early morning hours before breakfast).

Causes

Reactive or postprandial hypoglycemia may occur in several forms. In a patient with diabetes, it may result from the administration of too much insulin or, less commonly, from the administration of too much of an oral antidiabetic. It may result from delayed and excessive production of insulin after carbohydrate ingestion or from a sharp increase in insulin output after a meal (for example, after gastric surgery). This form usually can be prevented by reducing simple sugars and increasing protein in a meal. In some patients, reactive hypoglycemia has no known cause or may result from hyperalimentation as a result of gastric dumping syndrome or impaired glucose tolerance.

Fasting hypoglycemia usually results from an excess of insulin or insulin-like substances or from a decrease in counterregulatory hormones. It may also be exogenous (such as from the ingestion of alcohol or drugs) or endogenous (from organic problems such as tumors, liver disease, or small islet cell tumors).

Other endocrine causes include destruction of the pancreatic islet cells, adrenocortical insufficiency, and pituitary insufficiency. Nonendocrine causes include severe liver disease, such as hepatitis, liver cancer, cirrhosis, and liver congestion associated with heart failure.

Signs and symptoms

Reactive (postprandial) and fasting hypoglycemia cause fatigue, malaise, nervousness, irritability, trembling, tension, headache, hunger, diaphoresis, and rapid heart rate.

Fasting hypoglycemia may also cause CNS disturbances, such as altered level of consciousness, blurry or double vision, confusion, motor weakness, hemiplegia, seizures, or coma.

AGE ALERT

In infants and children, signs and symptoms are vague. A neonate's refusal to feed may be the primary clue to underlying hypoglycemia. Associated effects include tremors, twitching, a weak or high-pitched cry, diaphoresis, limpness (or weakness), seizures, and coma.

Treatment

Reactive (postprandial) hypoglycemia requires dietary modification to help delay glucose absorption and gastric emptying. Usually, this includes small, frequent, high-protein meals with added fiber and avoidance of simple carbohydrates. The patient may also receive an anticholinergic to slow gastric emptying and intestinal motility and inhibit vagal stimulation of insulin release.

For fasting hypoglycemia, surgery and drug therapy may be required. For patients with insulinoma, removal of the tumor is the treatment of choice. Drug therapy may include a nondiuretic thiazide (such as diazoxide) to inhibit insulin secretion, streptozocin and hormones (such as a glucocorticoid), and long-acting glycogen.

AGE ALERT

For neonates who have hypoglycemia, a hypertonic solution of dextrose 10% in water, calculated at 5 to 10 ml/kg of body weight, administered I.V. over 10 minutes and followed by 4 to 8 mg/kg/minute for maintenance, should reduce the chance of hypoglycemia. To reduce the chance of hypoglycemia in high-risk neonates, feedings of either breast milk or a solution of dextrose 5% to 10% in water should begin as soon after birth as possible. Infants and children older than age 1 should receive 1 ml/kg of dextrose 25% in water.

For severe hypoglycemia (producing confusion or coma), initial treatment is usually I.V. administration of a bolus of 25 or 50 g of glucose as a 50% solution. This treatment is followed by a constant infusion of glucose until the patient can eat a meal. A patient who has adrenergic reactions without CNS symptoms may receive oral carbohydrates; parenteral therapy is not required.

Nursing interventions

- Administer medications, as ordered.
- Avoid delays in mealtimes and provide a proper diet.
- Correct hypoglycemic episodes quickly. Measure the patient's blood glucose level to verify the presence and severity of hypoglycemia before taking steps to correct it.
- Monitor I.V. infusion of hypertonic glucose, circulatory overload, and cellular dehydration.

- Measure blood glucose levels, as ordered.
- Assess the effects of drug therapy and watch the patient for adverse reactions.

Hypovolemic shock

Potentially life-threatening hypovolemic shock is caused by reduced intravascular blood volume, which leads to decreased cardiac output and inadequate tissue perfusion. The subsequent tissue anoxia prompts a shift in cellular metabolism from aerobic to anaerobic pathways, resulting in an accumulation of lactic acid that produces metabolic acidosis. Without immediate treatment, hypovolemic shock can cause adult respiratory distress syndrome, acute tubular necrosis and renal failure, DIC, and multisystem organ dysfunction syndrome.

Causes

Hypovolemic shock usually results from acute blood loss—about 15% to 30% of total volume. Massive blood loss may result from GI bleeding, internal or external hemorrhage, or any condition that reduces circulating intravascular volume or causes significant loss of other body fluids.

Other causes include intestinal obstruction, peritonitis, acute pancreatitis, ascites, and dehydration as a result of excessive perspiration, severe diarrhea or protracted vomiting, diabetes insipidus, diuresis, and inadequate fluid intake.

Signs and symptoms

The patient's history includes a condition that reduces blood volume, such as GI hemorrhage, trauma, or severe diarrhea and vomiting. A patient with cardiac disease may have anginal pain.

Examination may show pale skin; decreased sensorium; and rapid, shallow respirations. Urine output is usually less than 25 ml/hour. Palpation may show rapid, thready peripheral pulses and cold, clammy skin. Auscultation of blood pressure usually detects a mean arterial pressure of less than 60 mm Hg and a narrowing pulse pressure.

Laboratory findings may include low hematocrit; decreased hemoglobin level, red blood cell count, and platelet count; elevated serum potassium, sodium, lactate dehydrogenase, creatinine, and blood urea nitrogen levels; increased urine specific gravity (greater than 1.020) and urine osmolality; decreased urine creatinine levels; decreased pH and partial pressure of arterial oxygen; and increased partial pressure of arterial carbon dioxide.

X-rays, gastroscopy, aspiration of gastric contents through a nasogastric (NG) tube, and tests for occult blood are used to identify internal bleeding sites. Coagulation studies may detect coagulopathy caused by DIC.

Treatment

Emergency treatment relies on prompt and adequate blood and fluid replacement to restore intravascular volume and raise blood pressure and maintain it above 60 mm Hg. Rapid infusion of normal saline or lactated Ringer's solution and possibly albumin or other plasma expanders may expand volume adequately until packed cells can be matched.

Other measures include administration of oxygen, control of bleeding, administration of dopamine or another inotropic drug, and, possibly, surgery. (To be effective, dopamine and other inotropic drugs must be used with vigorous fluid resuscitation.)

Nursing interventions

- Check for a patent airway and adequate circulation. If the patient experiences cardiac or respiratory arrest, start CPR.
- Begin an I.V. infusion with normal saline or lactated Ringer's solution.

- Monitor the patient's CVP, right atrial pressure, pulmonary artery pressure, pulmonary artery wedge pressure (PAWP), and cardiac output at least once hourly or as ordered.
- Monitor urine output hourly. If output falls below 30 ml/hour in an adult, increase the fluid infusion rate, but watch for signs of fluid overload such as elevated PAWP. Notify the physician if urine output does not increase.
- Obtain ABG samples, as ordered. Administer oxygen by face mask or through an established airway to ensure adequate tissue oxygenation. Adjust the oxygen flow rate according to the ABG measurements.
- Record the patient's blood pressure, pulse and respiratory rates, and peripheral pulse rates every 15 minutes and per facility protocol until they are stable. Monitor the patient's cardiac rhythm continuously.
- Notify the physician and increase the infusion rate if the patient has a progressive drop in blood pressure accompanied by a thready pulse.
- Obtain a complete blood count, electrolyte levels, typing and cross-matching, and coagulation studies, as ordered.
- During therapy, assess the patient's skin color and temperature, and note changes.
- Watch the patient for signs of impending coagulopathy.

Pneumothorax

Pneumothorax is characterized by an accumulation of air or gas between the parietal and visceral pleurae. The amount of air or gas trapped in the intrapleural space determines the degree of lung collapse. The most common types of pneumothorax are open, closed, and tension. Many factors contribute to pneumothorax. If left untreated, extensive pneumothorax and tension pneumothorax can lead to fatal pulmonary and circulatory collapse.

Causes

Open pneumothorax may be caused by penetrating chest injury (such as a gunshot or knife wound), insertion of a central venous catheter, chest surgery, transbronchial or closed pleural biopsy, or thoracentesis. Closed pneumothorax may be caused by blunt chest trauma, air leakage (from ruptured, congenital blebs adjacent to the visceral pleural space), rupture of emphysematous bullae, barotrauma as a result of mechanical ventilation, tubercular or cancerous lesions that erode into the pleural space, or interstitial lung disease. Tension pneumothorax may be caused by a penetrating chest wound treated with an airtight dressing, puncture of the lung or airway by a fractured rib, mechanical ventilation, high-level positive end-expiratory pressure that causes alveolar blebs to rupture, or occlusion or malfunction of a chest tube.

Signs and symptoms

The patient history shows sudden, sharp, pleural pain. The patient may report that the pain is exacerbated by chest movement, breathing, and coughing. He or she may also report shortness of breath.

Examination shows asymmetrical movement of the chest wall, with over-expansion and rigidity on the affected side. The patient may appear cyanotic. Patients with tension pneumothorax may have distended jugular veins, pallor, and may exhibit anxiety.

Palpation may show crackling beneath the skin, indicating subcutaneous emphysema and decreased vocal fremitus. If the patient has tension pneumothorax, palpation may show tracheal deviation away from the affected side (a late sign) and a weak and rapid pulse. Percussion may show hyperresonance on the affected side, and auscultation may disclose decreased or absent breath sounds over the collapsed lung. The patient may also be hypotensive. Spontaneous pneumothorax that releases only a small amount of air into the pleural space may not cause any signs or symptoms.

Treatment

Chest X-rays confirm the diagnosis. Other supportive diagnoses include an early decline in pulse oximetry readings and hypoxemia and respiratory acidosis, as shown by ABG studies. Treatment is conservative (bed rest, oxygen administration, aspiration of air with a large-bore needle, and, possibly, insertion of a Heimlich valve) for patients with spontaneous pneumothorax and no signs of increased pleural pressure, lung collapse of less than 30%, and no dyspnea or other indications of physiologic compromise.

For patients with lung collapse of more than 30%, treatment to reexpand the lung includes placing a thoracostomy tube in the second or third intercostal space in the midclavicular line. The tube is then connected to an underwater seal or low-pressure suction.

Recurring spontaneous pneumothorax requires thoracotomy and pleurectomy. Traumatic pneumothorax and tension pneumothorax require chest tube drainage; traumatic pneumothorax may also require surgical repair. An analgesic may be prescribed.

Nursing interventions

- Listen to the patient's fears and concerns, and offer reassurance, as appropriate.
- Keep the patient as comfortable as possible, and administer an analgesic, if necessary.

- Help the patient to a comfortable position. Many patients with pneumothorax feel most comfortable sitting upright.
- Monitor the patient for complications signaled by pallor, gasping respirations, and chest pain.
- Carefully monitor the patient's vital signs at least once every hour for indications of shock, increasing respiratory distress, or mediastinal shift. Auscultate breath sounds over both lungs.
- Make sure the suction setup is functioning appropriately. Monitor the patient for signs of tension pneumothorax. If he or she does not have a chest tube to suction, monitor him or her for recurrence of pneumothorax and recollapse of the lung.

Septic shock

Usually caused by a bacterial infection, septic shock causes inadequate blood perfusion and circulatory collapse. Unless treated promptly (preferably before symptoms fully develop), it progresses to multisystem organ dysfunction syndrome or death.

Causes

Many gram-positive and gram-negative bacteria as well as actinomycetes can cause septic shock. Preexisting infections caused by viruses, rickettsiae, chlamydiae, and protozoa may be complicated by septic shock. Other predisposing factors include immunodeficiency, advanced age, cirrhosis, trauma, burns, diabetes mellitus, and DIC.

Signs and symptoms

Clinical effects of septic shock vary according to the stage of the shock, the causative organism, and the age of the patient. Early signs and symptoms include oliguria, sudden fever (higher than 101° F [38.3° C]), chills, nausea, vomiting, diarrhea, and prostration.

Late signs and symptoms include restlessness, apprehension, irritability, thirst as a result of reduced perfusion of cerebral tissue, hypothermia, anuria, tachycardia, and tachypnea.

AGE ALERT

Hypotension, altered level of consciousness, and hyperventilation may be the only signs of septic shock in infants and elderly patients.

Treatment

The first goal of treatment is to monitor and reverse shock through volume expansion. I.V. fluids are administered, and a pulmonary artery catheter is inserted. Whole blood or plasma may be administered to raise the PAWP to a satisfactory level. An I.V. antibiotic is given, and a urinary catheter is inserted to monitor hourly output. Mechanical ventilation may be necessary.

If shock persists after fluid infusion, a vasopressor is given to help the patient maintain adequate blood perfusion. Other treatments may include giving I.V. bicarbonate to correct acidosis and administering drotrecogin alfa (activated) (Xigris) in progressing moderate or severe sepsis. Other treatments to combat infection include surgery to drain and excise abscesses and debridement.

Nursing interventions

- Remove I.V., intra-arterial, or urinary drainage catheters and send them to the laboratory for culture for causative organisms.
- Start an I.V. infusion of normal saline solution or lactated Ringer's solution.
- Administer an antibiotic I.V. to achieve effective blood levels rapidly. Monitor serum drug levels.

- Measure hourly urine output. Watch the patient for signs of fluid overload such as increased PAWP.
- If urine output is less than 30 ml/hour, increase the fluid infusion rate per facility protocol. Notify the physician if urine output does not improve. A diuretic may be ordered to increase renal blood flow and urine output.
- Monitor ABG studies. Administer oxygen by face mask or through an airway. Adjust the oxygen flow rate according to ABG measurements.
- If the patient's blood pressure drops below 80 mm Hg, increase the oxygen flow rate and notify the physician immediately.
- Record the patient's blood pressure, pulse and respiratory rates, and peripheral pulses every 5 minutes until his or her condition is stabilized. Record hemodynamic pressure readings every 15 minutes. Monitor cardiac rhythm continuously.
- Provide emotional support to the patient and his or her family.
- Document the occurrence of a nosocomial infection and report it to the infection-control nurse.

Spinal cord compression

Compression of the spinal cord can affect the patient's ability to perform activities of daily living. The onset and severity of symptoms vary with the etiology of the compression; onset may be acute (traumatic injury) or insidious (tumor growth). Outcome depends on the nature of the compression and how promptly the diagnosis is made.

Causes

Traumatic injury is the most common cause of spinal cord compression. Hyperflexion injuries usually result from sudden deceleration and usually affect the cervical region. Hyperextension injuries cause more damage because the spine swings through a larger arc, making cord compression more likely. Rotational injuries result from extreme lateral flexion. Compression injuries result from extreme vertical pressure, usually caused by a long fall.

Spinal cord tumors are less common than other types of tumors. They are usually benign, located in the thoracic region, and extradural.

Signs and symptoms

Clinical effects of spinal cord compression are related to the level of the injury. Usually, sudden, complete compression causes loss of movement, spinal reflexes, and pain sensation below the level of the lesion. Bowel and bladder dysfunction may also occur, along with inability to perspire and regulate body temperature below the level of the lesion. Incomplete, acute traumatic compression may result in any combination of these symptoms. (For more information, see *Functional loss from spinal cord injury.*)

With spinal cord tumors, the location of symptoms is related to the level of the lesion. Pain is the most common initial symptom, along with coldness and numbness. Motor weakness usually occurs along with sensory loss. Loss of sphincter control may occur; bladder control is usually affected before bowel control.

Treatment

For traumatic injury, treatment begins with immediate stabilization followed by the basic goals of decompression, realignment, and further stabilization. A 24-hour regimen of high-dose methylprednisolone (Medrol) is currently recommended to improve motor function and sensation by decreasing edema. Specific treatment depends on the type of injury and treatment may be surgical, nonsurgical, or a combination. If surgery is indicated, it is usually to decrease compression and stabilize the spine.

Treatment of spinal tumors—which may include radiation, chemotherapy, and surgery—depends on the type and location of the tumor as well as the rapidity of onset of symptoms.

Nursing interventions

- In patients with traumatic injury, perform physical assessments each time the vital signs are assessed and each time the patient is moved. Hypotension is common if the patient's head is raised above the level of his or her heart.
- Pay special attention to the patient's respiratory status, especially if he or she has a cervical lesion; measure the patient's vital capacity and tidal volume frequently.
- Maintain a patent airway and suction as needed; perform chest physiotherapy frequently.
- Instruct the patient to cough and perform deep-breathing exercises every 2 hours.
- Provide range-of-motion exercises and encourage the patient to participate as much as his or her function allows.
- Reposition the patient every 2 hours and provide meticulous skin care.
- Administer an analgesic and a muscle relaxant, as ordered. Monitor the patient for over sedation.
- Monitor the patient's intake and output to assess the fluid balance. Ensure adequate oral intake.
- Provide emotional support and encouragement to the patient and his or her family. Help enhance the patient's capabilities.
- Assist with arrangements and follow-up for rehabilitation.

Functional loss from spinal cord injury

Functional losses as a result of spinal cord injury include variable losses of motor function, deep tendon reflexes, sensory function, respiratory function, and bowel and bladder function, depending on which vertebral level is affected.

Level C1 to C4

- Complete loss of motor function below the neck
- No reflex loss
- Loss of sensory function in the neck and below
- Loss of involuntary and voluntary respiratory function
- Loss of bowel and bladder control

Level C5

- Loss of all motor function below the upper shoulders
- Loss of deep tendon reflexes in the biceps
- Loss of sensation below the clavicle and in most of the chest, abdomen, and upper and lower extremities
- Phrenic nerve intact but not the intercostal and abdominal muscles
- Loss of bowel and bladder control

Level C6

- Loss of all function below the shoulders; no elbow, forearm, or hand control
- Loss of deep tendon reflexes in the biceps
- Loss of sensation below the clavicle and in most of the chest, abdomen, and upper and lower extremities
- Phrenic nerve intact but not the intercostal and abdominal muscles
- Loss of bowel and bladder control

Level C7

- Loss of motor control to portions of the arms and hands
- Loss of deep tendon reflexes in the triceps
- Loss of sensation below the clavicle and in portions of the arms and hands

- Phrenic nerve intact but not the intercostal and abdominal muscles
- Loss of bowel and bladder function

Level C8

- Loss of motor control to portions of the arms and hands
- Loss of deep tendon reflexes in the triceps
- Loss of sensation below the chest and in portions of the hands
- Phrenic nerve intact but not the intercostal and abdominal muscles
- Loss of bowel and bladder function

Level T1 to T6

- Loss of all motor function below the midchest region, including the trunk muscles
- No reflex loss
- Loss of sensation below the midchest area
- Independent function of the phrenic nerve
- Some impairment of the intercostal and abdominal muscles
- Loss of bowel and bladder function

Level T6 to T12

- Loss of motor control below the waist
- No reflex loss
- Loss of all sensation below the waist
- No interference with respiratory function
- Impairment of the abdominal muscles, leading to diminished cough
- Loss of bowel and bladder control

Level L1 to L3

- Loss of control of most of the leg and pelvis
- Loss of the knee-jerk reflex
- Loss of sensation to portions of the lower legs, ankles, and feet
- No interference with respiratory function
- Loss of bowel and bladder control

(continued)

Functional loss from spinal cord injury *(continued)*

Level L3 to L4
- Loss of control of portions of the lower legs, ankles, and feet
- Loss of the knee-jerk reflex
- Loss of sensation to portions of the lower legs, ankles, and feet
- No interference with respiratory function
- Loss of bowel and bladder control

Level L4 to L5
- Varying extent of loss of motor control
- Loss of the ankle-jerk reflex (S1, S2)
- Loss of sensation in the upper legs and portions of the lower legs (lumbar sensory nerves) and in the lower legs, feet, and perineum (sacral sensory nerves)
- No interference with respiratory function
- Possible impairment of bowel and bladder control

Syndrome of inappropriate antidiuretic hormone secretion

Syndrome of inappropriate antidiuretic hormone (SIADH) secretion is marked by excessive release of antidiuretic hormone (ADH), which disturbs the fluid and electrolyte balance. Such disturbances result from an inability to excrete dilute urine, retention of free water, expansion of extracellular fluid volume, and hyponatremia. The syndrome occurs as a result of diseases that affect the osmoreceptors of the hypothalamus.

Causes

Most commonly, SIADH results from bronchogenic carcinoma of the lung; the tumor secretes excessive ADH or vasopressor-like substances. Other neoplastic diseases (such as pancreatic and prostatic cancer, Hodgkin's disease, and thymoma) may also trigger SIADH.

Additional causes include CNS disorders; pulmonary disorders; positive-pressure ventilation; drugs; and miscellaneous conditions, such as myxedema and psychosis.

Signs and symptoms

SIADH may cause weight gain despite appetite loss, nausea and vomiting, muscle weakness, restlessness, and, possibly, seizures and coma. Edema is rare unless water overload exceeds 4 L because much of the excess free water exists within cellular boundaries.

SIADH is suggested by a complete medical history that shows a positive water balance. The diagnosis is confirmed by the finding of serum osmolality of less than 280 mOsm/kg of water and a serum sodium level of less than 123 mEq/L. Other laboratory values that support the diagnosis include high urine sodium secretion (more than 20 mEq/L) without a diuretic. Other diagnostic studies show normal renal function and no evidence of dehydration.

Treatment

Treatment begins with restricted fluid intake (17 to 34 oz [503 to 1,005 ml]/day). With severe water intoxication, administration of 200 to 300 ml of 3% to 5% sodium chloride solution may be needed to increase the serum sodium level. If fluid restriction is ineffective, demeclocycline or lithium may be given to help block the renal response to ADH. When possible, treatment should include correcting the root cause of SIADH. If the syndrome is related to cancer, the water retention may be relieved by surgery, irradiation, or chemotherapy.

Nursing interventions

- Restrict fluids and provide comfort measures for thirst, including ice chips, mouth care, lozenges, and staggered water intake.
- Reduce unnecessary environmental stimuli and orient the patient, as needed.
- Provide a safe environment for the patient who has an altered level of consciousness. Take seizure precautions, as needed.
- Monitor the patient's serum osmolality and serum and urine sodium levels.
- Closely monitor and record the patient's intake and output, vital signs, and daily weight.
- Perform neurologic checks at least every 2 to 4 hours, depending on the patient's status. Look for and report early changes in level of consciousness.
- Observe the patient for signs and symptoms of heart failure, which may occur as a result of fluid overload.

Thyroid storm

Also known as thyrotoxic crisis, thyroid storm is an acute manifestation of hyperthyroidism. It usually occurs in patients with preexisting (although typically unrecognized) thyrotoxicosis. If thyroid storm is not treated promptly, hypotension, vascular collapse, coma, and death may occur.

Causes

Onset is almost always abrupt and is evoked by a stressful event, such as trauma, surgery, or infection. Less common causes include insulin-induced hypoglycemia or DKA, stroke, myocardial infarction, pulmonary embolism, sudden discontinuation of antithyroid medication, initiation of ^{131}I therapy, preeclampsia, and subtotal thyroidectomy with excess intake of synthetic thyroid hormone.

Signs and symptoms

Initially, the patient may have marked tachycardia, vomiting, and stupor. Other findings include irritability and restlessness, visual disturbances such as diplopia, tremors and weakness, angina, shortness of breath, cough, and swollen extremities. Palpation may show warm, moist, flushed skin and a high fever (101° F [38° C] or greater) that begins insidiously and rises rapidly to a lethal level.

Treatment

Treatment of thyroid storm includes administration of an antithyroid drug I.V., propranolol to block the sympathetic effects, a corticosteroid to inhibit conversion of the thyroid hormone thyroxine (T_4) to triiodothyronine and to replace depleted cortisol levels, and iodide to block the release of T_4. Supportive measures include administration of nutrients, vitamins, fluids, and a sedative.

Nursing interventions

- Monitor the patient's vital signs, electrocardiogram readings, and cardiopulmonary status continuously. Assess the patient for changes in level of consciousness.
- Expect to administer an antithyroid medication and a beta-adrenergic blocker to inhibit sympathetic effects. Monitor the patient's response to medications.
- Administer a corticosteroid to inhibit the conversion of T_4 and to replace

depleted cortisol, as ordered. Anticipate administering iodide to block the release of thyroid hormones.

- Monitor the patient's temperature closely. Apply cooling measures, if indicated, and administer acetaminophen, as ordered. Never administer aspirin because it may increase the patient's metabolic rate further.
- Institute safety measures, including seizure precautions, to protect the patient from injury.
- Provide supportive care and administer vitamins, nutrients, fluids, and a sedative, as ordered.

Tracheal erosion

Tracheal erosion is damage to the tracheal lumen that occurs through mechanical or chemical irritation. Tissue destruction usually progresses from interior to exterior tracheal structures, but it also may be caused or abetted by external pressure, especially to the posterior tracheal wall.

Causes

Chemical injury to the tracheal tissues occurs as epithelial cells and submucosal structures are destroyed by inhalation of toxic substances (such as smoke and corrosive gases) and by direct burn injury. Edema and inflammation also occur. Mechanical injury occurs when a foreign body is lodged in the airway; it may be accompanied by inflammation.

In the clinical setting, tracheal erosion usually results from traumatic intubation with a cuffed or uncuffed tracheal or endotracheal tube. High-pressure, low-volume cuffed tubes are most likely to cause damage.

Concomitant use of an NG tube places additional friction on the tracheal muscle, internally and externally, increasing the risk of tracheoesophageal fistula.

Signs and symptoms

Hemoptysis is the most common sign. Bleeding may be scant if only surface vessels are injured; it may be severe and can result in death if erosion penetrates the adjacent neck vessels. In patients receiving mechanical ventilation, a persistent air leak may indicate tracheal dilation and possible erosion. Tracheal erosion should be suspected when the patient aspirates food or fluid, especially during prolonged tracheal and NG intubation.

Treatment

Treatment is primarily limited to allowing the affected area to heal spontaneously. For injury caused by traumatic intubation, removal of the tube is desirable. Otherwise, pressure on the erosion site can be reduced by deflation of the cuff, recannulation with a smaller airway, or replacement of a standard tracheostomy tube with a dual cuffed or longer tube. Removal of an NG tube limits friction on the trachea. A gastric tube may be inserted to promote decompression or provide nutrition. An antibiotic may be given to treat infection and promote healing.

Nursing interventions

- Make sure that the endotracheal or tracheal tube is the correct size to avoid placing unnecessary pressure on the tracheal wall.
- Stabilize airway tubes to prevent irritation caused by movement.
- Maintain lateral wall pressures for nonatmospheric tubes at less than 18 mm Hg.
- Suction only as necessary, using a vacuum with less than 120 mm Hg of pressure. Never force a suction catheter against resistance.
- Use small-bore NG or gastric tubes to prevent erosion.
- If a fistula is suspected, discontinue NG intubation and notify the physician.

Selected references

Fischbach, F. T., & Fischbach, M. A. (2017). *Fischbach's manual of laboratory and diagnostic tests* (10th ed.). Philadelphia, PA: Wolters Kluwer.

Good, V. S., & Kirkwood, P. L. (2017). *Advanced critical care nursing* (2nd ed.). St. Louis, MO: Elsevier.

Lewis, S. L., Hagler, D., Bucher, L., Heitkemper, M. L., Harding, M. M., Kwong, J., & Roberts, D. (2016). *Medical surgical nursing: Assessment and management of clinical problems* (10th ed.). St. Louis, MO: Elsevier.

Papadakis, M. A., & McPhee, S. J. (2019). *Current medical diagnosis and treatment* (58th ed.). New York, NY: McGraw-Hill.

16

End-of-Life Care

Caring for the dying patient and the family

The experience of dying is unique for each patient and family. Nurses must discover what each dying patient and his or her family need. It is important to help both the patient and family prepare for the dying process.

The dying process

Death is the total failure of all body systems. Although each patient's death progresses differently, the dying process usually occurs over 10 to 14 days but may take as little as 24 hours. Occasionally, patients may seem to have an improvement in their strength, sensorium, and other symptoms in the days preceding death. The following summarizes the impact of the dying process on each body system.

Cardiovascular system

- Dehydration
- Initial increase in the heart rate, followed by a decrease as hypoxia develops
- Decrease in blood pressure and the volume of Korotkoff's sounds

Integumentary system

- Diaphoresis
- Cold, clammy skin
- Pale, ashen, or mottled skin
- Darkened skin at the sacrum and lower back
- Mottling of skin in the extremities and progressing proximally

Respiratory system

- Diminished or adventitious breath sounds
- Moist-sounding respirations
- Dyspnea or air hunger
- Tachypnea
- Irregular breathing patterns such as Cheyne-Stokes respirations

Musculoskeletal system

- Muscle weakness
- Difficulty swallowing

- Relaxation of the tissues of the soft palate
- Diminished gag reflex and reflexive clearing of the oropharynx

Renal system

- Decreased urine output

Other signs and symptoms

- Decreasing need or desire for food and drink
- Moaning and grunting with breathing
- Agitation and restlessness
- Decreased communication ("transitional withdrawal")
- Decreased hearing and vision
- Confusion
- Decreasing level of consciousness
- Visions of people and things not visible to others
- Bladder and bowel incontinence

Five signs of impending death

- Clouding of sensorium
- Audible respirations from secretions in airways ("death rattle")
- Mandibular movement on respiration
- Cyanosis or mottling of the extremities
- Absent radial artery pulse

Meeting patient and family needs

Palliative care and hospice care

Palliative care is an approach to care and a structured system of care delivery that aims to prevent and relieve distressing symptoms to improve quality of life for patients and their families. Palliative care emphasizes meeting physiologic needs such as pain control as well as the management of psychological, social, and spiritual needs. Palliative care may occur in hospital, outpatient, and long-term care settings. Palliative care is not limited to patients who have ceased

Meeting patient needs

Care of the dying patient should be individualized to meet each patient's unique needs. This chart identifies some specific interventions that may help the patient during the dying process.

Interventions	Rationales
• For acute air hunger or tachypnea, low-dose opioids such as morphine may be indicated.	• Morphine dilates the pulmonary vessels, decreases oxygen consumption, and decreases pulmonary congestion. This can reduce the patient's perception of dyspnea.
• Promote air movement with a fan or open windows. Provide space around the bed for air to move freely.	• Air movement can stimulate trigeminal nerve receptors in the cheek and nasopharynx that cause the brain stem to inhibit the sensation of difficulty breathing.
• Consider nursing interventions prior to suctioning such as repositioning the patient to a side-lying position, elevating the head of the bed, or administering prescribed anticholinergics.	• Secretions accumulate in the oropharynx or bronchi as death approaches. Suctioning may not relieve the loud, gurgling sound, or "death rattle." These secretions are hard to reach, and suctioning may cause discomfort. Repositioning may reduce airway obstruction, and anticholinergics may dry secretions.
• Perform frequent pain assessment, even during the patient's last hours. If possible, ask the patient what his or her goal for pain relief.	• Opioid requirements are unique for each patient and situation. Pain must be assessed and managed throughout the dying process. Titrate analgesics according to the goals of care, the severity of pain, the need for supplemental analgesics, the adverse side effects, the patient's functional abilities, the patient's emotional state, and the effect of pain on the patient's quality of life.
• When assessing the patient for delirium, review the onset of delirium symptoms with family members.	• In many cases, delirium may be reversible if the cause is identified. Medications can be a common cause of delirium. Other causes include sepsis, encephalopathy, central nervous system involvement by a tumor, metabolic changes, and multiple organ system failure. Delirium can be treated with cause-specific interventions, medications, or with palliative sedation, as appropriate.
• Accommodate changes in hearing and vision. Avoid whispering and do not say anything near the patient that you do not want him or her to hear. Provide dim lighting, but ensure that it is bright enough to allow the patient to recognize faces.	• Hearing is believed to be the last sense that is lost as dying occurs. Whispering may cause increased strain on the patient as his or her hearing diminishes. Changes in vision include increased sensitivity to light and loss of visual acuity.

life-prolonging therapies or for those with a limited life expectancy.

Hospice care provides coordinated interdisciplinary services to patients with serious progressive illness and a limited life expectancy, typically 6 months or less. Although the goal of hospice care is for patients to remain at home, hospice care may occur in a variety of settings such as a dedicated hospice facility, a hospital, or in the long-term care setting. The Centers for Medicare and Medicaid Services enforce conditions of participation, such as eligibility requirements, with hospice programs in the United States.

Meeting family needs

Meeting family needs can be as important as meeting the needs of the dying patient. In many cases, the family may not be prepared to lose their loved one, particularly in instances of accidents or the death of a young person. In other cases, the family may be more prepared, such as with prolonged illnesses. Regardless of the situation, ask the family members what their specific needs may be. It is best to do this early and to include all family members.

- Does the family have questions about the advantages and disadvantages of artificial nutrition and hydration?
- Do they have concerns about pain relief for the patient?
- Do they wish to be present at the time of death?
- How involved do they wish to be with the patient's physical care?
- What do they need to know about the processes before, during, and after the patient's death?

Teaching

- Discuss the signs of imminent death with the family before they occur.
- Encourage family members to stay with the patient if they wish.

- Support family members who do not wish to be present.
- Teach the family simple techniques to help keep the patient comfortable such as giving mouth care, assisting with positioning, and performing gentle massage. Offer this teaching only if the family is comfortable with it.
- When the patient's words and statements are unclear, work with the family members to determine what the patient is trying to communicate.
- Explain to the family that some dying patients may appear to see and hear someone or something that is not visible or audible to others in the room because dying patients often see visions of comforting figures.

Family care after patient death

- Ask if the family needs the support of a clergy member.
- Express sympathy for the family.
- Always treat the body with respect.
- Bathe and handle the body according to the family's wishes. Some cultures have rules and rituals for treatment of the body.
- Do not remove the body until the family is ready.
- Ask if the family needs assistance in contacting the funeral director.
- Ensure that the patient's personal possessions and valuables are given to the family.

Selected reference

Hinkle, J. L., & Cheever, K. H. (2014). End-of-life care. In J. Reifsnyder (Ed.), *Brunner & Suddarth's textbook of medical-surgical nursing* (13th ed., pp. 373–399). Philadelphia, PA: Wolters Kluwer.

17

Documentation Systems

Completing forms fully and concisely

Documentation refers to the preparation and maintenance of records that describe a patient's care. If you document with attention to detail, you will clearly show the quality of care your patient received, the outcome of that care, and the treatment that the patient still needs.

The detailed information you assemble will be scrutinized by many reviewers, including other health care team members; accrediting, certifying, and licensing organizations; performance improvement monitors; peer reviewers; and Medicare and insurance company reviewers. Attorneys and judges may also examine your documentation. Researchers and educators may use it to improve patient care and to provide continuing education.

Although each health care facility determines its own requirements for documentation and evaluation, those requirements must comply with legal, accreditation, and professional standards.

Similarly, a nursing department can select the documentation system it wants to use as long as the system demonstrates adherence to standards and care requirements. Regardless of the documentation system used, specific policies and procedures for documentation must be in place and known. Understanding them will help you document care accurately. It will also serve you well when evaluating or modifying your documentation system or when selecting a new one.

Depending on the policies of your health care facility, you will use one or more documentation systems to record your nursing interventions and evaluations and the patient's response.

Health care facilities may use traditional narrative charting or an alternative system, such as problem-oriented medical record (POMR), problem-intervention-evaluation (PIE), FOCUS, charting by exception (CBE), FACT, core, and outcome documentation systems. In addition, many heath care facilities use computerized charting systems.

Traditional narrative charting

Narrative charting is a straightforward chronological account of the patient's status, the nursing interventions performed, and the patient's response to those interventions that is suitable in any clinical setting. Documentation is usually included in the progress notes and is supplemented by flow sheets. The Joint Commission standards require all health care facilities to set policies on how frequently patients should be assessed. Document patient assessments as often as your institution requires and more frequently when you observe any of the following:

- change in the patient's condition
- patient's response to a treatment or medication
- lack of improvement in the patient's condition
- patient's or family member's response to teaching.

Document exactly what you hear, observe, inspect, do, or teach. Include as much specific, descriptive information as possible. Always document how your patient responds to care, treatments, and medications and progress toward the desired outcome. Also include notification to the physician for changes that have occurred. Document this communication, the physician's response, new orders that are followed, and the patient's response.

You can organize your notes by using a head-to-toe approach or by referring to the care plan and documenting the patient's progress in relation to the plan and any unresolved problems. Regardless of the way you organize your narrative note, be specific and document chronologically, recording exact times.

11/26/09	2255	Patient 4 hr postop; awakens easily, oriented X 3 but groggy, incision site in front of Ⓛ ear extending down and around the ear and into neck—approximately 6" in length—without dressing. No swelling or bleeding, bluish discoloration below Ⓛ ear noted, sutures intact. Jackson–Pratt drain in Ⓛ neck below ear with 20-ml bloody drainage measured. Drain remains secured in place with suture and anchored to Ⓛ anterior chest wall with tape. Pt. denied pain but stated she felt nauseated and promptly vomited 100 ml of clear fluid. Pt. attempted to get OOB to ambulate to bathroom with assistance, but felt dizzy upon standing. Assisted to lie down in bed. Voided 200 ml clear, yellow urine in bedpan. Pt. encouraged to deep breathe and cough q1hr, and turn frequently in bed. Lungs sound clear bilaterally. Antiembolism stockings applied to both lower extremities. Explanations given regarding these preventive measures. Pt. verbalized understanding. ———————————————— Bridget Smith, RN
	2300	Pt. continues to feel nauseated. Compazine 1 mg I.V. ———————————————— Bridget Smith, RN
	2335	Pt. states she's no longer nauseated. No further vomiting. Rating pain in incisional areas as 7/10, on a scale of 0 to 10. Medicated with morphine 2 mg I.V. ———————————————— Bridget Smith, RN
	2355	Pt. states pain as 1/10. Demonstrated taking deep breaths and coughing effectively. ———————— ———————————————— Bridget Smith, RN

Problem-oriented medical record

The POMR system focuses on specific patient problems. Developed by physicians and later adapted by nurses, POMR has five components: the database, problem list, initial plan, progress notes, and discharge summary.

Database

Subjective and objective data about the patient form the initial care plan. These data are collected during the initial assessment of the patient and include such information as reason for hospitalization or treatment, medical history, allergies, medications, physical and psychosocial findings, self-care abilities, educational needs, and discharge planning concerns.

Problem list

A numbered list of the patient's current problems in chronological order according to the date each was identified provides an overview of the patient's health status. You can refer to it by number when writing your notes. When a problem is resolved, note the date and time and highlight the problem with a felt-tip pen.

Initial plan

This includes expected outcomes and plans for further data collection, patient care, and teaching. Involve patients and significant others in planning and setting goals.

Progress notes

Typically, you must write a note for each current problem every 24 hours or when the patient's condition changes. SOAP, SOAPIE, or SOAPIER is used to structure progress notes. If you have nothing to record for a component, simply omit the letter from the note. The components of SOAPIER include:

- *Subjective data:* chief complaint or other information the patient or family members tell you
- *Objective data:* factual, measurable data, such as observable signs and symptoms, vital signs, or test values
- *Assessment data:* conclusions based on subjective and objective data and formulated as patient problems or nursing diagnoses
- *Plan:* strategy for relieving the patient's problems, including short- and long-term actions
- *Interventions:* measures you have taken to achieve expected outcomes
- *Evaluation:* analysis of the effectiveness of your interventions
- *Revision:* changes from the original care plan.

Discharge summary

This covers each problem on the list and notes whether it was resolved. Discuss any unresolved problems and specify plans for dealing with the problems after discharge. Also record communications with other facilities, home health agencies, and the patient.

11/26/09	2400	#1 Nausea related to anesthetic.
		S: Pt. states, "I feel nauseated."
		O: Pt. vomited 100 ml of clear fluid at 2255.
		A: Pt. is nauseated.
		P: Monitor nausea and give antiemetic as necessary.
		I: Pt. given Compazine 1 mg. I.V. at 2300.
		E: Pt. states she's no longer nauseated at 2335.
		#2 Risk for infection related to incision sites.
		O: Incision site in front of Ⓛ ear extending down and around the ear and into neck — approximately 6" in length — without dressing. No swelling or bleeding, bluish discoloration below Ⓛ ear noted, sutures intact. Jackson-Pratt drain in Ⓛ neck below ear with 20-ml bloody drainage. Drain remains secured in place with suture.
		A: No infection at present.
		P: Monitor incision sites for redness, drainage, and swelling. Monitor JP drain output. Teach pt. S&S of infection prior to discharge. Monitor temperature.
		#3 Delayed surgical recovery.
		O: Pt. oriented x 3 but groggy. Pt. attempted to get OOB at 2245 to ambulate to bathroom but felt dizzy upon standing. Lungs sound clear bilaterally.
		A: Pt. is dizzy when getting OOB. Pt. needs post-op education about mobility and coughing and deep-breathing exercises.
		P: Allowed pt. to use bedpan. Assist in getting OOB in 1 hour by dangling legs on side of bed for a few minutes before attempting to stand. Monitor blood pressure. Teach patient how to get out of bed slowly to prevent dizziness and to ask for assistance. Teach coughing and deep breathing, turning, use of antiembolism stockings.
		I: Allowed pt. to lie down in bed after feeling dizzy. Pt. used bedpan and voided 200 ml clear, yellow urine at 2245. Assisted in coughing and deep-breathing exercises and taught about turning, use of antiembolism stockings.
		E: Lungs remain clear bilaterally.
		#4 Acute pain related to surgical incision.
		S: 2245 pt. states "No" when asked if she has pain. At 2335 pt. states "It hurts."
		O: Pt. reports incisional pain as 7/10 on scale of 0 to 10.
		A: Pt. is in pain and needs pain medication.
		P: Give pain meds as ordered.
		I: Pt. given morphine 2 mg I.V. at 2335.
		E: Pt. states pain as 1/10. ———— Bridget Smith, RN

Problem-intervention-evaluation system

The PIE system organizes information according to patients' problems. It requires that you keep a daily assessment flow sheet and progress notes. Integrating the care plan into the nurses' progress notes eliminates the need for a separate care plan and provides a record that has a nursing—rather than medical—focus.

The daily assessment flow sheet includes areas for documenting assessment of major categories, such as respiration or pain, along with routine care and monitoring. It usually provides spaces to document times treatments were given as well as continued assessments of a specific area such as neurologic checks every hour. Progress notes are organized according to PIE:

Problem

Use data collected from your initial assessment to identify pertinent nursing diagnoses. Use the list of nursing diagnoses accepted by your facility, which usually corresponds to the diagnoses approved by the NANDA International. Some facilities use a separate problem list such as in the POMR. When

documenting a problem in the progress notes, label it as P and number it (for example, P#1). This way you can refer to it later by number without having to redocument the problem statement.

Intervention

Document the nursing actions you take for each nursing diagnosis. Label each entry as I followed by P and the problem number (for example, IP#1).

Evaluation

The patient's response to treatment makes up your evaluation. Use the label E followed by P and the problem number (for example, EP#1).

11/26/09	2400	P#1: Nausea related to anesthetic.
		IP#1: Pt. given Compazine 1 mg I.V. at 2300.
		EP#1: Pt. vomited 100-ml clear fluid at 2255. Pt. now states no nausea after given Compazine.
		P#2: Risk for infection related to incision sites.
		IP#2: Drainage from Jackson-Pratt drain measured. Site monitored for redness, drainage, and swelling. Temperature monitored.
		EP#2: Incision site in front of Ⓛ ear extending down and around the ear and into neck — approximately 6" in length — without dressing. No swelling or bleeding, bluish discoloration below Ⓛ ear noted, sutures intact. JP drain in Ⓛ neck below ear with 20 ml of bloody drainage. Drain remains secured in place with suture.
		P#3: Delayed surgical recovery.
		IP#3: At 2245, assisted patient getting back in bed and using bedpan after attempting to get up. Explained to pt. how to dangle legs and get OOB slowly. Assisted with and taught about coughing and deep-breathing exercises, turning, and use of antiembolism stockings. Assessed breath sounds.
		EP#3: Pt. reported feeling dizzy after first attempt to get OOB. Pt. did coughing and deep-breathing exercises effectively, and lungs sound clear bilaterally.
		P#4: Acute pain related to surgical incision.
		IP#4: Assessed pain as 7 on scale of 0 to 10. Gave pt. morphine 2 mg I.V. at 2335.
		EP#4: Prior to med. administration, pt. reported pain as 7/10. Now pt. reports pain as 1/10.
		— Bridget Smith, RN

FOCUS charting

FOCUS charting is organized into patient-centered topics or foci. It encourages you to use assessment data to evaluate these concerns.

Use a progress sheet with columns for the date, time, focus, and progress notes. In the focus column, write each focus as a nursing diagnosis, a sign or symptom, a patient's behavior, a special need, an acute change in the patient's condition, or a significant event. In the progress notes column, organize information using three categories: data (D), action (A), and response (R). In the data category, include subjective and objective information that describe the focus. In the action category, include immediate and future nursing actions based on your assessment of the patient's condition and any changes to the care plan you deem necessary based on your evaluation. In the response category, describe the patient's response to nursing or medical care. Using all three categories ensures concise documentation based on the nursing process. All other routine nursing tasks and assessment data can be documented on flow sheets and checklists.

Date	Time	Focus	Progress notes
11/26/09	2400	Nausea related to anesthetic	D: Pt. states she's nauseated. Vomited 100-ml clear fluid at 2255. ————
			A: Given Compazine 1 mg I.V. at 2300.
			R: Pt. reports no further nausea at 2335. No further vomiting. ————
		Risk for infection related to incision sites	D: Incision site in front of ℚ ear extending down and around the ear and into neck — approximately 6" in length — without dressing. Jackson-Pratt drain in ℚ neck below ear secured in place with suture. ————
			A: Assessed site and emptied drain. Taught patient S&S of infection. ————
			R: No swelling or bleeding; bluish discoloration below ℚ ear noted. JP drained 20-ml bloody drainage. Pt. states understanding of teaching.
		Delayed surgical recovery	D: Pt. reported dizziness after trying to get OOB to use the bathroom. ————
			A: Assisted patient back in bed and with use of bedpan. Taught pt. how to dangle legs and get OOB slowly. Also taught coughing and deep-breathing exercises, turning in bed, and use of antiembolism stockings. ————
			R: Pt. voided 200 ml in bedpan. Did coughing and deep breathing appropriately. Lungs clear bilaterally. Using antiembolism stockings. ————
		Acute pain related to surgical incision	D: Pt. reports pain as 7/10 on 0 to 10 scale.
			A: Given morphine 2 mg I.V. at 2335. ————
			R: Pt. reports pain as 1/10 at 2355. ————
			———————— Bridget Smith, RN

Charting by exception

CBE radically departs from traditional systems by requiring documentation of only significant or abnormal findings in the narrative portion of the record. To use CBE documentation effectively, you must know and adhere to established guidelines for nursing assessments and interventions and follow written standards of practice that identify the nurse's basic responsibilities. You document only deviations from the standards. Guidelines for interventions come from nursing diagnosis–based standardized care plans, patient care guidelines, physician's orders, incidental orders, and standards of nursing practice.

The CBE format involves the use of a nursing diagnosis–based standardized care plan and several types of flow sheets:

Nursing diagnosis–based standardized care plans

These preprinted care plans are used when you identify a nursing diagnosis. They allow members of the nursing team to share information about the patient's care needs, which helps to ensure that those needs are met. The care plans document changes in a patient's condition, adjustments or additions to nursing diagnoses, and the patient's response to treatment. Individualize your plan in the blank spaces provided.

Nursing care flow sheet

This form is used to document your assessments and interventions and is usually designed for a 24-hour period. After completing an assessment, compare your findings with the normal parameters defined in the printed guidelines on the form. Also compare your assessment findings with the previous nurse's notes to see if the patient's condition has changed. If your findings are within normal parameters and have not changed since the last nursing assessment, you can checkmark the category and add your initials. If your findings are not within normal limits or do not match the previous assessment, put an asterisk in the box and document your findings in the comment section or other designated area such as the progress notes. (See *Nursing care flow sheet for charting by exception*, page 686.)

Graphic record

This flow sheet is used to document trends in vital signs, weight, intake and output, and activity level. As with the nursing care flow sheet, use check marks and initials to indicate expected findings and use asterisks to indicate abnormal findings. Record abnormalities in the nurses' progress notes.

Patient-teaching record

Use this form to track and document patient teaching, including who and what is being taught, and document outcomes. Include teaching resources, social and behavioral measures, dates when goals are met, and other pertinent observations.

Patient discharge note

This form may be used to document ongoing discharge planning. A typical discharge form includes places to document patient instructions, appointments for follow-up care, medication and diet instructions, signs and symptoms to report, level of activity, and patient education.

Progress notes

The progress notes are used to document revisions to the care plan and interventions that do not lend themselves to any of the flow sheets. Because most flow sheets should have areas in which to document abnormal findings, the progress notes typically contain few assessment and intervention data. In addition, you may need to supplement your CBE documentation with nurses' progress notes.

FACT documentation

The FACT documentation system, which incorporates many CBE principles, has four key elements: **F**low sheets, **A**ssessments with baseline parameters, **C**oncise integrated progress notes and flow sheets documenting the patient's condition and responses, and **T**imely entries recorded when care is given. FACT requires that you document only exceptions to the norm or significant information about the patient. (See *Documenting with FACT*, page 688.)

Nursing care flow sheet for charting by exception

Hour		1400	1500	1600	1700	1800	1900	2000	2100	2200	2300	2400
ACTIVITY	Bed rest						BS	BS	BS			
	OOB									BS*		
	Ambulate (assist)											
	Ambulatory											
	Sleeping											
	BRP											
	HOB elevated											
	Cough, deep-breathe, turn						BS	BS	BS	BS	BS	BS
	ROM											
HYGIENE	Bath											
	Shave											
	Oral											
	Skin care											
	Perianal care — Active / Passive											
NUTRITION	Diet		*Sips of liquid*									
	% Eating											
	Feeding											
	Supplemental											
	S=Self, A=Assist, F=Feed											
BLADDER	Catheter											
	Incontinent											
	Voiding			*Clear yellow at 2245*								
	Intermittent cath.											
BOWEL	Stools (OB+, OB−)											
	Incontinent											
	Normal											
	Enema											
SPECIAL TREATMENTS	Special mattress											
	Special bed											
	Heel and elbow pads											
	Antiembolism stockings						BS	BS	BS	BS	BS	BS
	Traction: + = on, − = off											
	Isolation type											

Nursing care flow sheet for charting by exception *(continued)*

ASSESSMENT FINDINGS

	Day	Evening	Night	Key: ✓ = normal findings * = significant finding
Neurologic		✓ BS		
Cardiovascular		✓ BS		
Pulmonary		✓ BS		
Gastrointestinal		*		vomited X 1 at 2255. Given Compazine 1mg I.V. c̄ relief. ————
Genitourinary		✓ BS		
Surgical dressing and incision		* BS		Incision ⓛ ear around ear into neck 6" Jackson-Pratt drain, 20-ml bloody drainage.
Skin integrity		✓ BS		
Psychosocial		✓ BS		
Educational		* BS		Taught C&DB, use of antiembolism stockings, and OOB slowly c̄ legs dangling first. ———
Peripheral vascular		✓ BS		
Signatures	Bridget Smith, RN			

NORMAL ASSESSMENT FINDINGS

Neurologic
- Alert and oriented to time, place, and person
- Speech clear and understandable
- Memory intact
- Behavior appropriate to situation and accommodation
- Active range of motion (ROM) of all extremities; symmetrically equal strength
- No paresthesia

Cardiovascular
- Regular apical pulse
- Palpable bilateral peripheral pulses
- No peripheral edema
- No calf tenderness

Pulmonary
- Resting respirations 10 to 20 per minute, quiet and regular
- Clear sputum
- Pink nail beds and mucous membranes

Gastrointestinal
- Abdomen soft and nondistended
- Tolerates prescribed diet without nausea or vomiting
- Bowel movements within own normal pattern and consistency

Genitourinary
- No indwelling catheter in use
- Urinates without pain
- Undistended bladder after urination
- Urine clear yellow to amber color

Surgical dressing and incision
- Dressing dry and intact
- No evidence of redness, increased temperature, or tenderness in surrounding tissue
- Sutures, staples, Steri-Strips intact
- Sound edges well approximated
- No drainage present

Skin integrity
- Skin color normal
- Skin warm, dry, and intact
- Moist mucous membranes

Psychosocial
- Interacts and communicates in an appropriate manner with others

Educational
- Patient or significant others communicate understanding of the patient's health status, care plan, and expected response
- Patient or significant others demonstrate ability to perform health-related procedures and behaviors as taught

Peripheral vascular
- Affected extremity pink, warm, and movable within average ROM
- Capillary refill time <3 seconds
- Peripheral pulses palpable
- No edema: sensation intact without numbness or paresthesia
- No pain on passive stretch

Documenting with FACT

Developed in 1987 at Abbott Northwestern Hospital in Minneapolis, Minnesota, the FACT documentation system records nursing assessment findings and interventions that are exceptions to the norm. This sample shows portions of an assessment flow sheet and a postoperative flow sheet using the FACT format.

ASSESSMENT AND ACTION RECORD

	Date: 11/26/09 Time: 2245	11/26/09 2335	11/26/09 2355
Neurologic Alert and oriented to time, place, and person. PEARL. Symmetry of strength in extremities. No difficulty with coordination. Behavior appropriate to situation. Sensation intact without numbness or paresthesia.	✓ groggy	✓	✓
Orient patient.			
Refer to neurologic flow sheet.			
Pain No report of pain. If present, include patient statements about intensity (0 to 10 scale), location, description, duration, radiation, precipitating, and alleviating factors.	✓	7/10	1/10
Location		incision	incision
Relief measures		MSO4 2 mg I.V.	
Pain relief: Y = Yes N = No			y
Cardiovascular Apical pulse 60 to 100. S1 and S2 present. Regular rhythm. Peripheral (radial, pedal) pulses present. No edema or calf tenderness. Extremities pink, warm, movable within patient's range of motion (ROM).	✓	✓	✓
I.V. solution and rate			
Respiratory Respiratory rate 12 to 20 at rest, quiet, regular, and nonlabored. Lungs clear and aerated equally in all lobes. No abnormal breath sounds. Mucous membranes pink.	✓		✓
O₂ therapy			
TCDB/incentive spirometer	✓		✓
Musculoskeletal Extremities pink, warm, and without edema; sensation and motion present. Normal joint ROM, no swelling or tenderness. Steady gait without aids. Pedal, radial pulses present. Rapid capillary refill.	OOB→dizzy →BR	✓	
Activity (describe)		BR	BR
Nurse's signature and title	Bridget Smith, RN	Bridget Smith, RN	Bridget Smith, RN

Key: ✓ = Meets assessment criteria

FACT documentation begins with a complete initial baseline assessment on each patient using standardized parameters. This format involves an assessment-action flow sheet, a frequent assessment flow sheet, and progress notes. Flow sheets cover 24- to 72-hour periods. Always include the date and time and sign all entries.

Assessment-action flow sheet

Use this form to document ongoing assessments and interventions. Normal assessment parameters for each body system are printed on the form along with planned interventions. Individualize the flow sheet according to patient need. In the appropriate place on the form (next to "normal"), check off assessment or interventions done, or use the space provided to document abnormalities or completed interventions that are different from those printed on the form.

Frequent assessment flow sheet

Use this form to chart vital signs and frequent assessments. For example, on a surgical unit, this form would include a postoperative assessment section.

Progress notes

This form includes an integrated progress record on which you will use narrative notes to document the patient's progress and any significant incidents. As with FOCUS charting, write narrative notes using the data-action-response method. Update progress notes related to patient outcomes every 48 hours or as required by your facility.

11/26/09	2400	D: Pt. states she's nauseated. Vomited 100-ml clear fluid at 2255. A: Given Compazine 1 mg I.V. at 2300. R: Pt. reports no further nausea at 2335. No further vomiting. —Bridget Smith, RN

Core charting

Core charting focuses on the nursing process—the core or most important part of documentation. It consists of a database, a care plan, flow sheets, progress notes, and a discharge summary. Core charting requires that you assess and record a patient's functional and cognitive status within 8 hours of admission. The database and care plan are used as the initial assessment and focus on the patient's body systems and activities of daily living. They include a summary of the patient's problems and appropriate nursing diagnoses. Flow sheets are used to document the patient's activities and response to nursing interventions, diagnostic procedures, and patient teaching. Progress notes contain information for each problem organized in a data, action, evaluation or response (DAE) format. Finally, the discharge summary includes information related to nursing diagnosis, patient teaching, and follow-up care.

11/26/09	2400	D: Pt. states being nauseated. Vomited 100-ml clear fluid at 2255.
		A: Given Compazine 1 mg I.V. at 2300.
		E: Pt. reports no further nausea at 2335. No further vomiting.
		D: Incision site in front of ① ear extending down and around the ear and into neck — approximately 6" in length — without dressing. Jackson-Pratt drain in ① neck below ear secured in place with suture.
		A: Assessed site and emptied drain. Taught patient S&S of infection.
		E: No swelling or bleeding; bluish discoloration below ① ear noted. JP drained 20-ml bloody drainage. Pt. states understanding of teaching.
		D: Pt. reported dizziness after trying to get OOB to use the bathroom.
		A: Assisted patient back in bed and with use of bedpan. Taught pt. how to dangle legs and get OOB slowly. Also taught coughing and deep-breathing exercises, turning in bed, and use of antiembolism stockings.
		E: Pt. voided 200 ml in bedpan. Did coughing and deep breathing appropriately. Lungs clear bilaterally. Using antiembolism stockings.
		D: Pt. reports pain as 7/10 on 0 to 10 scale.
		A: Given morphine 2 mg I.V. at 2335.
		E: Pt. reports pain as 1/10 at 2345. ———— Bridget Smith, RN

Outcome documentation

Outcome documentation presents the patient's condition in relation to predetermined outcomes on the plan of care, focusing on desired outcomes rather than problems. This system uses progress notes, flow sheets, and plans of care. Some facilities use a separate teaching plan. (See *Multidisciplinary patient-family education record*.) Outcome documentation features these components:

Database

This includes subjective and objective data identifying the patient's problems and learning needs and is a foundation for ongoing evaluation.

Care plan

The care plan establishes priorities, identifies expected outcomes and nursing interventions, and documents the plan. Traditional handwritten plans, preprinted standardized plans, clinical pathways, and patient care guidelines can be used.

Expected outcome statements

Expected outcomes describe the desired results of nursing actions. Be specific and use outcome criteria that are measurable and include target dates or times. Learning outcomes focus on patient's behaviors that are measurable and observable. Outcomes are evaluated; if problems are resolved, outcomes are met. When outcomes are not met, the plan is reevaluated. (See *Writing expected outcomes and outcome criteria*, page 692.)

Multidisciplinary patient-family education record

This sample shows the features of a typical multidisciplinary patient-family education record.

INITIAL EDUCATIONAL EVALUATION

Date/Time _11/21/09_   _2255_

Motivational level: P = Patient   F = Family

_P/F_ Asks questions   _P/F_ Eager to learn   _____ Very anxious

_____ Uninterested   _____ Denies need for education   _____ Not appropriate for education

Barrier to education: _✓_ No barrier identified

_____ Visual deficit   _____ Auditory deficit   _____ Physical deficit

_____ Religious barrier   _____ Cultural barrier   _____ Dexterity deficit

_____ Language barrier   _____ Language spoken

Special learning needs _Care after surgery_

Community resources discussed:

_____ Cardiac support   _____ Twelve-step program   _____ Cancer support

_____ Hospice   _____ Achievement center   _____ Diabetic support

_____ Other _____

DATE/INITIAL	TOPIC	PT	FAM	RESPONSE CODE
11/22/09 BS	Pt. oriented to room postoperatively. ———	✓	✓	2, 6
11/22/09 BS	Explained purpose of Jackson-Pratt drain. ———	✓	✓	2, 6
11/22/09 BS	Instructed pt. on use of pain scale to report pain.	✓		
11/22/09 BS	Instructed pt. on coughing and deep-breathing exercises. ———	✓	✓	1, 3, 5
11/22/09 BS	Instructed pt. on use of antiembolism stockings, turning, & getting OOB slowly. ———	✓		5, 6
11/23/09 DR	Instructed pt. on how to empty JP drain herself. ——	✓	✓	2, 6
11/23/09 DR	Instructed pt. on S&S of infection to report to MD.	✓	✓	2, 6

Response codes:

1 Received literature

2 Communicates understanding

3 Requires reinforcement

4 Prior experience

5 Returned demo

6 Education achieved

7 Referral indicated

8 Refused/Uninterested

9 Inappropriate for education

Initials	Signature - Status	Initials	Signature - Status
BS	Bridget Smith, RN		
DR	Daniella Reams, RN		

Writing expected outcomes and outcome criteria

Here are two examples of how to develop patient-focused outcomes and outcome criteria based on selected nursing diagnoses.

Nursing diagnosis	Expected outcomes	Outcome criteria
Risk for infection related to incision	Patient will not develop postoperative wound infection.	• Patient states signs and symptoms to report to health care provider on discharge. • Patient demonstrates incision care. • Patient demonstrates emptying of Jackson-Pratt drain.
Acute pain related to effects of surgery	Pain will be reduced by time of discharge.	• Patient rates less pain using a numerical scale (for example, if patient had rated pain as 8 on scale of 1 to 10, any reduction in pain would be a rating of less than 8). • Patient expresses pain relief. • Patient can perform self-care activities without assistance. • Patient shows no facial mask of pain. • Patient does not guard incision site.

Computerized charting

Computerized nursing information systems (NISs) can increase efficiency and accuracy in all phases of the nursing process and can help nurses meet standards set by the American Nurses Association and The Joint Commission. Current NISs not only collect, transmit, and organize the information but also suggest nursing diagnoses and provide standardized patient status and nursing interventions that you can use for care plans and progress notes. They are also interactive, prompting you with questions and suggestions about the information you enter. Depending on your institution's software, you might use computers for these nursing processes:

Assessment

Admission data can be collected via computer terminals. After entering patient's data, such as health status, history, chief complaint, and other assessment data, the computer system can flag an entry if the data are outside the acceptable range.

Nursing diagnosis

Most current programs list standard diagnoses with associated signs and symptoms and can suggest one for your patient. You still need to use clinical judgment to determine if the suggested diagnosis is right for your patient.

Planning

To help nurses begin writing a care plan, computer programs can display recommended expected outcomes and interventions for the selected diagnoses. You can also use computers to compare and track patient outcomes for a selected group of patients.

Implementation

Use the computer to record actual interventions and patient-processing information, such as discharge or transfer instructions. Progress notes, medication administration, vital signs, and treatments can also be documented with the computer.

Evaluation

Use the computer to record evaluations and reevaluations and your patient's response to nursing care.

Nursing Minimum Data Set program

The Nursing Minimum Data Set (NMDS) program attempts to standardize nursing information. It contains three categories: nursing care, patient demographics, and service elements. The NMDS allows you to collect nursing diagnosis and intervention data and identify the nursing needs of various patient populations. It also lets you track patient outcomes. This system helps establish accurate estimates for nursing service costs and provides data about nursing care that may influence health care policy and decision making. With the NMDS, you can compare nursing trends locally, regionally, and nationally using data from various clinical settings, patient populations, and geographic areas. By comparing trends, you can set realistic outcomes for an individual patient as well as formulate accurate nursing diagnoses and plan

interventions. Also, NANDA International assigns numerical codes to all nursing diagnoses so those diagnoses can be used with the NMDS.

Nursing Outcomes Classification system

The Nursing Outcomes Classification (NOC) system provides the first comprehensive standardized method of measuring nursing-sensitive patient outcomes. The NOC has major implications for nursing administrative practices and the patient care delivery system. This system allows the nurse to compare patients' outcomes to the outcomes of larger groups according to parameters, such as age, diagnosis, or health care setting.

Voice-activated systems

Voice-activated systems are also available. They are most useful in hospital departments, such as the operating room, that have a high volume of structured reports. These software programs use a specialized knowledge base, nursing words, phrases, and report forms, combined with automated speech recognition (ASR) technology. ASR systems require little or no keyboard use and allow the user to record prompt and complete nursing notes by speaking into a telephone handset. The system displays the text on the computer screen. These systems increase the speed of reporting and free the nurse from paperwork.

Appendices
Index

Cultural considerations in patient care

As a health care professional, you interact with a diverse, multicultural patient population. If not handled properly, culture and language differences can lead to misunderstandings and a lack of compliance and can negatively affect patient outcomes.

To make sure that you give all your patients the best care, remember that a patient's cultural behaviors and beliefs may differ from yours. Learn the facts about diverse population groups, and keep your awareness of cultural differences and your skill with handling these differences up to date. Doing so will help avoid dangerous misunderstandings and ensure that you deliver effective, respectful care to all your patients.

Cultural competence

Cultural competence requires sensitivity to issues related to diverse cultures. You do not have to be an expert in other cultures to have cultural competence, but you must be willing to learn about and interact with patients and families from different cultures, social groups, and races.

Following these guidelines can help you provide culturally competent care:
- Identify your own values and beliefs.
- Realize that you may have stereotypes about people from countries you are not familiar with as well as people who speak a different primary language.
- Identify any biases and possible prejudices you may have.
- Seek and obtain information about different cultures and ethnic groups, including:
  - nonverbal and verbal communication practices
  - activities of daily living
  - food practices
  - symptom management
  - birth rituals and child care
  - death rituals
  - family relationships
  - spiritual and religious beliefs
  - illness beliefs
  - health practices.
- Look for opportunities to interact with patients from various cultures.
- Perform a cultural needs assessment at admission.
  - Determine the patient's ability to speak and read English, find out what his or her native language is, assess his or her ability to read lips (if appropriate), and decide if you will need an interpreter.
  - Ask the patient how he or she wants to be addressed.
  - Observe the patient's nonverbal communication style, assessing his or her eye contact, expressiveness, and ability to understand common signs and gestures.
  - Determine the patient's social orientation, including culture, race, ethnicity, family role, work, and religion.
  - Establish the patient's special comfort level, particularly in light of his or her conversation, proximity to others, body movement, and sense of personal space.
  - Ask about food preferences, family health history, religious and cultural health practices, and definitions of health and illness.
  - Identify the patient's major support people.
  - Determine if the patient is past oriented, present oriented, or future oriented.

The interpreter's role

Language assistance services should always be readily available to patients with limited English proficiency, often at all points of contact and during all hours of facility operation. Whenever possible, use a trained interpreter rather than a patient's family member or friend, according to your facility's policy. A family member or friend may have role conflicts or lack the necessary medical vocabulary; he or she may also change the message you are trying to convey based on his or her own perception of the situation or withhold vital information because it might be embarrassing.

Consider these tips when using an interpreter:

- Before beginning, meet with the interpreter to explain the purpose of the session.
- If appropriate, have the interpreter speak briefly with the patient beforehand to learn his or her educational level and needs.
- Instruct the interpreter to interpret exactly what the patient says and not to edit or summarize any information.
- Expect the session to move more slowly than a usual interchange because careful interpretation requires time.
- Speak in short sentences and avoid using complex medical terms, slang, and jargon.
- Speak clearly and a little more slowly than normal, but do not speak more loudly.
- During the interaction, look at and speak directly to the patient, not the interpreter. Look at and listen to the patient as he or she speaks.
- Avoid body language or gestures that may cause offense or be misinterpreted.
- Periodically assess the patient's understanding of what you have been discussing by asking him or her to repeat it back to you. Avoid asking, "Do you understand?"

Potential agents of bioterrorism

Listed below are examples of biological agents that may potentially be used as biological weapons and the major signs and symptoms associated with each.

Potential agents	Abdominal pain	Back pain	Blood pressure, decreased	Chest pain	Chills	Cough	Diarrhea, bloody	Diarrhea, watery	Diplopia	Dysarthria	Dysphagia	Dyspnea	Fever
Anthrax (cutaneous)													●
Anthrax (gastrointestinal)	●						●						●
Anthrax (inhalation)			●	●	●	●						●	●
Botulism									●	●	●	●	
Cholera			●					●					
Plague (septicemic)					●								●
Plague (pneumonic)				●	●	●						●	●
Smallpox	●	●											●
Tularemia				●	●	●						●	●

	Headache	Hematemesis	Hemoptysis	Lymphadenopathy	Malaise	Muscle spasms or muscle cramps	Myalgias	Nausea	Oliguria	Skin lesions	Ptosis	Skin turgor, decreased	Stridor, decreased	Tachycardia	Tachypnea	Vomiting	Weakness
	●			●	●					●							
		●						●								●	
													●				●
											●						●
						●			●			●	●			●	●
				●													
	●		●				●								●		
	●				●					●							
	●						●										

Web sites of selected organizations

Agency for Healthcare Research and Quality
www.ahrq.gov

American Association of Critical-Care Nurses
www.aacn.org

American Burn Association
www.ameriburn.org

American Cancer Society
www.cancer.org

American Diabetes Association
www.diabetes.org

American Heart Association
www.heart.org

American Holistic Nurses Association
www.ahna.org

American Lung Association
www.lung.org

American Nurses Association
www.nursingworld.org

American Pain Society
www.americanpainsociety.org

Centers for Disease Control and Prevention
www.cdc.gov

Centers for Medicare & Medicaid Services
www.cms.gov

Infusion Nurses Society
www.ins1.org

National Institute of Neurological Disorders and Stroke
www.ninds.nih.gov

National Kidney Foundation
www.kidney.org

National League for Nursing
www.nln.org

PubMed
www.ncbi.nlm.nih.gov/pubmed

Sigma Theta Tau International
www.sigmanursing.org

U.S. Department of Health & Human Services
www.hhs.gov

Wound, Ostomy and Continence Nurses Society
www.wocn.org

Dangerous abbreviations

The Joint Commission approved the following "minimum list" of dangerous abbreviations, acronyms, and symbols. Using this list should help protect patients from the effects of miscommunication in clinical documentation.

Abbreviation	Potential problem	Preferred term
U (for "unit")	Mistaken as "zero," "four," or "cc."	Write "unit."
IU (for "international unit")	Mistaken as "I.V." (intravenous) or "10" (ten).	Write "international unit."
Q.D., QD, q.d., qd (daily) Q.O.D., QOD, q.o.d., qod (every other day)	Mistaken for each other. The period after the Q can be mistaken for "I," and the "O" can be mistaken for "I."	Write "daily" and "every other day," respectively.
Trailing zero (X.0 mg), lack of leading zero (.X mg)	Decimal point is missed.	Never write a zero by itself after a decimal point (X mg), and always use a zero before a decimal point (0.X mg).
MS, MSO4, MgSO4	Mistaken for each other. Can mean "morphine sulfate" or "magnesium sulfate."	Write "morphine sulfate" or "magnesium sulfate."

© The Joint Commission, 2009. Reprinted with permission.

English-Spanish quick reference guide

anemia	la anemia	heart disease
angina	la angina	heart failure
appendicitis	la apendicitis	heart murmur
arteriosclerosis	la arteriosclerosis	hemorrhage
arthritis	la artritis	hemorrhoids
asthma	el asma	
backache	el dolor de espalda	hepatitis
blindness	la ceguera	hernia
bronchitis	la bronquitis	herpes
burn (first, second, or	la quemadura (de primer,	high blood pressure
third degree)	segundo, o tercer grado)	hives
bursitis	la bursitis	hoarseness
cancer	el cáncer	ill
chickenpox	la varicela, las viruelas locas	illness
chills	los escalofrios	immunization
cold	el catarro, el resfriado	infarct
cold sores	lasúlceras de la boca	infection
constipation	el estreñimiento	inflammation
convulsion	la convulsión	injury
cough	la tos	
cramps	los calambres	itch
deafness	la sordera	jaundice
diabetes	la diabetes	kidney stone
diarrhea	la diarrea	
discharge	el flujo	laryngitis
dizziness	el vértigo, el mareo	lesion
eczema	el eccema	leukemia
emphysema	el enfisema	lice
epilepsy	la epilepsia	lump
fainting spell	el desmayo	malignancy
fatigue	la fatiga	malignant
fever	la fiebre	measles
flu	la influenza, la gripe	meningitis
food poisoning	el envenenamiento por	menopause
	comestibles	metastasis
fracture	la fractura	migraine
gallbladder attack	el ataque de la vesícula biliar	multiple sclerosis
gallstone	el cálculo biliar	mumps
gastric ulcer	la úlcera gástrica	muscular dystrophy
glaucoma	el glaucoma	mute
gonorrhea	la gonorrea	obese
headache	el dolor de cabeza	overdose
heart attack	el ataque al corazón	overweight
heartbeat	el latido	pain
irregular	irregular	growing pain
rhythmical	rítmico	labor pain
slow	lento	phantom limb pain
fast (tachycardia)	taquicardia	
heartburn	las agruras (el ardor), acedía	referred pain

la enfermedad del corazón	sharp pain	el dolor agudo
el fallo cardíaco	shooting pain	el dolor punzante
el soplo del corazón	burning pain	el dolor que arde
la hemorragia	intense pain	el dolor intenso
las almorranas, las	severe pain	el dolor severo
hemorroides	intermittent pain	el dolor intermitente
la hepatitis	throbbing pain	el dolor palpitante
la hernia	palpitation	la palpitación
el herpes	paralysis	la parálisis
la presión alta	Parkinson's disease	la enfermedad de Parkinson
la urticaria	pneumonia	la pulmonía
la ronquera	psoriasis	la psoriasis
enfermo(a)	pus	el pus
la enfermedad	rash	la roncha, el salpullido, la
la inmunización		erupción
el infarto	relapse	la recaída
la infección	renal	renal
la inflamación	rheumatic fever	la fiebre reumática
el daño la lastimadura,	roseola	la roséola
la herida	rubella	la rubéola
la picazón, la comezón	rupture	la ruptura
la piel amarilla, la ictericia	scab	la costra
el cálculo en el riñón,	scar	la cicatriz
la piedra en el riñón	scratch	el rasguño
la laringitis	senile	senil
la lesión, el daño	shock	el choque
la leucemia	sore	la llaga
los piojos	spasm	el espasmo
el bulto	sprain	la torcedura
el tumor, la malignidad	stomachache	el dolor del estómago
maligno(a)	stomach ulcer	la úlcera del estómago
el sarampión	suicide	el suicidio
la meningitis	swelling	la hinchazón
la menopausia	syphilis	la sífilis
la metástasis	tachycardia	la taquicardia
la migraña, la jaqueca	toothache	el dolor de muela
la esclerosis múltiple	toxemia	la toxemia
las paperas	trauma	el trauma
la distrofia muscular	tuberculosis	la tuberculosis
mudo(a)	tumor	el tumor
obeso(a)	ulcer	la úlcera
la sobredosis	unconsciousness	la pérdida del conocimiento
el sobrepeso	virus	el virus
el dolor	vomit	el vómito, los vómitos
el dolor de crecimiento	wart	la verruga
el dolor de parto	weakness	la debilidad
el dolor de miembro	wheeze	el jadeo, la silba
fantasma	wound	la herida
el dolor referido	yellow fever	la fiebre amarilla

Crisis values of laboratory tests

Test	Low value	Common causes and effects	High value	Common causes and effects
Calcium, serum	<6 mg/dl (SI, <1.5 mmol/L)	Vitamin D or parathyroid hormone deficiency: tetany, seizures	>13 mg/dl (SI, >3.25 mmol/L)	Hyperparathyroidism: coma
Carbon dioxide	<6 mEq/L (SI, <6 mmol/L)	Complex pattern of metabolic and respiratory factors	>40 mEq/L (SI, >40 mmol/L)	Complex pattern of metabolic and respiratory factors
Creatinine, serum			>4 mg/dl (SI, >353.6 μmol/L)	Renal failure: coma
Glucose, blood	<40 mg/dl (SI, 2.2 mmol/L)	Excess insulin administration: brain damage	>400 mg/dl (SI, >22.2 mmol/L)	Diabetes: diabetic ketoacidosis
Hemoglobin	<5 g/dl (SI, <50 g/L)	Hemorrhage, vitamin B_{12} or iron deficiency: heart failure	>20 g/dl (SI, >200 g/L)	Chronic obstructive pulmonary disease: thrombosis, polycythemia vera
International Normalized Ratio			>3.6	Disseminated intravascular coagulation: uncontrolled oral anticoagulation
Partial pressure of arterial carbon dioxide	<20 mm Hg (SI, <2.7 kPa)	Complex pattern of metabolic and respiratory factors	>70 mm Hg (SI, >9.3 kPa)	Complex pattern of metabolic and respiratory factors
Partial pressure of arterial oxygen	<50 mm Hg (SI, <6.7 kPa)	Complex pattern of metabolic and respiratory factors		

Crisis values of laboratory tests *(continued)*

Test	Low value	Common causes and effects	High value	Common causes and effects
Partial thromboplastin time			>40 seconds (SI, >40 seconds) >70 seconds (SI, >70 seconds) (for patient on heparin)	Anticoagulation factor deficiency: hemorrhage
pH, blood	<7.2 (SI, <7.2)	Complex pattern of metabolic and respiratory factors	>7.6 (SI, >7.6)	Complex patterns of metabolic and respiratory factors
Platelet count	<50,000/μl	Bone marrow suppression: hemorrhage	>500,000/μl	Leukemia, reaction to acute bleeding: hemorrhage
Potassium, serum	<2.5 mEq/L (SI, <2.5 mmol/L)	Vomiting and diarrhea, diuretic therapy: cardiotoxicity, arrhythmia, cardiac arrest	>8 mEq/L (SI, >8 mmol/L)	Renal disease, diuretic therapy: cardiotoxicity, arrhythmia
Prothrombin time			>14 seconds (SI, >14 seconds) >20 seconds (SI, >20 seconds) (for patient on warfarin)	Anticoagulant therapy, anticoagulation factor deficiency: hemorrhage
Sodium, serum	<125 mEq/L (SI, <125 mmol/L)	Diuretic therapy: profuse sweating, gastrointestinal suctioning, diarrhea, vomiting, burns	>160 mEq/L (SI, >160 mmol/L)	Dehydration: vascular collapse
White blood cell count	<2,000/μl (SI, <2 × 10⁹/L)	Bone marrow suppression: infection	>20,000/μl (SI, 20 × 10⁹/L)	Leukemia: infection

Table of equivalents

Metric system equivalents

Metric weight

1 kilogram (kg or Kg)	= 1,000 grams (g or gm)
1 gram	= 1,000 milligrams (mg)
1 milligram	= 1,000 micrograms (μg or mcg)
0.6 g	= 600 mg
0.3 g	= 300 mg
0.1 g	= 100 mg
0.06 g	= 60 mg
0.03 g	= 30 mg
0.015 g	= 15 mg
0.001 g	= 1 mg

Metric volume

1 liter (l or L)	= 1,000 milliliters (ml)*
1 milliliter	= 1,000 microliters (μl)

Household metric

1 teaspoon (tsp)	= 5 ml
1 tablespoon (T or tbs)	= 15 ml
2 tablespoons	= 30 ml
8 ounces	= 236.6 ml
1 pint (pt)	= 473 ml
1 quart (qt)	= 946 ml
1 gallon (gal)	= 3,785 ml

Temperature conversions

Fahrenheit degrees	Celsius degrees	Fahrenheit degrees	Celsius degrees	Fahrenheit degrees	Celsius degrees
106.0	41.1	100.6	38.1	95.2	35.1
105.8	41.0	100.4	38.0	95.0	35.0
105.6	40.9	100.2	37.9	94.8	34.9
105.4	40.8	100.0	37.8	94.6	34.8
105.2	40.7	99.8	37.7	94.4	34.7
105.0	40.6	99.6	37.6	94.2	34.6
104.8	40.4	99.4	37.4	94.0	34.4
104.6	40.3	99.2	37.3	93.8	34.3
104.4	40.2	99.0	37.2	93.6	34.2
104.2	40.1	98.8	37.1	93.4	34.1
104.0	40.0	98.6	37.0	93.2	34.0
103.8	39.9	98.4	36.9	93.0	33.9
103.6	39.8	98.2	36.8	92.8	33.8
103.4	39.7	98.0	36.7	92.6	33.7
103.2	39.6	97.8	36.6	92.4	33.6
103.0	39.4	97.6	36.4	92.2	33.4
102.8	39.3	97.4	36.3	92.0	33.3
102.6	39.2	97.2	36.2	91.8	33.2
102.4	39.1	97.0	36.1	91.6	33.1
102.2	39.0	96.8	36.0	91.4	33.0
102.0	38.9	96.6	35.9	91.2	32.9
101.8	38.8	96.4	35.8	91.0	32.8
101.6	38.7	96.2	35.7	90.8	32.7
101.4	38.6	96.0	35.6	90.6	32.6
101.2	38.4	95.8	35.4	90.4	32.4
101.0	38.3	95.6	35.3	90.2	32.3
100.8	38.2	95.4	35.2	90.0	32.2

Weight conversions

1 oz = 28.35g   1 lb = 453.6 g   2.2 lb = 1 kg

*1 ml = 1 cubic centimeter (cc); however, ml is the preferred measurement term used today.

Index

Note: Page numbers followed by *f*, *t*, and *b* denote figures, tables, and boxes, respectively.